Clinical Management of Head and Neck Cancer

Clinical Management of Head and Neck Cancer

Editor: Agnes Carter

AMERICAN
MEDICAL PUBLISHERS
www.americanmedicalpublishers.com

AMERICAN
MEDICAL PUBLISHERS
www.americanmedicalpublishers.com

Cataloging-in-Publication Data

Clinical management of head and neck cancer / edited by Agnes Carter.
p. cm.
Includes bibliographical references and index.
ISBN 978-1-63927-997-5
1. Head--Cancer. 2. Neck--Cancer. 3. Head--Cancer--Treatment. 4. Neck--Cancer--Treatment.
5. Head--Cancer--Diagnosis. 6. Neck--Cancer--Diagnosis. I. Carter, Agnes.
RC280.H4 C55 2023
616.994 91--dc23

American Medical Publishers,
41 Flatbush Avenue,
1st Floor, New York,
NY 11217, USA

ISBN 978-1-63927-997-5 (Hardback)

Contents

Preface

The main aim of this book is to educate learners and enhance their research focus by presenting diverse topics covering this vast field. This is an advanced book which compiles significant studies by distinguished experts in the area of analysis. This book addresses successive solutions to the challenges arising in the area of application, along with it; the book provides scope for future developments.

Head and neck cancer includes any form of cancer that develops in the oral cavity, nasal cavity, paranasal sinuses, larynx, pharynx or salivary glands. Common symptoms of this type of cancer are persistent pain in the throat, a sensation of pain or difficulty when swallowing, jaw pain, a change in voice, persistent pain in the ear, etc. Diagnosis depends on specific signs and symptoms, and the results of blood tests. Computed tomography and magnetic resonance imaging are the imaging tests used to diagnose this disease. A histological examination and a microscopic inspection for the presence of cancerous cells can be performed through a biopsy of suspected cancerous lesions. Treatment for head and neck cancer is curated to the specific needs and general health of individual patients. Treatment and management may include surgery, chemotherapy, or radiation therapy. This book is a valuable compilation of topics, ranging from the basic to the most complex principles and practices in the clinical management of cancer of the head and neck. It will serve as a valuable source of reference for graduate and post graduate students.

It was a great honour to edit this book, though there were challenges, as it involved a lot of communication and networking between me and the editorial team. However, the end result was this all-inclusive book covering diverse themes in the field.

Finally, it is important to acknowledge the efforts of the contributors for their excellent chapters, through which a wide variety of issues have been addressed. I would also like to thank my colleagues for their valuable feedback during the making of this book.

Editor

1

Taiwanin E Induces Cell Cycle Arrest and Apoptosis in Arecoline/4-NQO-Induced Oral Cancer Cells Through Modulation of the ERK Signaling Pathway

Shih-Hao Wang [1,2], *Hsi-Chin Wu* [3], *Khan Farheen Badrealam* [4], *Yueh-Hsiung Kuo* [2,5,6], *Yun-Peng Chao* [7], *Hsi-Hsien Hsu* [8,9], *Da-Tian Bau* [4], *Vijaya Padma Viswanadha* [10], *Yi-Hui Chen* [11], *Pei-Jei Lio* [12], *Chung-Jen Chiang* [12*†] and *Chih-Yang Huang* [2,4,13,14,15*†]

[1] Department of Otolaryngology, Ditmanson Medical Foundation, Chiayi Christian Hospital, Chiayi, Taiwan, [2] Department of Biotechnology, Asia University, Taichung, Taiwan, [3] School of Medicine, China Medical University, Taichung, Taiwan, [4] Graduate Institute of Biomedicine, China Medical University and Hospital, Taichung, Taiwan, [5] Department of Chinese Pharmaceutical Sciences and Chinese Medicine Resources, China Medical University, Taichung, Taiwan, [6] Chinese Medicine Research Center, China Medical University, Taichung, Taiwan, [7] Department of Chemical Engineering, Feng Chia University, Taichung, Taiwan, [8] Division of Colorectal Surgery, Mackay Memorial Hospital, Taipei, Taiwan, [9] Mackay Medicine, Nursing and Management College, Taipei, Taiwan, [10] Department of Biotechnology, Bharathiar University, Coimbatore, India, [11] Department of M-Commerce and Multimedia Applications, Asia University, Taichung, Taiwan, [12] Department of Medical Laboratory Science and Biotechnology, China Medical University, Taichung, Taiwan, [13] Cardiovascular and Mitochondria Related Diseases Research Center, Hualien Tzu Chi Hospital, Hualien, Taiwan, [14] Center of General Education, Buddhist Tzu Chi Medical Foundation, Tzu Chi University of Science and Technology, Hualien, Taiwan, [15] Department of Medical Research, China Medical University Hospital, China Medical University, Taichung, Taiwan

***Correspondence:**
Chung-Jen Chiang
cjchiang@mail.cmu.edu.tw
Chih-Yang Huang
cyhuang@mail.cmu.edu.tw*

† These authors have contributed equally to this work

Taiwanin E is a bioactive compound extracted from *Taiwania cryptomerioides* Hayata. In this research endeavor, we studied the anti-cancer effect of Taiwanin E against arecoline and 4-nitroquinoline-1-oxide-induced oral squamous cancer cells (OSCC), and elucidated the underlying intricacies. OSCC were treated with Taiwanin E and analyzed through MTT assay, Flow cytometry, TUNEL assay, and Western blotting for their efficacy against OSCC. Interestingly, it was found that Taiwanin E significantly attenuated the cell viability of oral cancer cells (T28); however, no significant cytotoxic effects were found for normal oral cells (N28). Further, Flow cytometry analysis showed that Taiwanin E induced G1cell cycle arrest in T28 oral cancer cells and Western blot analysis suggested that Taiwanin E considerably downregulated cell cycle regulatory proteins and activated p53, p21, and p27 proteins. Further, TUNEL and Western blot studies instigated that it induced cellular apoptosis and attenuated the p-PI3K/p-Akt survival mechanism in T28 oral cancer cells seemingly through modulation of the ERK signaling cascade. Collectively, the present study highlights the prospective therapeutic efficacy of Taiwanin E against arecoline and 4-nitroquinoline-1-oxide-induced oral cancer.

Keywords: Taiwanin E, oral cancer, apoptosis, cell cycle arrest, therapeutics

INTRODUCTION

Over the years, complementary and alternative medicine therapies have garnered great attention all across the globe (1, 2). Accumulating evidences has highlighted the efficacy of various small molecule compounds/phytochemicals as effective therapeutic entities against various diseases and pathological conditions, including cancer (3–6). Previous reports from our group have ascertained the potential of several bioactive compounds against cancer together with providing an insight into their mechanisms of action (7–11).

Taiwania (*Taiwania cryptomerioides* Hayata) represents one of the most economically relevant plant species endemic to Taiwan. Numerous bioactive compounds have been derived from this plant species. Many of them have been demonstrated to exhibit potent activity against bacteria, fungi, termites, mites, and cancers (12–15). To this end, recently, we have provided convincing evidence for the efficacy of Taiwanin A against arecoline and 4-nitroquinoline-1-oxide-induced oral cancer (16–18). Nevertheless, to the best of our knowledge, the effect of Taiwanin E against oral cancer and the underlying mechanism remains poorly understood.

Despite advancement in the allied field of biomedical sciences, the repercussions that may arise from cancer represent a significant human toll. According to statistics, globally, oral cancer is amongst 10 most common cancers. Oral squamous cell carcinoma (OSCC) is the most common malignant epithelial neoplasm that can afflict the oral cavity. It is thought that more than 90% malignancies arising from the head and neck tissue section are OSCC (19). Despite the availability of treatment strategies, including surgery, radiation, and chemotherapy, the overall survival rate of patients remains poor (20, 21). Taking these into consideration, in the current research endeavor, we have studied the effect of Taiwanin E against oral cancer and elucidated the underlying mechanism for their efficacy against oral cancer.

Interestingly, it was found that Taiwanin E significantly attenuated the cell viability of oral cancer cells (T28) in a dose- and time-dependent fashion; nevertheless, no cytotoxic effects were found for normal oral cells (N28). Moreover, it was observed that Taiwanin E induces G1 cell cycle arrest in T28 cells, as was evident through Flow cytometry studies, and, further, Western blot analysis suggested that Taiwanin E considerably downregulated cell cycle regulatory proteins and activated p53, p21, and p27 proteins. In addition, TUNEL staining showed that Taiwanin E induced apoptosis in T28 oral cancer cells. Furthermore, it was found that the cell survival proteins, such as p-PI3K, p-Akt, and the antiapoptotic protein Bcl-xL, were considerably reduced following treatment with Taiwanin E; nevertheless, the pro-apoptotic proteins, such as Bax, Cyt C, and c Cas 3, were, however, considerably enhanced. Further, understanding the underlying intricacies; mechanistically, it was found that Taiwanin E modulated the expression of ERK and resulted in cellular apoptosis in T28 oral cancer cells. Taken together, the data convincingly ascertained the promising candidature of Taiwanin E against oral cancer.

MATERIALS AND METHODS

Chemicals and Reagents

All chemicals and reagents were procured from Sigma Aldrich Co. (MO, USA) unless otherwise mentioned.

Purification of Taiwanin E

Taiwanin E was obtained from freshly cut wood of *Taiwania cryptomerioides* Hayata. The procedures for isolation, purification, and characterization of Taiwanin E was performed following our previously published reports with slight modifications (22, 23). Finally, the as-purified Taiwanin E was dissolved in DMSO, filtered through 0.22 μm fluoropore filter (Millipore, MA, USA), and employed for subsequent studies.

Establishment of Cell Model for Oral Cancer

An OSCC model was established following the protocol described in our previous studies (16, 17). Basically, carcinogenesis was induced in C57BL/6J Narl male mice by daily oral administration of 0.5 mg/mL arecoline (Sigma Aldrich, MO, USA) and 0.2 mg/mL of 4-NQO (Sigma Aldrich, MO, USA) for 28 days. Thereafter, primary oral squamous carcinoma cells were derived from tumor (T28) tissue following 28 weeks of administration. In addition, primary oral squamous cells were also derived from a paired control group, i.e., non-tumor normal (N28), tissue, and these were used as normal control cells.

All the animal experimentation protocols performed in the study were strictly in accordance with the Animal Care and Use Committee of the China Medical University, Taichung, Republic of China (Taiwan).

N28 and T28 cells were cultured in Dulbecco's minimum essential medium (D7777) (Sigma Aldrich, MO, USA) supplemented with 10% charcoal-treated FBS (Characterized Fetal Bovine Serum, HyClone Inc., Utah, USA), 1% penicillin/streptomycin (Invitrogen Corp., California, USA), L-Glutamine, and $NaHCO_3$.

For treatment, cells were seeded in triplicate in cell culture plates and treated with varying concentrations of Taiwanin E (0, 1, 5, and 10 μM) for different time intervals (0, 3, 6, 12, 24, and 48 h), and thereafter, the cells were harvested and analyzed for respective parameters. For activator experiments, cells were treated with Taiwanin E (10 μM) and co-treated with increasing concentrations of ERK activator (0.5, 1.0, 2.5, and 5.0 μM) for 24 h. Thereafter, they were analyzed by MTT assay and Western blotting, following the standard procedures as described below.

Cell Viability Assay

Cell viability was assessed as reported in our previous studies (16). Basically, cells were seeded in triplicate in cell culture plates and treated with increasing concentrations of Taiwanin E (0, 1, 5, and 10 μM) for a 24 h time interval. In addition, cells were treated with Taiwanin E (10 μM) for different time intervals (0, 3, 6, 12, 24, and 48 h). Following incubation with Taiwanin E for varying concentrations and time periods, the cells were thereafter treated with 0.5 mg/mL of MTT reagent and incubated for 4 h in dark conditions. Finally, the formazan crystals were dissolved in 500 μL of DMSO (dimethyl sulfoxide), and the absorbance was acquired at 570 nm on a multi-well ELIZA plate reader. Cell viability was represented as the percentage of control.

Cell Cycle Analysis

Cell cycle study was performed with flow cytometry. Briefly, T28 oral cancer cells (1×10^5 cells/well) were seeded in tissue culture plates; thereafter, they were treated with varying doses of Taiwanin E (0, 1, 5, and 10 μM) for 24 h and treated with Taiwanin E (10 μM) for different time intervals (0, 3, 6, 12, 24, and 48 h). Following treatment, cells were harvested and subsequently fixed in chilled ethanol overnight at 4°C. Consequently, cells were washed with PBS, centrifuged at 600 ×g for 5 min and thereafter resuspended in PBS containing 10 mg/ml RNase A and incubated with 30 mg/ml of PI for 30 min at RT. Finally, the samples were acquired with flow cytometry (Becton Dickinson, CA, USA).

Western Blot Analysis

Western blot was executed as reported previously (16, 24). In brief, cells were lysed in RIPA lysis buffer containing 50 mM Tris, pH 7.5, 150 mM NaCl, 1% NP-40, 0.1% SDS, 0.5% sodium deoxycholate, phosphatase inhibitor cocktail, and a proteinase inhibitor cocktail and thereafter centrifuged at 12,000 × g for 30 min at 4°C to obtain the cell lysate (25). After this, the supernatants were obtained, and protein concentration was estimated through a Bio-RAD protein quantification reagent following the Bradford method. Thereafter, the samples were resolved through 8–12% sodium dodecyl sulfate polyacrylamide gel electrophoresis (SDS-PAGE) and blotted onto polyvinylidene difluoride (PVDF) membranes (Millipore, MA, USA). The membranes were thereafter blocked with blocking solution (5% skimmed milk in TBST) for 1 h at RT. Following the blocking steps, the membranes were washed with TBST thrice and finally incubated with primary antibodies against β-actin, Cyclin B1, Cyclin D1, Cyclin E, p21, p27, JNK, p-ERK, p-JNK, p38, Cytochrome C, Bcl-xL, and Bax from Santa Cruz (CA, USA); pS473-Akt, p-PI3K, cleaved caspase-3, pP53, and p-p38 from Cell Signaling (CA, USA); and ERK from BD Biosciences (CA, USA). Following the washing procedures, the membranes were then subsequently incubated with secondary antibodies for 1 h at RT. Finally, the Antigen–Antibody molecular intricacies were assessed with enhanced chemiluminescence (ECL) horseradish peroxidase (HRP) substrate (Millipore, MA, USA), and the signals were acquired by LAS 3,000 imaging system (Fujifilm, Tokyo, Japan). Membranes were stripped and reprobed with other antibodies for the subsequent detection of other proteins.

TUNEL Assay

Cellular apoptosis was analyzed by *in situ* terminal deoxynucleotide transferase-mediated dUTP nick end-labeling (TUNEL) assay following manufacturer-recommended procedures (26). In brief, cells were cultured in 24-well culture plates and treated with Taiwanin E, and, thereafter, the cells were harvested, washed with 1×PBS (Gibco BRL, Paisley, UK), and incubated with TUNEL assay reagents at RT for stipulated time intervals. After this, the samples were examined with flow cytometry (Becton Dickinson, CA, USA).

Statistical Analysis

Results are represented as mean ± SD. Statistical analysis was done with Graph Pad Prism5 statistical software (Graph-Pad, CA, USA). Multiple comparisons were assessed through ANOVA. *p* Values of ≤ 0.05 were regarded as statistically significant. All experiments were performed in triplicate in a blinded manner. Results were quantified with Image J software (NIH, Bethesda, MD, USA) and processed through Adobe Photoshop.

RESULTS

The Effect of Taiwanin E on Cell Viability and the Cell Cycle Process of Oral Cancer Cells Following Dose-Dependent Treatment

Normal oral cells N28 and cancer cells T28 were treated with increasing concentrations of Taiwanin E for a 24 h time interval; thereafter, cell viability was ascertained by MTT assay. MTT data showed that Taiwanin E exhibited cytotoxic effects on T28 oral cancer cells, especially at 10 μM concentration, whereas no cytotoxic effects were observed for N28 normal oral cells (**Figure 1A**). In addition, it was observed that Taiwanin E exhibited significant cytotoxicity against other squamous cell carcinoma cell lines SCC9 and SCC25 (data not shown). Considering the results, we further examined whether Taiwanin E treatment could modulate cell cycle progression in oral cancer cells T28. To this end, cells were treated with increasing concentrations of Taiwanin E for 24 h; thereafter, they were analyzed through flow cytometry. As evident from **Figure 1**, it was found that there were considerable increase in the G1 population (60.07% at 5 μM, 67.80% at 10 μM) in Taiwanin E-treated T28 cells as compared to control cells, wherein only 58.03% of cells were in the G1 population (**Figure 1B**). The data from the study suggested an accumulation in the G1 phase of the cell cycle following treatment with Taiwanin E.

The Effect of Taiwanin E on Cell Viability and the Cell Cycle Process of Oral Cancer Cells Following Time-Dependent Treatment

Further, N28 and T28 cells were treated with Taiwanin E (10 μM) for different time periods from 0 to 48 h, and cell viability was determined through MTT assay; interestingly, it was observed that Taiwanin E exhibited cytotoxic effects on T28 cells in a time-dependent manner. However, no such effects were observed for normal N28 oral cells (**Figure 2A**). Further, we also determined the effect of treatment of Taiwanin E for different time interval (0–48 h) on the cell progression; it was found that there were considerable increases in the G1 population in a time-dependent fashion (**Figure 2B**) (27).

Collectively, these results suggested that Taiwanin E exhibited cytotoxic manifestations toward tumor oral cells T28 in a dose- and time-dependent fashion; however, no cytotoxic effects were

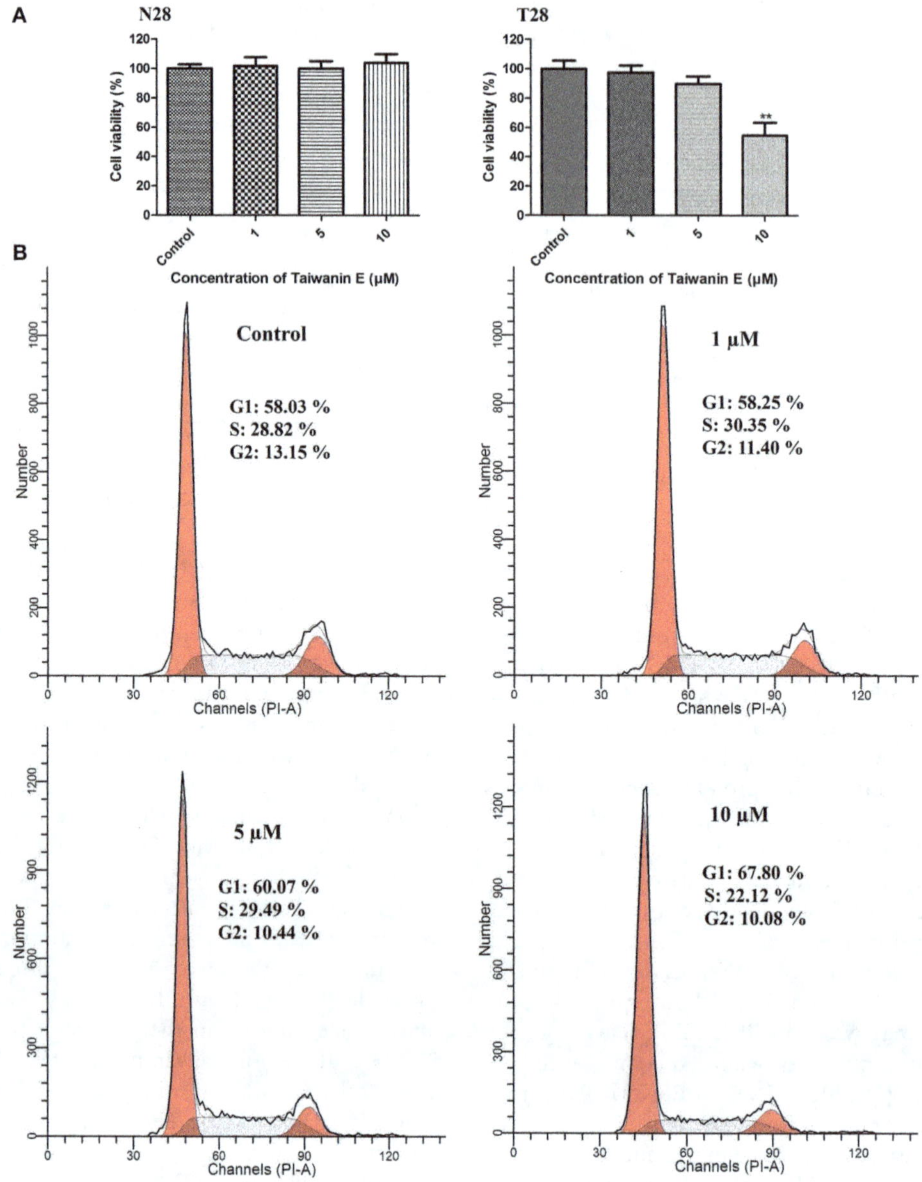

FIGURE 1 | Effect of Taiwanin E on cell viability and cell cycle progression of oral cells. Normal oral cells N28 and Cancer oral cells T28 were treated with varying concentrations of Taiwanin E (0, 1, 5, and 10 μM) for 24 h. The cell viability of N28 cells and T28 cells was assessed with MTT assay **(A)**. $^{**}p < 0.01$ represents significant differences compared with control. T28 cells were treated with varying concentrations of Taiwanin E (0, 1, 5, and 10) μM for 24 h, and the DNA content was assessed through flow cytometry. Results were represented as percentages of the cell population in G1, S, and G2 phases of the cell cycle **(B)**.

observed for normal oral cells N28. Moreover, Taiwanin E treatment in T28 cells modulated their normal regulation of cell cycle progression. Nevertheless, no significant effects were observed for normal oral cells N28 (data not shown).

The Effect of Taiwanin E on Cell Cycle-Related Proteins of Oral Cancer Cells

We further investigated whether Taiwanin E affects cell cycle-related proteins in T28 oral cancer cells. To this end, cells were treated with Taiwanin E (10 μM) for different time periods from 0 to 48 h and thereafter analyzed through Western blotting. Interestingly, it was found that the cell cycle regulatory proteins, such as cyclin B1, cyclin D1, and cyclin E, were considerably decreased (**Figure 3A**), whereas p53, p21, and p27 protein levels were substantially increased following treatment with Taiwanin E (**Figure 3B**).

The Effect of Taiwanin E on the Induction of Apoptosis in Oral Cancer Cells

We further investigated whether Taiwanin E could induce cellular apoptosis in T28 oral cancer cells. As evident through TUNEL assay, considerable apoptosis was observed following treatment with Taiwanin E (**Figure 4A**). To gain further insight

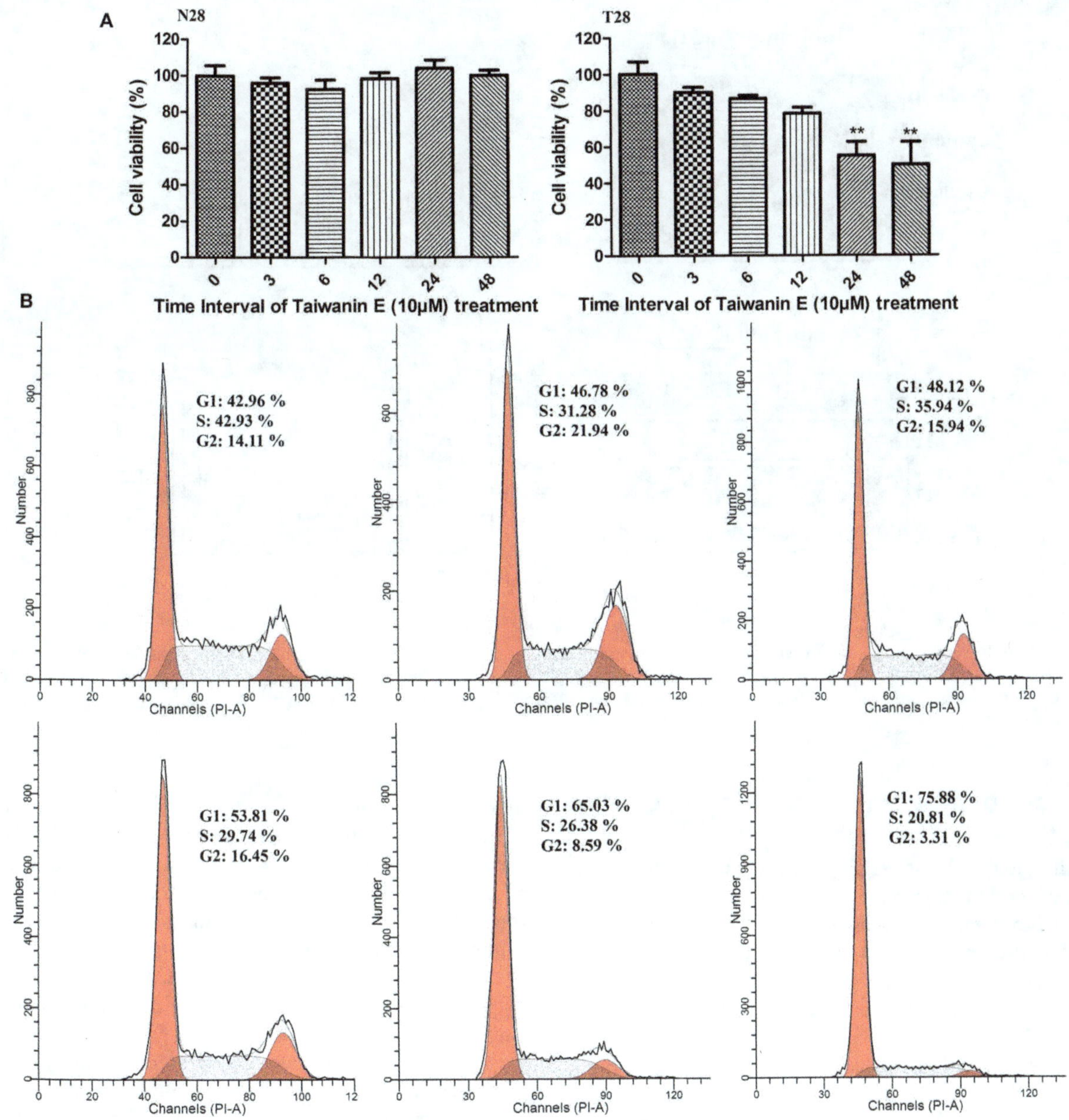

FIGURE 2 | Effect of Taiwanin E on cell viability and cell cycle progression of oral cells. Normal oral cells N28 and cancer oral cells T28 were treated with Taiwanin E (10 μM) for different time intervals. The cell viability of N28 cells and T28 cells was assessed with MTT assay **(A)**. $^{**}p < 0.01$ represents significant differences compared with control. T28 cells were treated with Taiwanin E (10 μM) for different time interval, and the DNA content was assessed through flow cytometry. Results were represented as a percentage of the cell population in G1, S, and G2 phases of the cell cycle **(B)**.

into the effect of Taiwanin E on T28 oral cancer cells, we examined the protein levels of p-PI3K, p-Akt, Bcl-xL, Bax, cytochrome C, and cleaved caspase 3. Intriguingly, it was observed that T28 cells, when treated with Taiwanin E, showed a significant decrement in survival-related proteins, including p-PI3K, p-Akt, and anti-apoptotic protein Bcl-xL, in a time-dependent manner; contrastingly, the levels of Bax, Cyt C, and cleaved-caspase 3 were considerably decreased accordingly (**Figure 4B**).

The Effect of Taiwanin E on the MAPK Signaling Cascade in Oral Cancer Cells

Further, the effect of Taiwanin E on the MAPK signaling cascade was investigated. As could be seen from the figure, following treatment with Taiwanin E, a considerable reduction in the p-ERK1/2 was observed; no significant effects, however, were observed for p-JNK and p-p38 proteins (**Figure 5**). Collectively, these results showed that Taiwanin E considerably regulated the MAPK signaling cascade.

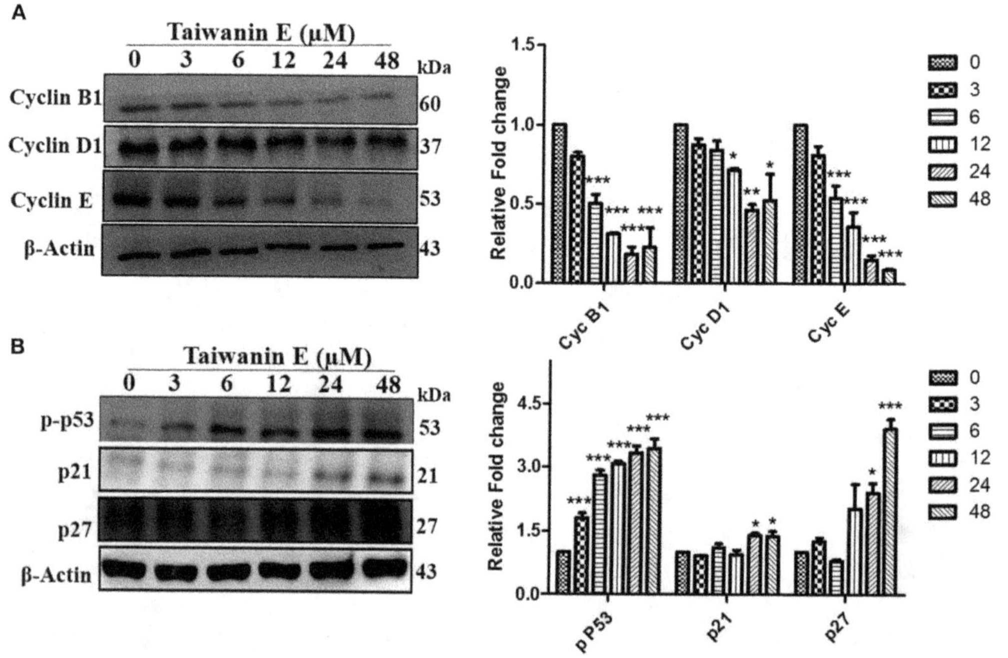

FIGURE 3 | Effect of Taiwanin E on cell cycle-related proteins in oral cancer cells. T28 cells were treated with Taiwanin E (10 μM) for different time intervals and thereafter analyzed through Western blotting. Samples were assessed for the expression of Cyclin B1, Cyclin D1, and Cyclin E **(A)** and p53, p21, and p27 **(B)**, respectively. Graphs represent mean values of three independent experiment in T28 cells. $^*p < 0.05$, $^{**}p < 0.01$, and $^{***}p < 0.001$ represent significant differences compared with control.

The Effects of Taiwanin E on ERK in Oral Cancer Cells

To further investigate the underlying intricacies of modulation of ERK in the efficacy of Taiwanin E, the effect of the ERK activator on T28 cell proliferation was ascertained. Intriguingly, it was observed that ERK activator co-treatment with Taiwanin E in T28 cells considerably reversed the effect of Taiwanin E in a dose-dependent fashion (**Figure 6A**). In addition, we further examined whether the ERK activator co-treatment could interfere with the signal transduction pathway of cellular apoptosis. Interestingly, the results showed that co-treatment with the ERK activator considerably increased Bcl-xL protein levels and reduced Cyt C protein levels (**Figure 6**). These results highlighted the role of ERK in the efficacy of Taiwanin E against T28 oral cancer cells.

Collectively, it could be envisaged that Taiwanin E considerably modulated ERK, which eventually led to the inhibition of cancer cell survival, induced cell cycle arrest at G1, and apoptosis in T28 oral cancer cells. Collectively, the data convincingly demonstrated that Taiwanin E may potentially become an effective small molecular drug against oral cancer in the near future.

DISCUSSION

Various bioactive compounds (lignans, flavones, sesquiterpenoids, diterpenoids, cyclitols, steroids, etc.) derived from Taiwania has been shown to be effective against various debilitating diseases. Accumulating evidences have shown their efficacy against various forms of cancers, including A-549 lung carcinoma, MCF-7 breast adenocarcinoma, and HT-29 colon adenocarcinoma (22). In this research endeavor, we investigated the anti-cancer effect of Taiwanin E against arecoline and 4-nitroquinoline-1-oxide-induced OSCC and elucidated the underlying mechanism thereof. Basically, OSCC were treated with Taiwanin E and analyzed for their bioactivities against OSCC. Collectively, the data of the present study suggest that Taiwanin E significantly attenuated the cell viability of oral cancer cells (T28) in a dose- and time-dependent fashion. Moreover, it was observed that Taiwanin E induced G1 cell cycle arrest in T28 cells, as was evident through Flow cytometry studies, and further Western blot analysis suggested that Taiwanin E considerably downregulated cell cycle regulatory proteins, including Cyclin B1, Cyclin D1, and Cyclin E, and activated p53, p21, and p27 proteins, respectively. Furthermore, TUNEL staining showed that Taiwanin E induced considerable apoptosis in T28 cells, and, in addition, it was found that the cell survival proteins, such as p-PI3K and p-Akt and the anti-apoptotic protein Bcl-xL, were considerably reduced following treatment with Taiwanin E The pro-apoptotic proteins, such as Bax, Cyt C, and c Cas-3, were, however, considerably enhanced. Furthermore, in understanding the underlying intricacies mechanistically, it was found that Taiwanin E seemingly modulated ERK and thereby attenuated cell survival and induced cellular apoptosis in T28 oral cancer cells.

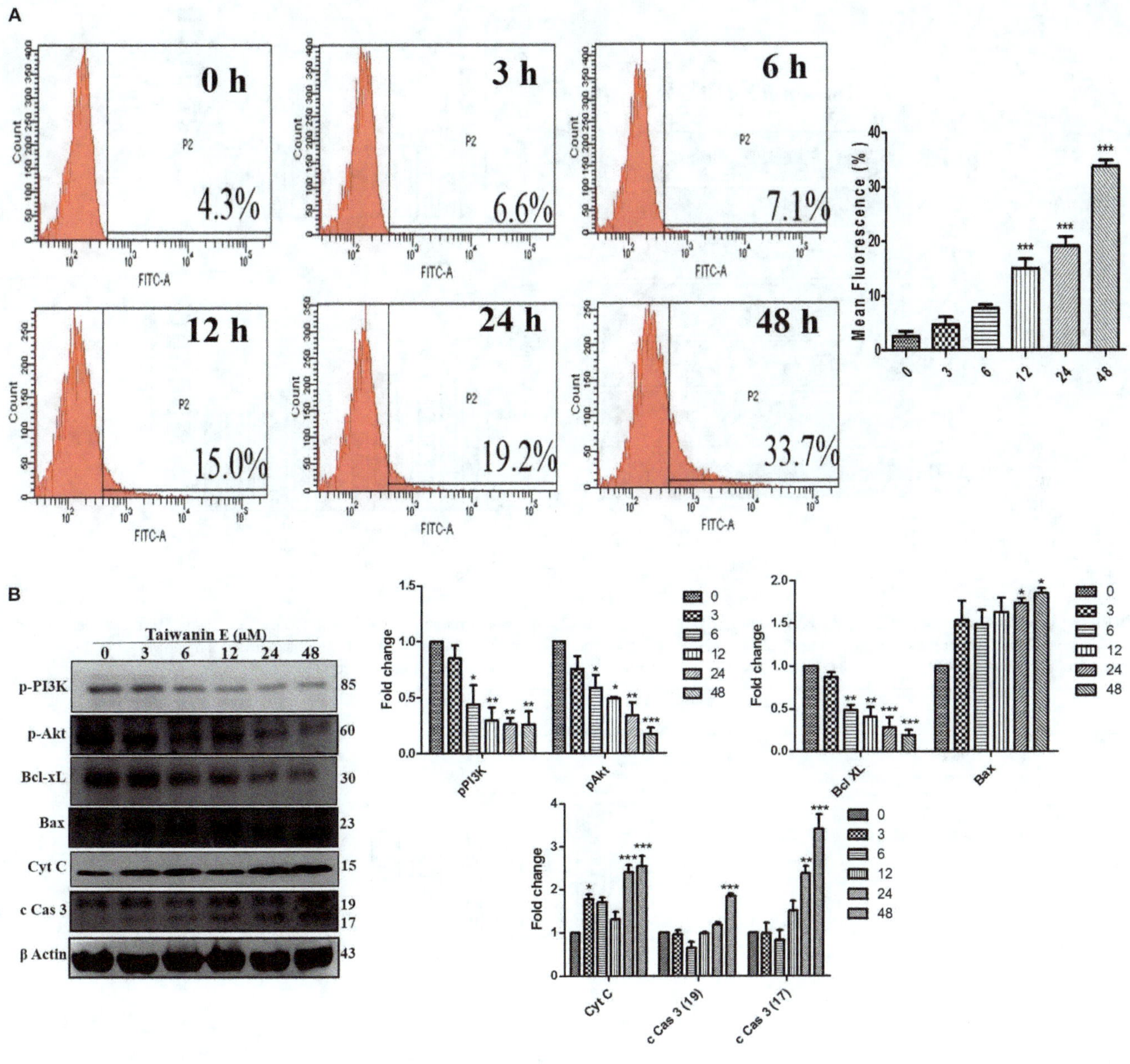

FIGURE 4 | Effect of Taiwanin E on the induction of cellular apoptosis in oral cancer cells. T28 cells were treated with Taiwanin E (10 μM) for different time periods The samples were stained with a TUNEL kit and analyzed through flow cytometry **(A)**. T28 cells were treated with Taiwanin E (10 μM) for different time periods. Cell lysates were analyzed for the expressions of p-PI3K, p-Akt, Bcl-xL, Bax, Cyt C, and c Cas 3 through Western blotting **(B)**. Graphs represents the mean value of three separate experiment in the T28 cells. *$p < 0.05$, **$p < 0.01$, and ***$p < 0.001$ represent significant differences compared with control group.

It is widely accepted that alteration in cell cycle progression causes severe cellular damage which eventually leads to apoptosis. It was found that Taiwanin E induces cell cycle arrest in OSCC in a dose and time dependent fashion. Analyzing the molecular intricacies underlying Taiwanin E-induced cell cycle arrest, it was observed that Taiwanin E treatment downregulated the expression of cell cycle regulatory proteins; in addition, Taiwanin E regulated the p53 tumor suppressor and increased the protein expression of p21 and p27. This is in concordance with the study by Shyur et al., wherein they demonstrated that Taiwanin A isolated from *Taiwania cryptomerioides* Hayata upregulated p53, phosphorylated p53, p21, and p27, and, contrastingly, downregulated the G(2)/M checkpoint mediators cyclins, leading to the induction of G(2)/M cell-cycle arrest in MCF-7 cells (13).

As a matter of fact, the apoptotic pathways are regulated through the orchestrated communication of diverse pro-apoptotic and anti-apoptotic signaling mediators. Essentially, the pro-apoptotic signaling mediators lead to the modulation of mitochondrial potential and subsequent release of mediators, which eventually triggers a cascade of events that lead to apoptosis. The data of the present study demonstrated that Taiwanin E treatment increased the amount of pro-apoptotic

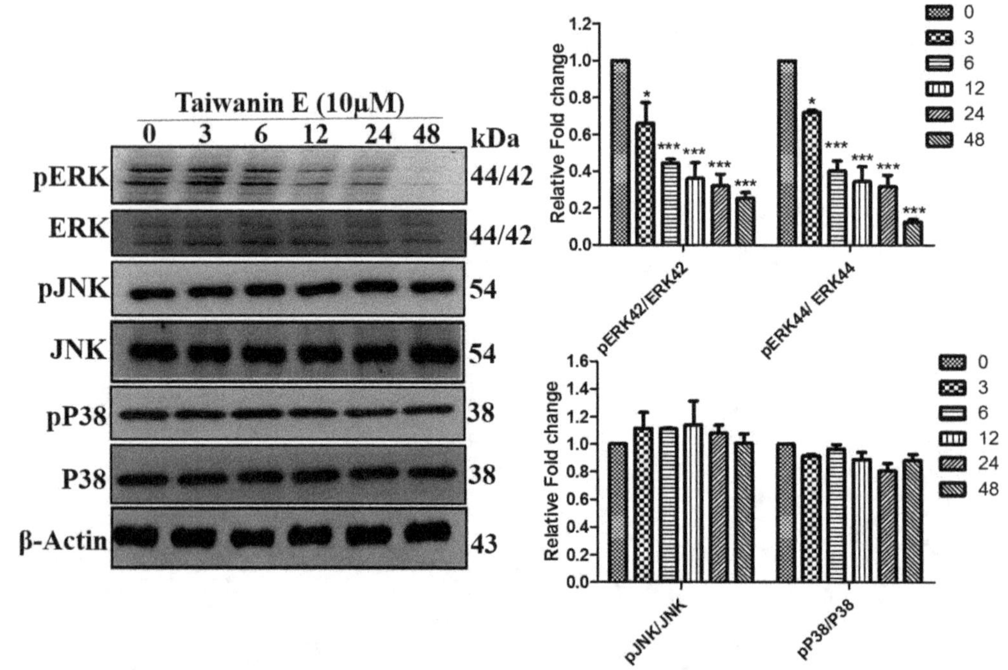

FIGURE 5 | Taiwanin E modulate the ERK signaling cascade in oral cancer cells. T28 cells were treated with Taiwanin E (10 µM) for different time periods. Thereafter, cell lysates were analyzed for the expression of ERK, pERK, JNK, pJNK, p38, and p-p38 through Western blotting. Graphs represents mean values of three independent experiment in T28 cells. *$p < 0.05$ and ***$p < 0.001$ represent significant differences compared with control.

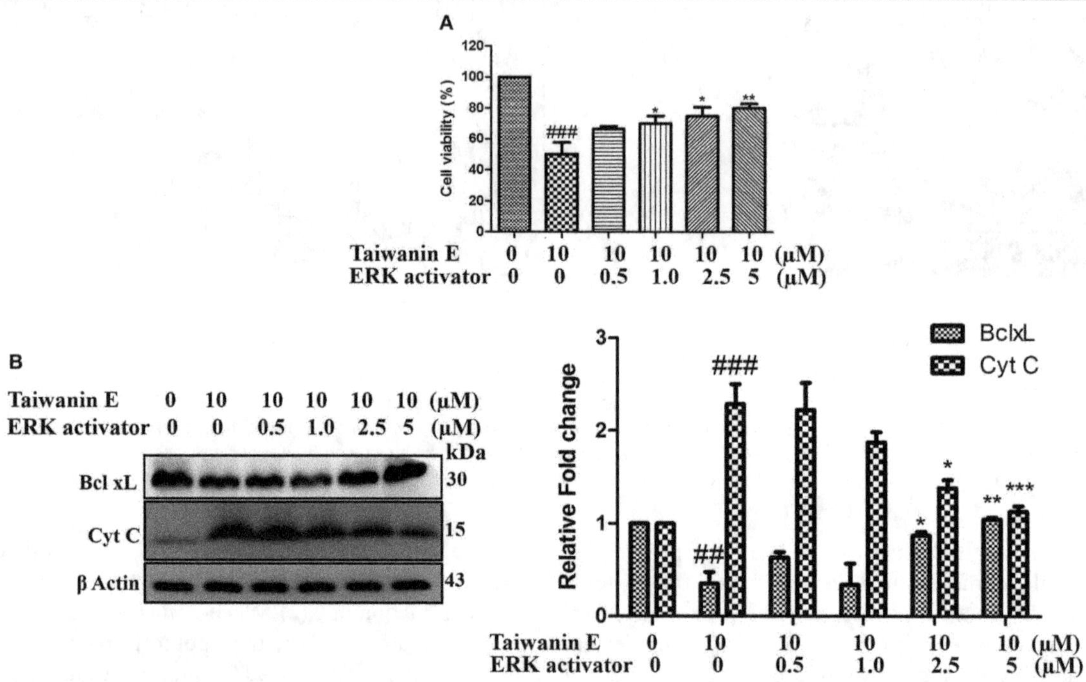

FIGURE 6 | Effect of Taiwanin E on ERK activation in oral cancer cells. T28 cells were co-treated with ERK activator and Taiwanin E for 24 h. Thereafter, cell viability was analyzed through MTT assay **(A)**. T28 cells were co-treated with ERK activator and Taiwanin E for 24 h. Thereafter, cell lysates were analyzed through Western blotting for the expression of Bcl-xL and Cyt C proteins through Western blotting **(B)**. Graphs represent mean value of three separate experiment in T28 cells. ##$p < 0.01$ and ###$p < 0.001$ represent significant differences compared with control group, whereas *$p < 0.05$, **$p < 0.01$, and ***$p < 0.001$ represent significant differences compared with the Taiwanin E-treated group.

proteins. Bax released cytochrome C from the mitochondria, induced Caspase activation, and downregulated the survival protein p-PI3K, p-Akt, and anti-apoptotic Bcl-xL, which is certainly suggestive of their promising anti-cancer potential against OSCC.

MAPK/ERK signaling cascades are crucial pathways that plays an imperative role in the orchestration of normal cell proliferation, survival, and differentiation. It is widely accepted that aberrant regulation of MAPK has been involved in various human diseases, including cancer. Thus, the MAPK/ERK signaling network has been the focus of various research endeavors in order to ascertain novel target-based approaches for cancer therapeutics (28). Intriguingly, our study demonstrated that Taiwanin E modulated ERK signaling for therapeutic efficacy (28). This is in concordance with the reports, wherein authors have implicated the role of the ERK signaling mediator in the efficacy of the anti-cancer compounds. To this end, Wang et al. reported that Geraniin inhibited migration and invasion of human osteosarcoma cancer cells, seemingly through the regulation of the PI3K/Akt and ERK1/2 signaling pathways (29). Furthermore, Fong et al., while demonstrating the efficacy of BPIQ-induced cell migration and apoptosis in human non-small cell lung cancer (NSCLC) cells, highlighted that MAPK kinases, in particular ERK mediators, were responsible for their anti-cancer potential (30). In addition, Kuo et al. have explicitly demonstrated that the a related compound of Taiwanin E, i.e., a novel derivative of Taiwanin A, inhibited dual key proliferation signaling transduction pathways in a Triple-Negative Breast Cancer model (31).

Collectively, keeping in mind the fact that various phytochemicals, such as taxol (from *Taxus brevifolia*) and camptothecin derivatives (from *Camptotheca acuminate*), are widely explored for cancer treatment, and, as Taiwanin E displayed lower cytotoxicity against normal oral cells, it could be envisaged as a promising drug to treat oral cancer in the near future, thus warranting future investigation.

AUTHOR CONTRIBUTIONS

S-HW and C-YH contributed toward the conception and design of the study. S-HW, H-CW, and KB performed the experiments and data analysis. KB, C-JC, and C-YH contributed to the manuscript writing, editing, and proofreading. Y-HK, Y-PC, H-HH, D-TB, VV, Y-HC, and P-JL supported the experiment design, data analysis, and the manuscript writing and proofreading.

REFERENCES

1. Chrysant SG, Chrysant GS. Herbs used for the treatment of hypertension and their mechanism of action. *Curr Hypertension Rep.* (2017) 19:77. doi: 10.1007/s11906-017-0775-5
2. Chiang JT, Badrealam KF, Shibu MA, Cheng SF, Shen CY, Chang CF, et al. Anti-apoptosis and anti-fibrosis effects of eriobotrya japonica in spontaneously hypertensive rat hearts. *Int J Mol Sci.* (2018) 19:E1638. doi: 10.3390/ijms19061638
3. Hedigan K. Cancer: herbal medicine reduces chemotherapy toxicity. *Nat Rev Drug Discov.* (2010) 9:765. doi: 10.1038/nrd3280
4. Efferth T, Li PC, Konkimalla VS, Kaina B. From traditional Chinese medicine to rational cancer therapy. *Trends Mol Med.* (2007) 13:353–61. doi: 10.1016/j.molmed.2007.07.001
5. Li-Weber M. Targeting apoptosis pathways in cancer by Chinese medicine. *Cancer Lett.* (2013) 332:304–12. doi: 10.1016/j.canlet.2010.07.015
6. Newman DJ, Cragg GM. Natural products as sources of new drugs over the last 25 years. *J Nat Prod.* (2007) 70:461–77. doi: 10.1021/np068054v
7. Abdelfadil E, Cheng YH, Bau DT, Ting WJ, Chen LM, Hsu HH, et al. Thymoquinone induces apoptosis in oral cancer cells through p38beta inhibition. *Am J Chinese Med.* (2013) 41:683–96. doi: 10.1142/S0192415X1350047X
8. Chen MC, Huang CY, Hsu SL, Lin E, Ku CT, Lin H, et al. Retinoic acid induces apoptosis of prostate cancer DU145 cells through Cdk5 overactivation. *Evid-Based Compl Altern Med.* (2012) 2012:580736. doi: 10.1155/2012/580736
9. Tsai KH, Hsien HH, Chen LM, Ting WJ, Yang YS, Kuo CH, et al. Rhubarb inhibits hepatocellular carcinoma cell metastasis via GSK-3-beta activation to enhance protein degradation and attenuate nuclear translocation of beta-catenin. *Food Chem.* (2013) 138:278–85. doi: 10.1016/j.foodchem.2012.10.038
10. Dung TD, Chang HC, Binh TV, Lee MR, Tsai CH, Tsai FJ, et al. Zanthoxylum avicennae extracts inhibit cell proliferation through protein phosphatase 2A activation in HA22T human hepatocellular carcinoma cells *in vitro* and *in vivo*. *Int J Mol Med.* (2012) 29:1045–52. doi: 10.3892/ijmm.2012.938
11. Dung TD, Chang HC, Chen CY, Peng WH, Tsai CH, Tsai FJ, et al. Zanthoxylum avicennae extracts induce cell apoptosis through protein phosphatase 2A activation in HA22T human hepatocellular carcinoma cells and block tumor growth in xenografted nude mice. *Int J Mol Med.* (2011) 28:927–36. doi: 10.3892/ijmm.2012
12. Ho PJ, Chou CK, Kuo YH, Tu LC, Yeh SF. Taiwanin a induced cell cycle arrest and p53-dependent apoptosis in human hepatocellular carcinoma HepG2 *Cells Life Sci.* (2007) 80:493–503. doi: 10.1016/j.lfs.2006.10.017
13. Shyur LF, Lee SH, Chang ST, Lo CP, Kuo YH, Wang SY. Taiwanin A inhibits MCF-7 cancer cell activity through induction of oxidative stress, upregulation of DNA damage checkpoint kinases, and activation of p53 and FasL/Fas signaling pathways. *Phytomedicine.* (2010) 18:16–24. doi: 10.1016/j.phymed.2010.06.005
14. Chang ST, Cheng SS, Wang SY. Antitermitic activity of essential oils and components from Taiwania (Taiwania cryptomerioides). *J Chem Ecol.* (2001) 27:717–24. doi: 10.1023/a:1010397801826
15. Chang ST, Chen PF, Wang SY, Wu HH. Antimite activity of essential oils and their constituents from Taiwania cryptomerioides. *J Med Entomol.* (2001) 38:455–7. doi: 10.1603/0022-2585-38.3.455
16. Tsai CY, Fang HY, Shibu MA, Lin YM, Chou YC, Chen YH, et al. Taiwanin C elicits apoptosis in arecoline and 4-nitroquinoline-1-oxide-induced oral squamous cell carcinoma cells and hinders proliferation via epidermal growth factor receptor/PI3K suppression. *Environ Toxicol.* (2019) 34:760–67. doi: 10.1002/tox.22742
17. Hsieh CH, Hsu HH, Shibu MA, Day CH, Bau DT, Ho CC, et al. Down-regulation of beta-catenin and the associated migration ability by Taiwanin C in arecoline and 4-NQO-induced oral cancer cells via GSK-3beta activation. *Mol Carcinogen.* (2017) 56:1055–67. doi: 10.1002/mc.22570
18. Lin KH, Shibu MA, Kuo YH, Chen YC, Hsu HH, Bau DT, et al. Taiwanin C selectively inhibits arecoline and 4-NQO-induced oral cancer cell proliferation via ERK1/2 inactivation. *Environ Toxicol.* (2017) 32:62–9. doi: 10.1002/tox.22212
19. Murugan AK, Munirajan AK, Tsuchida N. Ras oncogenes in oral cancer: the past 20 years. *Oral Oncol.* (2012) 48:383–92. doi: 10.1016/j.oraloncology.2011.12.006
20. Silverman S Jr. Demographics and occurrence of oral and pharyngeal cancers.

The outcomes, the trends, the challenge. *J Am Dental Assoc.* (2001) 132 (Suppl.):7s–11s. doi: 10.14219/jada.archive.2001.0382

21. Yu GP, Mehta V, Branovan D, Huang Q, Hashibe M, Zhang ZF, et al. Improved survival among patients with base of tongue and tonsil cancer in the United States. *Cancer Causes Control.* (2012) 23:153–64. doi: 10.1007/s10552-011-9864-y
22. Chang ST, Wang DS, Wu CL, Shiah SG, Kuo YH, Chang CJ. Cytotoxicity of extractives from Taiwania cryptomerioides heartwood. *Phytochemistry.* (2000) 55:227–32. doi: 10.1016/S0031-9422(00)00275-2
23. Hsu HH, Kuo WW, Day CH, Shibu MA, Li SY, Chang SH, et al. Taiwanin E inhibits cell migration in human LoVo colon cancer cells by suppressing MMP-2/9 expression via p38 MAPK pathway. *Environ Toxicol.* (2017) 32:2021–31. doi: 10.1002/tox.22379
24. Chao CN, Lai CH, Badrealam KF, Lo JF, Shen CY, Chen CH, et al. CHIP attenuates lipopolysaccharide-induced cardiac hypertrophy and apoptosis by promoting NFATc3 proteasomal degradation. *J Cell Physiol.* (2019) 234:20128–138. doi: 10.1002/jcp.28614
25. Khan BF, Hamidullah, Dwivedi S, Konwar R, Zubair S, Owais M. Potential of bacterial culture media in biofabrication of metal nanoparticles and the therapeutic potential of the as-synthesized nanoparticles in conjunction with artemisinin against MDA-MB-231 breast cancer cells. *J Cell Physiol.* (2018) 234:6951–64. doi: 10.1002/jcp.27438
26. Zhang X, Bommareddy A, Chen W, Khalifa S, Kaushik RS, Fahmy H, et al. Sarcophine-diol, a chemopreventive agent of skin cancer, inhibits cell growth and induces apoptosis through extrinsic pathway in human epidermoid carcinoma A431 Cells. *Transl Oncol.* (2009) 2:21–30. doi: 10.1593/tlo.08190
27. He X, Maimaiti M, Jiao Y, Meng X, Li H. Sinomenine Induces G1-Phase Cell Cycle Arrest and apoptosis in malignant glioma cells via downregulation of sirtuin 1 and induction of p53 acetylation. *Technol Cancer Res Treat.* (2018) 17:1533034618770305. doi: 10.1177/1533034618770305
28. Roberts PJ, Der CJ. Targeting the Raf-MEK-ERK mitogen-activated protein kinase cascade for the treatment of cancer. *Oncogene.* (2007) 26:3291–310. doi: 10.1038/sj.onc.1210422
29. Wang Y, Wan D, Zhou R, Zhong W, Lu S, Chai Y. Geraniin inhibits migration and invasion of human osteosarcoma cancer cells through regulation of PI3K/Akt and ERK1/2 signaling pathways. *Anti-Cancer Drugs.* (2017) 28:959–66. doi: 10.1097/CAD.0000000000000535
30. Fong Y, Wu CY, Chang KF, Chen BH, Chou WJ, Tseng CH, et al. Dual roles of extracellular signal-regulated kinase (ERK) in quinoline compound BPIQ-induced apoptosis and anti-migration of human non-small cell lung cancer cells. *Cancer Cell Int.* (2017) 17:37. doi: 10.1186/s12935-017-0403-0
31. Kuo YH, Chiang EI, Chao CY, Rodriguez RL, Chou PY, Tsai SY, et al. Dual inhibition of key proliferation signaling pathways in triple-negative breast cancer cells by a novel derivative of Taiwanin A. *Mol Cancer Therapeutics.* (2017) 16:480–93. doi: 10.1158/1535-7163.MCT-16-0011

2

Differentiation of Thyroid Nodules Difficult to Diagnose with Contrast-Enhanced Ultrasonography and Real-Time Elastography

Xuehua Xi [1†], Luying Gao [2†], Qiong Wu [2,3†], Shibao Fang [3], Jingzhu Xu [4], Ruyu Liu [2], Xiao Yang [2], Shenling Zhu [2], Ruina Zhao [2], Xingjian Lai [2], Xiaoyan Zhang [2], Bo Zhang [1,2] and Yuxin Jiang [2*]*

[1] Department of Ultrasound, China–Japan Friendship Hospital, Beijing, China, [2] Department of Ultrasound, Peking Union Medical College Hospital, Chinese Academy of Medical Sciences & Peking Union Medical College, Beijing, China, [3] Department of Ultrasound, Affiliated Hospital of Qingdao University, Qingdao, China, [4] Department of General Surgery, Peking Union Medical College Hospital, Chinese Academy of Medical Sciences & Peking Union Medical College, Beijing, China

***Correspondence:**
Bo Zhang
thyroidus@163.com
Yuxin Jiang
jiangyuxinxh@163.com

† These authors have contributed equally to this work and share first authorship

According to the 2015 American Thyroid Association (ATA), referred risk stratification and thyroid nodules with intermediate- and low-suspicion patterns are difficult to diagnose. The objective of this study is to evaluate the diagnostic performance of contrast-enhanced ultrasonography (CEUS) and elastosonography (ES) for the differentiation of these thyroid nodules. From November 2011 to June 2016, a total of 163 thyroid nodules with intermediate- and low-suspicion patterns in 150 consecutive patients at our hospital were studied before surgery. With surgical pathology as the standard, the diagnostic value of CEUS and ES was analyzed. There were 29 (17.8%) malignant lesions and 134 (82.2%) benign lesions. The enhancement patterns of CEUS, the echogenicity, and the elastography were significantly different between malignant and benign lesions ($P < 0.05$). Heterogenous enhancement was more common in malignant nodules, and the sensitivity, specificity, positive predictive value, negative predictive value, and odds ratio were 51.7, 88.1, 48.4, 89.4, and 10.1%, respectively. The diagnostic accuracy of CEUS was better than the conventional ultrasound [area under the curve (AUC), 0.729 vs. 0.616, $P = 0.021$]. The enhancement patterns of CEUS were helpful in the differential diagnosis of thyroid nodules with intermediate and low suspicion.

Keywords: thyroid carcinoma, contrast-enhanced ultrasonography, elastosonography, American Thyroid Association, intermediate- and low-suspicion patterns

INTRODUCTION

The 2015 American Thyroid Association Management Guidelines for Adult Patients with Thyroid Nodules and Differentiated Thyroid Cancer (1) (2015 ATA guidelines) proposed a risk stratification of thyroid nodules based on a series of studies on the ultrasonographic features of thyroid nodules. The guide classifies the sonographic appearance of the vast majority of thyroid nodules into the following categories of ultrasound patterns: high suspicion, intermediate suspicion, low suspicion, very low suspicion, and benign. Intermediate suspicion (malignancy risk 10–20%) nodules are hypoechoic solid nodules with smooth regular margins and without malignant features such as microcalcifications, extrathyroidal extension, or a taller-than-wide shape. Low-suspicion (malignancy risk, 5–10%) nodules are isoechoic or hyperechoic solid nodules or partially cystic nodules with eccentric uniformly solid areas without malignant features. These nodules have similar ultrasound features as nodules suspicious of follicular lesions in the "British Thyroid Association Guidelines for the Management of Thyroid Cancer" (2) (BTA guidelines). Despite the fact that the malignancy risk is not relatively high, differentiating malignant from benign lesions by conventional ultrasonography (CUS) is challenging.

Contrast-enhanced ultrasonography (CEUS) has been widely used to evaluate the microvessel perfusion of thyroid nodules. Elastosonography (ES) quantifies the firmness of the tissue and displays it as a color map on which the hardness of the tissues can be reflected. Many studies have concluded that the accuracy of the diagnosis of thyroid nodules can be increased by combining CEUS and ES with CUS (3–5). However, the value of CEUS and ES in evaluating nodules with intermediate- and low-suspicion patterns is unclear.

METHODS

This study was approved by the ethics committee of Peking Union Medical College Hospital (PUMCH), and informed consent was obtained from all patients before CEUS and ES.

Patients

A total of 604 patients with thyroid nodules admitted to PUMCH from November 2011 to June 2016 who met the following criteria were included in this study: (a) CUS indicated that the thyroid nodule was of intermediate or low suspicion according to the 2015 ATA guidelines for referred risk stratification, and (b) the largest diameter of the nodule was larger than 5 mm in size. The exclusion criteria were as follows: (a) patients who did not undergo surgery, (b) patients younger than 18 years of age, (c) women during pregnancy or lactation, and (d) patients who could not tolerate the intravenous injection of contrast agents because of heart, lung, kidney, or other vital organ dysfunction or severe allergies. A total of 163 thyroid nodules in 150 consecutive patients (mean age, 47.9; range, 18–83 years) were included. Two nodules in eight patients each and three nodules in three patients each were included. In six of those eight patients, the two nodules were located in different lobes. In two other patients, the two nodules were not near each other, although they were in the same lobe. In three patients, two of the three nodules were located in the same lobe, and the other was located in a different lobe. CUS, CEUS, and ES were performed in all patients, and the ultrasound-guided fine needle aspiration (FNA) was performed in nine patients before surgery.

Ultrasound Examination

All ultrasound (US) examinations were performed with a 5- to 12-MHz liner probe (iU22; Philips Medical System, Bothell, WA, United States). The CUS examination was performed with the standard equipment settings for thyroid glands. Standard machine settings for CEUS were used, and the contrast medium used was SonoVue (Bracco Imaging, Milan, Italy). With a 20- or 22-gauge peripheral intravenous cannula, SonoVue was injected intravenously as a bolus at a dose of 1.2 ml, followed by 5 ml of normal saline as a flush. The timer on the US machine was then started, and each contrast imaging acquisition lasted more than 2 min after the bolus injection; the imaging was digitally stored. During real-time elastography (RTE), the probe was positioned perpendicular to the skin, and no compression was applied at the skin above the targeted thyroid nodule. When there were two nodules in a patient, CEUS was performed on the second nodule after the first injected contrast agent was completely cleaned in the whole gland. CUS, RTE, and CEUS images and cine clips were analyzed by two radiologists with more than 5 years of experience in thyroid US. They were blinded to the patients' clinical data and pathological results. In cases of discrepancies between the two readers, a consensus was reached after discussion.

TABLE 1 | Clinical characteristics of nodules with intermediate and low suspicion.

Clinical characteristics	Malignant group ($n = 29$)	Benign group ($n = 121$)	*P*-value
Age (years)	44.0 ± 11.9	48.7 ± 11.8	0.706
Sex			0.054
Female	17 (58.6)	91 (75.2)	
Male	12 (41.4)	30 (24.8)	
Mixed with HT	1 (3.4)	19 (15.7)	0.081
Size (cm)*	2.1 ± 1.5	2.6 ± 1.4	0.675

HT, Hashimoto thyroiditis.
**For 163 nodules.*

TABLE 2 | Comparison of fine needle aspiration (FNA) cytopathology and histological pathology of nine nodules.

Nodule number	FNA cytopathology	Histological pathology
1	A small amount of thyroid follicular epithelial cells and no tumor cells	Thyroid atypical adenoma
2	Thyroid follicular epithelial cells and no tumor cells	Thyroid adenoma
3	Suspicious for a follicular neoplasm	Thyroid follicular carcinoma
4	Thyroid follicular epithelial cells and no tumor cells	Thyroid follicular carcinoma
5	No exception of follicular adenoma	Nodular goiter with adenomatous hyperplasia
6	Thyroid follicular adenoma	Nodular goiter with adenomatous hyperplasia
7	Tumor-like lesion from thyroid follicular epithelial cells. Tumor or adenomatous change cannot be distinguished because no specific capsule was seen.	Nodular hashimoto thyroiditis
8	Consistent with thyroid follicular neoplasm, and thyroid adenoma was considered	Nodular goiter with adenomatous hyperplasia
9	Thyroid follicular epithelial cells and no tumor cells	Nodular goiter

The CUS features of all thyroid nodules were recorded according to the halo, echogenicity, internal component, echotexture (homogenous or heterogenous), calcifications, and vascularity. Halos were classified as absent, regularly thin, or irregular (including thick halos, incomplete halos, and halos of different widths). Echogenicity was classified as hypoechogenicity, isoechogenicity, hyperechogenicity, or marked hyperechogenicity relative to the surrounding normal parenchyma. The internal component of a nodule was classified as solid (defined as composed entirely or nearly entirely of soft tissue, with only a few tiny cystic spaces) (6), predominantly solid, and predominantly cystic. Calcifications, when present, were categorized as microcalcifications, disrupted rim calcifications, and other types of calcifications. Microcalcifications were defined as calcifications that were ≤1 mm in diameter and visualized as tiny hyperechoic foci. Disrupted rim calcifications were defined as interrupted peripheral calcifications in association with a soft tissue rim outside the calcification. When a nodule had both microcalcifications and other types of calcifications, it was classified as having microcalcifications. The vascularity of nodules was classified into five types by Frates (7) as follows: 0 for no visible flow, 1 for minimal internal flow without a peripheral ring, 2 for a peripheral ring of flow (defined as >25% of the nodule's circumference) with minimal or no internal flow, 3 for a peripheral ring of flow with a small to moderate amount of internal flow, and 4 for extensive internal flow with or without a peripheral ring. We regarded type 4 as increased intranodular vascularity. CEUS characteristics included peak intensity (categorized as low, equal, or high) and enhanced pattern (categorized as homogenous, heterogenous, or ring enhancing). Elastography score elasticity was classified in five different patterns, adding elastography score (ESS) 0 to the version of Asteria criteria (8): ESS 0, red and blue, or blue and green, or red and green are layered distribution in cystic nodules or predominantly cystic nodules; ESS 1, homogenously in green (soft); ESS 2, predominantly in green with few blue areas/spots; ESS 3, predominantly in blue with a few green areas/spots; and ESS 4, completely in blue (hard).

TABLE 3 | Ultrasound (US) characteristics of benign and malignant thyroid nodules with intermediate and low suspicion.

US characteristics	Malignant nodules ($n = 29$)	Benign nodules ($n = 134$)	*P*-value
Halo			0.183
Absent	17 (58.6)	58 (43.3)	
Regular and thin	8 (27.6)	62 (46.3)	
Irregular	4 (13.8)	14 (10.4)	
Internal component			0.157
Solid	20 (69.0)	74 (55.2)	
Predominantly solid	9 (31.0)	47 (35.1)	
Predominantly cystic	0 (–)	13 (9.7)	
Echogenicity			0.033
Hyperechogenicity	1 (3.4)	18(13.4)	
Isoechogenicity	5 (17.2)	53 (39.6)	
Hypoechogenicity	20 (69.0)	57 (42.5)	
Marked hypoechogenicity	3 (10.3)	6 (4.5)	
Homogeneity			0.762
Homogenous	7 (24.1)	36 (26.9)	
Heterogenous	22 (75.9)	98 (73.1)	
Calcification			0.746
Absent	18 (62.1)	95 (70.9)	
Microcalcification	1 (3.4)	3 (2.2)	
Disrupted rim calcification	0 (0)	0 (0)	
Other types of calcification	10 (34.5)	36 (26.9)	
Vascularity type			0.429
Type 0	0 (0)	0 (0)	
Type 1	2 (6.9)	0 (-)	
Type 2	3 (10.3)	1 (0.7)	
Type 3	4 (13.8)	27 (20.1)	
Type 4	20 (69.0)	106 (79.1)	
Risk stratification			<0.001
Intermediate suspicion	21 (72.4)	45 (33.6)	
Low suspicion	8 (27.6)	89 (66.4)	

Review of Histopathology

An experienced pathologist who was blinded to the clinical information reviewed the histopathology of all the specimens. The papillary thyroid carcinomas (PTCs) were divided into classical PTC and follicular variants of the PTC (FVPTC).

Statistical Analysis

The statistical analysis was performed with the SPSS statistical package (Version 19.0, SPSS Chicago, IL, United States)

TABLE 4 | Contrast-enhanced ultrasonography (CEUS) and elastosonography (ES) characteristics of malignant and benign thyroid nodules.

CEUS and ES characteristics	Malignant nodules ($n = 29$)	Benign nodules ($n = 134$)	*P*-value
Enhanced pattern			<0.001
Ring enhancing	11 (37.9)	89 (66.4)	
Homogenous	2 (6.9)	24 (17.9)	
Heterogenous	15 (51.7)	16 (11.9)	
No enhancement	1 (3.4)	5 (3.7)	
Peak intensity*			0.289
High	10 (34.5)	55 (41.0)	
Equal	9 (31.0)	51 (38.1)	
Low	9 (31.0)	21 (15.7)	
Elastography score†			0.015
0	1 (3.8)	13 (9.7)	
1	0 (–)	12 (9.0)	
2	11 (42.3)	68 (50.7)	
3	9 (34.6)	36 (26.9)	
4	5 (19.2)	5 (3.7)	

**The peak intensity of two nodules was not determined because the nodules were too large and the surrounding thyroid parenchyma could not be displayed in the same plane for reference.*

†The ES of the three nodules was not determined because the nodules were too close to the carotid artery and the results were unreliable.

and MedCalc 11.4.2.0 software (MedCalc Software, Ostend, Belgium). The quantitative data were expressed as the mean ± standard deviation. The Student's t-test was used for comparing the groups. The χ^2 test or Fisher's exact test was used to compare categorical data. The sensitivity, specificity, positive predictive value (PPV), negative predictive value (NPV), and accuracy were calculated through a comparison with the pathological findings. A receiver operating characteristic (ROC) curve analysis was used to compare CEUS, ES, and CUS. A $P < 0.05$ was considered statistically significant.

RESULTS

Clinical Characteristics

The clinical characteristics are summarized in **Table 1**. The age, gender, nodule size, and incidence of coexistence with Hashimoto thyroiditis (HT) did not significantly differ between the benign and malignant groups ($P > 0.05$). The results of the cytopathology and histopathology of the nine nodules that underwent FNA are summarized in **Table 2**. Histological pathology demonstrated that 29 lesions (17.8%) were malignant, and 134 lesions (82.2%) were benign. One hundred one nodular goiters (75.4%) constituted the majority of benign lesions, 18 of the 134 lesions were adenomatous nodules (ANs). The remainder of the benign lesions consisted of six follicular adenomas (FAs, 25.4%) and nine HTs (6.7%). Of the malignant lesions, 21 cases were PTCs, with 17 classical variant and 4 follicular variants, 7 cases were follicular carcinomas (FCs), and 1 case was medullary carcinoma (MC). Cervical lymph node metastasis was confirmed in one FC and six PTCs. Metastatic lesions were found in cervical striated muscles and fibrous connective tissues in another FC.

US Characteristics

The CUS characteristics are summarized in **Table 3**. No significant difference was observed in the US features of absent or irregular halos (a solid internal component, a heterogenous echo

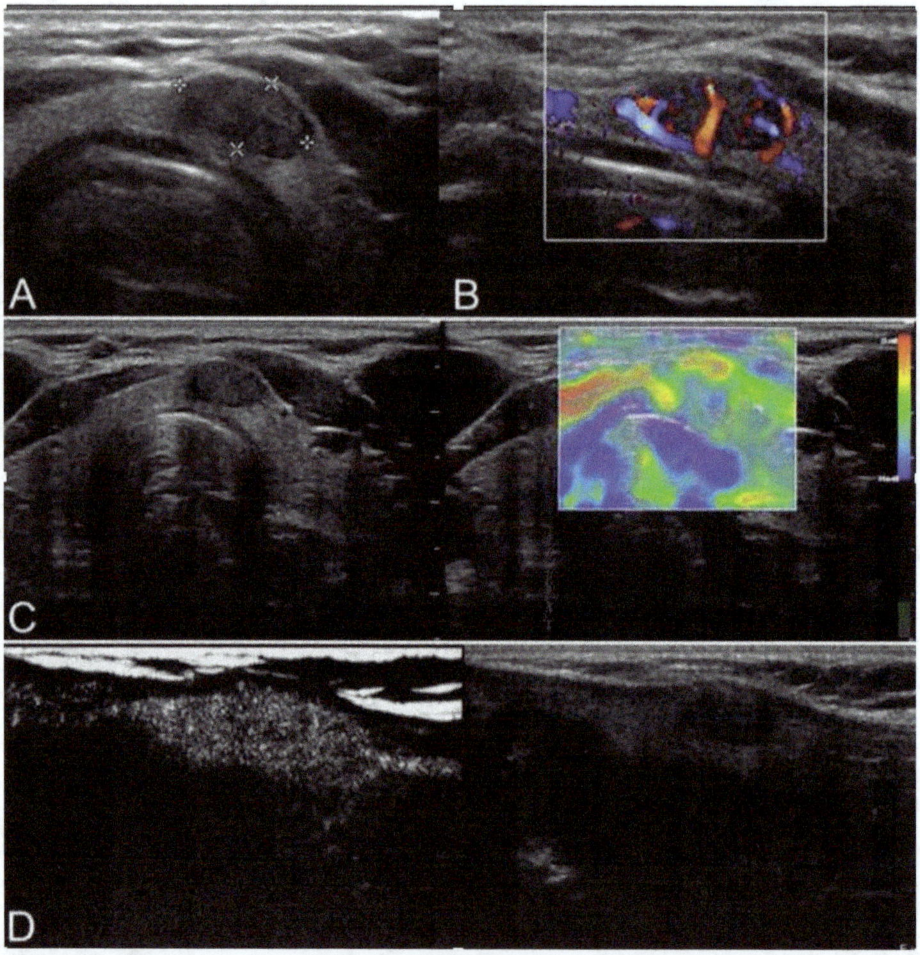

FIGURE 1 | Ultrasound of a 42-year-old man who incidentally detected a thyroid nodule is shown. **(A)** Conventional ultrasonography (CUS) showed that there was a solid hypoechoic nodule with a regular margin in the isthmus of the thyroid. The nodule was of intermediate suspicion. **(B)** Color Doppler showed intranodular and peripheral vascularity. **(C)** The elastography score was 2, indicating that the nodule was soft. **(D)** Contrast-enhanced ultrasonography (CEUS) revealed heterogenous enhancement. The nodule was a papillary thyroid carcinoma (PTC) confirmed by histological pathology.

texture, and microcalcification or disrupted rim calcification between benign and malignant lesions). Moderate or abundant blood flow (Frates type 3 or 4) was detected in the majority of the nodules with intermediate- and low-suspicion patterns. The difference in increased intranodular vascularity (Frates type 4) between benign and malignant lesions was not statistically significant ($P > 0.05$). Of the malignant nodules, two PTCs showed peripheral vascularity without intranodular vascularity, and four PTCs showed partial hypervascularity with perforating vessels into the nodule. Regular peripheral and intranodular vascularity was found in the other 15 malignant lesions.

The CEUS characteristics and ES of the nodules are shown in **Table 4** and **Figures 1–4**. Heterogenous enhancement was significantly ($P < 0.001$) associated with a malignant outcome with a 10.1 odds ratio [OR; 95% confidence interval (CI) ranging from 3.9 to 25.7]. The sensitivity, specificity, positive predictive value, and negative predictive value were 51.7, 88.1, 48.4, and 89.4%, respectively. The enhancement patterns of 12 PTCs and 2 FCs and 1 MC were heterogenous, 2 PTCs were homogenous, 1 PTC had no enhancement, and the remaining 6 PTCs and 5 FCs exhibited a ring-enhancing pattern. Among the benign nodules, 89 cases (66.4%) showed a ring-enhancing pattern; 24 cases (17.9%) showed homogenous enhancement, including 18 nodular goiters and 3 HT; and 16 cases (11.9%) showed heterogenous enhancement, including 10 nodular goiter, 2 FAs, and 4 HTs. The intensity of enhancement was not significantly different ($P = 0.289$). Most of the nodules showed soft texture in elasticity imaging, and the difference in the ES between the benign and malignant groups was significant ($P = 0.015$).

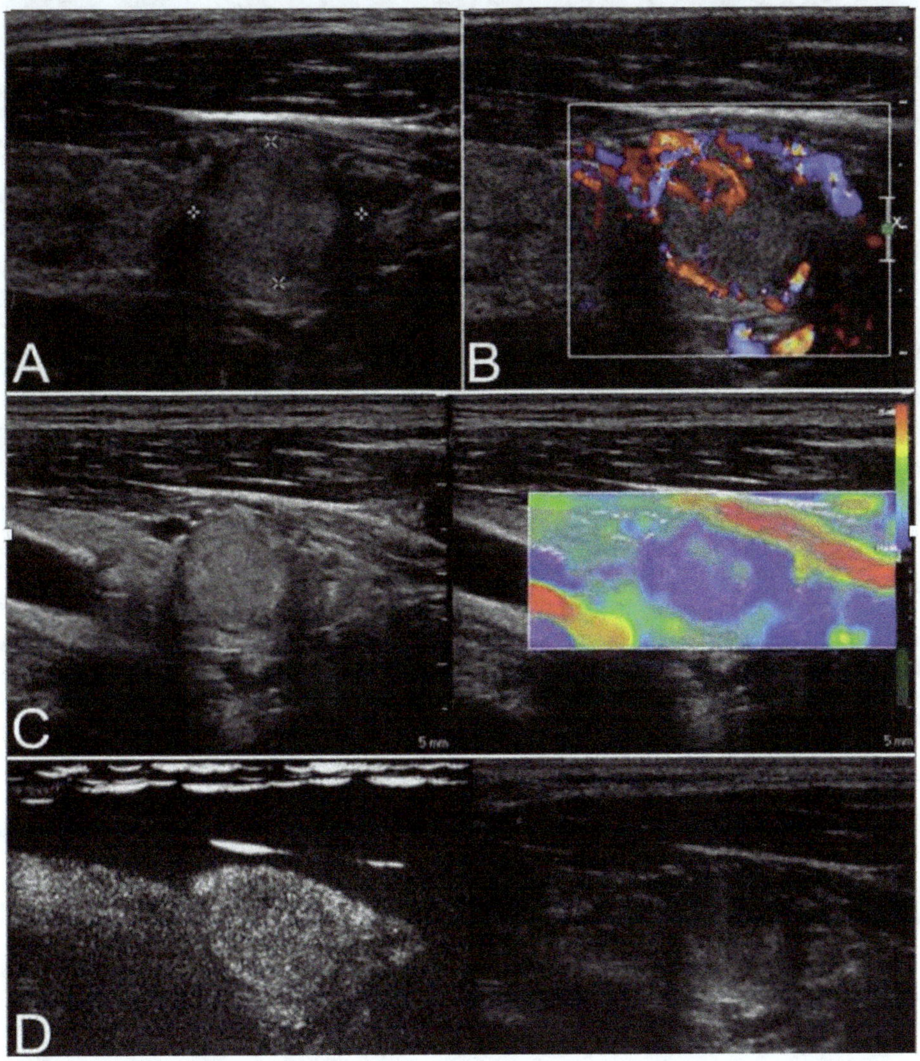

FIGURE 2 | This case is a 27-year-old man with an follicular carcinoma (FC) nodule. **(A)** Conventional ultrasonography (CUS) showed a solid hyperechoic nodule in the left lobe that was associated with a regular thin halo and an inside area that was hypoechoic, which is indicative of low suspicion. **(B)** Abundant intranodular and peripheral vascularity was detected. **(C)** The elastography score was 2, indicating a soft stiffness. **(D)** Contrast-enhanced ultrasonography (CEUS) revealed heterogenous enhancement.

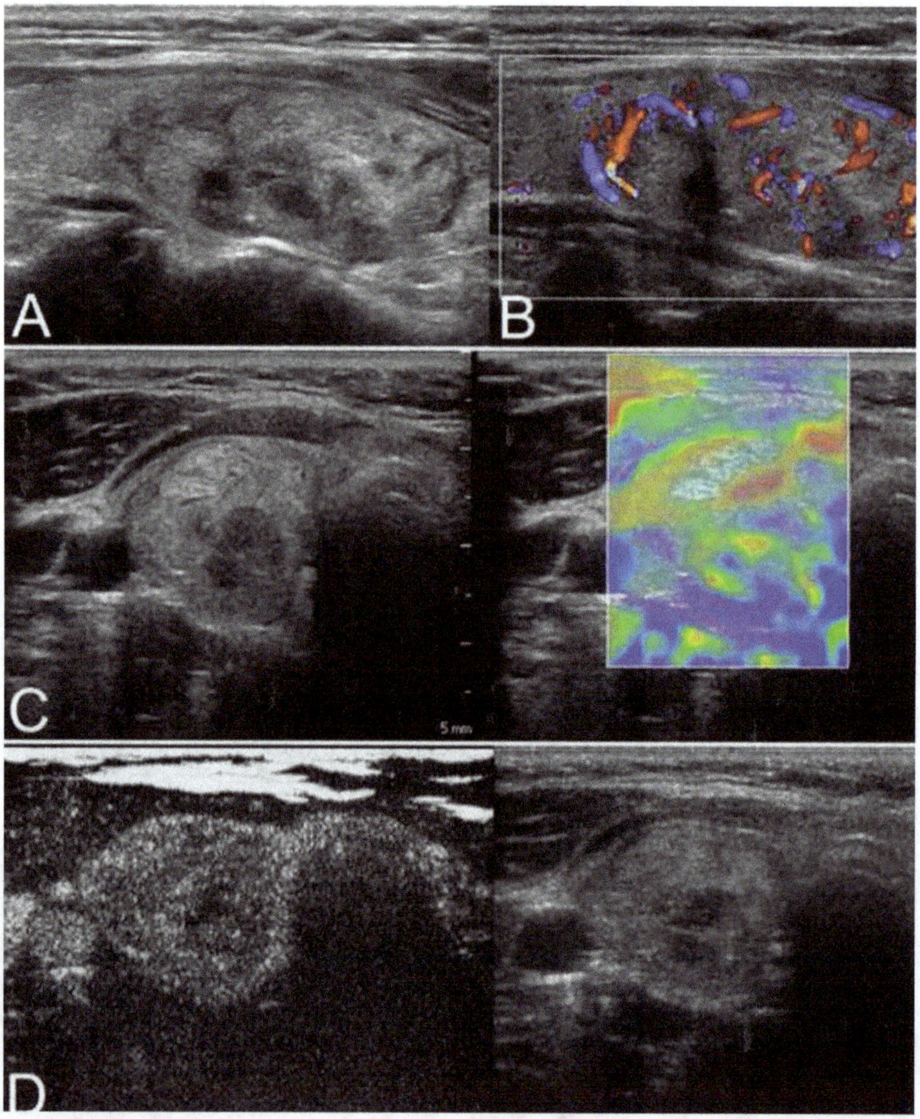

FIGURE 3 | (A) The isoechoic solid nodule with a regular thin halo was evaluated as low suspicion by conventional ultrasonography (CUS) in a 38-year-old man. **(B)** Color Doppler showed intranodular and peripheral vascularity. **(C)** The elastography score was 3, indicating a hard stiffness. **(D)** Contrast-enhanced ultrasonography (CEUS) revealed ring enhancement. The nodule was a follicular adenoma.

Diagnostic Performance of the CEUS and ES

Sensitivity, specificity, PPV, NPV, accuracy, and area under the curve (AUC) of CUS were 69.0, 57.5, 26.0, 89.5, 59.5, and 0.61% (95% CI, 0.53–0.69), respectively. Nodules with the CEUS patterns of heterogenous enhancement was considered malignant. The sensitivity, specificity, PPV, NPV, accuracy, and AUC for CEUS were 51.7, 88.1, 48.4, 89.4, 81.6, and 0.73% (95% CI, 0.65–0.80), respectively. The ROC curves demonstrated that the best cutoff value for ES was 3. The sensitivity, specificity, PPV, NPV, accuracy, and AUC for ES were 53.8, 69.4, 25.5, 88.6, 66.9, and 0.62% (95% CI, 0.54–0.69), respectively (**Table 5**). The CEUS showed a higher AUC than CEUS and ES (0.729 vs. 0.616, P = 0.021; 0.729 vs. 0.608, P = 0.046). We added this in *Result* and *Abstract* and emphasized in red color (lines 37 and 88–99).

DISCUSSION

High-resolution neck ultrasonography is the most important method for the evaluation of a thyroid nodule. The latest ATA guidelines have proposed criteria for risk stratification that categorizes the thyroid nodules and stratify the risk of malignancy. However, the differential diagnosis of nodules with intermediate and low suspicion is difficult. In the "British Thyroid Association Guidelines for the Management of Thyroid Cancer" (2), these nodules are defined as suspicious of follicular lesions on ultrasound and classified as indeterminate/equivocal.

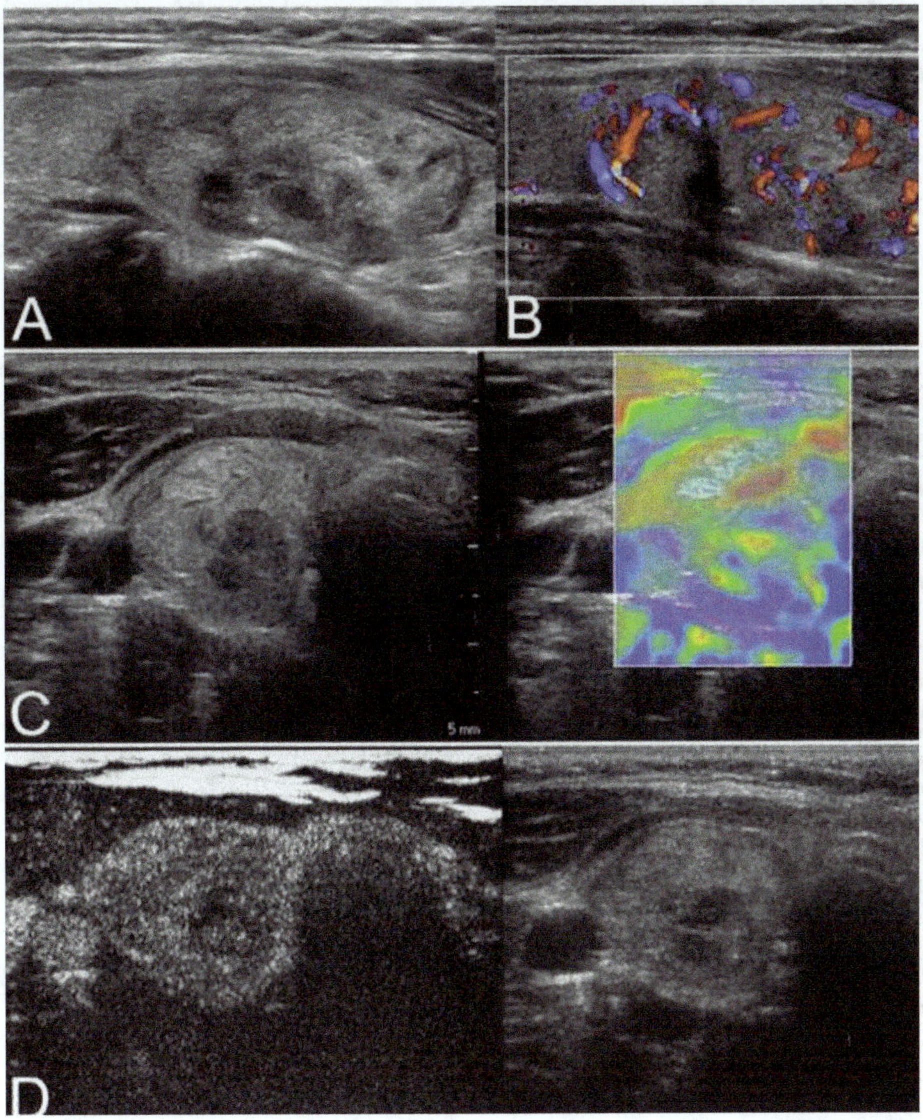

FIGURE 4 | A nodular goiter with adenomatous hyperplasia in a 59-year-old woman is shown. **(A)** Conventional ultrasonography (CUS) showed that the solid hyperechoic nodule in the right lobe was heterogenous in echotexture and had regular margins, indicative of low suspicion. **(B)** Color Doppler showed intranodular and peripheral vascularity. **(C)** The elastography score was 2, indicating a soft stiffness. **(D)** Contrast-enhanced ultrasonography (CEUS) revealed ring-enhancement.

A total of 71.4% of the nodules were thyroid tumors with a follicular growth pattern. Our study showed that the enhancement pattern was a significant factor for differentiating benign and malignant nodules with intermediate and low suspicion. Some researchers have revealed that age, sex, and tumor size are predictive parameters of malignancy in follicular neoplasms of the thyroid (diagnosed by intraoperative frozen section or FNA) (9, 10). The male gender, ages <45 years, and nodules larger than 4 cm were risk factors for malignancy. In our study, 15.7% of women and 28.6% of men had malignant nodules. Sixteen patients (10.7%) younger than 45 years of age and 13 patients (8.7%) older than 45 years of age were diagnosed with malignant lesions, with no statistically significant differences observed. Of the 29 malignant nodules, only 3 (10.3%) were larger than 4 cm. Therefore, using sex, age, and nodule size as the predictive malignant parameters may result in missed diagnoses and misdiagnoses.

Conventional ultrasound features such as a solid internal component, hypoechogenicity, irregular margins, a taller-than-wide shape, and microcalcification are predictive of thyroid carcinoma (11, 12). However, these features are classical malignant characteristics for non-follicular neoplasms. Koike et al. (13) found that the sensitivity of preoperative US diagnosis was 18.2% for follicular neoplasms. Multiple logistic regression analyses revealed that conventional ultrasound could not identify FC and FA (13). The results of this study were similar to these previous results.

TABLE 5 | Diagnostic efficiency of the contrast-enhanced ultrasonography (CEUS), elastosonography (SE) and conventional ultrasonography (CUS).

	Se (%)	Sp (%)	PPV (%)	NPV (%)	Ac (%)	AUC (95% CI)*
CUES	51.7	88.1	48.4	89.4	81.6	0.729 (0.653–0.796)
SE	53.8	69.4	25.5	88.6	66.9	0.616 (0.536–0.692)
CUS	69.0	57.5	26.0	89.5	59.5	0.608 (0.528–0.685)

CEUS, contrast-enhanced ultrasonography; ES, elastosonography; CUS, conventional ultrasonography; Se, sensitivity; Sp, specificity; PPV, positive predictive value; NPV, negative predictive value; AUC, area under the curve; CI, confidence interval.

CEUS can reflect the state of microcirculation perfusion of nodules. Three meta-analyses showed that both the sensitivity and specificity of CEUS were more than 85% (14–16). Most research have suggested that a heterogenous enhancement pattern is a reliable index for predicting malignancy and that a ring-enhancement pattern is a feature of benign nodules. Our study has revealed that the predictivity of malignancy of ATA risk stratification is improved by adding CEUS. The malignancy risk of the intermediate and low suspicious nodules is 5–20%. The risk can increase to 38.5% when the nodule shows heterogenous enhancement. Despite the low sensitivity (51.7%), it has a very high specificity and OR for malignancy. Of the 29 malignant nodules, 12 PTCs and 2 FCs and MC presented with heterogenous enhancement, which might be due to the more heterogenous growth of malignant nodules and the more imbalanced blood distribution, with the coexistence of areas of rich and poor microvasculature. In addition, malignant nodules contain regions of complicated morphological collagen degeneration, which have either no small vessels or vessels whose caliber is so small that microbubbles cannot enter, resulting in heterogenous enhancement. However, the other six PTCs and five FCs presented with ring enhancement. Two FVPTC nodules were 3.8 and 4.0 cm in ultrasound images, but the pathological size of the cancer area was only 0.4 and 0.5 cm, respectively, with the surrounding tissue presenting with nodular goiter. This finding may result in a benign enhancement pattern. The reason that malignant nodules showed ring enhancement may be that the nodules were surrounded by vessels or that vessels existed in the capsule of the nodule, which is consistent with the color Doppler features.

Elastosonography provided an estimation of tissue stiffness. In our study, only 14 malignant nodules were hard, with 3–4 elastography scores. The other 15 malignant nodules were relatively soft. This result was different from most studies, which reported that malignant thyroid nodules were often stiff. The most likely reason is that the constitution of the cases was vastly different. In this study, 24.1% of the malignant nodules were FCs, and 13.8% of the nodules were FVPTCs. Pathological changes in these nodules showed that follicular cells containing colloid were abundant, making the texture soft. Therefore, real-time elastography was not able to distinguish benign and malignant nodules with intermediate and low suspicion.

FNA is the best preoperative diagnostic method for thyroid nodules but is indeterminate in 15–20% of the cases especially when follicular neoplasms are involved. When a follicular neoplasm is suspected, the histological possibilities include an AN, FA, or FC. FVPTC will also sometimes fall into this category when the nuclear features are more subtle. These features cannot be distinguished by the use of cytology alone because the evaluation of morphology is subjective (17, 18) and the sample is too limited to represent the entire heterogenous lesion. In addition, the presence of capsule or vessel invasion for diagnosing FC cannot be evaluated by FNA (19). One FC in this study was suspicious for a follicular neoplasm, and the other FC exhibited only thyroid follicular epithelial cells and no tumor cells. Another lesion that was suspicious for FC by FNA was a nodular goiter with adenomatous hyperplasia confirmed by surgical pathology.

A limitation of our study is selective bias. This study is a retrospective study, and the subjects included were patients undergoing surgery. Whether the results are applicable to all clinical conditions remains to be verified. In addition, the strain ratio was not evaluated with ES. Further large studies using more indicators are needed to obtain a more accurate value.

CONCLUSIONS

The CEUS enhancement pattern is helpful for differentiating between benign and malignant nodules with an intermediate or low suspicion. Heterogenous enhancement is associated with malignant nodules, a finding that could modify the clinical decision to avoid the misdiagnosis of FC in some patients. CUS characteristics, other qualitative CEUS indices, ES, and FNA have limited value.

ETHICS STATEMENT

This prospective study was approved by the ethics committee of Peking Union Medical College Hospital, and informed consent was obtained. The patients/participants provided their written informed consent to participate in this study. Written informed consent was obtained from the individual(s) for the publication of any potentially identifiable images or data included in this article.

AUTHOR CONTRIBUTIONS

BZ and YJ conceived and designed the study. JX, RL, and RZ collected the data. XY and SZ performed the analysis. XL and XZ prepared all the figures and tables. XX, LG and QW were major contributors in writing the manuscript. SF edited the manuscript. All authors read and approved the final manuscript.

REFERENCES

1. Haugen BR, Alexander EK, Bible KC, Doherty GM, Mandel SJ, Nikiforov YE, et al. 2015 American thyroid association management guidelines for adult patients with thyroid nodules and differentiated thyroid cancer: the American thyroid association guidelines task force on thyroid nodules and differentiated thyroid cancer. *Thyroid.* (2016) 26:1–133. doi: 10.1089/thy.2015.0020
2. Perros P, Boelaert K, Colley S, Evans C, Evans RM, Gerrard Ba G, et al. Guidelines for the management of thyroid cancer. *Clin Endocrinol.* (2014) 811:1–122. doi: 10.1111/cen.12515
3. Giusti M, Campomenosi C, Gay S, Massa B, Silvestri E, Monti E, et al. The use of semi- quantitative ultrasound elastosonography in combination with conventional ultrasonography and contrast-enhanced ultrasonography in the assessment of malignancy risk of thyroid nodules with indeterminate cytology. *Thyroid Res.* (2014) 7:9. doi: 10.1186/s13044-014-0009-8
4. Cantisani V, Consorti F, Guerrisi A, Guerrisi I, Ricci P, Di Segni M, et al. Prospective comparative evaluation of quantitative-elastosonography (Q-elastography) and contrast-enhanced ultrasound for the evaluation of thyroid nodules: preliminary experience. *Eur J Radiol.* (2013) 82:1892–8. doi: 10.1016/j.ejrad.2013.07.005
5. Liang XN, Guo RJ, Li S, Zheng ZM, Liang HD. Binary logistic regression analysis of solid thyroid nodules imaged by high-frequency ultrasonography, acoustic radiation force impulse, and contrast-enhanced ultrasonography. *Eur Rev Med Pharmacol Sci.* (2014) 18:3601–10.
6. Grant EG, Tessler FN, Hoang JK, Langer JE, Beland MD, Berland LL, et al. Thyroid ultrasound reporting lexicon: white paper of the ACR thyroid imaging, reporting and data system (TIRADS) committee. *J Am Coll Radiol.* (2015) 12:1272–9. doi: 10.1016/j.jacr.2015.07.011
7. Frates MC, Benson CB, Doubilet PM, Cibas ES, Marqusee E. Can color doppler sonography aid in the prediction of malignancy of thyroid nodules? *J Ultrasound Med.* (2003) 22:127–31. doi: 10.7863/jum.2003.22.2.127
8. Asteria C, Giovanardi A, Pizzocaro A, Cozzaglio L, Morabito A, Somalvico F, et al. US- elastography in the differential diagnosis of benign and malignant thyroid nodules. *Thyroid.* (2008) 18:523–31. doi: 10.1089/thy.2007.0323
9. Paramo JC, Mesko T. Age, tumor size, and in-office ultrasonography are predictive parameters of malignancy in follicular neoplasms of the thyroid. *Endocr Pract.* (2008) 14:447–51. doi: 10.4158/EP.14.4.447
10. Baloch ZW, Fleisher S, LiVolsi VA, Gupta PK. Diagnosis of "follicular neoplasm": a gray zone in thyroid fine-needle aspiration cytology. *Diagn Cytopathol.* (2002) 26:41–4. doi: 10.1002/dc.10043
11. Kwak JY, Han KH, Yoon JH, Moon HJ, Son EJ, Park SH, et al. Thyroid imaging reporting and data system for US features of nodules: a step in establishing better stratification of cancer risk. *Radiology.* (2011) 260:892–9. doi: 10.1148/radiol.11110206
12. Choi YJ, Yun JS, Kim DH. Clinical and ultrasound features of cytology diagnosed follicular neoplasm. *Endocr J.* (2009) 56:383–9. doi: 10.1507/endocrj.K08E-310
13. Koike E, Noguchi S, Yamashita H, Murakami T, Ohshima A, Kawamoto H, et al. Ultrasonographic characteristics of thyroid nodules: prediction of malignancy. *Arch Surg.* (2001) 136:334–7. doi: 10.1001/archsurg.136.3.334
14. Yu D, Han Y, Chen T. Contrast-enhanced ultrasound for differentiation of benign and malignant thyroid lesions: meta-analysis. *Otolaryngol Head Neck Surg.* (2014) 151:909–15. doi: 10.1177/0194599814555838
15. Ma X, Zhang B, Ling W, Liu R, Jia H, Zhu F, et al. Contrast-enhanced sonography for the identification of benign and malignant thyroid nodules: systematic review and meta-analysis. *J Clin Ultrasound.* (2016) 44:199–209. doi: 10.1002/jcu.22311
16. Sun B, Lang L, Zhu X, Jiang F, Hong Y, He L. Accuracy of contrast-enhanced ultrasound in the identification of thyroid nodules: a meta analysis. *Int J Clin Exp Med.* (2015) 8:12882–9.
17. Olson MT, Boonyaarunnate T, Aragon Han P, Umbricht CB, Ali SZ, Zeiger MA. A tertiary center's experience with second review of 3885 thyroid cytopathology specimens. *J Clin Endocrinol Metab.* (2013) 98:1450–7. doi: 10.1210/jc.2012-3898
18. Olson MT, Clark DP, Erozan YS, Ali SZ. Spectrum of risk of malignancy in subcategories of atypia of undetermined significance. *Acta Cytol.* (2011) 55:518–25. doi: 10.1159/000333232
19. Wang CC, Friedman L, Kennedy GC, Wang H, Kebebew E, Steward DL, et al. A large multicenter correlation study of thyroid nodule cytopathology and histopathology. *Thyroid.* (2011) 21:243–51. doi: 10.1089/thy.2010.0243

3

Delayed Response After Confirmed Progression (DR) and Other Unique Immunotherapy-Related Treatment Concepts in Cutaneous Squamous Cell Carcinoma

*Annette M. Lim[1,2], Karda Cavanagh[3], Rodney J. Hicks[4], Luke McLean[1], Michelle S. Goh[5], Angela Webb[6] and Danny Rischin[1,2]**

[1] Department of Medical Oncology, Peter MacCallum Cancer Centre, Melbourne, VIC, Australia, [2] Sir Peter MacCallum Department of Oncology, Faculty of Medicine, Dentistry and Health Sciences, The University of Melbourne, VIC, Australia, [3] Department of Cancer Imaging, Peter MacCallum Cancer Centre, Melbourne, VIC, Australia, [4] Department of Nuclear Medicine, Peter MacCallum Cancer Centre, Melbourne, VIC, Australia, [5] Department of Dermatology, Peter MacCallum Cancer Centre, Melbourne, VIC, Australia, [6] Department of Plastic Surgery, Peter MacCallum Cancer Centre, Melbourne, VIC, Australia

***Correspondence:**
Danny Rischin
Danny.Rischin@petermac.org*

Non-melanoma skin cancers are one of the most common cancers diagnosed worldwide, with the highest incidence in Australia and New Zealand. Systemic treatment of locally advanced and metastatic cutaneous squamous cell carcinomas has been revolutionized by immune checkpoint inhibition with PD-1 blockade. We highlight treatment issues distinct to the management of the disease including expansion of the traditional concept of pseudoprogression and describe delayed responses after immune-specific response criteria confirmed progressive disease with and without clinical deterioration. We term this phenomenon "delayed response after confirmed progression (DR)". We also discuss the common development of second primary tumors, heterogeneous disease responses, and expanding clinical boundaries for immunotherapy use.

Keywords: immunotherapy, PD-1 inhibition, pseudoprogression, cutaneous squamous carcinoma, second primary tumors (SPTs)

INTRODUCTION

Non-melanoma skin cancers (NMSC) predominantly basal cell carcinomas (BCC) and cutaneous squamous cell carcinomas (CSCC) are the most frequently diagnosed cancer in North America and Australia/New Zealand (1). Although most are resectable, the morbidity related to disease is significant and accounts for the most common cancer-related cause for hospitalization in Australia exacerbated by the multiplicity of skin cancer excisions (2–4). Approximately 5% of CSCC recur or metastasize leading to death or management associated with significant morbidity due to disease occurrence on sun-exposed areas such as the face, head and neck (5, 6).

In 2018, the first report of the efficacy of cemiplimab, a PD-1 inhibitor, was published for the treatment of patients with locally advanced or metastatic CSCC who were not candidates for curative surgery or radiation. The objective response rate (ORR) to therapy was 47% (range: 34-61), leading to Food and Drug Administration (FDA) and European Medicines Agency (EMA) approval and a paradigm shift in the management of these tumors (7, 8). Updated data indicates that the median duration of response and median overall survival (OS) have not been reached, with estimated 24 month-OS being 73.3% (95% CI: 66.1-79.2) (9). The KEYNOTE-629 study showed that pembrolizumab is also efficacious (ORR 34%; 95% CI: 25- 44) (10), which also led to FDA approval. First line pembrolizumab in the CARSKIN trial for locally advanced or metastatic CSCC (including radiotherapy naive patients, n=20/57) achieved a week 15 ORR of 41% (95% CI: 26-58%) (11). Therefore, the use of PD-1 blockade for the treatment of advanced CSCC represents a major breakthrough in the management of these common epithelial cancers.

We report our immunotherapy management experiences unique to CSCC that challenge and expand current clinical concepts in practice.

EXPANDING ON THE CONCEPT OF PSEUDOPROGRESSION – "DELAYED RESPONSES AFTER CONFIRMED PROGRESSION (DR)" AND RESPONSE AFTER CLINICAL DETERIORATION

The Response Evaluation Criteria in Solid Tumors (RECIST) criteria is a validated measure for the standardized evaluation of cancer therapies, determined by the assessment of the change of tumor burden with treatment (12). There are notable limitations of the RECIST guidelines in patients treated with immunotherapy, given that "pseudoprogression" can occur with an increase in tumor size due to inflammatory cell infiltrates followed by tumor reduction (13), and improved OS can occur without RECIST defined reduction in tumor measurements (14–16). Thus, RECIST criteria have been modified to include immune-related response criteria (irRC), immune-related response evaluation criteria in solid tumors (irRECIST), modified RECIST1.1 for immunotherapy (iRECIST), and immune-modified RECIST (imRECIST) (17–20).

Pseudoprogression occurs in under 10% of all cancers treated with immunotherapy, with an incidence in head and neck cancer of approximately 1% (21–24). To address pseudoprogression, the irRC, irRECIST and iRECIST require the use of confirmatory imaging at least 4 weeks after initial progression is documented (we will refer to this collectively as iCPD, immune confirmed disease progression as per iRECIST), a minimum size increase of $>5x5mm^2$ or 10mm, an increase in the sum of tumor measurements from the nadir of 20-25%, and incorporation of new lesions in the sum of tumor dimension measurements before confirmation of progressive disease (PD) (17–19). The imRECIST criteria is similar, but permits the best response assessment to occur after observation of progressive disease, which avoids underestimation of survival rates (20). All criteria recommend that treatment beyond progression should only occur if a patient's performance status and disease-related symptomatology are stable.

We describe two cases to redefine our understanding of pseudoprogression, with delayed disease response observed after iCPD and after observation of clinical deterioration. We introduce new terminology to capture the phenomenon as "delayed response after confirmed progression (DR)". We also discuss a case of tumor response observed in a patient with clinical deterioration, with treatment beyond progression.

Case One

This case illustrates the observation of DR. Patient One was diagnosed with a T2N0M0 occipital scalp/vertex CSCC excised with clear margins in September 2017. In July 2018, a 35mm in-transit recurrence was resected with an involved margin. Re-excision and ipsilateral neck dissection demonstrated a 2.5mm residual CSCC 1.2mm from the deep margin, and 1/41 nodes involved with extranodal extension to the surgical margin. Adjuvant radiotherapy of 66 Gy/33# was completed in October 2018. Within three weeks, biopsy of multiple new in-field in-transit CSCC and an out-of-field intramuscular lesion confirmed recurrent disease. Following multidisciplinary meeting (MDM) discussion, he was referred for consideration of immunotherapy for his recurrent CSCC.

The patient was enrolled on the NCT02760498 to receive cemiplimab 400mg Q4W, with RECIST 1.1 measurements determined by radiological assessments as per protocol. The progression of lesions documented by photography, and radiological assessments are summarized in **Figures 1A, B**. Four weeks after initial dose, Patient One reported worsening disease-related pain. The largest CSCC lesion had increased by 10mm with new ulceration (black arrow), other baseline lesions had also increased in size with ulceration, while at least three new lesions greater than 10mm had developed with multiple other smaller lesions visible. This corresponded to unconfirmed progressive disease (iUPD). Four weeks later prior to his third dose, ongoing progression was noted with further ulceration and coalescence of lesions (white checked arrow), and increasing size of new nodules by more than 10mm (black spotted arrow) confirming iCPD. At that time point, RECIST 1.1 assessment by imaging confirming PD (**Figure 1B**). Approval for treatment beyond progression was granted. By the next visit, all lesions had improved clinically with a reduction in size and improvement in pain. The patient completed 12 months of therapy with a complete clinical response. To date, the patient remains in clinical and radiological remission.

Case Two

This case illustrates DR. Patient Two had a long history of multiple NMSC lesions being excised from the head, neck, and chest, including a Merkel cell carcinoma (MCC). Patient Two had a CSCC lesion from the left clavicular area that required multiple re-excisions over a six-month period before clear margins were achieved in January 2018. In May 2018, a left infraclavicular chest recurrent CSCC was excised that involved

A

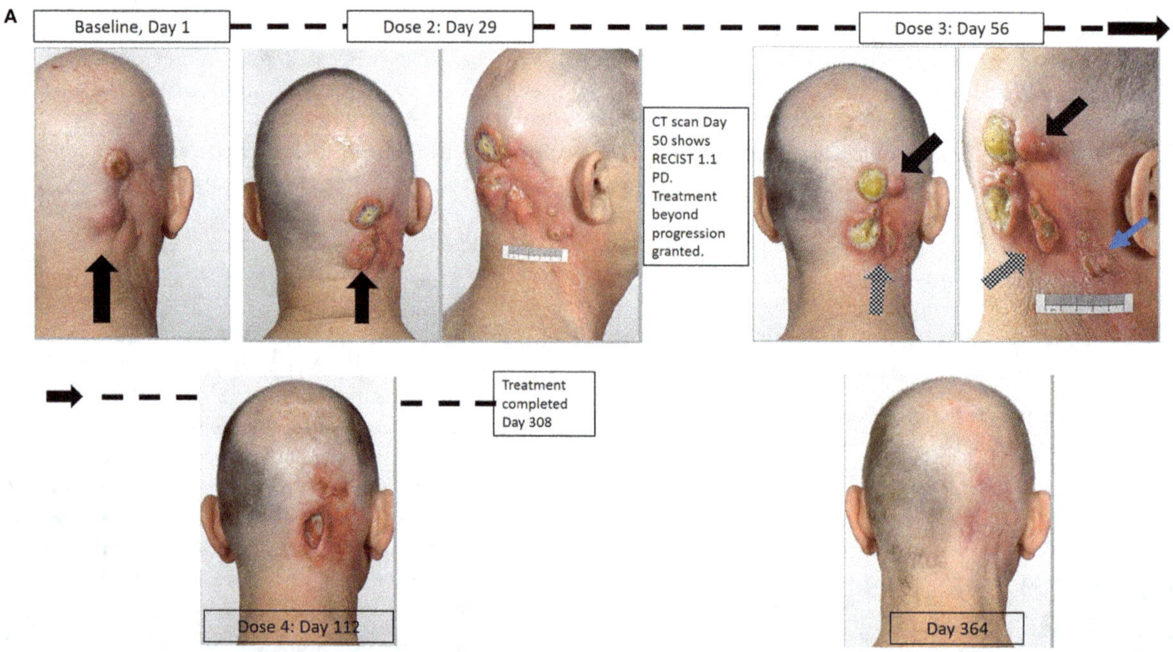

B

Target Lesion Site (in mm)		Baseline RECIST	Clinic review Dose 2 Day 28	CT Day 50	Clinic review Dose 3 Day 56	CT Day 108	CT Day 167	CT Day 335	CT Day 386 Follow up 2 months	CT Day 442 Follow up 4 months
A	Right paraoccipital subcutaneous lesion	31x21	Progression, ulceration, increased pain	37x29	Progression, ulceration, increased pain	29 x 20	25x18	16x6	Too small to measure default 5mm	Too small to measure default 5mm
B	Right neck intramuscular deposit	14 x10	Confluent progression with other lesions	17 x 15	Progression, ulcerated, increased pain	12 x 12	0	0	0	0
Total (Target) mm		**45**		**54**		**41**	**25**	**16**	5	5
% change from baseline **% change from re-baseline after iUPD**		NA		+20		-9 -24	-44 -53	-64 -70	-89 -91	-89 -91
Non-Target Lesion Site			**Present (P) or Absent (A)**							
1 Dermal deposits right neck		Present		Present		Present	Absent	Absent	Absent	Absent
New lesions			At least 3x10mm	Yes, multiple new scalp and neck	Increased further by >20mm but no new lesions	No	No	No	No	No
Overall Response RECIST 1.1			**PD**	**PD**	**PD**	**PD**	**PD**	**PD**	**PD**	**PD**
Including clinical assessments iRECIST irRECIST imRECIST			**iUPD iUPD iUPD**	**iCPD iCPD iCPD**	**iCPD iCPD iCPD**	**iCPD iCPD iSD**	**iCPD iCPD iPR**	**iCPD iCPD iPR**	**iCPD iCPD iPR**	**iCPD iCPD iPR**

FIGURE 1 | Continued

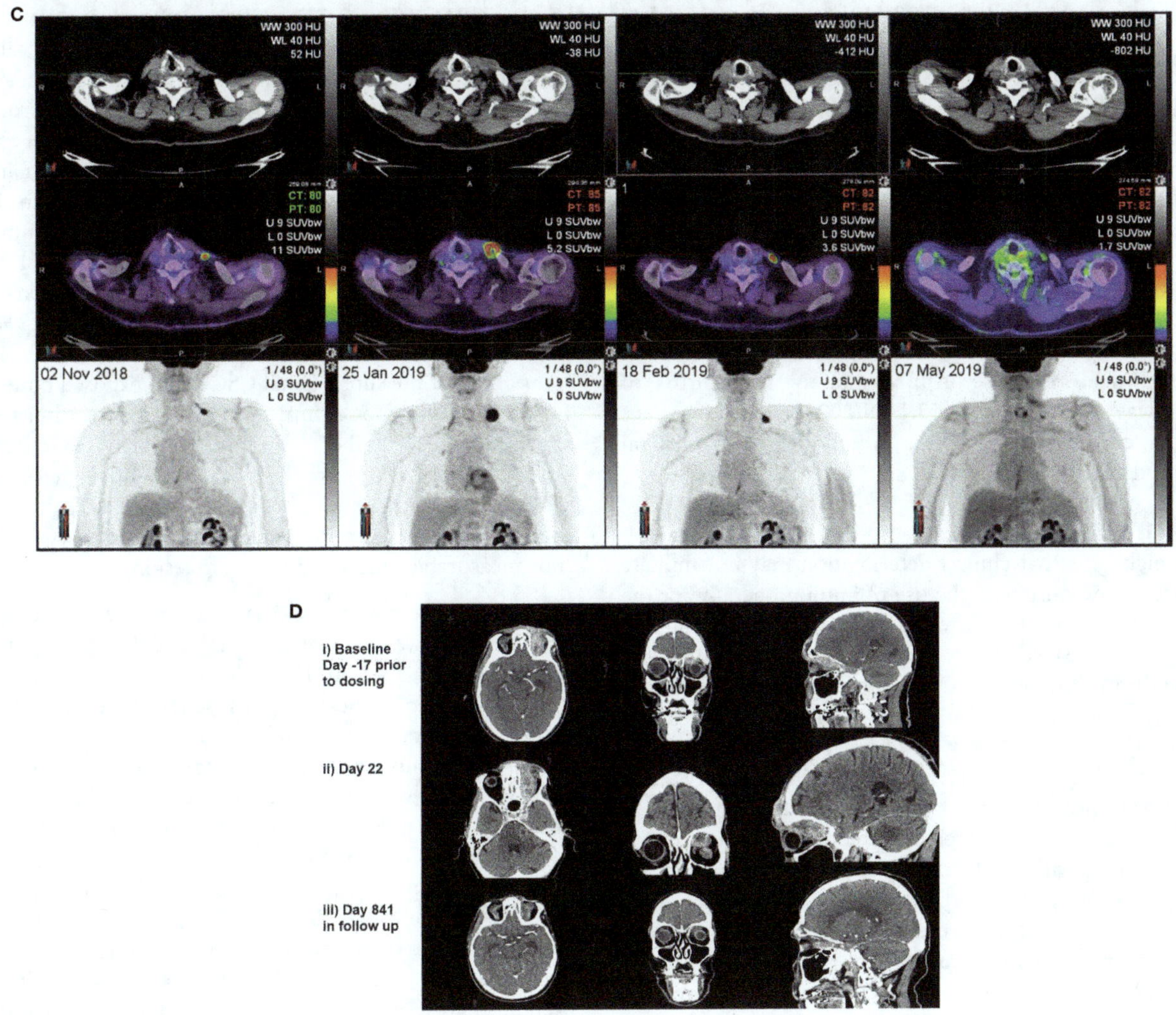

FIGURE 1 | Correlative clinical photographs, tumor response measurements according to time, and fluorodeoxyglucose - positron emission tomography (FDG-PET) and CT scan images of discussed patient cases. **(A, B)** Patient One's photographic images demonstrating iUPD and iCPD, with accompanying tumor response measurements according to RECIST 1.1 and immune based criteria at key time points. **(C)** Patient Two's FDG-PET images over time with low dose axial CT, fused axial CT, and maximal intensity projection (MIP) images in each column from 02/NOV/2018, 25/JAN/2019, 18/FEB/2019, and 07/MAY/2019, demonstrating evidence of progression and regression with ongoing immunotherapy. **(D)** Patient Three's representative images of disease at baseline, at progression and with response. Images i) Baseline (Day-17 prior to dosing) Post contrast CT: (axial, coronal, sagittal) demonstrates enhancing soft tissue extending from the cutaneous left forehead along the roof of the left orbit in the distribution of V1, involving the cavernous sinus, Meckel's cave, nerve root entry zone of the left trigeminal nerve and likely involvement of the trigeminal nuclei with soft tissue at the left pons. ii) Day 22 Post contrast CT: (axial, coronal, sagittal) demonstrates increasing volume of enhancing soft tissue extending from the cutaneous left forehead along the roof of the left orbit in the distribution of V1, involving the cavernous sinus, Meckel's cave, nerve root entry zone of the left trigeminal nerve and involvement of the trigeminal nuclei with soft tissue at the left pons. iii) Day 841 (in follow up) Post contrast CT: (axial, coronal, sagittal) demonstrates small volume residual non-enhancing soft tissue extending from the cutaneous left forehead along the roof of the left orbit. The remaining soft tissue has resolved on CT.

the clavicular head of the pectoralis major muscle and pathologically measured 32mm with a deep margin of 0.7mm and evidence of perineural invasion. Re-excision demonstrated no residual disease but another 0.3mm central chest poorly differentiated carcinoma of uncertain origin was concurrently excised with clear margins. Adjuvant radiotherapy of 60Gy/30# was completed on August 2018. Two months later, a biopsy of a nodule over the medial aspect of the left clavicle confirmed recurrent CSCC. Magnetic resonance imaging (MRI) and computer tomography (CT) scans were unable to define the lesion, but fluorodeoxyglucose positron emission tomography (FDG-PET) scan identified an ~13mm left supraclavicular lesion (**Figure 1C**). After MDM discussion, Patient Two was referred for consideration of immunotherapy. Given his history of MCC, he was ineligible for trial participation and self-funded pembrolizumab 200mg Q3W which commenced on 28/NOV/2018. At review prior to the second dose (19/DEC/2018), his lesion had increased by more than 10mm to ~40x30mm with purpuric discoloration of the intact skin consistent with iUPD. By review prior to the third dose (08/JAN/2019), the lesion had fungated through the skin. A restaging FDG-PET scan (25/JAN/2019) performed after administration of three doses of pembrolizumab demonstrated marked interval progression with increase in size of disease to 33mm confirming iCPD (+254%). On 29/JAN/2019, iCPD was confirmed clinically and the fourth dose of immunotherapy was abandoned and surgical salvage was planned. Two weeks later prior to surgery, the patient reported clinical improvement and repeat imaging performed (18/FEB/2019) demonstrated reduction in tumor size to 15mm (-55% from previous). Pembrolizumab was resumed and by the subsequent visit, he had obtained a complete clinical response. Approximately 12 months of treatment was completed on 02/JAN/2020 and the patient remains in complete metabolic, radiological and clinical response to date.

Case Three

This case highlights that clinical deterioration may not militate against disease response with the use of immunotherapy for the treatment of CSCC. Patient Three had a long history of multiple NMSC and at age 81 years was diagnosed with a T4N0M0 left supraorbital/intraorbital CSCC with perineural disease that involved all branches of the left trigeminal nerve to the cisternal portion. Despite 54Gy in 27 fractions of radiotherapy completed on December 2017, MRI scan in February 2018 revealed disease progression with increasing tumor anterior to the left frontal bone, new marrow infiltration of the floor of the left cranial fossa with nodular dural enhancement and no response in the pre-existing orbital disease (**Figure 1D**). After MDM discussion, he was referred for consideration of immunotherapy. He consented to trial participation in the NCT02760498 (cemiplimab 3 mg/kg Q2W). At Day 1 review, his ECOG performance status was assessed as 1, and examination demonstrated a 25mm left supraorbital mass, complete left eyelid proptosis, complete opthalmoplegia of his left eye, decreased sensation in the trigeminal nerve distribution with patient report of neuropathic pain. At Day 15 his pain had improved but he reported falls at home on the background of worsening balance, resulting in local trauma to the forehead. Clinical examination demonstrated no obvious abnormalities compared to baseline, however ECOG performance status was assessed as 2. Patient Three was referred for allied health management and received his second dose of cemiplimab. Two days later, he was admitted to hospital following a fall with a head strike with loss of consciousness, and reported nausea. CT brain (Day 21) identified disease progression (+44%, iUPD) with enhancement of the left trigeminal nerve disease into the cerebellar peduncle and left-sided pons with surrounding edema. The patient was discharged mobilizing on a wheeled frame the following day. At Day 29 review, the patient reported a significant improvement in his neuropathic pain, the supraorbital mass was clinically smaller but his ECOG performance status was assessed as 2. Restaging CT scans performed (Day 50) identified ongoing disease progression with an increase in size in all target lesions (+42% from baseline, RECIST 1.1 PD, iUPD). MRI brain demonstrated progression with increased diffuse skin thickening, increased enhancement of the orbital and periorbital disease, new destruction of the bones associated with the left frontal and ethmoid sinus and left orbit, soft tissue intracranial extension into the left anterior and middle cranial fossa, with increased trigeminal perineural invasion into the left brainstem. In clinic on Day 57, he reported a complete absence of trigeminal nerve pain and a reduction of the left supraorbital mass to 15mm was noted. Treatment beyond progression was approved. By Day 104, imaging demonstrated ongoing RECIST PD (+28%, iUPD) with subsequent review confirming regression of the exophytic component of the supraorbital CSCC and exposed bone. Patient Three went on to complete 659 days on therapy after experiencing a number of immune-related (≤Grade 2) and other medical adverse events (not treatment-related). His most recent imaging of his target lesions (**Figure 1D**) demonstrated complete resolution of the pons lesion, stable orbital lesion and "not measurable" ulcerated left scalp lesion.

Two of the patient cases presented introduce a new phenomenon we have defined as a "delayed response after confirmed progression (DR)". That is, the observation of a clinical and radiological response after iCPD. In both cases, clinical deterioration was observed early in treatment but after treatment beyond progression, durable clinical and radiological improvement was obtained. In one case, change of tumor evolution with the cessation of new lesions developing may have been the only indication to herald DR. Review of our institutional experience of patients treated with cemiplimab on trial (up to 15/SEP/2020) in the advanced setting who have received more than one dose, demonstrates an estimated incidence of 2/39 (5%) of DR without any cases of "traditional pseudoprogression". We have observed DR occurring late in treatment courses and "traditional pseudoprogression" for non-trial patients. We also raise the concept that clinical deterioration may not militate against tumor response. In distinction to the three cases discussed where all patients experienced disease-related deterioration, the KEYNOTE-629 study which used RECIST 1.1 criteria for response evaluation reported that 29 *clinically stable* patients received treatment beyond progression (10). Of these, 12 patients continue on therapy and eight patients have developed responses (1 complete response, 7 partial responses according to irRECIST; FIG S4 (10)).

Therefore, our observation of DR and scenarios discussed further below, caution against a nihilistic approach to CSCC patient management when using immunotherapy. These cases highlight the important consideration of the timing and method of disease response assessments and the limitations of most criteria to capture pseudoprogression/DR, response rates and best overall response (BOR) assessments as part of clinical trial reporting. Use of the RECIST 1.1 framework will have not accurately reflected BOR for these patients, with the known limitation of most frameworks to act as a surrogate for progression-free and overall survival (25). Although the timing of imaging assessments are necessarily at a time point to permit sufficient receipt of therapy to assess response, these scans may not contemporaneously reflect disease evolution and response. Further, data from trials that utilize immunotherapy in the neoadjuvant setting prior to definitive surgery suggests that complete pathological responses may be seen only as partial response on imaging (26–29). This highlights the clinical need for research into the predictive and prognostic role of imaging techniques in patients treated with immunotherapy for CSCC and the need to identify relevant molecular liquid biopsy biomarkers for disease surveillance (30–32).

SECOND PRIMARY TUMORS ON IMMUNOTHERAPY

Multiplicity is common for patients with NMSC, with ~74% of all skin cancers being excised from patients with multiple NMSC lesions particularly involving the head and neck region (2, 3). We have observed that patients on immunotherapy can develop both CSCC and BCC as second primary tumors (SPT) despite responsive disease elsewhere, likely due to field cancerization (33). The mechanism by which SPT escape treatment control have not yet been elucidated and are likely to illuminate molecular mechanisms behind immune escape.

From a clinical management perspective, it is critical that SPT development is not mistaken as treatment failure given that these lesions can resolve with ongoing therapy or can be managed with local therapy. As a general principle, the SPT should be observed for a period whilst continuing immunotherapy and if regression or stability does not occur then local therapy can be pursued with a view of continuing systemic therapy for control of the other immunotherapy-responsive disease. On retrospective review of our patients treated with cemiplimab on trial, of eight patients who developed biopsy proven SPT resistant to immunotherapy, seven patients with CSCC and six with BCC required formal excision and/or radiotherapy for local management with all but one patient having more than one lesion. We have not identified any situation for which the new SPT has resulted in metastatic disease or has heralded the development of disease progression in existing lesions. Molecular profiling of these SPTs that develop on immunotherapy is important to define disease heterogeneity and to identify the likely numerous mechanisms of immune escape.

HETEROGENEOUS RESPONSES ON IMMUNOTHERAPY

Discordant immunotherapy responses can be observed between existing lesions, where concurrent local therapy for immunotherapy-resistant lesions may be warranted to secure control. Given the common multiplicity of NMSCs occurring in the same patient (2), awareness of response heterogeneity is key to avoid inappropriate early cessation of immunotherapy.

Case Four

This case demonstrates heterogeneous responses of two baseline lesions to immunotherapy. Patient Four was a 70 year old man with a multiply recurrent CSCC of his left forearm which had required six re-excisions. The largest resected recurrence was a 70x50mm spindled/poorly differentiated CSCC, up to 8mm in depth, with lymphovascular and perineural invasion. Adjuvant 56Gy/28# of radiotherapy was completed in September 2018, with a truncated course due to toxicity. In May 2019, Patient Four developed a painful locally recurrent CSCC of his left elbow with bone on view that measured 41x32mm on MRI scan, and a small right cheek lesion suspected to be a separate primary CSCC. Following MDM discussion, surgery for the cheek lesion was planned prior to immunotherapy for the elbow lesion. Wide local excision of the cheek lesion on the 26/JUN/2019 revealed three areas containing moderately differentiated CSCC spanning over 26mm, 32mm and 40mm with a transected deep margin, multiple CSCC tissue deposits of 2mm to 8mm, with perineural invasion abutting the margin. Re-excision was performed on 03/JUL/2019 revealing multiple foci of moderately differentiated CSCC deposits with perineural invasion, vascular tumor emboli, and tumor 0.2mm from a margin. Patient Four consented to participation the NCT02760498. At baseline, the exophytic left elbow lesion clinically measured 70x35mm. Prior to the third dose (Day 57), a near complete clinical response of the left elbow CSCC was observed with a residual superficial ulcer measuring 10mm accompanied by an improvement in pain. MRI scan confirmed the lesion had reduced to 32x13mm. A month later (Day 87) a right cheek nodule recurred and given its persistence, resection was performed on Day 106 demonstrating an 11mm CSCC with ≤1mm margins. Ongoing immunotherapy secured a complete clinical response for the left elbow lesion by Day 141 with imaging showing no identifiable tumor (nominal RECIST measurement of 5mm). However, three further excisions (Day 147, Day 188, Day 218) were required to manage the cheek lesion which recurred twice during adjuvant radiotherapy planning. Palliative radiotherapy of 36Gy in 6# to the cheek lesion was completed on Day 283. Most recent imaging demonstrated a complete metabolic response (Day 335) and ongoing radiological PR (nominal 5mm, Day 447) of the left elbow disease. However, since Day 394 clinical recurrence of the right cheek nodule has been progressive. Due to the absence of local therapies available to effectively treat the recurrent right cheek CSCC, Patient Four decided to cease further immunotherapy to pursue best supportive care.

Tumoral heterogeneity leading to discordant treatment response is a known therapeutic hurdle that can contribute to disease progression with the development of clonal resistance (34–38). In the era of immunotherapy which can secure durable disease control, understanding the contribution of local therapy towards overall disease control and survival is crucial but poorly understood. It has been observed in patients with melanoma treated with immunotherapy who received local therapy to progressive lesions in order to achieve no evidence of disease, that those who had local therapy to new lesions had poorer survival compared to those who had local therapy to progressive pre-existing metastases (PFS 6% vs 70%, p=0.001) (39). Consideration of the anatomical site of oligoclonal resistant disease will have clinical (e.g. brain versus lung) and therapeutic implications (e.g. surgery versus radiotherapy). Patient Four's case demonstrates that discordant immunotherapy responses can be observed between lesions, where concurrent local therapy may be warranted in an attempt to secure control of immunotherapy-resistant lesions.

EXPANDING CLINICAL BOUNDARIES - ACTIVITY IN ADVANCED, FUNGATING, DISFIGURING DISEASE AND GOOD TOLERANCE DESPITE MULTIPLE COMORBIDITIES

It is essential to consider patient factors, treatment morbidity and goals of management in oncological care. Comorbidities and

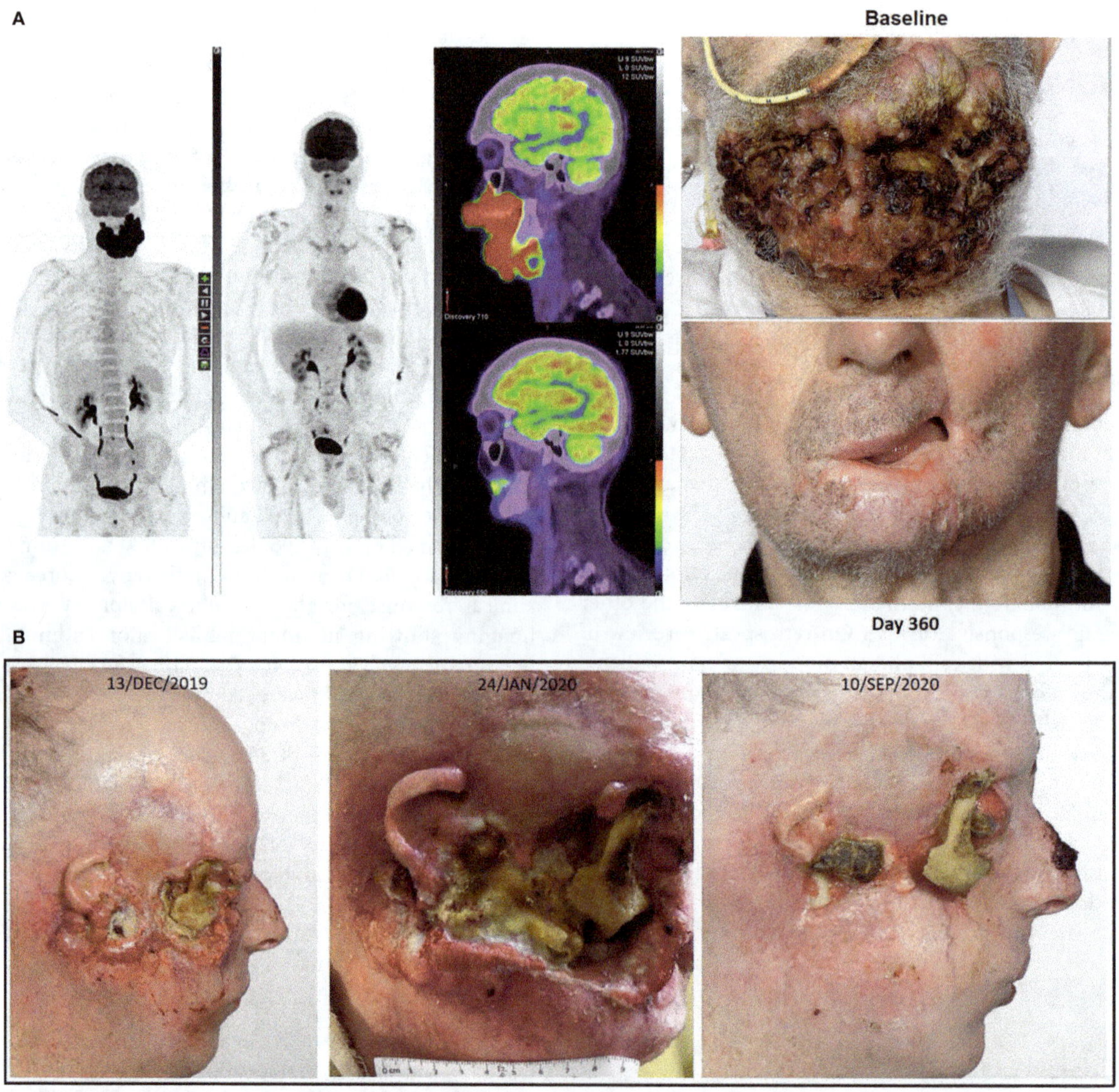

FIGURE 2 | (A) This figure illustrates the FDG-PET matched MIP and fused axial images with photographs at baseline and after receipt of cemiplimab of a 75-year-old male who had declined investigation and treatment of CSCC originating from his chin. After 18 months of pursuing alternative treatment, he accepted immunotherapy when the disease had become so advanced it mechanically impacted his ability to eat. He consented to participation in the NCT02760498, and after receipt of two doses clinical regression of the lesion was noted. His disease remains in complete remission after two years of therapy completed more than 12 months ago. **(B)** This figure illustrates re-epithelialization occurring during the receipt of compassionate access cemiplimab in a 45-year-old patient with more than a 20 year history of multiple NMSC including synchronous CSCC, BCC and MCC. The patient ceased vismodegib to commence cemiplimab on 13/DEC/2019 but required recommencement of vismodegib on 19/APR/2020 due to recurrence of multiple BCC lesions. He remains on dual therapy given the symptomatic improvement achieved with good pain control and resolution of right cheek CSCC-related trismus.

ECOG performance status guide management to optimize patient outcomes that may focus on quality of life or may be driven to obtain survival benefits or both. It is well recognized that a large disparity exists between trial patients versus "real-world" patients, who often are older, of minority groups, and with comorbidities that may interfere with assessment of therapeutic efficacy or toxicity (40) (41, 42). In the context of the functionally and cosmetically sensitive anatomical region of the head and neck, it is crucial to define that immunotherapy is generally tolerable and associated with improved quality of life (22, 43, 44). In CSCC, Maubec et al. have reported improved health-related quality of life for patients with immunotherapy-responsive disease (11), and use of PD-1 blockade has been demonstrated to be tolerable with side effects reported similar to other checkpoint inhibitors and with the ability to secure durable disease control (7, 9, 45). Noteworthy in the trial reports, is the median age of patients being 71-80 years with the oldest patients being 99 years old (7, 10, 11).

Our institutional experience in the trial and "real-world" setting is that checkpoint inhibitor therapy is exceptionally well tolerated by patients with CSCC. Generally, few treatment contraindications exist and few comorbidities raise concern including extreme age, dialysis, other synchronous malignancies requiring treatment, and poor ECOG performance status. This is a paradigm change in our approach to patients with CSCC and is paramount given the dramatic response rates achieved by therapy, providing symptomatic and durable control. This is in stark contradistinction to our approach with mucosal head and neck cancer patients. As illustrated in **Figure 2**, there are not many clinical situations in which disease is considered "too advanced" for immunotherapy. That is, the stage of disease, location of disease, and extent of disease does not militate against response to immunotherapy. Anecdotally, the extent of re-epithelialization following response can be impressive creating complexity around the timing of reconstructive surgery if pursued.

CONCLUSION AND FUTURE DIRECTIONS

Use of immunotherapy has revolutionized the care of patients with advanced CSCC, leading to a paradigm shift in the selection of patients for treatment with the expectation of response and durable control even in the advanced recurrent or metastatic setting. We have focused on describing unique clinical concepts related to the treatment of CSCC with immunotherapy including the phenomenon of delayed response after confirmed progression (DR), observation of tumor responses despite clinical deterioration in iCPD, and the need to consider flexible treatment approaches in patients with multiple NMSC.

An improved understanding of CSCC will undoubtedly enhance patient selection for therapy as ongoing clinical research efforts investigate the role of immunotherapy in the adjuvant and neoadjuvant settings. Few cancer registries collect data on CSCC or advanced CSCC, limiting our understanding of the spectrum of disease, burden of need, morbidity and costs related to treatment. The therapeutic advances necessitate rapid development of real-time methods to assess tumor response (e.g. liquid biopsy, imaging or combination approaches) that are more informative than current imaging modalities and response criteria. Translational research will be crucial to molecularly define the clinical spectrum of CSCC (46, 47), and identify reliable predictive and prognostic markers to therapy, including mechanisms of immune evasion. Specifically, comprehensive profiling of immunotherapy exposed tumors, including single cell sequencing approaches, will be important to further clarify inter-tumoral, intra-tumoral and tumor microenvironment molecular processes that underpin the described clinical concepts (48, 49).

ETHICS STATEMENT

The studies involving human participants were reviewed and approved by Peter MacCallum Cancer Centre Ethics Committee. Written consent has been provided by the patient with reidentifiable images.

AUTHOR CONTRIBUTIONS

Concept and design – AL, DR. All authors contributed to the article and approved the submitted version.

ACKNOWLEDGMENTS

Regeneron and Sanofi have reviewed the manuscript prior to publication but have not contributed or modified the manuscript in any substantial way. We thank all the patients and families, who have received treatment at our center. We thank our clinical trial team members who have contributed significantly to patient care.

REFERENCES

1. Bray F, Ferlay J, Soerjomataram I, Siegel RL, Torre LA, Jemal A. Global cancer statistics 2018: GLOBOCAN estimates of incidence and mortality worldwide for 36 cancers in 185 countries. *CA Cancer J Clin* (2018) 68(6):394–424. doi: 10.3322/caac.21492
2. Pandeya N, Olsen CM, Whiteman DC. The incidence and multiplicity rates of keratinocyte cancers in Australia. *Med J Aust* (2017) 207(8):339–43. doi: 10.5694/mja17.00284
3. Richmond-Sinclair NM, Pandeya N, Ware RS, Neale RE, Williams GM, van der Pols JC, et al. Incidence of Basal Cell Carcinoma Multiplicity and Detailed Anatomic Distribution: Longitudinal Study of an Australian Population. *J Invest Dermatol* (2009) 129(2):323–8. doi: 10.1038/jid.2008.234
4. Australian Institute of Health and Welfare 2019. *Cancer in Australia 2019. Cancer series no.119. Cat. no. CAN 123.* Canberra: AIHW (2019).
5. Brantsch KD, Meisner C, Schonfisch B, Trilling B, Wehner-Caroli J, Rocken M, et al. Analysis of risk factors determining prognosis of cutaneous squamous-cell carcinoma: a prospective study. *Lancet Oncol* (2008) 9 (8):713–20. doi: 10.1016/S1470-2045(08)70178-5

6. Nakamura K, Okuyama R, Saida T, Uhara H. Platinum and anthracycline therapy for advanced cutaneous squamous cell carcinoma. *Int J Clin Oncol* (2013) 18(3):506–9. doi: 10.1007/s10147-012-0411-y
7. Migden MR, Rischin D, Schmults CD, Guminski A, Hauschild A, Lewis KD, et al. PD-1 Blockade with Cemiplimab in Advanced Cutaneous Squamous-Cell Carcinoma. *N Engl J Med* (2018) 379(4):341–51. doi: 10.1056/NEJMoa1805131
8. Migden MR, Khushalani NI, Chang ALS, Lewis KD, Schmults CD, Hernandez-Aya L, et al. Cemiplimab in locally advanced cutaneous squamous cell carcinoma: results from an open-label, phase 2, single-arm trial. *Lancet Oncol* (2020) 21(2):294–305. doi: 10.1016/s1470-2045(19)30728-4
9. Rischin D, Khushalani NI, Schmults CD, Guminski AD, Chang ALS, Lewis KD, et al. Phase II study of cemiplimab in patients (pts) with advanced cutaneous squamous cell carcinoma (CSCC): Longer follow-up. *J Clin Oncol* (2020) 38(15_suppl):10018-. doi: 10.1200/JCO.2020.38.15_suppl.10018
10. Grob JJ, Gonzalez R, Basset-Seguin N, Vornicova O, Schachter J, Joshi A, et al. Pembrolizumab Monotherapy for Recurrent or Metastatic Cutaneous Squamous Cell Carcinoma: A Single-Arm Phase II Trial (KEYNOTE-629). *J Clin Oncol Off J Am Soc Clin Oncol* (2020) 38(25):2916–25. doi: 10.1200/JCO.19.03054
11. Maubec E, Boubaya M, Petrow P, Beylot-Barry M, Basset-Seguin N, Deschamps L, et al. Phase II Study of Pembrolizumab As First-Line, Single-Drug Therapy for Patients With Unresectable Cutaneous Squamous Cell Carcinomas. *J Clin Oncol Off J Am Soc Clin Oncol* (2020) 38(26):3051–61. doi: 10.1200/JCO.19.03357
12. Eisenhauer EA, Therasse P, Bogaerts J, Schwartz LH, Sargent D, Ford R, et al. New response evaluation criteria in solid tumours: revised RECIST guideline (version 1.1). *Eur J Cancer* (2009) 45(2):228–47. doi: 10.1016/j.ejca.2008.10.026
13. Di Giacomo AM, Danielli R, Guidoboni M, Calabrò L, Carlucci D, Miracco C, et al. Therapeutic efficacy of ipilimumab, an anti-CTLA-4 monoclonal antibody, in patients with metastatic melanoma unresponsive to prior systemic treatments: clinical and immunological evidence from three patient cases. *Cancer Immunol Immunother* (2009) 58(8):1297–306. doi: 10.1007/s00262-008-0642-y
14. Llovet JM, Ricci S, Mazzaferro V, Hilgard P, Gane E, Blanc JF, et al. Sorafenib in advanced hepatocellular carcinoma. *N Engl J Med* (2008) 359(4):378–90. doi: 10.1056/NEJMoa0708857
15. Choi H, Charnsangavej C, Faria SC, Macapinlac HA, Burgess MA, Patel SR, et al. Correlation of computed tomography and positron emission tomography in patients with metastatic gastrointestinal stromal tumor treated at a single institution with imatinib mesylate: proposal of new computed tomography response criteria. *J Clin Oncol Off J Am Soc Clin Oncol* (2007) 25(13):1753–9. doi: 10.1200/JCO.2006.07.3049
16. Wolchok JD, Hoos A, O'Day S, Weber JS, Hamid O, Lebbé C, et al. Guidelines for the Evaluation of Immune Therapy Activity in Solid Tumors: Immune-Related Response Criteria. *Clin Cancer Res* (2009) 15(23):7412–20. doi: 10.1158/1078-0432.Ccr-09-1624
17. Seymour L, Bogaerts J, Perrone A, Ford R, Schwartz LH, Mandrekar S, et al. iRECIST: guidelines for response criteria for use in trials testing immunotherapeutics. *Lancet Oncol* (2017) 18(3):e143–e52. doi: 10.1016/S1470-2045(17)30074-8
18. Wolchok JD, Hoos A, O'Day S, Weber JS, Hamid O, Lebbe C, et al. Guidelines for the evaluation of immune therapy activity in solid tumors: immune-related response criteria. *Clin Cancer Res* (2009) 15(23):7412–20. doi: 10.1158/1078-0432.CCR-09-1624
19. Nishino M, Giobbie-Hurder A, Gargano M, Suda M, Ramaiya NH, Hodi FS. Developing a common language for tumor response to immunotherapy: immune-related response criteria using unidimensional measurements. *Clin Cancer Res* (2013) 19(14):3936–43. doi: 10.1158/1078-0432.Ccr-13-0895
20. Hodi FS, Ballinger M, Lyons B, Soria JC, Nishino M, Tabernero J, et al. Immune-Modified Response Evaluation Criteria In Solid Tumors (imRECIST): Refining Guidelines to Assess the Clinical Benefit of Cancer Immunotherapy. *J Clin Oncol Off J Am Soc Clin Oncol* (2018) 36(9):850–8. doi: 10.1200/JCO.2017.75.1644
21. Chiou VL, Burotto M. Pseudoprogression and Immune-Related Response in Solid Tumors. *J Clin Oncol Off J Am Soc Clin Oncol* (2015) 33(31):3541–3. doi: 10.1200/JCO.2015.61.6870
22. Ferris RL, Blumenschein GJr, Fayette J, Guigay J, Colevas AD, Licitra L, et al. Nivolumab for Recurrent Squamous-Cell Carcinoma of the Head and Neck. *N Engl J Med* (2016) 375(19):1856–67. doi: 10.1056/NEJMoa1602252
23. Seiwert TY, Burtness B, Mehra R, Weiss J, Berger R, Eder JP, et al. Safety and clinical activity of pembrolizumab for treatment of recurrent or metastatic squamous cell carcinoma of the head and neck (KEYNOTE-012): an open-label, multicentre, phase 1b trial. *Lancet Oncol* (2016) 17(7):956–65. doi: 10.1016/S1470-2045(16)30066-3
24. Long GV, Weber JS, Larkin J, Atkinson V, Grob J-J, Schadendorf D, et al. Nivolumab for Patients With Advanced Melanoma Treated Beyond Progression: Analysis of 2 Phase 3 Clinical Trials. *JAMA Oncol* (2017) 3 (11):1511–9. doi: 10.1001/jamaoncol.2017.1588
25. Mushti SL, Mulkey F, Sridhara R. Evaluation of Overall Response Rate and Progression-Free Survival as Potential Surrogate Endpoints for Overall Survival in Immunotherapy Trials. *Clin Cancer Res* (2018) 24(10):2268–75. doi: 10.1158/1078-0432.Ccr-17-1902
26. Tarhini A, Lin Y, Lin H, Rahman Z, Vallabhaneni P, Mendiratta P, et al. Neoadjuvant ipilimumab (3 mg/kg or 10 mg/kg) and high dose IFN-α2b in locally/regionally advanced melanoma: safety, efficacy and impact on T-cell repertoire. *J immunother Cancer* (2018) 6(1):112–. doi: 10.1186/s40425-018-0428-5
27. Rozeman EA, Menzies AM, van Akkooi ACJ, Adhikari C, Bierman C, van de Wiel BA, et al. Identification of the optimal combination dosing schedule of neoadjuvant ipilimumab plus nivolumab in macroscopic stage III melanoma (OpACIN-neo): a multicentre, phase 2, randomised, controlled trial. *Lancet Oncol* (2019) 20(7):948–60. doi: 10.1016/s1470-2045(19)30151-2
28. Blank CU, Rozeman EA, Fanchi LF, Sikorska K, van de Wiel B, Kvistborg P, et al. Neoadjuvant versus adjuvant ipilimumab plus nivolumab in macroscopic stage III melanoma. *Nat Med* (2018) 24(11):1655–61. doi: 10.1038/s41591-018-0198-0
29. Amaria RN, Reddy SM, Tawbi HA, Davies MA, Ross MI, Glitza IC, et al. Neoadjuvant immune checkpoint blockade in high-risk resectable melanoma. *Nat Med* (2018) 24(11):1649–54. doi: 10.1038/s41591-018-0197-1
30. Tan AC, Emmett L, Lo S, Liu V, Kapoor R, Carlino MS, et al. FDG-PET response and outcome from anti-PD-1 therapy in metastatic melanoma. *Ann Oncol* (2018) 29(10):2115–20. doi: 10.1093/annonc/mdy330
31. Tie J, Wang Y, Tomasetti C, Li L, Springer S, Kinde I, et al. Circulating tumor DNA analysis detects minimal residual disease and predicts recurrence in patients with stage II colon cancer. *Sci Transl Med* (2016) 8(346):346ra92. doi: 10.1126/scitranslmed.aaf6219
32. Bensch F, van der Veen EL, Lub-de Hooge MN, Jorritsma-Smit A, Boellaard R, Kok IC, et al. 89Zr-atezolizumab imaging as a non-invasive approach to assess clinical response to PD-L1 blockade in cancer. *Nat Med* (2018) 24 (12):1852–8. doi: 10.1038/s41591-018-0255-8
33. Christensen SR. Recent advances in field cancerization and management of multiple cutaneous squamous cell carcinomas. *F1000Res* (2018) 7:F1000 Faculty Rev–690. doi: 10.12688/f1000research.12837.1
34. Wolf Y, Bartok O, Patkar S, Eli GB, Cohen S, Litchfield K, et al. UVB-Induced Tumor Heterogeneity Diminishes Immune Response in Melanoma. *Cell* (2019) 179(1):219–35.e21. doi: 10.1016/j.cell.2019.08.032
35. Aslan K, Turco V, Blobner J, Sonner JK, Liuzzi AR, Núñez NG, et al. Heterogeneity of response to immune checkpoint blockade in hypermutated experimental gliomas. *Nat Commun* (2020) 11(1):931. doi: 10.1038/s41467-020-14642-0
36. Lu LC, Hsu C, Shao YY, Chao Y, Yen CJ, Shih IL, et al. Differential Organ-Specific Tumor Response to Immune Checkpoint Inhibitors in Hepatocellular Carcinoma. *Liver Cancer* (2019) 8(6):480–90. doi: 10.1159/000501275
37. Seiwert TY, Kiess AP. Time to Debunk an Urban Myth? The "Abscopal Effect" With Radiation and Anti–PD-1. *J Clin Oncol Off J Am Soc Clin Oncol* (2021) 39(1):1–3. doi: 10.1200/jco.20.02046
38. McBride S, Sherman E, Tsai CJ, Baxi S, Aghalar J, Eng J, et al. Randomized Phase II Trial of Nivolumab With Stereotactic Body Radiotherapy Versus

Nivolumab Alone in Metastatic Head and Neck Squamous Cell Carcinoma. *J Clin Oncol Off J Am Soc Clin Oncol* (2021) 39(1):30–7. doi: 10.1200/jco.20.00290

39. Klemen ND, Wang M, Feingold PL, Cooper K, Pavri SN, Han D, et al. Patterns of failure after immunotherapy with checkpoint inhibitors predict durable progression-free survival after local therapy for metastatic melanoma. *J ImmunoTher Cancer* (2019) 7(1):196. doi: 10.1186/s40425-019-0672-3
40. Leonardi GC, Gainor JF, Altan M, Kravets S, Dahlberg SE, Gedmintas L, et al. Safety of Programmed Death–1 Pathway Inhibitors Among Patients With Non–Small-Cell Lung Cancer and Preexisting Autoimmune Disorders. *J Clin Oncol* (2018) 36(19):1905–12. doi: 10.1200/jco.2017.77.0305
41. Murthy VH, Krumholz HM. Gross CP. Participation in Cancer Clinical TrialsRace-, Sex-, and Age-Based Disparities. *JAMA* (2004) 291(22):2720–6. doi: 10.1001/jama.291.22.2720
42. Ludmir EB, Mainwaring W, Lin TA, Miller AB, Jethanandani A, Espinoza AF, et al. Factors Associated With Age Disparities Among Cancer Clinical Trial Participants. *JAMA Oncol* (2019) 5(12):1769–73. doi: 10.1001/jamaoncol.2019.2055
43. Cohen EEW, Soulieres D, Tourneau CL, Dinis J, Licitra LF, Ahn M-J, et al. Health-related quality of life (HRQoL) of pembrolizumab (pembro) vs standard of care (SOC) for recurrent/metastatic head and neck squamous cell carcinoma (R/M HNSCC) in KEYNOTE-040. *J Clin Oncol* (2018) 36 (15_suppl):6013–. doi: 10.1200/JCO.2018.36.15_suppl.6013
44. Cohen EEW, Bell RB, Bifulco CB, Burtness B, Gillison ML, Harrington KJ, et al. The Society for Immunotherapy of Cancer consensus statement on immunotherapy for the treatment of squamous cell carcinoma of the head and neck (HNSCC). *J immunother Cancer* (2019) 7(1):184–. doi: 10.1186/s40425-019-0662-5
45. Rischin D, Migden MR, Lim AM, Schmults CD, Khushalani NI, Hughes BGM, et al. Phase 2 study of cemiplimab in patients with metastatic cutaneous squamous cell carcinoma: primary analysis of fixed-dosing, long-term outcome of weight-based dosing. *J Immunother Cancer* (2020) 8(1). doi: 10.1136/jitc-2020-000775
46. Ji AL, Rubin AJ, Thrane K, Jiang S, Reynolds DL, Meyers RM, et al. Multimodal Analysis of Composition and Spatial Architecture in Human Squamous Cell Carcinoma. *Cell* (2020) 182(2):497–514.e22. doi: 10.1016/j.cell.2020.05.039
47. Frazzette N, Khodadadi-Jamayran A, Doudican N, Santana A, Felsen D, Pavlick AC, et al. Decreased cytotoxic T cells and TCR clonality in organ transplant recipients with squamous cell carcinoma. *NPJ Precis Oncol* (2020) 4 (1):13. doi: 10.1038/s41698-020-0119-9
48. Stewart CA, Gay CM, Xi Y, Sivajothi S, Sivakamasundari V, Fujimoto J, et al. Single-cell analyses reveal increased intratumoral heterogeneity after the onset of therapy resistance in small-cell lung cancer. *Nat Cancer* (2020) 1:423–36. doi: 10.1038/s43018-019-0020-z
49. Wang R, Dang M, Harada K, Han G, Wang F, Pool Pizzi M, et al. Single-cell dissection of intratumoral heterogeneity and lineage diversity in metastatic gastric adenocarcinoma. *Nat Med* (2021) 27(1):141–51. doi: 10.1038/s41591-020-1125-8

4

SIX1 Activates STAT3 Signaling to Promote the Proliferation of Thyroid Carcinoma via EYA1

Deguang Kong [1], Anping Li [2], Yu Liu [3], Qiuxia Cui [4], Kun Wang [5], Dan Zhang [5], Jianing Tang [4], Yaying Du [5], Zhisu Liu [1], Gaosong Wu [4] and Kongming Wu [2*]*

[1] Department of General Surgery, Zhongnan Hospital of Wuhan University, Wuhan, China, [2] Department of Medical Oncology, The Affiliated Cancer Hospital of Zhengzhou University and Henan Cancer Hospital, Zhengzhou, China, [3] Department of Geriatrics, Tongji Hospital of Tongji Medical College, Huazhong University of Science and Technology, Wuhan, China, [4] Department of Thyroid and Breast Surgery, Zhongnan Hospital of Wuhan University, Wuhan, China, [5] Department of Thyroid and Breast Surgery, Tongji Hospital of Tongji Medical College, Huazhong University of Science and Technology, Wuhan, China

***Correspondence:**
Gaosong Wu
wugaosongtj@163.com
Kongming Wu
wukm_lab@163.com

As a critical member of the Retinal Determination Gene Network (RDGN), SIX1 has been regarded as a tumor promoter in various types of cancer. However, its role in papillary thyroid carcinoma (PTC) has never been investigated. In this study, thyroid carcinoma tissue microarray staining was employed to identify the expression patterns of SIX1 and its co-activator EYA1. Papillary thyroid cancer cell lines, BCPAP, and TPC-1 cells were used to investigate the potential mechanism of SIX1 *in vitro* and *in vivo*. Flow cytometry analysis, MTT assay, the growth curve assay, colony formation assay, EdU incorporation and xenograft assay were performed to demonstrate the role of SIX1 in the malignant change of PTC cells. Western blot and Real-time PCR were used to detect the interaction among the SIX1, EYA1, and STAT3 signaling. In comparison with normal tissue, high expressions of SIX1 and EYA1 were associated with a malignant tumor. Importantly, SIX1 strongly correlated with EYA1 in thyroid carcinoma tissue microarray. Functional assays indicated SIX1 increased EYA1 expression by stabilizing EYA1 at the post-transcriptional level. Besides, SIX1 promoted the proliferation and invasion of thyroid carcinoma via activation of STAT3 signaling and its downstream targets in an EYA1-dependent manner. SIX1 can integrate with EYA1 to contribute to PTC development via activation of the classical STAT3 signaling. These data suggested targeting the abnormal activation of the SIX1/EYA1 complex may represent a novel therapeutic strategy for advanced PTC patients.

Keywords: SIX1, EYA1, STAT3 signal, thyroid papillary carcinoma, tumor growth

INTRODUCTION

The incidence of thyroid cancer is rapidly increasing in recent two decades, and it has become the most common endocrine malignancy worldwide (1, 2). As the predominant pathological type of thyroid carcinoma, papillary thyroid carcinoma (PTC) accounts for more than 80% of the total (3). For most of PTC patients, conventional surgical thyroidectomy with radioactive iodine ablation and thyrotropin hormone-suppressive levothyroxine can obtain a satisfactory outcome (4). However, about 10% of cases suffer from a locally advanced or metastatic disease at diagnosis, which are the most frequent causes of thyroid cancer-related death (5). Understanding the molecular basis of thyroid cancer is essential for developing effective strategies for advanced PTC patients (6).

The development of therapeutic agents that target tumor driver genes is the fundament for precision medicine (7). Exciting discoveries like the genetic duet of *BRAF* ^{V600E} and *RAS* mutations have led to significant progress in targeted therapies. Several *BRAF* tyrosine kinase inhibitors are either approved or undergoing investigation for patients with malignancies carrying *BRAF* mutations (8). However, the complexity in molecular subtypes of PTCs is still a challenge in exploring novel biomarker for guiding personal treatment in advanced stage (9). Meanwhile, alterations of critical signaling pathways in thyroid development like MAPK and PI3K-AKT can initiate tumorigenesis and promote tumor metastasis (10). Targeting the aberrant expression of development related genes or signaling may provide an opportunity for the molecular-based treatment of thyroid cancer.

In this respect, the *retinal determination gene network* (RDGN) family is required for organismal development in mammalian (11). This regulatory network mainly consists of *dachshund* (*dac*/Dach), the Six family transcription factor *sine oculis* (*so*/Six) and a tyrosine phosphatase *eyes absent* (*eya*/Eya). The balance of Dach/Eya/Six network governs the tissue differentiation (11). Recently, the abnormal activation SIX1 and EYA family have been proved to be involved in the development of multiple cancers. SIX1 promoted malignant transformation of mammary epithelial cells, including increased proliferation and anchorage independent growth by activating cyclin A1 (12). Via activation of TGF-β and MAPK signal, SIX1 enhanced the accumulation of cancer stem cells (CSCs) as well as induced epithelial-mesenchymal transition (EMT), and even switched the role of TGF-β/SMAD signal from tumor suppressors to oncogenic proteins in breast cancer (13–16). SIX1 can inhibit p53 by upregulating microRNA-27a-3p and downregulating ribosomal protein L26 (RPL26) to diminish the p53-mediated tumor suppression across different cancer types (7). Most recent study found the microRNA-548a-3p/SIX1 axis strongly linked aerobic glycolysis to carcinogenesis (17). SIX1 and EYA can integrate with other signal pathways to modulate the apoptosis, cell proliferation and tumor growth (18). To date, the profiles of SIX1 and EYA1 have been independently identified as a prognostic biomarker in breast cancer (13, 19). However, the functional relationship of SIX1 and EYA1 in thyroid cancer remains to be discovered.

Abnormal re-activation of embryological genes can trigger the tumorigenesis. A previous study has indicated that the Eyal and Sixl were required for the morphogenesis of mammalian thyroid (20). Given these observations, the role of SIX1 and EYA1 in tumorigenesis and progression of PTC deserves further investigation. In this study, we explored the role of SIX1 in PTC through *in vitro* and *in vivo* experiments, which implicated SIX1 coordinated with EYA1 to drive neoplastic growth and invasion via activation of the classical STAT3 signaling.

MATERIALS AND METHODS

PTC Tissue Microarray and Immunohistochemistry

Commercially available tissue microarray (TMA) slides (TH8010 and TH802a, US Biomax, Inc.) were purchased for immunohistochemistry (IHC) analysis. Specific primary antibodies against SIX1 (Sigma, USA) and EYA1 (Proteintech, China) were used for IHC with a 2-step protocol (21). Whole slide image capture was performed on the EVOS auto cell image system (Life technology, USA). For semi-quantitative evaluation of protein level in tissue, the staining intensity was graded as previously described (22). The immunohistochemical score were assessed by two experienced pathologists without knowledge of patients' characteristics. Scores were calculated on intensity and percentage of positive staining tumor cell nuclei or cytoplasm in the whole tissue stains were evaluated according to Fromowitz Standard. Briefly, the staining intensity was graded as follows: no staining, 0; weakly positive, 1; moderately positive, 2; and strongly positive, 3. The percentage of positive cells was into four grades: 0–25% staining, 1; 26–50% staining, 2; 51–75% staining, 3; and 76–100% staining, 4. The multiplication of the intensity and percentage scores was used to calculate the final staining score. For quantification, all stains were assessed at 200×magnifications and at least three fields from each core were counted.

Cells Culture and Transfection

Human papillary thyroid cancer cell lines BCPAP, NPA and TPC-1 were provided by Dr. Du (Tongji Hospital of Tongji Medical College) and cultured in recommended condition. Cell line authenticity was confirmed by Short Tandem Repeat (STR) DNA profiling (the STR profiles were shown in **Supplementary Materials**). All experiments were performed using cell lines from passage 6 to 25. Cells were seeded at 50% confluence in 6 cm plate on the day before transduction. HEK 293T cells were transfected with pLV vector or pLV-SIX1 expression plasmid with package plasmids by Lipofectamine™ 2000 (Invitrogen, Carlsbad CA, USA). The supernatant was collected and polybrene (1:1,000) was added into the supernatant. The mixed supernatant was applied to recipient cells for infection. The expression of SIX1 was verified by quantitative reverse transcription-PCR (qRT-PCR) and Western blot. For small interfering RNA (siRNA)-mediated downregulation of EYA1, BCPAP-Vector and BCPAP-SIX1 cells were seeded in 6-well plates and transfected with siRNA or scramble control (Ribobio Company, Guangzhou, China) duplexes using Lipofectamine™ 2000 (Invitrogen, Carlsbad CA, USA). EYA1 siRNA: (sense) 5′-CAGGAAAUAAUUCACUCACAAdTdT-3′; (antisense) 5′-UUGUGAGUGAAUUAUUUCCUGdTdT- 3′.

Western Blot Analysis

Cell and tissue lysates were extracted using ice-cold RIPA buffer and measured using a bicinchoninic acid (BCA) protein assay kit (Promoter, China). Proteins were resolved on 10% SDS-polyacrylamide gels and transferred to PVDF membranes. The antibodies used in Western blot were as follows: SIX1, EYA1, C-MYC (Santa Cruz, USA), STAT3 (Cell Signaling Technology, USA), p-STAT3 (Tyr705) (Cell Signaling Technology, USA), BCL-XL (Cell Signaling Technology, USA), Caspase 3 (Proteintech, China), Cleaved PARP1 (Ruiying Bio, China), Cleaved Caspase 9 (Ruiying Bio, China), β-tublin (Cell Signaling Technology, USA), GAPDH (Cell Signaling Technology, USA) and VINCULIN (Sigma, USA).

Quantitative Reverse Transcription-PCR (qRT-PCR)

RNA was prepared from PTC cells with the TRIzol reagent (Invitrogen, USA). cDNA was reversed from 1 μg total RNA using a reverse transcription kit (TOYOBO, Japan). RT-qPCR was performed with the SYBR® Green Real-time PCR Master Mix Kit (TOYOBO, Japan). Gene expression was normalized to GAPDH. The primer sequences for real-time RT-PCR were as follows: SIX1: (forward) 5′-ACAAGAACGAGAGCG TACTCA-3′, (reverse) 5′-CTCCACGTAATGCGCCTTCA-3′; EYA1: (forward) 5′-GTTCATCTGGGACTTGGA-3′, (reverse) 5′-GCTTAGGTCCTGTCCGTT-3′; GAPDH: (forward) 5′-CAATGACCCCTTCATTGACC-3′, (reverse) 5′-GATCTCGC TCCTGGAAGATG-3′.

Cell Proliferation Assays

For MTT assay, 2,000 cells were seeded into 96-well plates and analyzed by adding MTT (tetrazolium bromide, 5 mg/mL, GE Healthcare) as previously described (22). To measure the growth curve, 2.5×10^3 cells were seeded in 24-well culture plates and the numbers of viable cells were serially counted for 6–7 days. Colony formation assay was performed as previously described (23). Two weeks later, cells were fixed with 4% paraformaldehyde and stained by 0.5% crystal violet for visualization and counting on the plate.

Cell-Cycle Analysis

About 3×10^5 cells were seeded into a 6 cm Petri dish. After 24 h incubation, the cells were collected and fixed with 75% cold ethanol at −20°C overnight. DNA was incubated with 200 μL RNase A (1 mg/mL) and 500 μL propidium iodide (PI, 100 μg/mL) for 30 min at room temperature in the dark and analyzed by using the FACSort flow cytometer (Becton, Dickinson Company, USA). The data were analyzed with ModFit LT V2.0 software (Becton, Dickinson Company, USA).

Transwell Migration and Invasion Assay

Transwell chambers (pore size 8.0 μm) (Corning Inc., USA) were either uncoated (migration assay) or coated (invasion assay) with Matrigel as previously described (23). All experiments were conducted in triplicate.

Annexin V-FITC/PI Assay

The apoptosis was determined by the Annexin V-FITC/PI apoptosis detection kit (BD Biosciences, USA). Briefly, cells were treated with 200 μM H_2O_2 (Sigma, USA) for 24 h. The cells were collected, and then resuspended in 200 μL of binding buffer. After incubation of Annexin V-FITC and PI for 15 min at room temperature, 300 μL binding buffer was added to the cells and the results were analyzed by flow cytometry (Beckman-Coulter Inc., USA). The experiment was repeated in triplicate.

Ethynyl-20-deoxyuridine (EdU) Incorporation Assay

EdU incorporation assay was performed with EdU assay kit (Ribobio, China). Briefly, 1×10^3 cells per well were culture in 96-well plates for 48 h, and then 50 μM of EdU was added to each well and cultured for additional 2 h. The cells were fixed with 4% formaldehyde for 15 min and treated with 0.5% Triton X-100 for 20 min. After washing with PBS, 100 μl of 1 × Apollo reaction cocktail was added and incubated for 30 min. After staining with 100 μl of Hoechst 33342 for 30 min, the cells were visualized under EVOS cell image system. The results were analyzed by Image-Pro Plus 6.0 software (Media Cybernetics, USA). All experiments were done in triplicate and three independent repeating experiments were performed.

Immunofluorescent Labeling of SIX1 and EYA1

Cells were seeded in a 24-well plate (5×10^4cells/well) and cultured for 48 h, then fixed with 4% paraformaldehyde. Next, cells were permeabilized with 0.1% Triton X-100 and blocked using 5% goat serum for 30 min. Cells were further incubated overnight with primary antibodies against SIX1 (anti-mouse, 1:100, Santa Cruz, USA), EYA1 (anti-rabbit, 1:100, Proteintech, China). Next day, cells were incubated with either Alexa Fluor 594 or Alexa Fluor 488 for 1 h. Nuclei were visualized with DAPI stain. The stained cells were examined with EVOS cell image system.

Tumor Formation Assay

Five- to 6-week-old female NOD/SCID mice were purchased from Beijing HFK Bioscience Limited Company and maintained under the Specific Pathogen-Free (SPF) conditions at Laboratory Animal Centre. All the protocols were reviewed and approved by the Institutional Ethics Committee and performed in accordance with national guidelines. All mice were randomly divided into two groups: TPC1-shControl ($n = 20$) and TPC1-shSIX1 ($n = 20$). Cells were counted and serially diluted in 100 ml of 1:1 PBS/Matrigel, and injected subcutaneously. The mice were monitored every 3 days. At 3 weeks post-injection, all mice were euthanized and analyzed for tumor formation. Tumors were collected for further Western Blot analysis.

Statistical Analysis

GraphPad Prism 6.0 software was used for the statistical analyses. The IHC scores were tested whether the data matched normal distribution or not. If it was, then the difference between groups were conducted by using parametric statistics (*Student t*-test), otherwise performing non-parametric statistics (*Mann-Whitney* test). The correlations between clinicopathological and immunohistochemical variables were calculated according to *Person* χ^2-test. Cell culture experiments differences between the groups were evaluated by the *Student t*-test, including EdU assays, MTT activity, growth curve assays, colony formation assay, Transwell migration, and invasion assays, Annexin V-FITC/PI assays, PCR and western blot assays. All data were expressed as mean ± standard error. $P < 0.05$ were considered statistically significant.

RESULTS

Both SIX1 and EYA1 Were Increased in PTC Patients

To identify the expression pattern of SIX1 and EYA1 in human thyroid tissue as well as tumor, we performed IHC analysis by using two tissue microarrays (TH8010 and TH802a). After excluding the duplicated reports ($n = 6$) and detached sample ($n = 9$), two tissue microarrays contained 145 samples, including normal thyroid tissue ($n = 10$), atypical adenoma ($n = 1$), oncocytoma ($n = 4$), colloid adenoma ($n = 15$), fetal adenoma ($n = 10$), follicular adenoma ($n = 10$), follicular carcinoma (FTC, $n = 18$), medullary carcinoma (MTC, $n = 5$), papillary carcinoma (PTC, $n = 66$), and anaplastic carcinoma (ATC, $n = 6$). The IHC score for each type was shown in **Figure 1A**. In comparison with normal tissue, SIX1 and EYA1 kept low expression in benign tumor and no statistic difference was found for either SIX1 or EYA1 between groups. However, a significant increase in SIX1 and EYA1 was detected in malignant tumor, including FTC ($p = 0.011$, $p = 0.038$; respectively), MTC ($p = 0.006$, $p = 0.043$; respectively), PTC ($p < 0.001$, $p < 0.001$; respectively) and ATC samples ($p = 0.002$, $p < 0.001$; respectively) (**Figure 1A**). The representative images of IHC staining for normal and cancerous tissue were shown in **Figure 1B**. Intriguingly, SIX1 was tightly linked to EYA1 in malignant tumor. The analysis from Spearman correlation based on all malignant sample in these tissue microarrays indicated that SIX1 had a strongly positive relationship with EYA1 (**Figure 1C**). BRAF mutation is the most common mutation in PTC (8). To test whether there was relationship between SIX1/EYA1 and $BRAF^{V600E}$ mutation, the GEO database (GSE54958) was applied to analyze. There was no difference in the expression of SIX1/EYA1 and $BRAF^{V600E}$ mutation (Data not shown).

Since PTC is the most common type of thyroid carcinoma and also occupied the majority of the tissue microarrays in this study, we next examined the association of SIX1 and EYA1

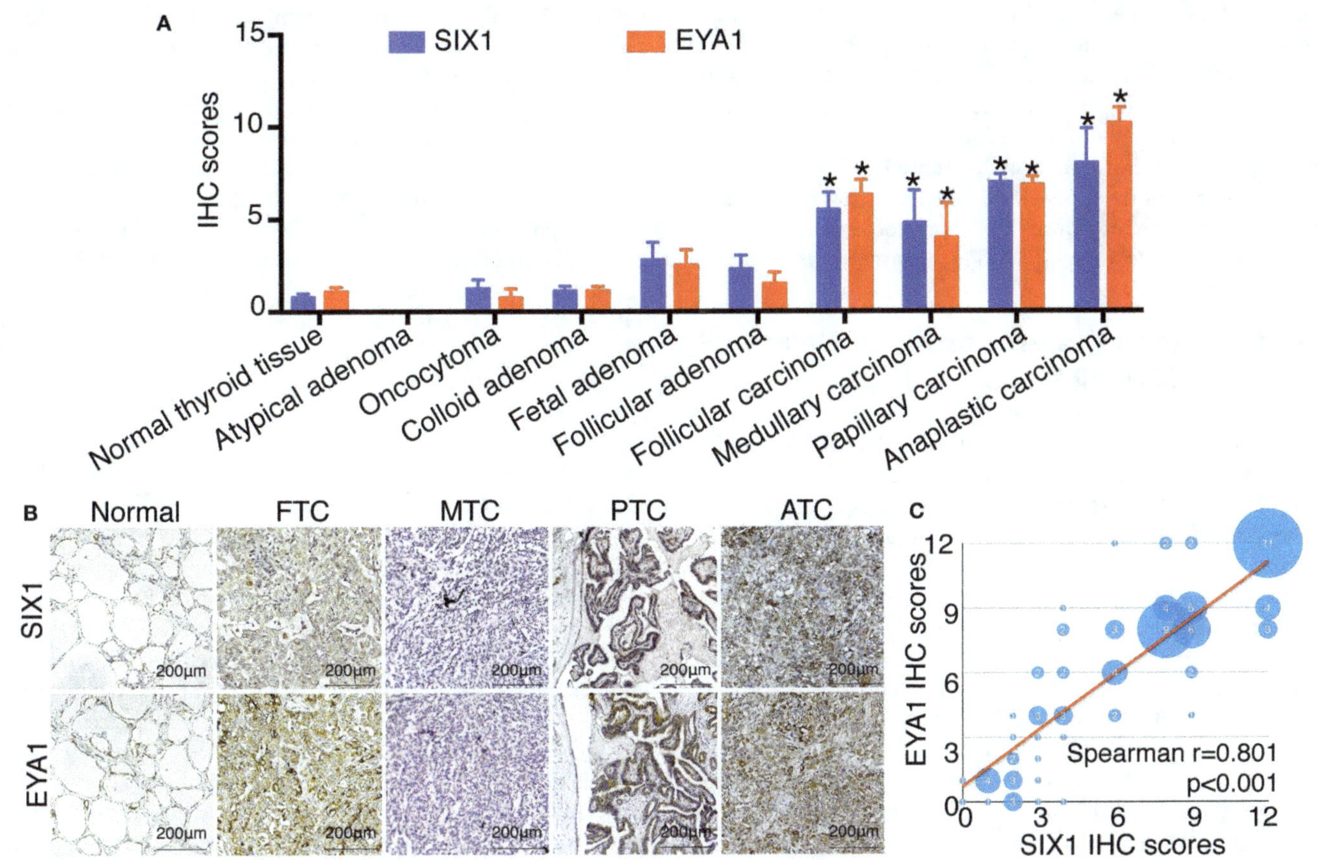

FIGURE 1 | The expression of SIX1 and EYA1 in PTC tissues. The semi quantitative results displayed as median ± stand error **(A)**. The relative expression of SIX1 and EYA1 in thyroid carcinoma tissue microarray, including normal thyroid tissue, atypical adenoma, oncocytoma, colloid adenoma, fetal adenoma, follicular adenoma, follicular carcinoma, medullary carcinoma, papillary carcinoma, and anaplastic carcinoma, *represents a statistical difference was found compared with normal tissue. **(B)** Representative immunohistochemistry images of SIX1 and EYA1 expression in normal thyroid, papillary thyroid carcinoma (PTC), follicular thyroid carcinoma (FTC), medullary thyroid carcinoma (MTC), and anaplastic thyroid cancer (ATC). **(C)** The positive relationship between SIX1 and EYA1 in thyroid malignant carcinoma.

TABLE 1 | Association between SIX1/EYA1 expression and clinicopathologic factors in papillary carcinoma (TH8010 + TH802a).

Characteristics	SIX1 expression			EYA1 expression		
	Low (≤6)	High (>6)	*p*	Low (≤6)	High (>6)	*p*
Sex			0.481*			0.177*
Male	4	8		3	9	
Female	24	30		25	29	
Age (y)	38.96 ± 2.429	49.63 ± 2.662	0.006†	39.5 ± 2.434	49.24 ± 2.7	0.012†
Tumor size			0.347*			0.145*
≤4 cm (T1 + T2)	12	12		13	11	
>4 cm (T3 + T4)	16	26		15	27	
Lymph node metastasis			0.043*			0.030*
Absent	23	23		24	22	
Present	4	14		4	14	
Stage			0.015*			0.015*
I + II	24	22		24	22	
III + IVA	4	16		4	16	

*Person chi-square test.
†Independent-sample t-test.

expression with clinicopathological parameters. Based on the semi-quantitative criteria, we defined IHC score over 6 (>6) was higher and scores under 6 (≤6) was lower expression. We found that the levels of SIX1 and EYA1 expression were significantly associated with age, lymph node metastasis (two sample missed this information, tissue ID: Etg030430 and Etg030007) and clinical stage, but not tumor size (**Table 1**). Based on these data, high expressions of SIX1 and EYA1 are closely correlated with thyroid malignant tumor. SIX1 may cooperate with EYA1 and play a key role in lymph node metastasis via a BRAF-independent manner.

SIX1 Increased the Proportion of Cells in S Phase in PTC Cell Lines

Since SIX1 is a DNA-specific transcriptional factor, whereas EYA1 basically acts as a co-factor to increase SIX1-dependent function (11), we mainly focused on the functional role of SIX1 in thyroid cancer for first. The base line expressions of SIX1 were detected by western blot in PTC cell lines, including BCPAP, TPC-1, and NPA, with HEK 293T cell as a positive control. The results showed that SIX1 were barely expressed in BCPAP cells, whereas highly enriched in TPC-1 cells (**Figure 2A**). The next step was establishing the thyroid cell lines with either overexpression or knockdown of SIX1 by employing lentivirus-mediated gene transfer system. BCPAP cells stably overexpressing SIX1 were successfully transduced by pLV-SIX1 (BCPAP-SIX1) and pLV empty vector (BCPAP-Vector). Meanwhile, lentivirus shRNA expression vector for SIX1 or scramble control were transduced into TPC-1 cells (**Figure 2B**).

To assess the role of SIX1 in cell cycle regulation, propidium iodide staining and flow cytometry were performed. Overexpression of SIX1 significantly decreased the percentage of cells in the G0/G1 phase (78.47 ± 2.37% vs. 67.31 ± 1.56%, $p = 0.017$) and increased the subpopulation in the S phases (16.33 ± 2.44% vs. 27.68 ± 1.72%, $p = 0.019$) in BCPAP cells (**Figures 2C,D**). Conversely, knockdown SIX1 in TPC-1 cells induced a significant increase of G0/G1 phase (53.73 ± 0.87% vs. 64.79 ± 1.46%, $p = 0.003$) and a decrease in the S-phase population (34.42 ± 0.61% vs. 22.77 ± 1.32%, $p = 0.001$) compared with control group (**Figures 3A,B**). To further evaluate the effect of SIX1 in cell cycle regulation, EdU incorporation assay was examined. In accordance with results of flow cytometry, the proportion of EdU positive cells was increased by 2.84-folds induced by SIX1 overexpressing in BCPAP cells (**Figure 2E**). And the number of EdU positive cells in TPC-1-shSIX1 group was reduced by 40% in comparison with TPC1-shControl (**Figure 3C**). Taken together, these data demonstrate that SIX1 promoted cell cycle progression in thyroid cancer cells.

SIX1 Overexpression Induced Proliferation, Cell Migration, and Invasion in PTC

To examine the effect of SIX1 on PTC cellular proliferation, MTT assays, cell growth curve, and colony formation assays were performed to assess the proliferative ability. MTT assays showed the tumor cell growth rate significantly increased after ectopic expression of SIX1 (**Figure 2F**) and decreased after silencing the endogenous SIX1 expression (**Figure 3D**), which were in accord with the findings from cell growth curve (**Figures 2G, 3E**). Transfecting the exogenous *SIX1* gene into BCPAP cells can increase both colony number and size (**Figure 2H**), and SIX1 knockdown otherwise resulted in approximately 50% colony growth inhibition in the TPC-1 cells (**Figure 3F**). Furthermore, cell migration and invasion were significantly increased in BCPAP cells with SIX1 overexpression (**Figure 2I**) and decreased by half in TPC-1 cells after knockdown of SIX1 (**Figure 3G**). These data suggested that SIX1 induced the oncogenic properties of PTC.

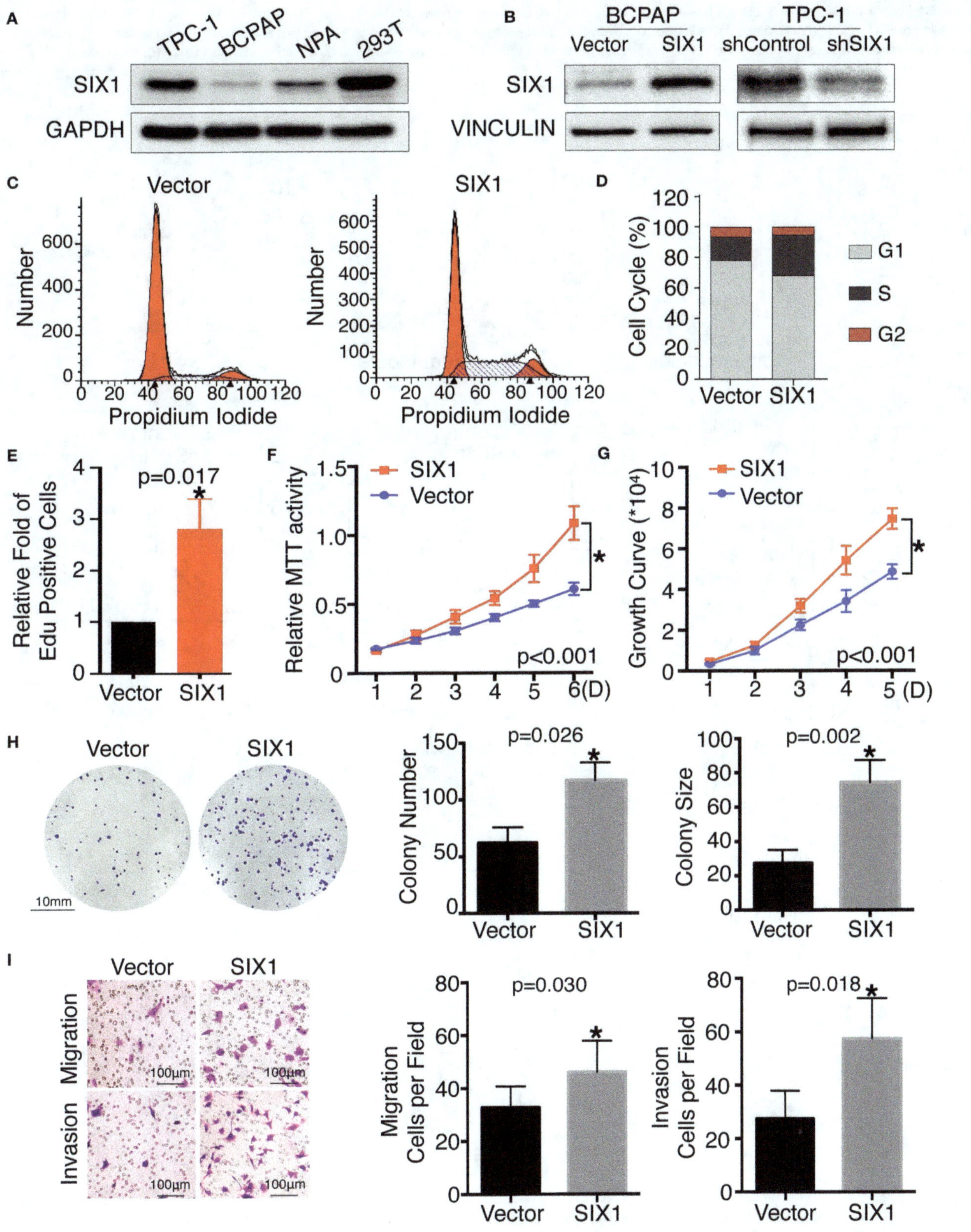

FIGURE 2 | Ectopic expression of SIX1 increased the proportion of cells in S phase and promoted proliferation, migration and invasion in BCPAP cell lines. Protein abundance of SIX1 in PTC cell lines by western blot analysis **(A)**. Western blot analysis confirmed the efficiency of ectopic expressing SIX1 in BCPAP cells or silencing SIX1 in TPC-1 cells **(B)**. Representative images of cell cycle plot **(C)** and quantitative results ($n = 3$) **(D)**. Quantitative results of EdU staining of cells with SIX1

(Continued)

FIGURE 2 | overexpression ($n = 3$) **(E)**. MTT assays of BCPAP cells with ectopic expression of SIX1 ($n = 5$) **(F)**. Growth curve assays of BCPAP cells with ectopic expression of SIX1 ($n = 5$) **(G)**. Representative images of colony formation assays of BCPAP cells with ectopic expression of SIX1 and quantitative results ($n = 3$) **(H)**. The representative images of migration and invasion assay in BCPAP cells with SIX1 overexpression and quantitative analysis ($n = 3$) **(I)**. $^*p < 0.05$.

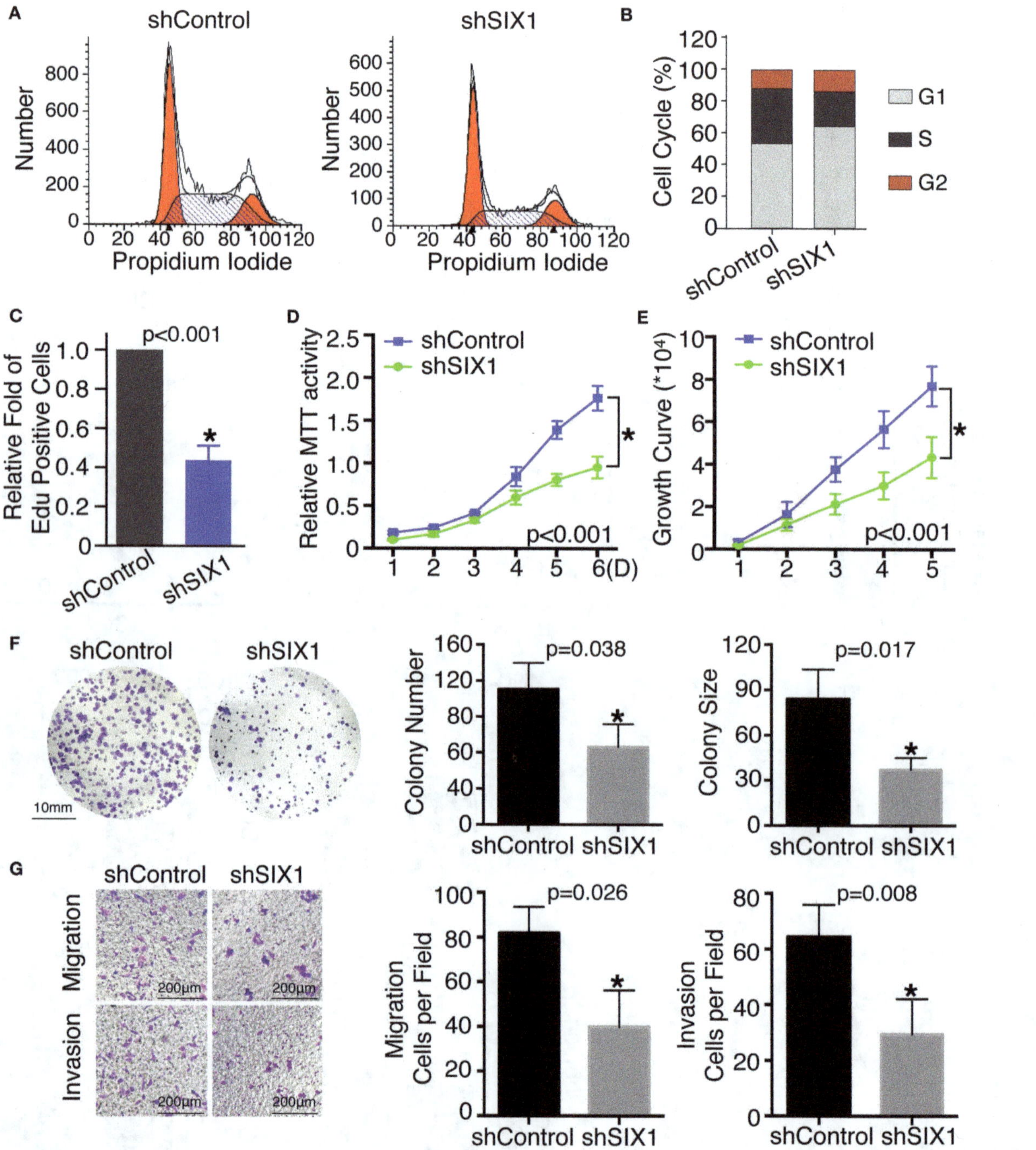

FIGURE 3 | Knockdown SIX1 decreased the proportion of cells in S phase and inhibited proliferation, migration, and invasion in TPC-1 cell lines. Representative images of cell cycle plot **(A)** and quantitative results ($n = 3$) **(B)**. Quantitative results of EdU staining of cells with SIX1 knockdown ($n = 3$) **(C)**. MTT assays of TPC-1 cells after silencing SIX1 ($n = 5$) **(D)**. Growth curve assays of TPC-1 cells after silencing SIX1 ($n = 5$) **(E)**. Representative images of colony formation assays of TPC-1 cells after silencing SIX1 and quantitative results ($n = 3$) **(F)**. The representative images of migration and invasion assay in TPC-1 cells after silencing SIX1 and quantitative analysis ($n = 3$) **(G)**. $^*p < 0.05$.

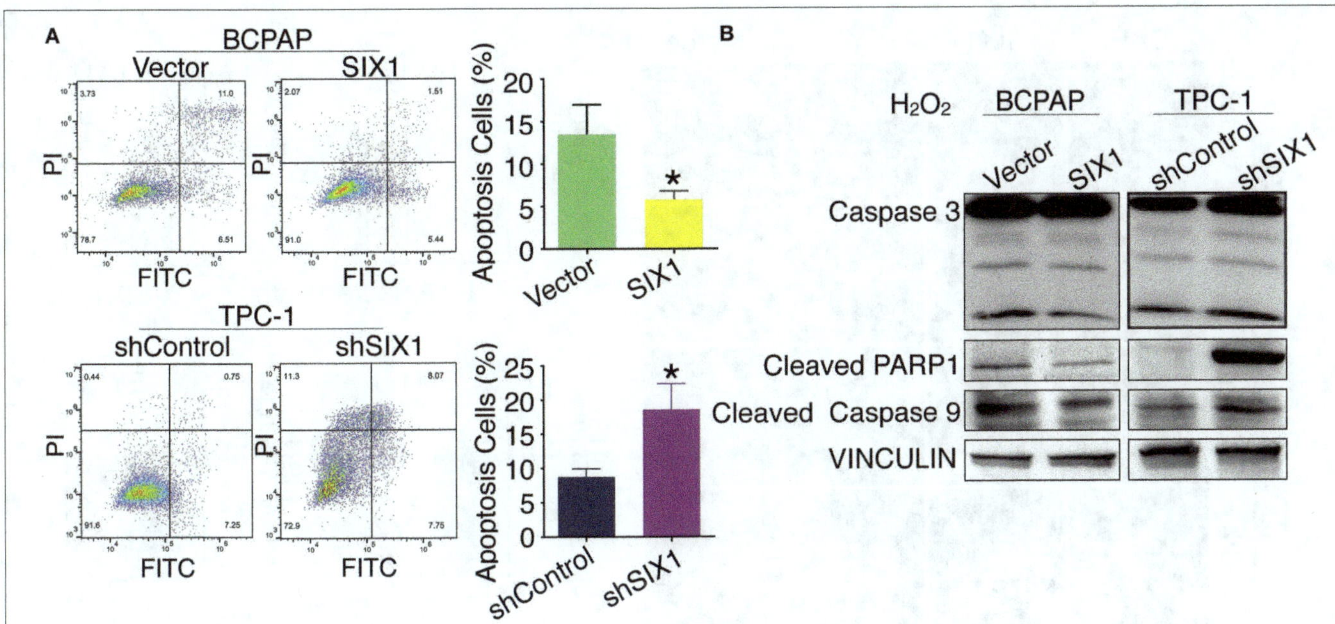

FIGURE 4 | SIX1 attenuated H_2O_2-induced apoptosis in PTC cell lines. PTC cell lines were incubated for 24 h, and then exposed to 200 μM H_2O_2 for 24 h. Annexin V-FITC/PI assay was used to evaluate the apoptosis. Representative image of apoptosis assay and quantitative analysis (n = 3) **(A)**. The protein expression of caspase 3, cleaved PARP1 and cleaved caspase 9 in PTC cell lines was detected by Western blotting **(B)**. $^*p < 0.05$.

SIX1 Protected PTC Cells Against H_2O_2-Induced Apoptosis

Increased proliferation and reduced apoptosis are the fundamental feature of cancer cells. Next, we evaluated whether SIX1 protected PTC cell lines from apoptosis assessed by Annexin V-FITC/PI staining. Flow cytometric analysis results indicated that H_2O_2 induced apoptosis in PTC cell lines. The proportion of apoptotic cells in BCPAP-SIX1 group was significantly reduced from 13.46 to 5.82% in comparison with BCPAP-Vector (p = 0.022) (**Figure 4A**). The proportion of apoptotic cells in TPC1-shSIX1 group was increased significantly from 8.75 to 18.56% in comparison with TPC1-shControl (p = 0.0133) (**Figure 4A**). The protein expression levels of caspase 3, cleaved PARP1 and cleaved caspase 9 were detected by Western blotting. The results showed that SIX1 significantly attenuated H_2O_2-induced upregulation of cleaved Caspase 3, cleaved PARP1 and cleaved Caspase 9 protein expression (**Figure 4B**).

STAT3 Signal Is Responsible for the SIX1-Induced Proliferation of PTC Cells in an EYA1-Dependent Manner

Although there is a consensus that EYA functions as a co-activator in SIX1-associated malignant properties, little is known about whether and how SIX1 modulates EYA1 expression. Immunofluorescence assay showed the positive relationship and co-localization of SIX1 and EYA1 (**Figure 5A**). Moreover, we carried out qRT-PCR to examine the mRNA change. However, the mRNA of *EYA1* did not change when *SIX1* was overexpressed in BCPAP or *SIX1* was knocked down in TPC-1 cells (**Figure 5B**), indicating that SIX1 induces the protein abundance of EYA1 at post-transcriptional level, rather than directly involves in the transcriptional regulation of EYA1 mRNA.

Cell cycle proteins regulated by SIX1 might be responsible for the proliferation in PTC. To address the underlying mechanisms, cell cycle elements were screened by western blot. SIX1 significantly promoted the abundance of C-MYC (**Figure 5C**). Since C-MYC is the downstream target of STAT3 signaling and other group has reported SIX1 can induce p-STAT3 expression in human keratinocytes (24), we hypothesized that SIX1 might promote C-MYC abundance via activation of STAT3 signaling. Ectopic expression of SIX1 could significantly upregulate the expression of p-STAT3 (Try705) as well as its downstream target BCL-XL. As expected, knockdown SIX1 in TPC-1 cell showed the opposite (**Figure 5C**).

To further determine whether EYA1 was required for the SIX1-induced STAT3 signaling activation. siRNA was used to transiently knock down EYA1 in BCPAP-vector and BCPAP-SIX1 cells. Intriguingly, the upregulation of p-STAT3, C-MYC, and BCL-XL induced by SIX1 was abolished after silencing EYA1. Additionally, knocking down EYA1 in BCPAP-Vector cells diminished endogenous expression of STAT3 signal and its downstream targets (**Figure 5D**). We evaluated the effects of EYA1 knock-down in TPC-1 cells which had higher endogenous expression of SIX1. The expressions of SIX1, p-STAT3, C-MYC, and BCL-XL abundance were down regulated after silencing EYA1 by siRNA in TPC-1 cells (**Figure 5E**).

Next, we compared the functional significance of SIX1/EYA1 interaction. Both colony formation assay and MTT showed that the proliferation ability was significantly reduced when

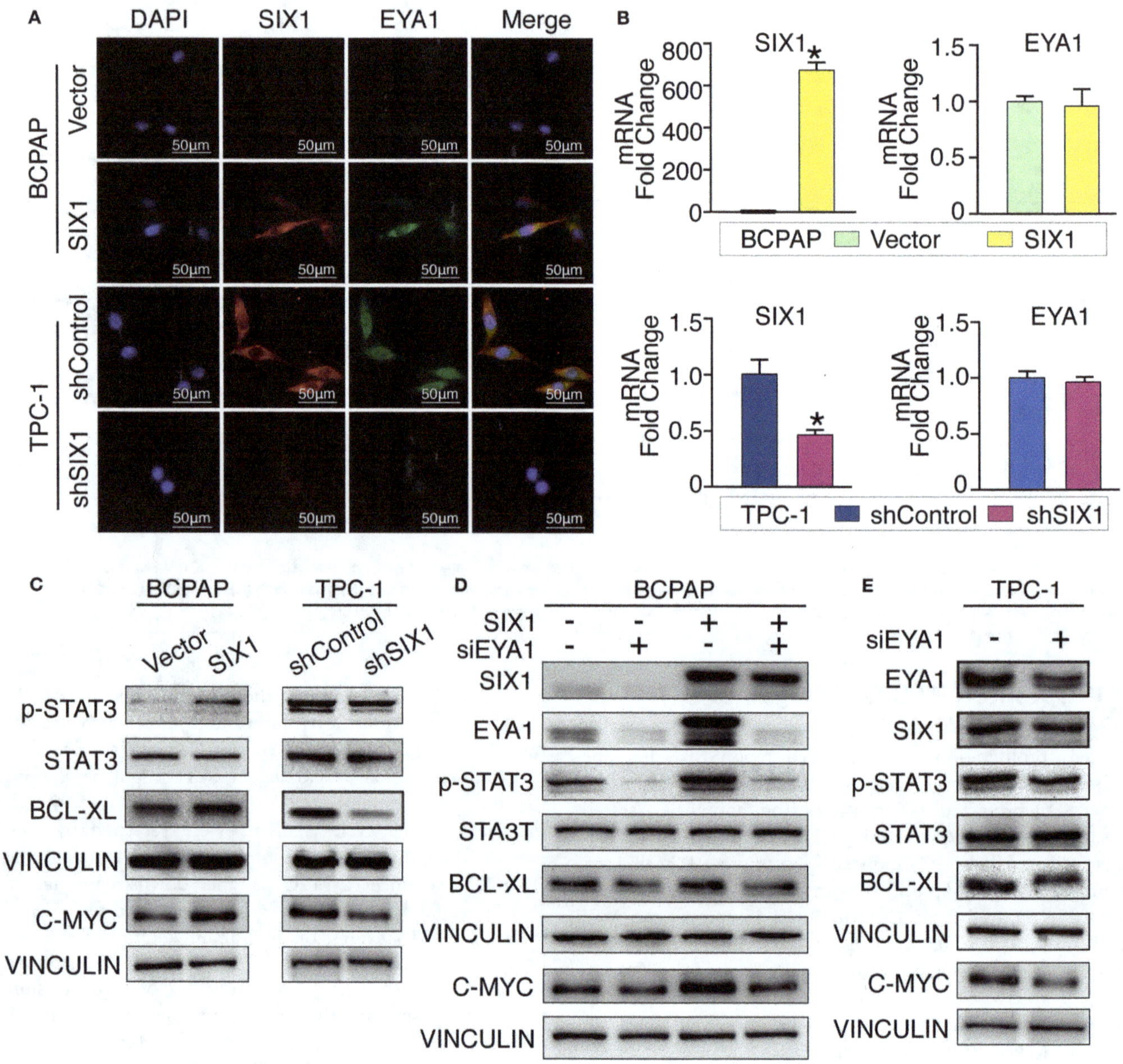

FIGURE 5 | SIX1 activated STAT3 signaling pathway to promote PTC cells proliferation via EYA1. Immunofluorescence show the co-localization of SIX1 (red) and EYA1 (green) **(A)**. The relative mRNA level of SIX1 and EYA1 in PTC cell lines with SIX1 overexpression or silencing **(B)**. Western blot analysis of indicated protein from PTC cells with SIX1 overexpression or silencing **(C)**. Western blot analysis of indicated protein from BCPAP cells with SIX1 and/or EYA1 silencing **(D)**. Western blot analysis of indicated protein from TPC-1 cells with EYA1 silencing **(E)**. *$p < 0.05$.

EYA1 was knocked down in SIX1-overexpressing BCPAP cells (**Figures 6A,B,E**). In agreement, SIX1-induced DNA synthesis was inhibited by knock down EYA1, as evaluated by EdU incorporation assay (**Figures 6G,H**). On the other side, colony formation assay and MTT demonstrated that knockdown endogenous EYA1 can inhibit TPC-1 cell growth (**Figures 6C,D,F**). Together, these data suggest that the activation of STAT3 signaling induced by SIX1 is dependent on the presence of EYA1 in PTC cells.

Silencing SIX1 Suppressed Tumor Growth as Well as STAT3 Signal Activation *in vivo*

To test whether blocking the expression of SIX1 abolished the PTC cell proliferation *in vivo*, 2×10^6 TPC1-shControl or TPC1-shSIX1 cells were injected, respectively, into the subcutaneous fat of immunodeficient mice. Downregulation of the endogenous SIX1 by shRNA in TPC-1 cells not only showed a trend of slowing down the tumor associated weight loss (**Figure 7A**), but also significantly reduced the volume as well as the weight of

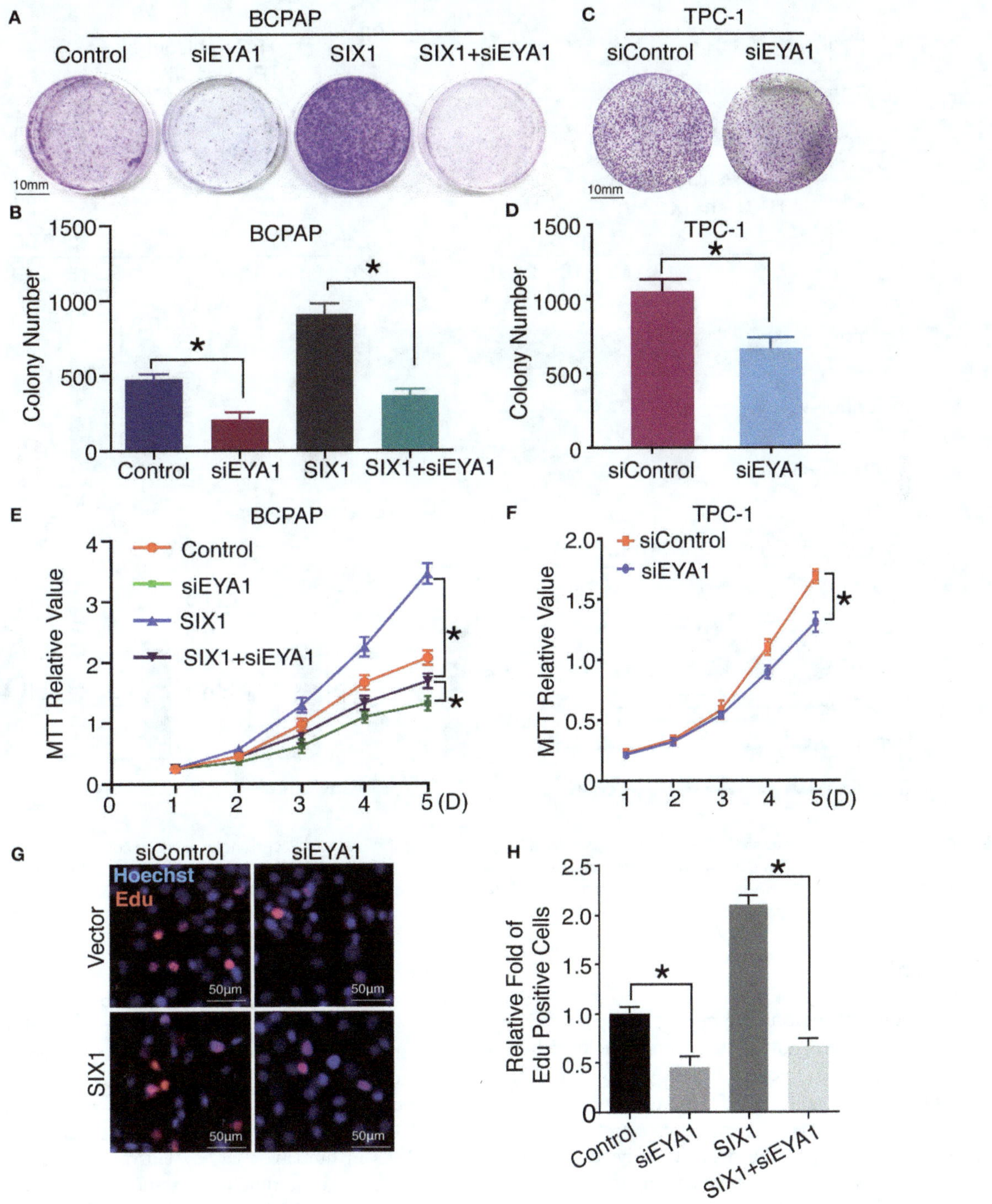

FIGURE 6 | Interaction of SIX1 and EYA1 determined PTC cells proliferation. Representative image of colony formation from BCPAP cells with SIX1 overexpression and/or siEYA1 **(A)** and quantitative analysis ($n = 3$) **(B)**. Representative image of colony formation from TPC-1 cells with siEYA1 **(C)** and quantitative analysis ($n = 3$) **(D)**. MTT assay of BCPAP cells with SIX1 overexpression and/or siEYA1 ($n = 5$) **(E)**. MTT assay of TPC-1 cells with siEYA1($n = 5$) **(F)**. Representative images of EdU assay of BCPAP cells with SIX1 overexpression and/or siEYA1 **(G)** and quantitative analysis ($n = 3$) **(H)**. $^{*}p < 0.05$.

xenografted tumors (**Figures 7B–D**). At the time of sacrifice, xenograft tumors were harvested and examined by western blot. Consistent with these findings *in vitro,* the tumors in TPC1-shSIX1 group retained SIX1 lower-expression *in vivo* and the levels of EYA1, p-STAT3 (Try705) and C-MYC were significantly decreased compared with shControl group (**Figures 7E,F**). Taken together, these results highlight the potential for targeting SIX1 in the comprehensive therapy for PTC patients.

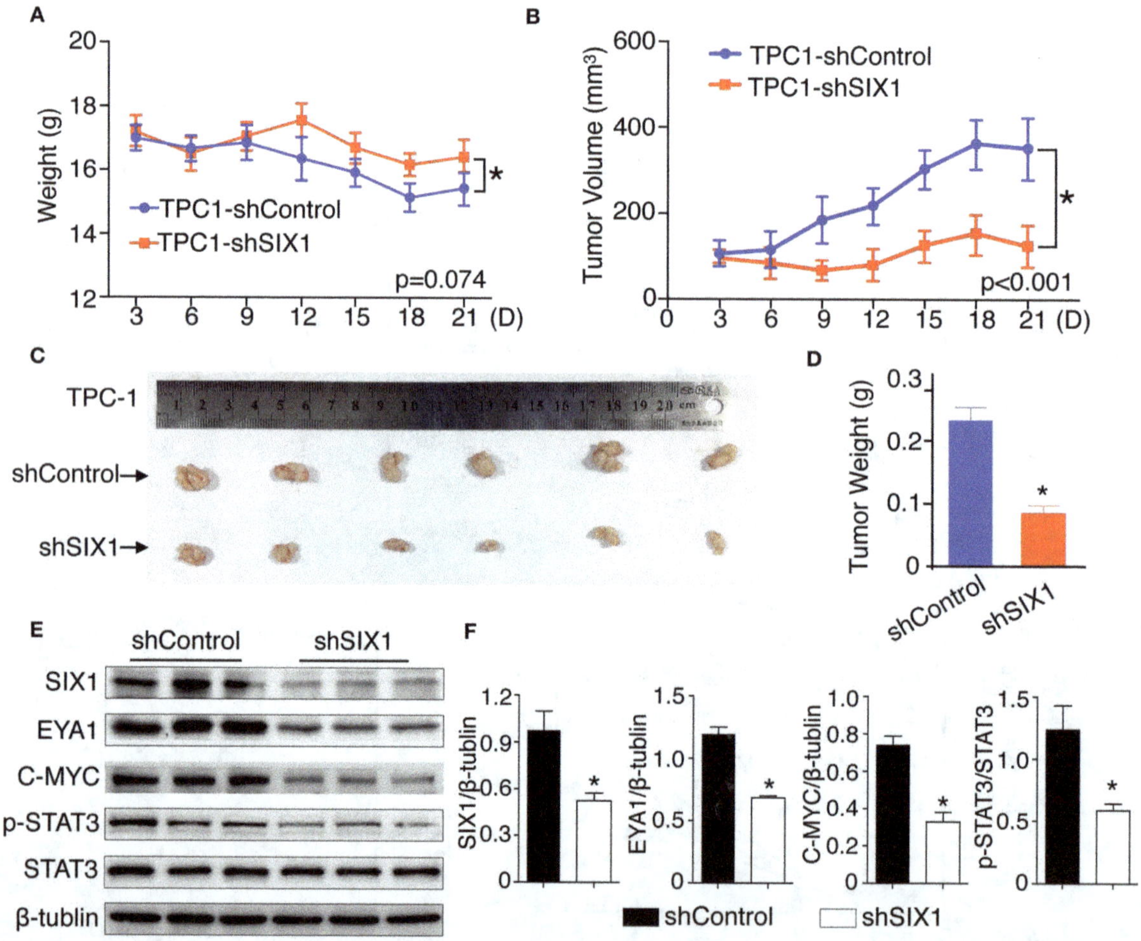

FIGURE 7 | Silencing SIX1 suppressed tumor growth as well as STAT3 signal *in vivo*. TPC-1 cells with SIX1 silencing or vector control were implanted into immunodeficiency mice, the body weight **(A)** and tumor volume **(B)** was monitored ($n = 20$). Representative tumor image **(C)** and quantitative analysis ($n = 20$) **(D)** were showed. Western blot analysis of total protein from tumor tissue **(E)** and relative quantitative analysis ($n = 3$) **(F)**. $^{*}p < 0.05$.

DISCUSSION

Exciting outcome of molecular targeting therapy is driving the need for better understanding the tumor biological features of each patient (7). Recent evidence has linked RDGN family with the progression of various cancers, indicating it might be a potential therapeutic target for precision medicine (11–18, 25). In the present study, our results first showed that SIX1 protein elevated in thyroid malignant tumor. In papillary thyroid carcinoma, high expressions of SIX1 and EYA1 were associated with advanced age, lymph node metastasis and clinical stage. Functional assays suggested SIX1 not only enhanced PTC proliferation, but also provided significant protection against apoptosis, which relied on the activation of STAT3 signaling. The analysis of patients' samples indicated EYA1 was positively correlated with SIX1. Not only the ectopic expression of SIX1 increased EYA1, but also STAT3 signaling activation induced by SIX1 depended on EYA1.

Although Six1 had intrinsic transcriptional domain, its activation required Eya family to be the co-activator (26). Co-transfection of Six/*so* and Eya/*eya* induced a huge synergistic activation of the downstream targets, whereas Six or Eya alone showed a low level of transcription. Therefore, it generally recognized that Six1-Eya function as a transcriptional complex (11). However, the coordinated mechanism between SIX1 and EYAs in human is largely elusive. Current studies are mainly focused on the functional association between SIX1 and EYAs. It has been reported SIX1 bound to EYA by a single amphipathic helical structure, an essential part for SIX1-associated metastatic phenotypes (27). One significant finding in our study was that SIX1 induced EYA1 protein expression in PTC and modulated its abundance at the post-transcriptional level. Recent evidence indicated that cyclin-dependent kinase 6 (CDK6) bound to and promoted degradation of the EYA2 protein, and SIX1 partially stabilized EYA2 against CDK6 induced degradation (28), which is in support of our finding. Our results also showed EYA1 was necessary for STAT3 signaling activation as well as the cellular proliferation induced by SIX1. Based on these data, it indicates SIX1 might stabilize the EYA1 protein rather than activate the gene transcription directly, suggesting a reciprocal regulation between SIX1 and EYA family.

Another intriguing finding is STAT3 signaling is involved in the regulation of SIX1 in PTC. This is consistent with a previous report demonstrating that SIX1 can increase the phosphorylation of STAT3 in HPV16-immortalized human keratinocytes (24). Given the role of STAT3 signaling in regulating cell proliferation, vascular formation and immune response associated with cancer progression, it is important to explore novel targets that inhibit the ectopic activation of STAT3 signaling (29). By activating pro-proliferative and pro-survival genes, including C-MYC and Cyclin D1, and anti-apoptotic BCL-2 or BCL-XL, STAT3 mediated tumorigenesis by protecting cells from apoptotic stress, and promoting cell-cycle progression and inflammation response in multiple cancers (30). STAT3 phosphorylated on Try705 in the carboxyl-terminal transactivation domain is regarded as the key to amplify STAT3 signal. In thyroid, STAT3 pathway was found to be involved in the onset and invasion of tumor (31). STAT3 interacted with the sonic hedgehog (SHH) pathway, which can predict the prognosis or guiding the personal therapy against PTC (32). Ekpe-Adewuy et al. revealed that growth factor receptor-alpha (PDGFRα) promoted EMT of PTC cells via provoking STAT3 signal pathway (33). Our study found SIX1 activated STAT3 signaling in an EYA1-dependent manner by increased the level of phospho-Try705. *In vitro* experiments indicated that SIX1 increased the phosphorylation of STAT3, leading to an increasing of C-MYC and BCL-XL to promote cell proliferation and anti-apoptosis. In addition, the activation of STAT3 signaling induced by SIX1 relied on EYA1. Silencing EYA1 expression abolished the SIX1-medicated STAT3 signaling activation in cell proliferation. Our mouse xenograft model also confirmed that decreased SIX1 abundance was associated with significantly reduced tumor volume and suppression of STAT3 signaling. These findings suggest that STAT3 signaling plays a crucial role in the functional significance of SIX1 in thyroid cancer, and it may raise a possibility that JAK/STAT3 inhibitors can be treated in those PTC patients with high expression of SIX1.

Our study indicated that SIX1 and EYA1 might be used as malignancy hallmarks in papillary thyroid cancer. Higher levels of SIX1 and EYA1 were found correlated with advanced age and lymph node metastasis, which are well-known poor prognostic factors in PTC. Although the tumor size showed no significant relationship with SIX1 or EYA1 expression, the functional assays identified that overexpression of SIX1 contribute to the proliferation of PTC cells, whereas knockdown SIX1 showed the opposite. Moreover, the success of lipid nanoparticles (LNP)-formulated siRNA targeting VEGF and kinesin spindle protein (KSP) in cancer patients with liver metastasis raised a hope that silencing SIX1 expression using shRNA or miRNA maybe a potential cancer treatment strategy (34). For example, microRNA-185 translationally represses SIX1 and thereby sensitizes SIX1-overexpressing cancer cells to TRAIL-induced apoptosis (35). It is known that EYAs mediate the transcriptional activation of SIX1 (27). Our study also showed that EYA1 is responsible for SIX1-induced STAT3 signaling activation, indicating disruption of EYA1 function may suppress the SIX1-mediate tumor growth in PTC. To date, Benzbromarone and its derivative, Benzarone were also found to be well-recognized EYA inhibitors (36). The major metabolite of Benzbromarone, 6-hydroxy Benzbromarone, is a more powerful inhibitor of EYAs, and may block tumor growth by inhibiting angiogenesis (37). Therefore, a combination treatment with either SIX1 or EYA1 inhibitors may provide benefit in a properly selected group of PTC patients.

ETHICS STATEMENT

This study was approved by the Institutional Review Board of Tongji Hospital.

AUTHOR CONTRIBUTIONS

GW and KWu developed the hypothesis and designed the experiments. DK, AL, YL, QC, KWa, DZ, JT, and YD performed the experiments. DK prepared the manuscript. ZL contributed to the pathology review and interpretation.

REFERENCES

1. Mao Y, Xing M. Recent incidences and differential trends of thyroid cancer in the USA. *Endocr Relat Cancer.* (2016) 23:313–22. doi: 10.1530/ERC-15-0445
2. Tufano RP, Noureldine SI, Angelos P. Incidental thyroid nodules and thyroid cancer: considerations before determining management. *JAMA Otolaryngol Head Neck Surg.* (2015) 141:566–72. doi: 10.1001/jamaoto.2015.0647
3. Zhang S, Wang Y, Chen M, Sun L, Han J, Elena VK, et al. CXCL12 methylation-mediated epigenetic regulation of gene expression in papillary thyroid carcinoma. *Sci Rep.* (2017) 7:44033. doi: 10.1038/srep44033
4. Haugen BR, Alexander EK, Bible KC, Doherty GM, Mandel SJ, Nikiforov YE, et al. 2015 American thyroid association management guidelines for adult patients with thyroid nodules and differentiated thyroid cancer: the american thyroid association guidelines task force on thyroid nodules and differentiated thyroid cancer. *Thyroid.* (2016) 26:1–133. doi: 10.1089/thy.2015.0020
5. Valerio L, Pieruzzi L, Giani C, Agate L, Bottici V, Lorusso L, et al. Targeted therapy in thyroid cancer: state of the art. *Clin Oncol.* (2017) 29:316–24. doi: 10.1016/j.clon.2017.02.009
6. Lan X, Xu J, Chen C, Zheng C, Wang J, Cao J, et al. The landscape of circular RNA expression profiles in papillary thyroid carcinoma based on RNA sequencing. *Cell Physiol Biochem.* (2018) 47:1122–32. doi: 10.1159/000490188
7. Biankin AV, Piantadosi S, Hollingsworth SJ. Patient-centric trials for therapeutic development in precision oncology. *Nature.* (2015) 526:361–70. doi: 10.1038/nature15819
8. Jiao X, Zhang H, Xu X, Yu Y, Zhang H, Zhang J, et al. S100A4 knockout sensitizes anaplastic thyroid carcinoma cells harboring BRAFV600E/Mt to vemurafenib. *Cell Physiol Biochem.* (2018) 49:1143–62. doi: 10.1159/000493296

9. Xing M. Molecular pathogenesis and mechanisms of thyroid cancer. *Nat Rev Cancer.* (2013) 13:184–99. doi: 10.1038/nrc3431
10. Jin Z, Cheng X, Feng H, Kuang J, Yang W, Peng C, et al. Apatinib inhibits angiogenesis via suppressing Akt/GSK3beta/ANG signaling pathway in anaplastic thyroid cancer. *Cell Physiol Biochem.* (2017) 44:1471–84. doi: 10.1159/000485583
11. Liu Y, Han N, Zhou S, Zhou R, Yuan X, Xu H, et al. The DACH/EYA/SIX gene network and its role in tumor initiation and progression. *Int J Cancer.* (2016) 138:1067–75. doi: 10.1002/ijc.29560
12. Coletta RD, Christensen KL, Micalizzi DS, Jedlicka P, Varella-Garcia M, Ford HL. Six1 overexpression in mammary cells induces genomic instability and is sufficient for malignant transformation. *Cancer Res.* (2008) 68:2204–13. doi: 10.1158/0008-5472.CAN-07-3141
13. Iwanaga R, Wang CA, Micalizzi DS, Harrell JC, Jedlicka P, Sartorius CA, et al. Expression of Six1 in luminal breast cancers predicts poor prognosis and promotes increases in tumor initiating cells by activation of extracellular signal-regulated kinase and transforming growth factor-beta signaling pathways. *Breast Cancer Res.* (2012) 14:R100. doi: 10.1186/bcr3219
14. Micalizzi DS, Christensen KL, Jedlicka P, Coletta RD, Barón AE, Harrell JC, et al. The Six1 homeoprotein induces human mammary carcinoma cells to undergo epithelial-mesenchymal transition and metastasis in mice through increasing TGF-beta signaling. *J Clin Invest.* (2009) 119:2678–90. doi: 10.1172/JCI37815
15. Micalizzi DS, Wang CA, Farabaugh SM, Schiemann WP, Ford HL. Homeoprotein Six1 increases TGF-beta type I receptor and converts TGF-beta signaling from suppressive to supportive for tumor growth. *Cancer Res.* (2010) 70:10371–80. doi: 10.1158/0008-5472.CAN-10-1354
16. Xu H, Zhang Y, Altomare D, Pena MM, Wan F, Pirisi L, et al. Six1 promotes epithelial-mesenchymal transition and malignant conversion in human papillomavirus type 16-immortalized human keratinocytes. *Carcinogenesis.* (2014) 35:1379–88. doi: 10.1093/carcin/bgu050
17. Li L, Liang Y, Kang L, Liu Y, Gao S, Chen S, et al. Transcriptional regulation of the Warburg effect in cancer by SIX1. *Cancer Cell.* (2018) 33:368–85.e367. doi: 10.1016/j.ccell.2018.01.010
18. Kong D, Liu Y, Liu Q, Han N, Zhang C, Pestell RG, et al. The retinal determination gene network: from developmental regulator to cancer therapeutic target. *Oncotarget.* (2016) 7:50755–65. doi: 10.18632/oncotarget.9394
19. Wu K, Li Z, Cai S, Tian L, Chen K, Wang J, et al. EYA1 phosphatase function is essential to drive breast cancer cell proliferation through cyclin D1. *Cancer Res.* (2013) 73:4488–99. doi: 10.1158/0008-5472.CAN-12-4078
20. Xu PX, Zheng W, Laclef C, Maire P, Maas RL, Peters H, et al. Eya1 is required for the morphogenesis of mammalian thymus, parathyroid and thyroid. *Development.* (2002) 129:3033–44.
21. Liu Q, Li A, Yu S, Qin S, Han N, Pestell RG, et al. DACH1 antagonizes CXCL8 to repress tumorigenesis of lung adenocarcinoma and improve prognosis. *J Hematol Oncol.* (2018) 11:53. doi: 10.1186/s13045-018-0597-1
22. Chu Q, Han N, Yuan X, Nie X, Wu H, Chen Y, et al. DACH1 inhibits cyclin D1 expression, cellular proliferation and tumor growth of renal cancer cells. *J Hematol Oncol.* (2014) 7:73. doi: 10.1186/s13045-014-0073-5
23. Liu Y, Zhou R, Yuan X, Han N, Zhou S, Xu H, et al. DACH1 is a novel predictive and prognostic biomarker in hepatocellular carcinoma as a negative regulator of Wnt/β-catenin signaling. *Oncotarget.* (2015) 6:8621–34. doi: 10.18632/oncotarget.3281
24. Xu HW, Pirisi L, Creek KE. Six1 overexpression at early stages of HPV16-mediated transformation of human keratinocytes promotes differentiation resistance and EMT. *Virology.* (2015) 474:144–53. doi: 10.1016/j.virol.2014.10.010
25. Towers CG, Guarnieri AL, Micalizzi DS, Harrell JC, Gillen AE, Kim J, et al. The Six1 oncoprotein downregulates p53 via concomitant regulation of RPL26 and microRNA-27a-3p. *Nat Commun.* (2015) 6:10077. doi: 10.1038/ncomms10077
26. Blevins MA, Towers CG, Patrick AN, Zhao R, Ford HL. The SIX1-EYA transcriptional complex as a therapeutic target in cancer. *Expert Opin Ther Targets.* (2015) 19:213–25. doi: 10.1517/14728222.2014.978860
27. Patrick AN, Cabrera JH, Smith AL, Chen XS, Ford HL, Zhao R. Structure-function analyses of the human SIX1-EYA2 complex reveal insights into metastasis and BOR syndrome. *Nat Struct Mol Biol.* (2013) 20:447–53. doi: 10.1038/nsmb.2505
28. Kohrt D, Crary J, Zimmer M, Patrick AN, Ford HL, Hinds PW, et al. CDK6 binds and promotes the degradation of the EYA2 protein. *Cell Cycle.* (2014) 13:62–71. doi: 10.4161/cc.26755
29. Frank DA. STAT3 as a central mediator of neoplastic cellular transformation. *Cancer Lett.* (2007) 251:199–210. doi: 10.1016/j.canlet.2006.10.017
30. Furtek SL, Backos DS, Matheson CJ, Reigan P. Strategies and approaches of targeting STAT3 for cancer treatment. *ACS Chem Biol.* (2016) 11:308–18. doi: 10.1021/acschembio.5b00945
31. Zhang J, Gill A, Atmore B, Johns A, Delbridge L, Lai R, et al. Upregulation of the signal transducers and activators of transcription 3 (STAT3) pathway in lymphatic metastases of papillary thyroid cancer. *Int J Clin Exp Pathol.* (2011) 4:356–62.
32. Dong W, Cui J, Tian X, He L, Wang Z, Zhang P, et al. Aberrant sonic hedgehog signaling pathway and STAT3 activation in papillary thyroid cancer. *Int J Clin Exp Med.* (2014) 7:1786–93.
33. Ekpe-Adewuyi E, Lopez-Campistrous A, Tang X, Brindley DN, McMullen TP. Platelet derived growth factor receptor alpha mediates nodal metastases in papillary thyroid cancer by driving the epithelial-mesenchymal transition. *Oncotarget.* (2016) 7:83684–700. doi: 10.18632/oncotarget.13299
34. Tabernero J, Shapiro GI, LoRusso PM, Cervantes A, Schwartz GK, Weiss GJ, et al. First-in-humans trial of an RNA interference therapeutic targeting VEGF and KSP in cancer patients with liver involvement. *Cancer Discov.* (2013) 3:406–17. doi: 10.1158/2159-8290.CD-12-0429
35. Imam JS, Buddavarapu K, Lee-Chang JS, Ganapathy S, Camosy C, Chen Y, et al. MicroRNA-185 suppresses tumor growth and progression by targeting the Six1 oncogene in human cancers. *Oncogene.* (2010) 29:4971–9. doi: 10.1038/onc.2010.233
36. Tadjuidje E, Wang TS, Pandey RN, Sumanas S, Lang RA, Hegde RS. The EYA tyrosine phosphatase activity is pro-angiogenic and is inhibited by benzbromarone. *PLoS ONE.* (2012) 7:e34806. doi: 10.1371/journal.pone.0034806
37. Pandey RN, Wang TS, Tadjuidje E, McDonald MG, Rettie AE, Hegde RS. Structure-activity relationships of benzbromarone metabolites and derivatives as EYA inhibitory anti-angiogenic agents. *PLoS ONE.* (2013) 8:e84582. doi: 10.1371/journal.pone.0084582

5

Apatinib Inhibits Cell Proliferation and Induces Autophagy in Human Papillary Thyroid Carcinoma via the PI3K/Akt/mTOR Signaling Pathway

Xiangrui Meng [1†], Huijuan Wang [2†], Jingzhu Zhao [2], Linfei Hu [2], Jingtai Zhi [2], Songfeng Wei [2], Xianhui Ruan [2], Xiukun Hou [2], Dapeng Li [2], Jun Zhang [2], Weiwei Yang [3], Biyun Qian [4], Yu Wu [2,5], Yuan Zhang [6], Zhaowei Meng [7], Lizhao Guan [8], Huilai Zhang [1], Xiangqian Zheng [2*] and Ming Gao [2*]*

[1] Key Laboratory of Cancer Prevention and Therapy, Department of Lymphoma, National Clinical Research Center for Cancer, Tianjin's Clinical Research Center for Cancer, Tianjin Medical University Cancer Institute and Hospital, Tianjin, China, [2] Key Laboratory of Cancer Prevention and Therapy, Department of Thyroid and Neck Tumor, National Clinical Research Center for Cancer, Tianjin's Clinical Research Center for Cancer, Tianjin Medical University Cancer Institute and Hospital, Tianjin, China, [3] Department of Otolaryngology-Head and Neck Surgery, Tianjin First Center Hospital, Tianjin, China, [4] Department of Epidemiology, School of Public Health, Shanghai Jiao Tong University, Shanghai, China, [5] Department of Head and Neck Surgery, Fujian Cancer Hospital, Fujian Medical University Cancer Hospital, Fujian, China, [6] Department of Head and Neck Surgery, Jiangsu Cancer Hospital, Jiangsu Institute of Cancer Research, Nanjing Medical University Affiliated Cancer Hospital, Nanjing, China, [7] Department of Nuclear Medicine, Tianjin Medical University General Hospital, Tianjin, China, [8] Department of Biochemistry and Molecular Biology, School of Basic Medical Sciences, Tianjin Medical University, Tianjin, China

Correspondence:
Huilai Zhang
zhlwgq@126.com
Xiangqian Zheng
xiangqian_zheng@163.com
Ming Gao
headandneck2008@126.com

† These authors have contributed equally to this work

Background: Patients with metastatic radioiodine-refractory papillary thyroid carcinoma (PTC) have limited treatment options and a poor prognosis. There is an urgent need to develop new drugs targeting PTC for clinical application. Apatinib, a novel small-molecule tyrosine kinase inhibitor (TKI), is highly selective for vascular endothelial growth factor receptor-2 (VEGFR2) and exhibits antitumor effects in a variety of solid tumors. Although apatinib has been shown to be safe and efficacious in radioiodine-refractory differentiated thyroid cancer, the mechanism underlying its antitumor effect is unclear. In this report, we explored the effects of apatinib on PTC *in vitro* and *in vivo*.

Methods: VEGFR2 expression levels were evaluated by immunohistochemistry (IHC), qPCR, and western blotting (WB). The effects of apatinib on cell viability, colony formation, and migration in the Transwell assay were assessed *in vitro*, and its effect on tumor growth rate was assessed *in vivo*. In addition, the levels of proteins in signaling pathways were determined by WB. Finally, the autophagy level was assessed by WB, immunofluorescence (IF), and transmission electron microscopy.

Results: We found that high VEGFR2 expression is associated with tumor size, T stage, and lymph node metastasis in patients with PTC and that apatinib inhibits PTC cell growth, promotes apoptosis, and induces cell cycle arrest through the PI3K/Akt/mTOR signaling pathway. Moreover, apatinib induces autophagy, and pharmacological inhibition of autophagy or small interfering RNA (siRNA)-mediated targeting of autophagy-associated gene 5 (ATG5) can further increase PTC cell apoptosis.

Conclusion: Our data suggest that apatinib can induce apoptosis and autophagy via the PI3K/Akt/mTOR signaling pathway for the treatment of PTC and that autophagy is a potential novel target for future therapy in resistant PTC.

Keywords: apatinib, papillary thyroid carcinoma, PI3K, apoptosis, autophagy

INTRODUCTION

Thyroid cancer is the most common endocrine system tumor, and 53,990 new cases were predicted in 2018 (1). Standard treatments for papillary thyroid carcinoma (PTC), the most common type of thyroid cancer, include surgery, thyroid-stimulating hormone suppression, and radioiodine treatment. With these standard treatments, most patients have a good prognosis; however, 5% of patients present with radioiodine-refractory thyroid cancer and distant metastasis (2, 3). Currently, few treatment options are available for these patients. Therefore, new therapeutic strategies are urgently needed for PTC patients with advanced disease.

With an improved understanding of the molecular mechanisms of thyroid cancer, several important tumorigenic factors have been identified as new targets for antitumor therapy (4–6). A series of antitumor drugs, especially multiple targeted tyrosine kinase inhibitors (TKIs), have been developed for clinical treatment. Among them, sorafenib and vandetanib have been approved as standard therapies for advanced PTC (7, 8). In addition, an increasing number of TKIs are undergoing clinical trials. Apatinib is a new oral TKI that inhibits vascular endothelial growth factor receptor-2 (VEGFR2) with high selectivity. Apatinib has been approved as a safe and effective drug for patients with advanced gastric cancer for whom standard chemotherapy has failed (9, 10). In addition, apatinib has shown antitumor effects in various types of solid tumors in a number of ongoing phase II and III clinical trials (11, 12). Lin et al. (13) reported that apatinib showed promising efficacy in a small number of patients with radioiodine-refractory differentiated thyroid cancer. However, the antitumor mechanism of apatinib in PTC is unclear.

Drug resistance, a perpetual theme in the field of cancer treatment, is associated with multiple mechanisms. A series of studies have shown that autophagy activity plays an important role in TKI resistance. Autophagy is a catabolic process that is prevalent in eukaryotic cells that provides energy to support metabolism and survival by degrading proteins and organelles and maintains cell homeostasis (14). Accumulating evidence associates autophagy with adaptive drug resistance in multiple tumors. Patients with chronic lymphocytic leukemia who presented a higher level of autophagy were reported to exhibit a shorter survival time after treatment with imatinib than those who presented a lower level of autophagy, and imatinib treatment was more efficacious in patients with a higher level of autophagy. The same phenomenon was observed in the treatment of differentiated thyroid cancer with vemurafenib (15). Vemurafenib, a selective RAF inhibitor, did not achieve good results in the treatment of B-Raf mutant thyroid cancer, and the mechanism of drug resistance was shown to be related to autophagy induced by vemurafenib. Therefore, autophagy inhibition has become a potential target for TKI-resistant cancers.

In this study, we found that apatinib had an antitumor effect on PTC *in vitro* and *in vivo*. We also discovered that apatinib could induce protective autophagy. Notably, we investigated the relationship between apoptosis and autophagy induced by apatinib and inferred that targeting apatinib-induced autophagy has potential therapeutic benefit in the treatment of PTC.

Abbreviations: PTC, papillary thyroid carcinoma; VEGFR2, vascular endothelial growth factor receptor-2; ATG5, autophagy-associated gene 5; TKIs, tyrosine kinase inhibitors.

MATERIALS AND METHODS

Reagents

Apatinib was kindly provided by Jiangsu Hengrui Medicine Company (Jiangsu, China). The following primary antibodies were used: anti-VEGFR2, anti-Akt, anti-phospho-Akt (anti-p-Akt), anti-mTOR, anti-phospho-mTOR (anti-p-mTOR), anti-P70S6K, anti-phospho-P70S6K (anti-p-P70S6K), anti-ULK1, anti-phospho-ULK1 [anti-p-ULK1 (Ser 757)], anti-cyclin D1, anti-Bcl-2, anti-cleaved caspase3, anti-P21, anti-Bax, anti-ATG5, anti-P62/SQSTM1, anti-LC3B, and anti-Ki-67 antibodies (Cell Signaling Technology, Danvers, MA, USA), and anti-GAPDH and anti-cleaved PARP antibodies (GeneTex, Irvine, CA, USA). Hydroxychloroquine (HCQ) and SC79 were purchased from Selleck Chemicals (Houston, TX, USA).

Cell Lines and Cell Culture

Four PTC cell lines (BCPAP, K1, KTC-1, and TPC-1 cells), two ATC cell lines (CAL-62 and 8505C cells), and one normal follicular epithelial cell line (Nthy-oris-3 cells; N9) were used in this study. K-1, TPC-1, and N9 cells were purchased from American Type Culture Collection (ATCC, USA), and the other cell lines were purchased from the Type Culture Collection of the Chinese Academy of Sciences (Shanghai, China). All the cell lines used in our experiments were routinely authenticated with short tandem repeat DNA profiling analysis by us or the investigator from which we received the cells, and the passage number of the cells used for experiments was ~20–30 in our laboratory. The cells were cultured in RPMI-1640 or DMEM supplemented with 10% FBS and 1% antibiotics (penicillin and streptomycin). All the cells were maintained in a humidified incubator at 37°C with 5% CO_2. All culture reagents were purchased from Gibco (Grand Island, NY, USA).

Clinical Data and Tissue Samples

A total of 187 patients diagnosed with PTC between January 2013 and June 2013 at Tianjin Medical University Cancer were enrolled in the study. Paraffinized blocks of cancer tissue were used to generate tissue microarrays (TMAs), with a random selection of 43 adjacent normal thyroid follicular tissues used as a control. Fresh cancer and adjacent normal thyroid follicular tissue specimens were collected from 22 PTC patients. All patients provided informed consent. This study was performed with the approval of the Tianjin Medical University Institutional Review Board.

Animals

Twenty 4-week-old female NSG mice weighing 20 to 22 g purchased from SPF Biotechnology (Beijing, China) were used for the K-1 cell xenografts. All mice were housed under pathogen-free conditions. All animal experiments were carried out with the approval of the Ethics Committee of the Tianjin Medical University Cancer Institute and Hospital.

Immunohistochemistry

The 3 μm sections on the TMA and from the paraffin block were subjected to immunohistochemical staining for

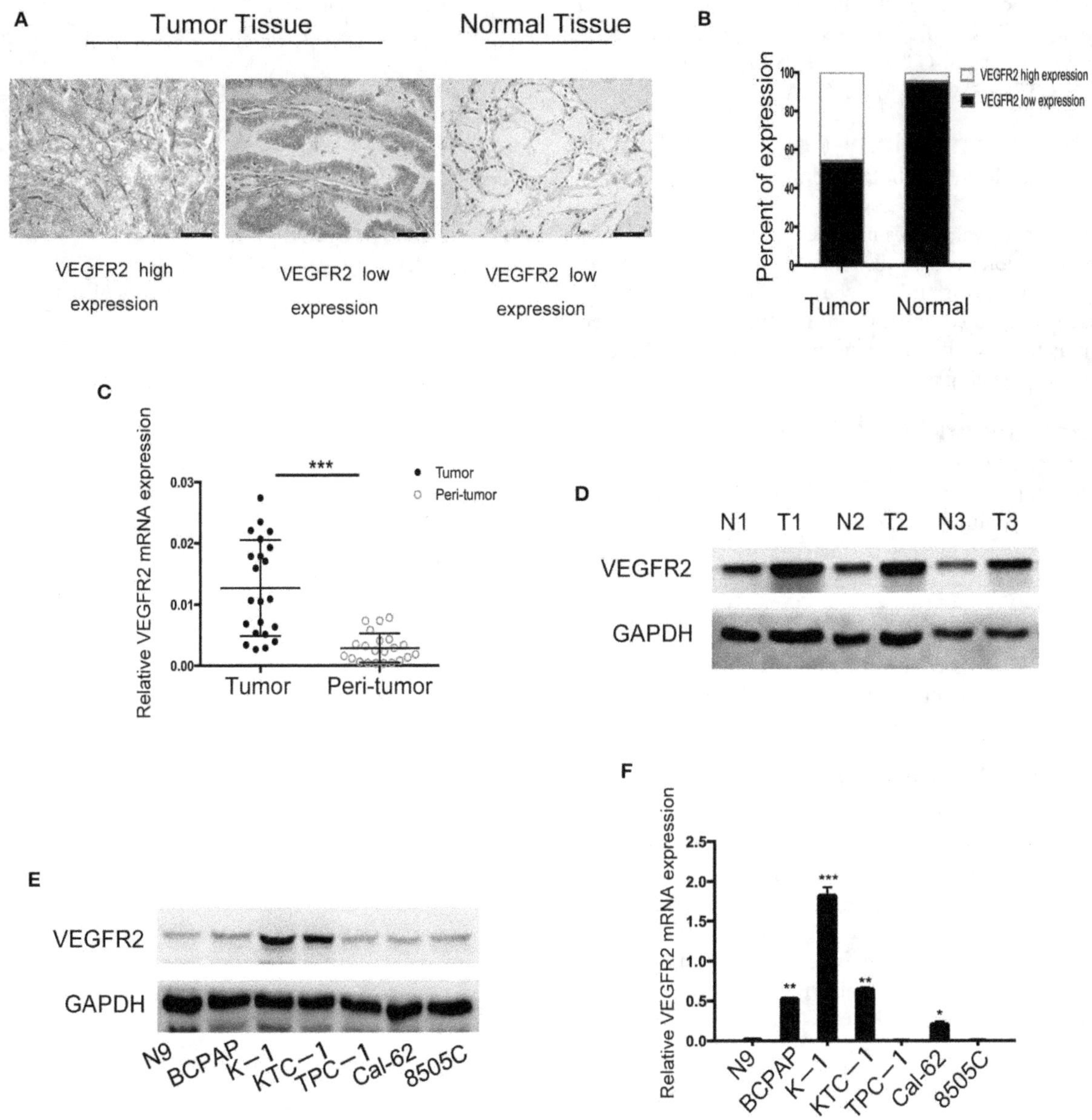

FIGURE 1 | VEGFR2 expression is elevated in PTC. **(A)** Immunohistochemical staining of a TMA containing PTC and normal thyroid follicular tissue specimens for VEGFR2. **(B)** VEGFR2 expression in PTC and normal thyroid follicular tissue. **(C)** VEGFR2 mRNA levels in PTC and normal thyroid follicular tissue. **(D)** Western blot assay showing increased VEGFR2 expression in PTC tissue compared to normal thyroid tissue. **(E)** Western blot assay of VEGFR2 expression in thyroid cell lines. **(F)** VEGFR2 mRNA levels in thyroid cell lines. Data are expressed as the mean ± SD (*$P < 0.05$, **$P < 0.01$, ***$P < 0.001$ vs. N9 cells).

VEGFR2, cleaved caspase3, and Ki-67 according to standard immunohistochemistry (IHC) protocol. Signals were amplified using a DAB substrate kit. Images were taken with an Olympus BX51 microscope. The results were evaluated independently by two experienced pathologists and scored with the H-score method.

RNA Extraction and Quantitative RT-PCR

Total RNA was extracted from tissues and cells by using a TRIzol reagent (Invitrogen, Carlsbad, CA, USA), and total RNA was reverse-transcribed to cDNA using PrimeScript RT Master Mix (TaKaRa, Tokyo, Japan). To quantify VEGFR2 and actin mRNA levels, quantitative RT-PCR was performed on the reverse-transcribed products with SYBR Premix Ex Taq II (TakaRa, Tokyo, Japan) and specific primers. The sequences of the primers were as follows: 5′-GTGATCGGAAATGACACTGGAG-3′ and 5′-CATGTTGGTCACTAACAGAAGCA-3′.

Cell-Viability and Colony-Formation Assays

The cell counting kit-8 (CCK8, Dojindo, Japan) assay was used as previously described to assess cell viability. The IC50 was calculated from survival curves using GraphPad Prism 7.0. For the colony-formation assay, cells were seeded at 500 cells per well in 6-well plates on the day before the experiment and then cultured in a medium containing apatinib at different concentrations for 2 weeks. Cell colonies were stained with 0.1% crystal violet before being photographed.

Cell Apoptosis and Cell Cycle Analyses

Cells were treated with apatinib at different concentrations for 24 h, collected by trypsinization, washed twice with PBS, and stained with staining solution from an Annexin V/FITC detection kit. The samples were analyzed by flow cytometry according to the kit's instructions.

Cells were treated with apatinib at different concentrations for 24 h, collected by trypsinization, and washed twice with PBS. The harvested cells were fixed with 70% cold ethanol at −20°C overnight and stained with a propidium iodide (PI) solution containing RNase. Samples were analyzed by flow cytometry.

Protein Extraction and Western Blotting (WB)

Proteins were extracted from different cells by using protease and phosphatase inhibitors according to the manufacturer's instructions, and the protein concentration was quantified using the BCA method. Equal amounts of protein were resolved by 8%–12% SDS-PAGE and transferred to PVDF membranes. Primary antibodies against the following proteins were used: VEGFR2, Akt, p-Akt, mTOR, p-mTOR, P70S6K, p-P70S6K, ULK1, p-ULK1 (Ser 757), cleaved PARP, Bcl-2, Bax, cleaved caspase3, cyclin D1, P21, P62, ATG5, and LC3B.

Immunofluorescence (IF) Staining

Cells were cultivated on coverslips, incubated with 5 μM apatinib for 24 h, fixed in 4% paraformaldehyde for 20 min, and then permeabilized with 0.2% Triton X-100 for 5 min. After being blocked with 5% BSA for 1 h, the cells were incubated with anti-LC3B primary antibody overnight at 4°C. Then, the cells were washed, incubated with secondary antibody, and stained with 4',6-diamidino-2-phenylindole (DAPI) (Solarbio, Beijing, China). Cells mounted on coverslips were observed by confocal microscopy.

Cells were incubated with apatinib with or without HCQ in the above steps.

Transmission Electron Microscopy

The ultrastructure of autophagosomes in the treated cells was identified by transmission electron microscopy as described previously (16).

RNA Interference

Small interfering RNA (siRNA) targeting ATG5 was designed and synthesized by GenePharma (Shanghai, China). K-1 cells were transfected with ATG5 siRNA with Lipofectamine 2000 according to the manufacturer's instructions. The total protein was extracted 48 h after transfection as described previously (17).

TABLE 1 | VEGFR2 expression in thyroid cancer and normal thyroid follicular tissue.

VEGFR2 expression	Tumor tissue	Normal tissue	χ^2	*p*-value
Low	101 (54%)	41 (95.4%)		
High	86 (46%)	2 (4.6%)	23.571	0.000

TABLE 2 | Relationship between clinicopathological features and VEGFR2 expression in PTC ($n = 187$).

Clinicopathological feature	VEGFR2 expression		χ^2	*p*-value
	Low	High		
Age				
<55	81 (52.6%)	73 (47.4%)	0.702	0.402
≥55	20 (60.6%)	13 (39.4%)		
Gender				
Male	22 (41.5%)	31 (58.5%)	4.654	0.031
Female	79 (59.0%)	55 (41.0%)		
Tumor size				
>1	47 (40.2%)	70 (59.8%)	24.102	0.000
≤1	54 (77.1%)	16 (22.9%)		
Multifocality				
Absent	65 (50.8%)	63 (49.2%)	1.703	0.192
Present	36 (61.0%)	23 (39.0%)		
T stage				
I–II	98 (58.0%)	71 (42.0%)	11.182	0.001
III–IV	3 (16.7%)	15 (83.3%)		
Lymph node metastasis				
Absent	70 (76.9%)	21 (23.1%)	37.464	0.000
Present	31 (32.3%)	65 (67.7%)		
TNM stage				
I–II	98 (56.3%)	76 (43.6%)	5.382	0.02
III–IV	3 (23.1%)	10 (76.9%)		

Xenograft Model

All mice were housed under pathogen-free conditions. All animal experiments were carried out with the approval of the Ethics Committee of the Tianjin Medical University Cancer Institute and Hospital. K1 cells (5×10^6 in 0.1 ml of serum-free medium/mouse) were injected subcutaneously into the right buttock of each mouse. When the tumor grew to $3 \times 3\,mm^2$, the mice were randomly assigned to four groups, and the five mice in each group were administered dimethyl sulfoxide (DMSO), apatinib (100 mg/kg/day orally), HCQ (60 mg/kg/day interperitoneally), or a combination of apatinib and HCQ for 28 days. The mice were then monitored for an additional 14 days. The tumors were measured every 4 days with digital calipers.

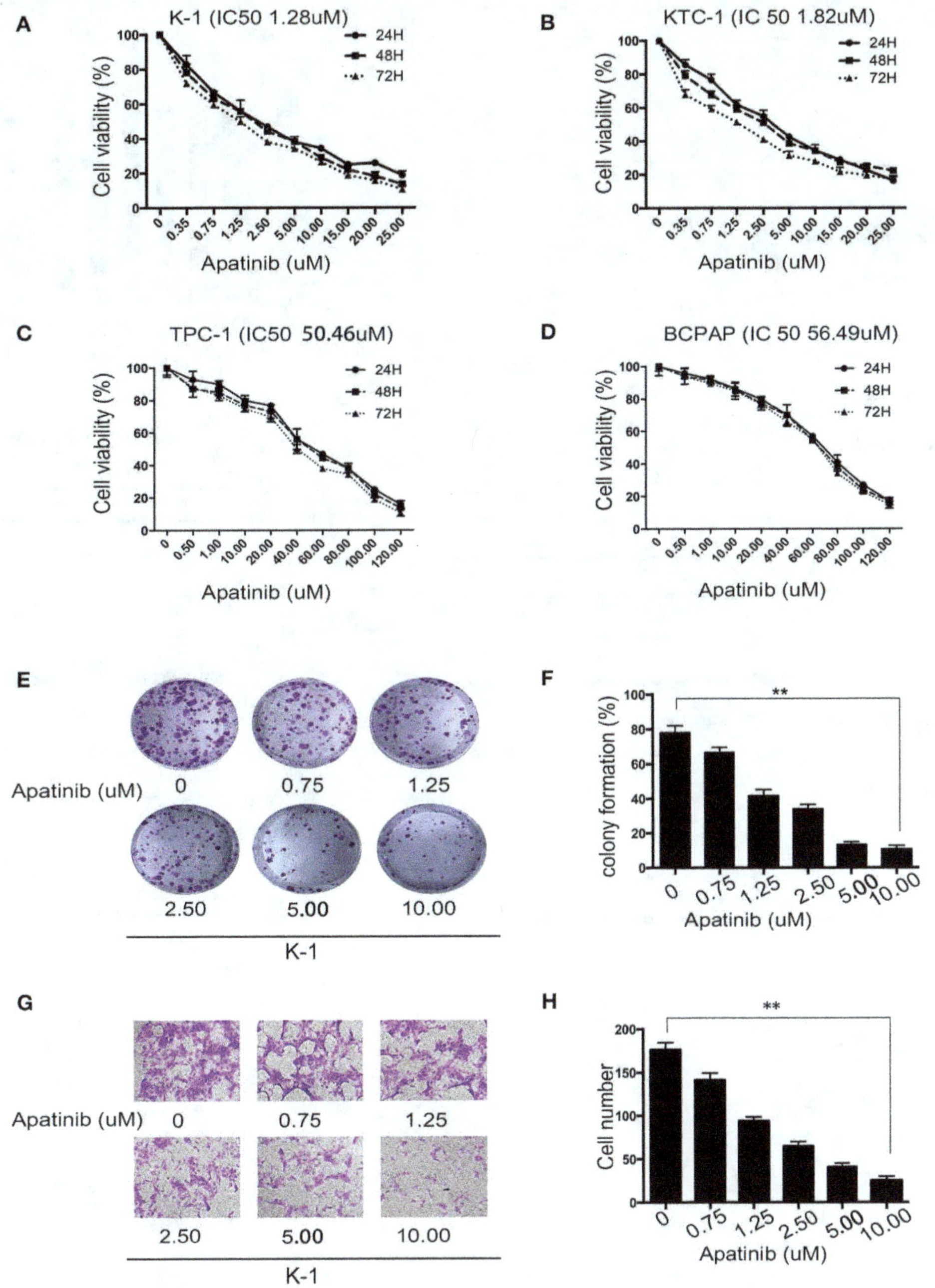

FIGURE 2 | Apatinib inhibits the proliferation and migration of PTC cell lines. **(A–D)** K-1, KTC-1, TPC-1, and BCPAP cells were incubated with apatinib at various concentrations for 24, 48, and 72 h. Then, cell viability was detected by CCK8 assay, and the IC50 values of apatinib at 24 h are shown in brackets behind the name of the cell line. **(E,F)** Apatinib inhibited the long-term proliferation of K-1 cells, as measured by colony-formation assay. **(G,H)** Apatinib suppressed the migration of K-1 cells, and the migration index was measured by Transwell assay. Each experiment was performed three times. Data are expressed as the mean ± SD (*P < 0.05, **P < 0.01, ***P < 0.001).

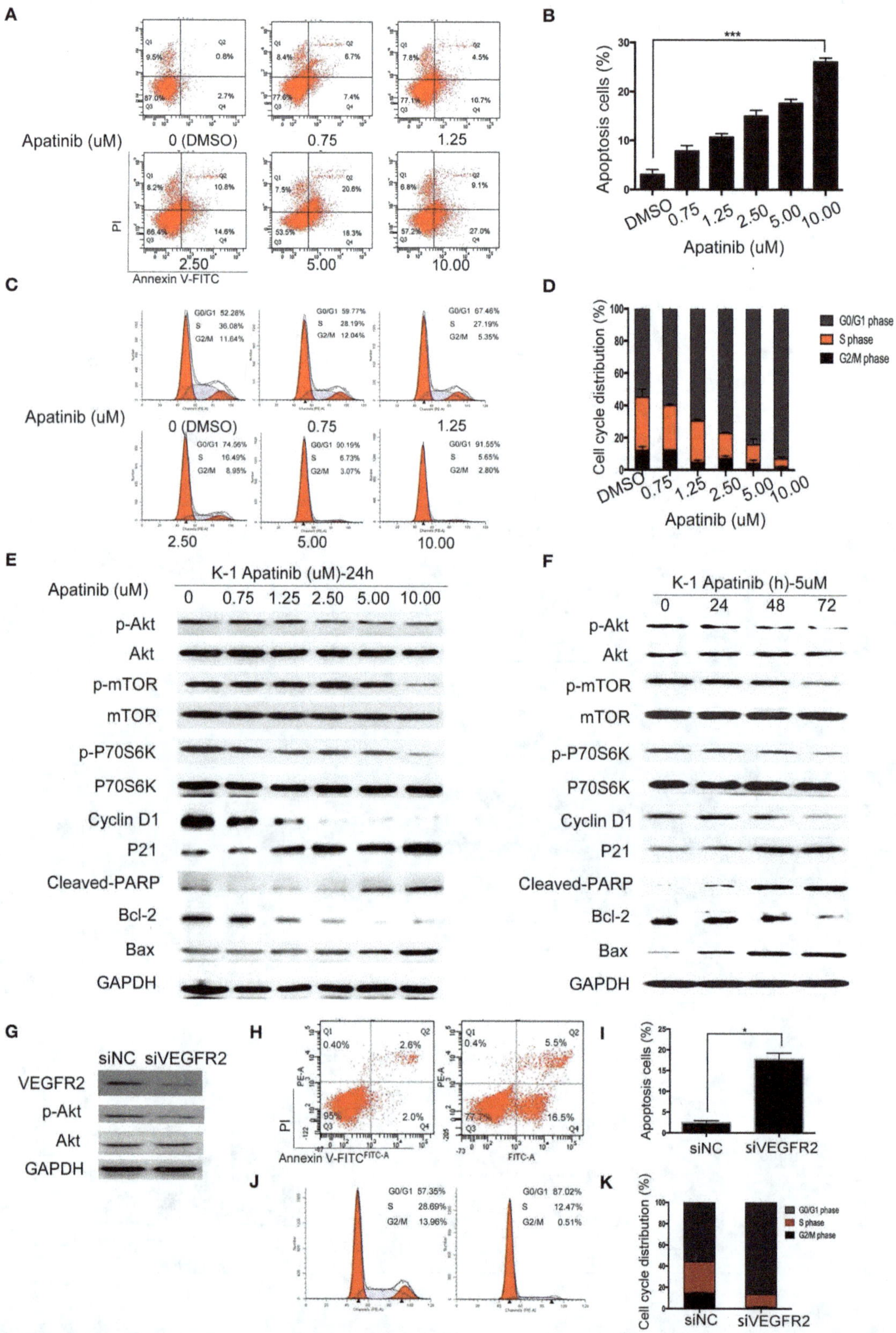

FIGURE 3 | Apatinib induces apoptosis and cell cycle arrest *in vitro*. **(A,B)** Annexin V-FITC/PI staining to detect apoptosis in PTC cells induced by apatinib at various concentrations. Apoptotic cells were analyzed by flow cytometry; (AnV+) (PI−) cells were considered early apoptotic, while (AnV+) (PI+) cells were considered late

(Continued)

FIGURE 3 | apoptotic. **(C,D)** Apatinib at various concentrations caused G0/G1 arrest in PTC cells. After PI staining, the cell cycle distribution was assessed by flow cytometry. **(E,F)** The expression of proteins related to apoptosis, the cell cycle, and cell signaling pathways was determined by western blotting. **(G)** K-1 cells were transfected with VEGFR2 siRNA, the protein expression level of VEGFR2; p-Akt and Akt were detected by western blot. **(H,I)** After VEGFR2 was downregulated, the percentage of apoptotic cells were analyzed by flow cytometry; (AnV+) (PI–) cells were considered early apoptotic, while (AnV+) (PI+) cells were considered late apoptotic. **(J,K)** After VEGFR2 was downregulated, the cell cycle distribution was assessed by flow cytometry. Data are expressed as the mean ± SD ($^{*}P < 0.05$, $^{**}P < 0.01$, $^{***}P < 0.001$).

Statistical Analysis

GraphPad Prism version 7.0 (La Jolla, CA, USA) was used for statistical analyses. Differences among variants were assessed by the chi-square test, and comparisons between groups were analyzed by one-way ANOVA. *P*-values indicating significant differences are shown in the figures as follows: $^{***}p < 0.001$, $^{**}p < 0.01$, $^{*}p < 0.05$.

RESULTS

VEGFR2 Expression Was Elevated in PTC

VEGFR2 expression was evaluated in 187 cases of PTC and 43 adjacent normal thyroid follicular epithelial tissues through IHC. The expression of VEGFR2 at the plasma membrane and in the cytoplasm was detected. We observed that most signals were detected from cancer cells (numerous true papillae and ground glass nuclei compared with follicular epithelial cells), as shown in **Figure 1A**. VEGFR2 expression was higher in thyroid cancer tissue than in normal thyroid follicular tissue (**Figure 1B** and **Table 1**). Meanwhile, a high level of VEGFR2 expression was associated with tumor size, T stage, lymph node metastasis, and tumor node metastasis (TNM) stage (**Table 2**). To further explore VEGFR2 expression in PTC, RT-PCR was used to detect VEGFR2 mRNA levels in fresh specimens from 22 PTC patients; these mRNA levels were obviously higher in PTC tissues than in normal thyroid follicular tissues (**Figure 1C**). Three of the 22 patients were randomly selected for an analysis of VEGFR2 protein expression in tissue by WB, the results of which showed that VEGFR2 expression was higher in cancer tissue than in normal tissue (**Figure 1D**). Next, we examined VEGFR2 protein and mRNA levels in seven thyroid cell lines, including normal thyroid follicular epithelial cells, PTC cell lines, and anaplastic thyroid cancer cell lines. VEGFR2 expression in the K-1 and KTC-1 PTC cell lines was higher than that in the other cell lines (**Figures 1E,F**). These data suggest that VEGFR2 expression is elevated in PTC.

Apatinib Inhibited the Proliferation and Migration of PTC Cell Lines

To assess the effects of apatinib on the growth of PTC cells, we used the K-1, KTC-1, TPC-1, and BCPAP cell lines. We treated the cell lines with apatinib at increasing concentrations for 24, 48, and 72 h and used the CCK8 assay to determine cell viability. Apatinib effectively inhibited the growth of PTC cells in a dose-dependent manner (**Figures 2A–D**). The IC50 values for apatinib in K-1 and KTC-1 cells, which highly expressed VEGFR2, were 1.28 and 1.82 μM, respectively, at 24 h. The IC50 value for apatinib in TPC-1 and BCPAP cells, which exhibited low VEGFR2 expression, were 50.46 and 56.49 μM at 24 h, respectively. Based on these results, we used the K-1 and KTC-1 cell lines for further investigation. To further examine the effects of apatinib on PTC cell proliferation, a colony-formation assay was performed with K-1 and KTC-1 cells. Apatinib reduced the colony-formation ability of K-1 (**Figures 2E,F**) and KTC-1 cells (**Figures S1A,B**) in a dose-dependent manner. These data confirmed that apatinib suppressed the proliferation of PTC cells *in vitro*.

To examine the effects of apatinib on the migration and invasion of PTC cells, Transwell assays were carried out with K-1 and KTC-1 cells. We found that apatinib inhibited the migration and invasion of K-1 (migration assay shown in **Figures 2G,H**; invasion assay shown in **Figures S1E,F**) and KTC-1 (migration assay shown in **Figures S1C,D**; invasion assay shown in **Figures S1G,H**) cells in a dose-dependent manner. These data suggested that apatinib inhibits PTC cell migration and invasion.

Apatinib Induced Apoptosis and Cell Cycle Arrest in PTC Cells

To confirm the effect of apatinib on PTC cells, K-1 and KTC-1 cells were treated with apatinib at various concentrations for 24 h, stained with Annexin V/FITC and PI, and analyzed by flow cytometry. The results confirmed that apatinib induced apoptosis in both K-1 (**Figures 3A,B**) and KTC-1 (**Figures S2A,B**) cells in a concentration-dependent manner. Moreover, PTC cells treated with apatinib at various concentrations for 24 h in G0/G1 phase of the cell cycle accumulated, as shown in **Figures 3C,D** and **Figures S2C,D**. To ascertain the mechanism of this effect, we examined the expression of proteins related to cell signaling (Akt, mTOR, and P70S6K), the cell cycle (cyclin D1 and P21), and apoptosis signaling (cleaved PARP, Bax, and Bcl-2) by WB. Apatinib decreased cyclin D1 expression and increased P21 expression in a dose- and time-dependent manner. Meanwhile, apatinib upregulated cleaved PARP and Bax levels and downregulated Bcl-2 levels in a dose- and time-dependent manner. Apatinib also downregulated p-Akt, p-mTOR, and p-P70S6K levels, shown in **Figures 3E,F** and **Figures S3A–C**. To verify whether the antitumor effect of apatinib is governed by the VEGFR2-mediated pathways, we knocked down in K-1 cells using siRNA. K-1 cells were transfected with VEGFR2 siRNA for 24 h. As shown in **Figure 3G**, VEGFR2 siRNA inhibited the expression of VEGFR2 and p-Akt. Compared with the control group, VEGFR2 downregulated group-induced apoptosis and cell cycle arrest, shown in **Figures 3H–K**. Therefore, all the data confirmed that apatinib can regulate the PI3K/Akt/mTOR signaling pathway and induce apoptosis and cell cycle arrest in PTC cells.

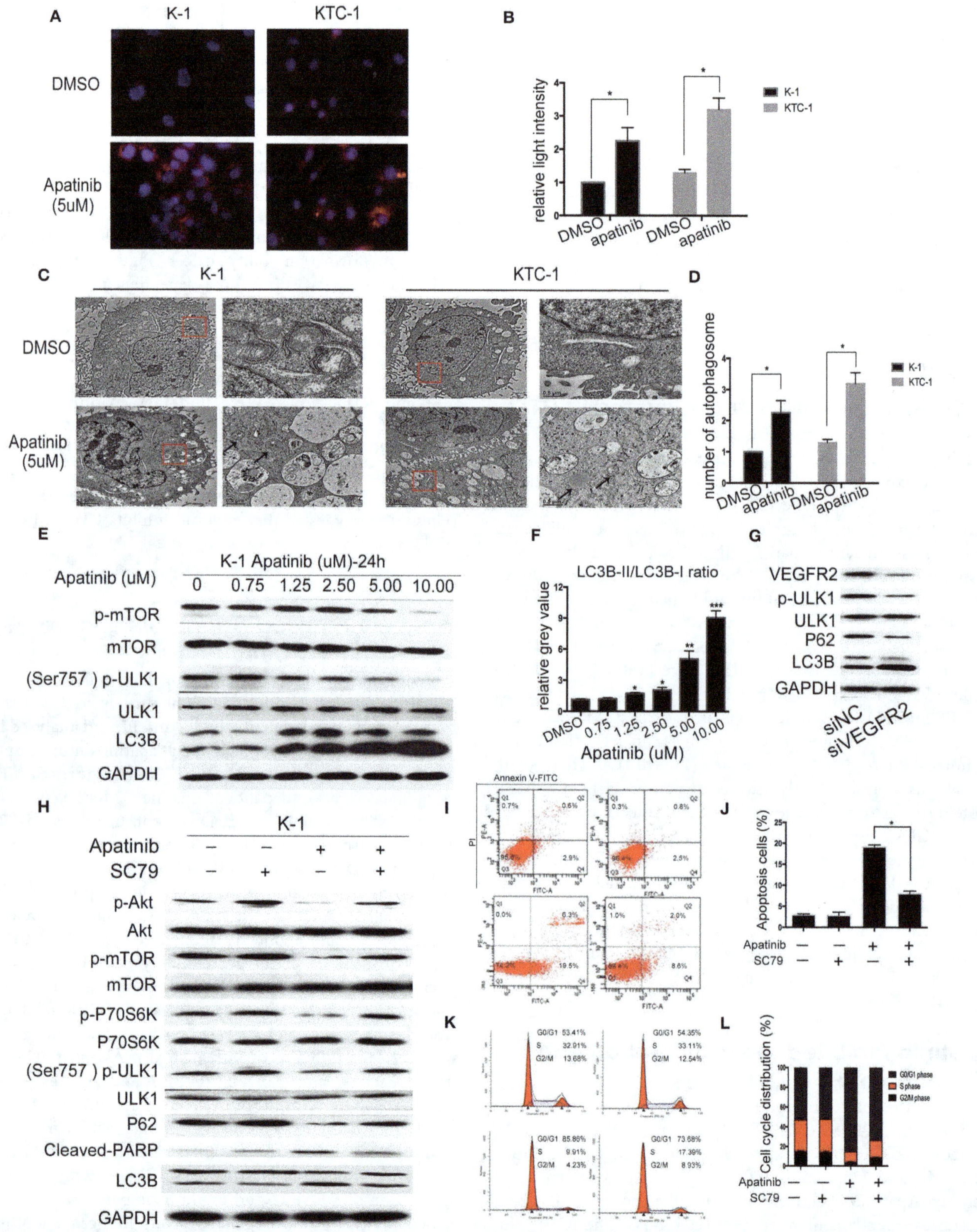

FIGURE 4 | Apatinib induces autophagy in PTC cell lines via the Akt/mTOR signaling pathway. **(A,B)** Immunofluorescence images of K-1 and KTC-1 cells treated with or without 5 μM apatinib for 24 h. Original images were taken at 400× magnification. There were more LC3B puncta in the apatinib-treated group than in the control

(Continued)

FIGURE 4 | group. **(C,D)** Transition electron microscopy images of K-1 and KTC-1 cells treated with or without apatinib for 24 h. More autophagic vacuoles (AVs) were observed in the apatinib-treated group than in the control group. Arrows: autophagosomes. **(E)** The expression of proteins related to cell signaling pathways and autophagy. **(F)** The relative gray value of LC3B-II/LC3B-I. **(G)** K-1 cells were transfected with VEGFR2 siRNA, the protein expression level of VEGFR2; p-ULK1, ULK1, P62, and LC3B were detected by western blot. **(H)** K-1 cells were treated with apatinib with or without SC79 for 24 h. The expression of proteins related to apoptosis, the cell cycle, and cell signaling pathways was determined by western blotting. **(I,J)** K-1 cells were treated as **(H)**; the percentage of apoptotic cells was analyzed by flow cytometry; (AnV+) (PI−) cells were considered early apoptotic, while (AnV+) (PI+) cells were considered late apoptotic. **(K,L)** K-1 cells were treated as **(H)**; the cell cycle distribution was assessed by flow cytometry. Data are expressed as the mean ± SD ($^{*}P < 0.05$, $^{**}P < 0.01$, $^{***}P < 0.001$).

Apatinib Induced Autophagy in PTC Cell Lines via the Akt/mTOR Signaling Pathway

Autophagy is a double-edged sword in tumors, as it can cause tumor survival or death. A number of studies have found that the mechanism of TKI resistance is closely related to autophagy. Therefore, we next examined whether apatinib causes autophagy in PTC. First, we measured the expression of LC3B, a key marker in the initial stage of autophagy, using an IF assay. As shown in **Figures 4A,B**, apatinib-treated cells showed LC3B accumulation. Furthermore, we used transmission electron microscopy to assess the formation of autophagic vacuoles (autophagosomes). As shown in **Figures 4C,D**, the formation of autophagosomes in apatinib-treated cells was dramatically increased compared with that in untreated cells. Finally, we performed WB to measure protein expression, and as shown in **Figures 4E,F**, after treatment with apatinib at various concentrations, the expression of p-mTOR and p-ULK1 decreased, while that of LC3B increased, further confirming that apatinib induces autophagy in PTC cells.

To explore whether apatinib-induced autophagy is governed by the VEGFR2-mediated pathways, we knocked down in K-1 cells using siRNA. K-1 cells were transfected with VEGFR2 siRNA for 24 h. As shown in **Figure 4G**, after VEGFR2 was downregulated, the expression of VEGFR2, p-ULK1, and P62 were decreased, and the expression of LC3B was increased. The data suggested that apatinib-induced autophagy was governed by VEGFR2-mediated pathways. Many recent reports (18, 19) have indicated that the PI3K/Akt/mTOR signaling pathway negatively regulates autophagy and apoptosis in many tumors. As shown in **Figure 3**, apatinib could regulate the Akt/mTOR signaling pathway and induce apoptosis. To further investigate whether the Akt/mTOR signaling pathway is involved in apatinib-induced autophagy in PTC cells, we treated K-1 cells with apatinib and SC79, an agonist of AKT. As shown in **Figure 4H**, the expression of p-Akt, p-mTOR, p-P70S6K, p-ULK1, and P62 was increased in cells treated with both SC79 and apatinib compared with apatinib-treated cells, and the expression of cleaved PARP and LC3B was decreased, suggesting that apoptosis and autophagy were inhibited. Meanwhile, flow cytometry data showed that cells treated with both apatinib and SC79 have a lower apoptotic rate and a lower cell cycle arrest rate than cells treated with the apatinib signal group, shown in **Figures 4I–L**. Thus, activation of the Akt pathway could rescue the apoptosis and autophagy induced by apatinib. Taken together, these results confirmed that apatinib induces apoptosis and autophagy in PTC cells via the PI3K/Akt/mTOR signaling pathway.

Inhibition of Autophagy Sensitized PTC Cells to Apatinib

To determine whether LC3B accumulation induced by apatinib is due to inhibited autophagosome degradation or enhanced autophagosome formation, we treated K-1 cells with DMSO or apatinib with/without HCQ. HCQ inhibits the final stage of autophagy, preventing the degradation of autophagosomes by increasing lysosomal pH. As shown in **Figures 5A,B**, among both K-1 and KTC-1 cells, LC3B expression was decreased in the cotreated group compared with the apatinib-treated group. Similarly, among K-1 and KTC-1 cells, compared with the apatinib-treated groups, the cotreated groups showed increased autophagic vacuole formation (**Figures 5C,D**). These data suggested that autophagy was inhibited by HCQ treatment.

To explore the role of apatinib-induced autophagy in PTC cells, we treated K-1 cells with DMSO, apatinib, HCQ, or both apatinib and HCQ and found that combination treatment was the most effective at inducing apoptosis, as evidenced by the significantly higher ratio of apoptotic cells than that in the group treated with apatinib alone (**Figures 5E,F**), and the same result was observed in the KTC-1 cell line (**Figures S4A,B**). In apatinib-treated cells, LC3B-II expression increased, and the expression of P62, a substrate of autophagosome degradation, decreased. In the cotreatment group, LC3B-II and P62 expression levels were further increased; as shown in **Figure 5G**, autophagy was inhibited in the cotreated group, which exhibited increased cleaved PARP and Bax expression levels and decreased Bcl-2 expression levels. Taken together, these results suggested that apatinib-induced autophagy was cytoprotective and that inhibiting autophagy could increase apoptosis.

To further determine whether HCQ functions by inhibiting autophagy rather than through an unknown mechanism, we inhibited autophagy using genetic tools. ATG5, a key gene in the formation of autophagic vacuoles, was knocked down in K-1 cells using siRNA. K-1 cells were transfected with ATG5 siRNA for 24 h and then treated with or without apatinib for another 24 h. As shown in **Figures 5H–J**, ATG5 siRNA inhibited the expression of ATG5 and LC3B, suggesting that autophagy had been inhibited. Compared with the group treated with negative control siRNA, the group treated with ATG5 siRNA and the apatinib combination treatment group showed significant increased cleaved PARP levels. Overall, these results demonstrated that autophagy inhibitors enhance the efficacy of apatinib in PTC cells.

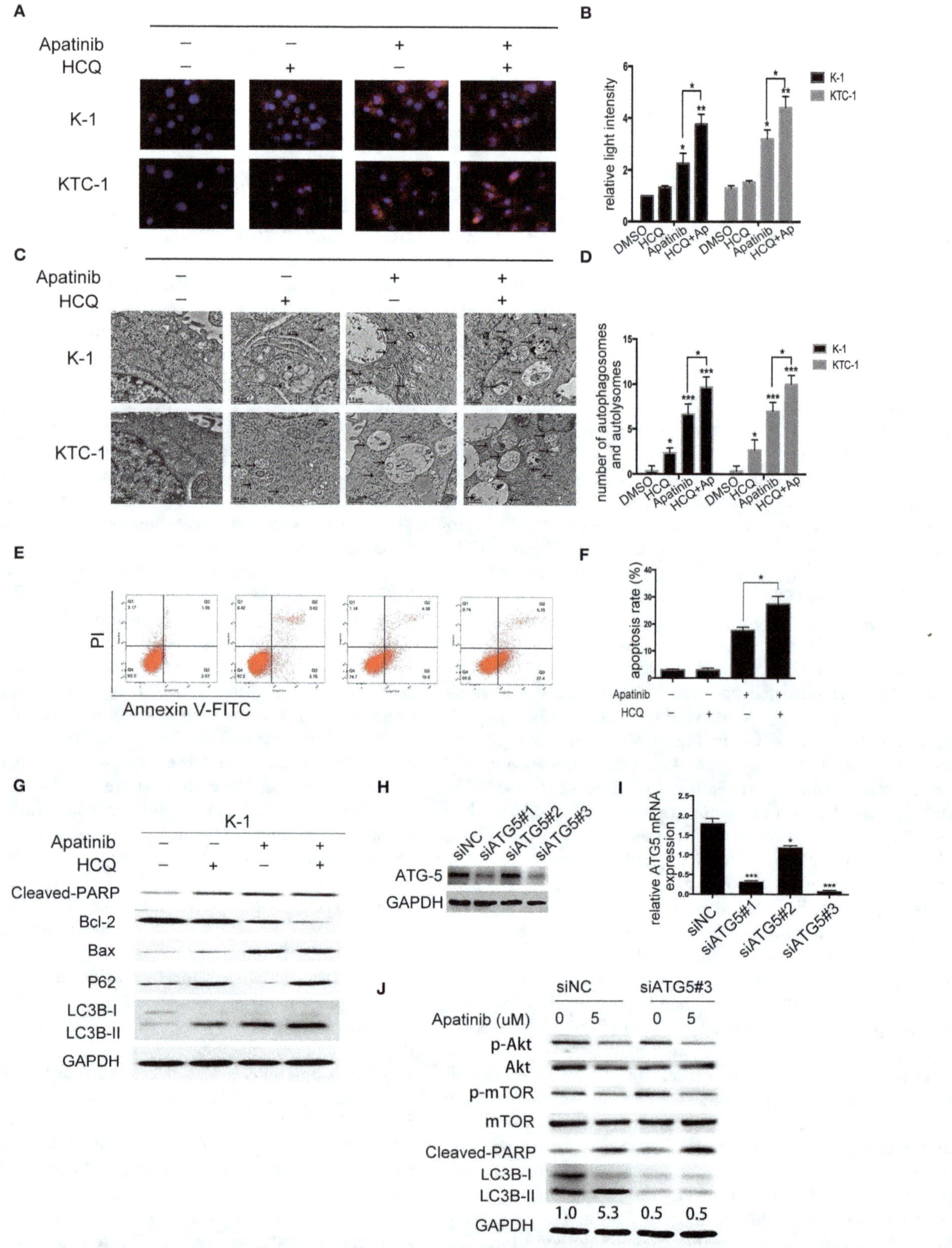

FIGURE 5 | Inhibition of autophagy enhances apatinib-induced apoptosis in PTC cells. **(A, B)** Representative immunofluorescence images of K-1 and KTC-1 cells treated with DMSO, HCQ, apatinib, or a combination of apatinib and HCQ. **(C, D)** Representative transition electron microscopy images of K-1 and KTC-1 cells

(Continued)

FIGURE 5 | treated with DMSO, HCQ, apatinib, or a combination of apatinib and HCQ. Arrows: autophagosomes and autolysosomes. **(E, F)** Inhibition of autophagy with HCQ enhanced the apoptosis of apatinib-treated PTC cells. **(G)** The expression levels of autophagy- and apoptosis-related proteins were detected by western blotting after the treatment of K-1 cells with apatinib with or without HCQ. **(H)** K-1 cells were transfected with ATG5 siRNA, the protein expression levels of ATG5. **(I)** K-1 cells were transfected with ATG5 siRNA, the mRNA expression levels of ATG5. **(J)** After ATG5 downregulation, the expression levels of p-Akt, p-mTOR, cleaved PARP, and LC3B in K-1 cells with or without apatinib treatment were determined by western blotting. Data are expressed as the mean ± SD (*$P < 0.05$, **$P < 0.01$, ***$P < 0.001$).

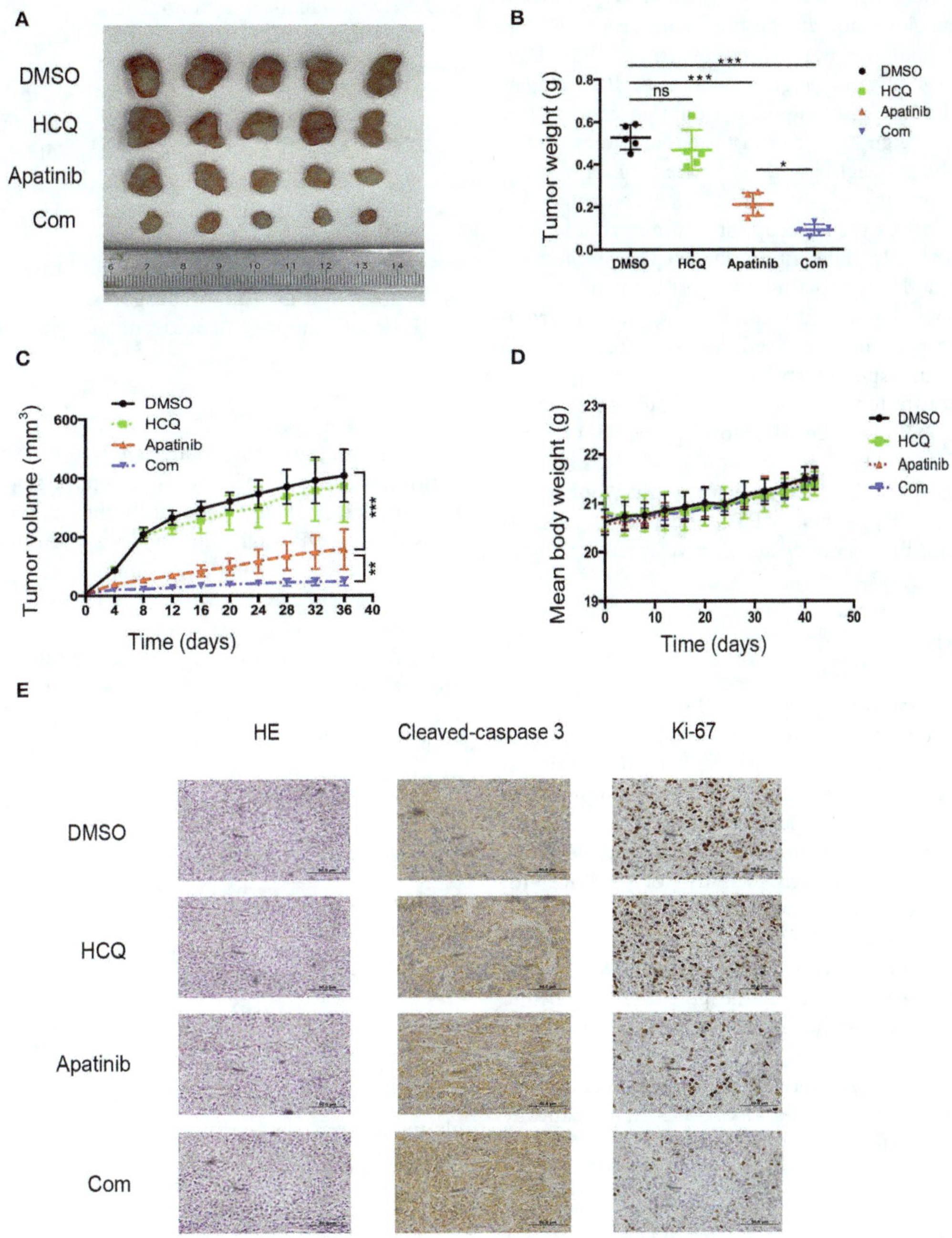

FIGURE 6 | Inhibition of autophagy enhanced the suppression of PTC growth by apatinib *in vivo.* **(A)** Images of tumors dissected from mice in the four groups (DMSO control group, HCQ single-treatment group, apatinib single-treatment group, and apatinib and HCQ combined treatment group) inoculated with K-1 cells. **(B)** Tumor weights in the four groups. **(C)** Tumor volumes in the four groups. **(D)** Mouse weights in the four groups. **(E)** HE and IHC staining to detect cleaved caspase 3 and Ki-67 in the four groups. Data are expressed as the mean ± SD (*$P < 0.05$, **$P < 0.01$, ***$P < 0.001$).

Inhibition of Autophagy Enhanced the Suppression of PTC Growth Induced by Apatinib *in vivo*

To confirm the effect of apatinib-induced apoptosis and autophagy on PTC *in vivo*, we used K-1 cells to generate an *in vivo* xenograft model. The xenograft mice were divided into the following four groups: group A (a DMSO control group), group B (a HCQ single-treatment group), group C (an apatinib single-treatment group), and group D (an apatinib and HCQ combination treatment group). Based on our results, the DMSO control group and the HCQ single-treatment group did not show significant differences in tumor volume or tumor weight. In contrast, the apatinib single-treatment group showed significantly decreased tumor volume and tumor weight compared with the DMSO control group and the HCQ single-treatment group, and tumor volume and weight were significantly different in the HCQ combination treatment group and the apatinib single-treatment group. Moreover, Ki-67 expression in the combined treatment group was significantly decreased, and cleaved caspase3 expression was increased, implying that apoptosis was enhanced in these tumors. These results demonstrated that apatinib-mediated suppression of tumor growth and blockade of autophagy could improve the antitumor effect on PTC *in vivo*, as shown in **Figure 6**. Taken together, these results suggested that autophagy inhibitors enhance the efficacy of apatinib in PTC and that given their low toxicity, these inhibitors can be an effective curative therapy in PTC.

DISCUSSION

PTC is the most common type of thyroid cancer and has a favorable prognosis. However, a small proportion of PTC patients develop metastatic disease and are resistant to conventional therapies, including thyrotropin-suppressive therapy and radioactive iodine; the outlook in these patients is therefore dim, as current treatment options for these patients are limited. Apatinib is a novel TKI highly selective for VEGFR2 with good antitumor effects in various types of solid tumors. Apatinib was shown to be safe and highly efficacious in a small number of patients with radioiodine-refractory differentiated thyroid cancer (13). In this report, we investigated the potential therapeutic effect of apatinib on PTC and the mechanism of apatinib *in vitro* and *in vivo*.

Apatinib was reported to suppress angiogenesis in anaplastic thyroid carcinoma by blocking the Akt/GSK3/ANG pathway (20–22); however, the effect of apatinib in PTC is unclear. In this report, we discovered that apatinib could inhibit PTC cell growth and migration and the induction of apoptosis. The PI3K/Akt signaling pathway plays an important role in a variety of tumors, including thyroid cancer, and is closely related to tumorigenesis, proliferation, invasion, apoptosis, and autophagy. Our data showed that p-Akt levels were decreased after apatinib treatment in a dose- and time-dependent manner.

Thus, we suggest that apatinib promotes apoptosis through the PI3K/Akt/mTOR signaling pathway. Autophagy is a ubiquitous cellular mechanism for the maintenance of homeostasis. In tumor cells, autophagy plays a dual role as it can promote death or survival. Some studies have confirmed that TKI resistance is associated with increased autophagic activity (23–25). In this report, we found that apatinib induced autophagy in PTC, as it does in other types of tumors. Moreover, we used HCQ, an autophagy inhibitor, in combination with apatinib to inhibit autophagic flux and increase apoptosis, further confirming that apatinib-induced autophagy is a protective mechanism in tumor cells. Moreover, the same results were obtained in ATG5-knockdown PTC cells, and these results were further confirmed at the genetic level. The Akt signaling pathway closely interacts with mTOR to influence autophagy, and in this study, we found that after apatinib treatment, the levels of p-mTOR, p-P70S6K, and p-ULK1 were decreased. Moreover, apatinib cotreatment with SC79, an activator of Akt, reduced apoptosis and autophagy. Thus, we demonstrated that apatinib can induce apoptosis and autophagy via the PI3K/Akt/mTOR signaling pathway and that this pathway might be a novel mechanism of drug resistance. Furthermore, the blockade of autophagy could enhance the sensitivity of PTC to apatinib.

In summary, our data show that apatinib exerted antitumor effects in PTC by suppressing tumor growth, promoting apoptosis, and inhibiting migration through the PI3K/Akt/mTOR signaling pathway. Additionally, apatinib could induce autophagy. Importantly, apatinib-induced autophagy was cytoprotective in PTC cells, and the blockade autophagy could improve apoptosis *in vitro* and *in vivo*. Thus, these findings reinforce our research findings and the clinical application of apatinib and indicate that autophagy is a new molecular therapeutic target in PTC. Combination treatment with apatinib and an autophagy inhibitor may be a useful therapeutic strategy for refractory PTC, and our data provide support for future clinical trials of autophagy inhibitors.

ETHICS STATEMENT

The studies involving human participants were reviewed and approved by Ethics Committee of Tianjin Cancer Institute and Hospital. The patients/participants provided their written informed consent to participate in this study. The animal study was reviewed and approved by Ethics Committee of Tianjin Cancer Institute and Hospital. Written informed consent was obtained from the individual(s) for the publication of any potentially identifiable images or data included in this article.

AUTHOR CONTRIBUTIONS

Conceptualization: XZ. Data curation and investigation: XM and HW. Formal analysis: JZhao and LH. Funding acquisition: XZ, JZhi, SW, XR, DL, YZ, ZM, WY, and LG. Methodology: BQ and MG. Project administration: HZ and MG. Resources: XZ and

MG. Software: XH, JZhang, YW, HZ, XZ, and MG. Writing—original draft and writing—review and editing: XM.

Tumor Hospital Foundation for Clinical Trials, China (No. C1701), and the Jiangsu Provincial Key Research Development Program (BE2016796).

REFERENCES

1. Siegel RL, Miller KD, Jemal A. Cancer statistics. *CA Cancer J Clin.* (2018) 68:7–30. doi: 10.3322/caac.21442
2. Tuttle RM, Haddad RI, Ball DW, Byrd D, Dickson P, Duh QY, et al. Thyroid carcinoma, version 2.2014. *J Natl Compr Canc Netw.* (2014) 12:1671–80. doi: 10.6004/jnccn.2014.0169
3. Antonelli A, Fallahi P, Ferrari SM, Carpi A, Berti P, Materazzi G, et al. Dedifferentiated thyroid cancer: a therapeutic challenge. *Biomed Pharmacother.* (2008) 62:559–63. doi: 10.1016/j.biopha.2008.07.056
4. Bible KC, Ryder M. Evolving molecularly targeted therapies for advanced-stage thyroid cancers. *Nat Rev Clin Oncol.* (2016) 13:403–16. doi: 10.1038/nrclinonc.2016.19
5. Spitzweg C, Bible KC, Hofbauer LC, Morris JC. Advanced radioiodine-refractory differentiated thyroid cancer: the sodium iodide symporter and other emerging therapeutic targets. *Lancet Diabetes Endocrinol.* (2014) 2:830–42. doi: 10.1016/S2213-8587(14)70051-8
6. Harris PJ, Bible KC. Emerging therapeutics for advanced thyroid malignancies: rationale and targeted approaches. *Expert Opin Investig Drugs.* (2011) 20:1357–75. doi: 10.1517/13543784.2011.614230
7. Schlumberger M, Tahara M, Wirth LJ, Robinson B, Brose MS, Elisei R, et al. Lenvatinib versus placebo in radioiodine-refractory thyroid cancer. *N Engl J Med.* (2015) 372:621–30. doi: 10.1056/NEJMoa1406470
8. Brose MS, Nutting CM, Jarzab B, Elisei R, Siena S, Bastholt L, et al. Sorafenib in radioactive iodine-refractory, locally advanced or metastatic differentiated thyroid cancer: a randomised, double-blind, phase 3 trial. *Lancet.* (2014) 384:319–28. doi: 10.1016/S0140-6736(14)60421-9
9. Li J, Qin S, Xu J, Guo W, Xiong J, Bai Y, et al. Apatinib for chemotherapy-refractory advanced metastatic gastric cancer: results from a randomized, placebo-controlled, parallel-arm, phase II trial. *J Clin Oncol.* (2013) 31:3219–25. doi: 10.1200/JCO.2013.48.8585
10. Li J, Qin S, Xu J, Xiong J, Wu C, Bai Y, et al. Randomized, double-blind, placebo-controlled phase iii trial of apatinib in patients with chemotherapy-refractory advanced or metastatic adenocarcinoma of the stomach or gastroesophageal junction. *J Clin Oncol.* (2016) 34:1448–54. doi: 10.1200/JCO.2015.63.5995
11. Hu X, Zhang J, Xu B, Jiang Z, Ragaz J, Tong Z, et al. Multicenter phase II study of apatinib, a novel VEGFR inhibitor in heavily pretreated patients with metastatic triple-negative breast cancer. *Int J Cancer.* (2014) 135:1961–9. doi: 10.1002/ijc.28829
12. Hu X, Cao J, Hu W, Wu C, Pan Y, Cai L, et al. Multicenter phase II study of apatinib in non-triple-negative metastatic breast cancer. *BMC Cancer.* (2014) 14:820. doi: 10.1186/1471-2407-14-820
13. Lin Y, Wang C, Gao W, Cui R, Liang J. Overwhelming rapid metabolic and structural response to apatinib in radioiodine refractory differentiated thyroid cancer. *Oncotarget.* (2017) 8:42252–61. doi: 10.18632/oncotarget.15036
14. Rabinowitz JD, White E. Autophagy and metabolism. *Science.* (2010) 330:1344–8. doi: 10.1126/science.1193497
15. Wang W, Kang H, Zhao Y, Min I, Wyrwas B, Moore M, et al. Targeting autophagy sensitizes BRAF-Mutant thyroid cancer to vemurafenib. *J Clin Endocrinol Metab.* (2017) 102:634–43. doi: 10.1210/jc.2016-1999
16. Shen Y, Yang J, Zhao J, Xiao C, Xu C, Xiang Y. The switch from ER stress-induced apoptosis to autophagy via ROS-mediated JNK/p62 signals: a survival mechanism in methotrexate-resistant choriocarcinoma cells. *Exp Cell Res.* (2015) 334:207–18. doi: 10.1016/j.yexcr.2015.04.010
17. Fan Q, Meng X, Liang H, Zhang H, Liu X, Li L, et al. miR-10a inhibits cell proliferation and promotes cell apoptosis by targeting BCL6 in diffuse large B-cell lymphoma. *Protein Cell.* (2016) 7:899–912. doi: 10.1007/s13238-016-0316-z
18. Viola G, Bortolozzi R, Hamel E, Moro S, Brun P, Castagliuolo I, et al. MG-2477, a new tubulin inhibitor, induces autophagy through inhibition of the Akt/mTOR pathway and delayed apoptosis in A549 cells. *Biochem Pharmacol.* (2012) 83:16–26. doi: 10.1016/j.bcp.2011.09.017
19. Harashima N, Inao T, Imamura R, Okano S, Suda T, Harada M. Roles of the PI3K/Akt pathway and autophagy in TLR3 signaling-induced apoptosis and growth arrest of human prostate cancer cells. *Cancer Immunol Immunother.* (2012) 61:667–76. doi: 10.1007/s00262-011-1132-1
20. Jin Z, Cheng X, Feng H, Kuang J, Yang W, Peng C, et al. Apatinib inhibits angiogenesis via suppressing Akt/GSK3beta/ANG signaling pathway in anaplastic thyroid cancer. *Cell Physiol Biochem.* (2017) 44:1471–84. doi: 10.1159/000485583
21. Manfredi GI, Dicitore A, Gaudenzi G, Caraglia M, Persani L, Vitale G. PI3K/Akt/mTOR signaling in medullary thyroid cancer: a promising molecular target for cancer therapy. *Endocrine.* (2015) 48:363–70. doi: 10.1007/s12020-014-0380-1
22. Motti ML, Califano D, Troncone G, De Marco C, Migliaccio I, Palmieri E, et al. Complex regulation of the cyclin-dependent kinase inhibitor p27kip1 in thyroid cancer cells by the PI3K/AKT pathway: regulation of p27kip1 expression and localization. *Am J Pathol.* (2005) 166:737–49. doi: 10.1016/S0002-9440(10)62295-X
23. Liu K, Ren T, Huang Y, Sun K, Bao X, Wang S, et al. Apatinib promotes autophagy and apoptosis through VEGFR2/STAT3/BCL-2 signaling in osteosarcoma. *Cell Death Dis.* (2017) 8:e3015. doi: 10.1038/cddis.2017.422
24. Calabretta B, Salomoni P. Inhibition of autophagy: a new strategy to enhance sensitivity of chronic myeloid leukemia stem cells to tyrosine kinase inhibitors. *Leuk Lymphoma.* (2011) 52(Suppl. 1):54–9. doi: 10.3109/10428194.2010.546913
25. Li YY, Lam SK, Mak JC, Zheng CY, Ho JC. Erlotinib-induced autophagy in epidermal growth factor receptor mutated non-small cell lung cancer. *Lung Cancer.* (2013) 81:354–61. doi: 10.1016/j.lungcan.2013.05.012

6

MRI-Based Radiomics to Differentiate Between Benign and Malignant Parotid Tumors with External Validation

Francesca Piludu [1], Simona Marzi [2], Marco Ravanelli [3], Raul Pellini [4], Renato Covello [5], Irene Terrenato [6], Davide Farina [3], Riccardo Campora [3], Valentina Ferrazzoli [7] and Antonello Vidiri [1]*

[1] Radiology and Diagnostic Imaging Department, IRCCS Regina Elena National Cancer Institute, Rome, Italy, [2] Medical Physics Laboratory, IRCCS Regina Elena National Cancer Institute, Rome, Italy, [3] Department of Radiology, University of Brescia, Brescia, Italy, [4] Department of Otolaryngology & Head and Neck Surgery, IRCCS Regina Elena National Cancer Institute, Rome, Italy, [5] Department of Pathology, IRCCS Regina Elena National Cancer Institute, Rome, Italy, [6] Biostatistics-Scientific Direction, IRCCS Regina Elena National Cancer Institute, Rome, Italy, [7] Department of Biomedicine and Prevention, University of Rome "Tor Vergata", Rome, Italy

***Correspondence:**
Simona Marzi
simona.marzi@ifo.gov.it

Background: The differentiation between benign and malignant parotid lesions is crucial to defining the treatment plan, which highly depends on the tumor histology. We aimed to evaluate the role of MRI-based radiomics using both T2-weighted (T2-w) images and Apparent Diffusion Coefficient (ADC) maps in the differentiation of parotid lesions, in order to develop predictive models with an external validation cohort.

Materials and Methods: A sample of 69 untreated parotid lesions was evaluated retrospectively, including 37 benign (of which 13 were Warthin's tumors) and 32 malignant tumors. The patient population was divided into three groups: benign lesions (24 cases), Warthin's lesions (13 cases), and malignant lesions (32 cases), which were compared in pairs. First- and second-order features were derived for each lesion. Margins and contrast enhancement patterns (CE) were qualitatively assessed. The model with the final feature set was achieved using the support vector machine binary classification algorithm.

Results: Models for discriminating between Warthin's and malignant tumors, benign and Warthin's tumors and benign and malignant tumors had an accuracy of 86.7%, 91.9% and 80.4%, respectively. After the feature selection process, four parameters for each model were used, including histogram-based features from ADC and T2-w images, shape-based features and types of margins and/or CE. Comparable accuracies were obtained after validation with the external cohort.

Conclusions: Radiomic analysis of ADC, T2-w images, and qualitative scores evaluating margins and CE allowed us to obtain good to excellent diagnostic accuracies in differentiating parotid lesions, which were confirmed with an external validation cohort.

Keywords: head and neck (H&N) cancer, salivary gland (SG) tumors, radiomics, MRI, DWI

INTRODUCTION

Salivary gland tumors represent about 3-6% of head and neck tumors, with different incidences among tumor histotypes (1). Imaging is commonly used to determine the anatomic origin of the lesions (superficial vs. deep) and the extent of the tumor, in the differentiation between benign and malignant lesions and in the evaluation of neck nodes. This information is crucial to defining the treatment plan, which highly depends on the histology of the tumor. For example, a superficial parotidectomy is performed in cases of pleomorphic adenomas when sited in the superficial portion of the gland, while a total parotidectomy is performed in cases of malignant tumors, and conservative management is the preferred choice for Warthin's tumors with low potential for malignancy (2).

Fine needle aspiration cytology with or without ultrasonography is an important technique for the pre-surgical evaluation the salivary gland masses. However, considering the rarity and variety of salivary gland neoplasms, particularly malignant lesions, this technique requires great experience and may be inconclusive due to inadequate samples (1, 2).

Ultrasonography (US) and magnetic resonance imaging (MRI) are useful in the evaluation of parotid gland tumors (3, 4). Morphologic features of the lesion can help to separate benign from malignant lesions, including the shape, margins, signal characteristics on T1-weighted and T2-weighted (T2-w) images, type of contrast enhancement (CE), and perineural spread (4, 5). The apparent diffusion coefficient (ADC) derived from diffusion-weighted imaging (DWI) and the enhancement pattern from dynamic contrast-enhanced MRI have also been demonstrated to improve the ability to discriminate benign and malignant lesions (6).

Although the use of multiparametric imaging has increased in recent years, the results are controversial in regard to the role of morphologic and functional parameters derived from multimodal MRI in the differential diagnosis of parotid gland tumors (4, 5, 7, 8). Some studies indicate that sharp margins do not indicate malignancy (7, 8), while others found that heterogeneous CE cannot be used to distinguish benign from malignant lesions (4). An overlap of the mean ADC values between low-grade malignant lesions and benign lesions has also been described (4, 9).

Radiomics is a rapidly emerging field that was proposed a few years ago to extract mineable quantitative features from medical images such as CT, MR, and PET-CT images *via* dedicated algorithms and methodologies (10). The outputs of these analysis are parametric variables that could be correlated with genomic and clinical parameters, particularly in oncologic applications, which provide a more comprehensive tumor description and improve diagnostic accuracy and clinical predictions (11).

Innumerable radiomic features can be calculated in relation to the shape, pixel intensity histogram, and distribution of pixel intensities inside or in the neighborhood of a region of interest (texture analysis), which are potentially useful in predicting the pathological characteristics, response to treatment, and overall survival (12, 13). The purpose of this study is to evaluate the role of MRI-based radiomic analysis using both T2-w images and ADC maps in the differentiation of parotid lesions, and to develop predictive models with validation using an external patient cohort.

MATERIALS AND METHODS

Patients

This study was approved by the institutional review board and was conducted in accordance with the ethical statements of the Declaration of Helsinki. The requirement for informed consent was waived by the institutional review board. This study involved a retrospective evaluation of MRI examinations of 69 patients with parotid gland lesions, consecutively identified in our Institute between 2015 and 2019.

Histopathology diagnosis was obtained in all cases on surgical specimens, by a pathologist who is dedicated to the evaluation of head and neck tumors and has more than 10 years of experience. The exclusion criteria were: recurrence, unsatisfactory image quality, lesions with diameter <5 mm to avoid bias due to partial volume effects.

All patients underwent pre-treatment MRI studies. The patient group included 41 men and 28 women with an average age of 61.1 ± 14.8 years (range 27-90 years). A total of 69 parotid lesions were evaluated, of which 37 were benign, including 13 (18.8%) Warthin's tumors and 18 (26.1%) cases of pleomorphic adenoma. The other 32 lesions were malignant. Of the 10 parotid metastases, six were from previous cutaneous squamous cell carcinoma and four from previous cutaneous melanoma. The patient and tumor characteristics are provided in more detail in **Table 1**.

TABLE 1 | Patients' characteristics of training and validation cohort.

Characteristic	Training cohort	External Validation cohort
Patient Number	69	44
Age (years)		
Mean ± standard deviation	61.1 ± 14.8	57.5 ± 15
Sex (male/female)	41/28 (59.4%/40.6%)	26/18 (59.1%/40.9%)
Tumor type, n (%)	69 (100%)	44(100%)
Benign	37 (53.6%)	24 (38.6%)
Pleomorphic adenoma	18 (26,1%)	17 (38.6%)
Basal cell adenoma	2 (2.9%)	-
Adenomyoepithelioma	1 (1.5%)	-
Myoepithelial	2 (2.9%)	-
Oncocytoma	1 (1.5%)	-
Warthin tumor	13 (18,8%)	7 (15.9%)
Malignant	32 (36.4%)	20 (45.5%)
Mucoepidermoid carcinoma	5 (7.2%)	3
Acinic cell carcinoma	2 (2.9%)	3
Ductal carcinoma	4 (5.8%)	3
Adenoidocystic carcinoma	6 (8.7%)	4
Lymphoepithelial carcinoma	3 (4.4%)	7 others (3 high grade, 1 cystadenocarcinoma, 3 myoepithelial)
Carcinoma ex pleomorphic adenoma	1 (1.5%)	
Squamous cell carcinoma	1 (1.5%)	
Metastasis	10 (14.5%)	

This population was used as a training cohort and divided into three groups: benign tumors with the exclusion of Warthin's tumors (24 cases), Warthin's tumors (13 cases), and malignant tumors (32 cases). Three predictive models were built to compare these groups in pairs. Furthermore, another 44 patients were recruited at the Department of Radiology of the University of Brescia (Italy) and used as an external validation cohort. The tumor characteristics of this cohort are reported in **Table 1**.

MRI Acquisition Protocols

In Rome, for the training cohort, MRI was performed on a 1.5-T system (Optima MR 450w, GE Health-care, Milwaukee, WI, USA) with dedicated 16-channel receive-only radiofrequency coils: a head coil, a surface neck coil, and a spine coil. The MRI examination included fast spin-eco (FSE) T2-weighted images on the coronal plane (acquisition matrix 288 × 256, field of view 27 x 27 cm, TR/TE 5901 ms/102, slice thickness 4 mm). Next, axial FSE T2-weighted images were obtained (TR/TE 6844 ms/105 ms, field of view 26 cm, in-plane spatial resolution 0.47 mm × 0.47 mm, slice thickness 3 mm, spacing between slices 3.3 mm) along with pre-contrast T1-weighted images (acquisition matrix 288 × 256, field of view 20 cm, TR/TE 617 ms/8.1, slice thickness 3 mm) on the axial plane, which were acquired from the level of the skull base to the thoracic inlet.

DWI was obtained *via* single-shot spin-echo and echo-planar imaging (field of view 26–28 cm, in-plane spatial resolution 2-2.2 mm × 2-2.2 mm TR/TE 4500 ms/77 ms, slice thickness 4 mm, spacing between slices 5 mm, bandwidth 1953 Hz/pixel). Three different b values were used (b = 0, 500, and 800 s/mm^2) with diffusion-sensitizing gradients applied in three orthogonal directions to obtain trace-weighted images. ADC maps of the training set were generated using the commercial software package Ready View (GE Advantage Workstation, READYView, Palo Alto, CA, USA). The imaging protocol also included post-contrast (Gadolinium 0.1 mmol/kg) T1-w images with liver acquisition with volume acceleration (LAVA) sequences (acquisition matrix 288 × 288, field of view 26-26 cm, TR/TE 9.8 ms/min, slice thickness 1 mm, 214 slices) in axial and coronal planes as required for the routine examination.

In Brescia, for the validation cohort, MRI was performed on a 1.5-T system (Aera, SIEMENS Healthineers Medical Solutions, Knoxville, TN, USA) with dedicated head and neck coils. The parameters of T2-w images were similar to those used for the training cohort (TR/TE 52 20 ms/105 ms, in-plane spatial resolution 0.43 mm × 0.43 mm, slice thickness 3 mm, spacing between slices 4.5 mm). DWI was obtained *via* single-shot spin-echo and echo-planar imaging (field of view, 25 cm in-plane spatial resolution 1.8 mm × 1.8 mm, TR/TE 3900 ms/60 ms, bandwidth 1455 Hz/pixel, slice thickness 3 mm, spacing between slices 4.5 mm). Two different b values were used (b = 50 and 800 s/mm^2) with diffusion-sensitizing gradients applied in three orthogonal directions to obtain trace-weighted images. ADC maps of the validation cohort were automatically generated by the software MR Syngo (SIEMENS, Healthineers Medical Solutions).

Extraction of Radiomic Features

The extraction of the radiomic features was performed using S-IBEX software (14). S-IBEX is a standardized version of IBEX (image biomarker explorer) software (15) that was recently adapted and validated according to the guidelines of the Image Biomarker Standardization Initiative (IBSI) (16). The entire tumor volume was delineated by consensus between two radiologists with more than 20 and 10 years of experience in head and neck (A.V. and F.P) using T2-w images.

First- and second-order features were derived from a volumetric analysis of T2-w images, including morphological features (29 features), intensity histogram features (23 features), intensity-volume histogram features (7 features), and grey level co-occurrence matrix or GLCM (25 features). Only first-order features from the intensity direct analysis (9 features) were extracted from ADC maps for a total of 93 features for each lesion. The IBSI reference manual (16) suggests not using some morphological features because they do not have reference values (i.e., the minimum volume enclosing ellipsoid volume and area density, as well as the oriented minimum bounding box volume and area density). Thus, these four features were not included in the statistical analyses, leaving a total of 89 features that were finally evaluated for each lesion.

A description of each feature family is reported in **Supplemental Data**. The formulas used for the calculation are described the IBSI reference manual (16). Details on the image pre-processing, including interpolation, re-segmentation and intensity discretization, are indicated in **Supplemental Data**.

Qualitative Evaluation of Margins and Contrast Enhancement Type

Two radiologists who have more than 10 years of experience in head and neck and were unaware of the pathological results examined all pre-surgery MRI examinations in relation to the type of margins (regular if the lesion border was well-defined in any sequence or irregular if the lesion border was ill-defined) on both T2- and T1-w images, and the type of CE (1 homogeneous, 2 inhomogeneous, 3 absent) in post contrast T1-w images. The results were obtained by establishing a consensus between the radiologists. The qualitative scores were also included in the feature selection and model building.

Statistical Analysis

The feature selection and modeling were performed in the Matlab environment. The relationships between categorical variables (type of CE and margins) and the classification response were evaluated using the chi-squared test. The initial selection of the most significant features was carried out using the Mann-Whitney test with a cutoff for p of 0.10. Before further selection of the remaining features, the training and validation datasets were standardized using the z-score normalization method as indicated by Haga et al. (17). Based on this method, each feature was normalized as z=(x-)/std, where x, and std are the feature value, mean value, and standard deviation, respectively. Thus, a *neighborhood component analysis (NCA)* was applied through the Matlab function *fscnca* to further reduce the number of significant variables. To perform NCA, the regularization parameter lambda was tuned to find the optimal lambda value that produces the best classification performance.

In the case of high correlation between the selected features (Spearman correlation coefficient Rho >0.7, p <0.05), the one with the highest accuracy was chosen. The model with the final feature set was achieved using the support vector machine (SVM) binary classification algorithm. A five-fold cross-validation was applied to avoid overfitting due to the small dataset. The classification performance is reported in terms of the accuracy, sensitivity, specificity, positive predictive value (PPV), and negative predictive value (NPV).

RESULTS

The volumes of benign, Warthin's, and malignant lesions were 2.7 cm^3 (range, 0.2-21.1 cm^3), 5.2 cm^3 (range, 0.6-69.2 cm^3), and 5.1 cm^3 (range, 0.5-114 cm^3), respectively.

Relevant features included in the predictive models are reported in **Table 2**. The predictive performance of the three models on the training cohort and those tested on the validation cohort is reported in **Tables 3** and **4**, respectively. In the training cohort, the model for discriminating between Warthin's and malignant tumors reached the best accuracy of 86.7% (sensitivity 87.5%, specificity 84.6%) with a combination of four parameters: the 25th percentile of ADC (P25), the morphological feature of the volume density of the approximate enclosing ellipsoid (AEE) from T2-w images, and the type of margins and enhancement. When this model was tested on the validation cohort, it produced an accuracy of 77.8% (sensitivity 90%, specificity 42.9%).

In the training cohort, the model for discriminating between benign and Warthin's tumors showed a high accuracy of 91.9% (sensitivity 84.6%, specificity 95.8%) with a combination of four parameters: P25 of ADC, volume density AEE, minimum histogram gradient from T2-w images, and the type of enhancement. When this model tested on the validation cohort, it produced a comparable accuracy of 91.7% (sensitivity 85.7%, specificity 94.1%).

In the training cohort, the model for discriminating between benign tumors and malignant tumors had an accuracy of 80.4% (sensitivity 84.4%, specificity 75%) with a combination of four

TABLE 2 | Relevant features included in the predictive models.

	Warthin's Tumors		Malignant Tumors		*P value**
	Median	***IQR***	***Median***	***IQR***	
P25 of ADC (× 10^{-6} mm^2/s)	911	190	1058	379	0.054
Volume Density AEE	1.29	0.07	1.26	0.10	0.011
	Benign Tumors		Warthin's Tumors		
	Median	*IQR*	*Median*	*IQR*	*P value**
P25 of ADC (× 10^{-6} mm^2/s)	1506.88	612.00	911.00	189.75	<0.001
Volume Density AEE	1.26	0.07	1.29	0.07	0.0481
Minimum Histogram Gradient	-7.25	15.25	-16.00	18.63	0.0582
	Benign Tumors		Malignant Tumors		
	Median	*IQR*	*Median*	*IQR*	*P value**
P25 of ADC (× 10^{-6} mm^2/s)	1507	612	1058	379	<0.001
P10 of T2	9.00	3.00	6.50	4.00	0.007

**P values refer to Mann-Whitney test. P25, 25th percentile of the ADC distribution inside the lesion; P10 of T2, 10th percentile of the T2-weighetd signal intensity distribution inside the lesion; AEE, approximate enclosing ellipsoid.*

TABLE 3 | Predictive Performance of the three models on the training cohort.

End-point	Selected Features	Accuracy(%)	Sensitivity(%)	Specificity(%)	PPV(%)	NPV(%)
Warthin's versus Malignant Tumors	*ADC P25*	86.7	87.5	84.6	93.3	73.3
	Volume Density AEE	[73.2, 95.0]	[71.0, 96.5]	[54.5,98.1]	[79.5, 98.1]	[51.7, 87.6]
	Margins					
	Gd					
Benign* versus Warthin's Tumors	*ADC P25*	91.9	84.6	95.8	91.7	92.0
	Volume Density AEE	[78.1, 98.3]	[54.6, 98.1]	[78.9, 99.9]	[61.4, 98.7]	[76.2, 97.6]
	MinimumHistogramGradient					
	Gd					
Benign* versus Malignant Tumors	*ADC P25*	80.4	84.4	75.0	81.8	78.2
	T2 P10	[67.6, 89.8]	[67.2, 94.7]	[53.3, 90.2]	[68.9, 90.1]	[60.9, 89.3]
	Gd					
	Margins					

**Benign tumors with exclusion of Warthin's tumors. Abbreviations as in previous tables. In squared brackets the 95% confidence interval is reported.*

TABLE 4 | Predictive Performance of the three models tested on the validation cohort.

End-point	Selected Features	Accuracy(%)	Sensitivity(%)	Specificity(%)	PPV(%)	NPV(%)
Warthin's versus Malignant Tumors	*ADC P25* *Volume Density AEE* Margins Gd	81.5 [61.9,93.7]	90.0 [68.3,98.8]	57.1 [18.4,90.1]	85.7 [71.6,93.5]	66.7 [31.7, 89.6]
Benign* versus Warthin's Tumors	*ADC P25* *Volume Density AEE* *MinimumHistogramGradient* Gd	91.7 [73.0,99.0]	85.7 [42.1,99.6]	94.1 [71.3, 99.9]	85.7 [46.7,97.6]	94.1 [72.2, 99.9]
Benign* versus Malignant Tumors	*ADC P25* *T2 P10* Gd Margins	89.2 [74.6,97.0]	85.0 [62.1,96.8]	94.1 [71.3,99.9]	94.4 [71.6,99.1]	84.2 [65.1, 93.8]

**Benign tumors with exclusion of Warthin's tumors. Abbreviations as in previous tables. In squared brackets the 95% confidence interval is reported.*

parameters: P25 of ADC, P10 from T2-w images, and the types of margins and of CE. When this model was tested on the validation cohort, it produced an accuracy of 89.2% (sensitivity 85%, specificity 94.1%).

The results of chi-squared tests performed on the qualitative variables (type of margins and type of CE) included in the model building are reported in **Table 5**. **Figure 1** shows three correct classified lesions in the training dataset and three misdiagnosed cases in the validation set (a Warthin's tumor, a pleomorphic adenoma, and a malignant tumor, respectively).

The values of the most significant features initially selected by the Mann-Whitney test for each group and box plots of the features finally included in the models are shown in **Supplemental Data**.

TABLE 5 | Chi-square Test performed on qualitative variables, Type of Margins (a) and Type of Contrast Enhancement (b) in the three patient groups.

a. **Type of Enhancement**	**Homogeneous**	**Inhomogeneous**	**Absent**	**P value**
Warthin's Tumors	0	7	6	
			(28.9%)	
Malignant Tumors	1	25	6	
			(71.1%)	0.151
	(2.2%)	(71.1%)	(26.7%)	
Benign Tumors	11	12	1	
			(64.9%)	
Warthin's Tumors	0	7	6	
			(35.1%)	0.001
	(29.7%)	(51.4%)	(18.9%)	
Benign Tumors	11	12	1	
			(42.9%)	
Malignant Tumors	1	25	6	
			(57.1%)	0.0004
	(21.4%)	(66.1%)	(12.5%)	

b. **Type of Margins**	**Irregular Margins**	**Regular Margins**	**P value**
Warthins' Tumors	0	13	
		(28.9%)	0.009
Malignant Tumors	19	13	
		(71.1%)	
	(42.2%)	(57.8%)	
Benign Tumors	4	20	
		(64.9%)	0.315
Warthins' Tumors	0	13 (35.1%)	
	(10.8%)	(89.2%)	
Benign Tumors	4	20	
		(42.9%)	0.003
Malignant Tumors	19	13 (57.1%)	
	(41.1%)	(58.9%)	

DISCUSSION

In the evaluation of parotid gland tumors, there is overlap of the imaging signs between different neoplastic histologies (6, 8, 18), which represents a major limitation in the pre-surgical work-up of these lesions. Some recent studies report that texture analysis of MRI may provide a useful and objective description of signal patterns, which contribute to accurate diagnosis between tumors that look alike by a visual inspection (11, 13). The value of a computer-assisted discrimination of benign and malignant tumors has been explored in various organs (19–21), but only a few studies have assessed the contribution in parotid masses (12, 22–26).

In the present investigation, we identified the most discriminative features from pre-surgery MRI examinations based on first- and second-order texture analyses of T2-w images and first-order texture analysis of ADC maps for the separation of benign and malignant parotid lesions. All the three proposed models had good to excellent predictive performance, in combination with qualitative scores related to the type of margins or CE. This suggests that the texture analysis should be used as an additional tool for supporting radiologists' decisions and not in isolation (22).

Consistent with prior studies, we found significantly lower ADC values for Warthin's tumors than those of benign and malignant tumors (27, 28). Among the ADC-derived parameters, the 25th percentile (P25) of the ADC distribution inside the lesion was found to be the most relevant and was selected in all three models. This confirms the important role of DWI for the differential diagnosis of parotid lesions, as reported in previous studies (4, 9, 22, 29, 30). The P25 of ADC represents the ADC value associated with the tumor sub-volume with the most

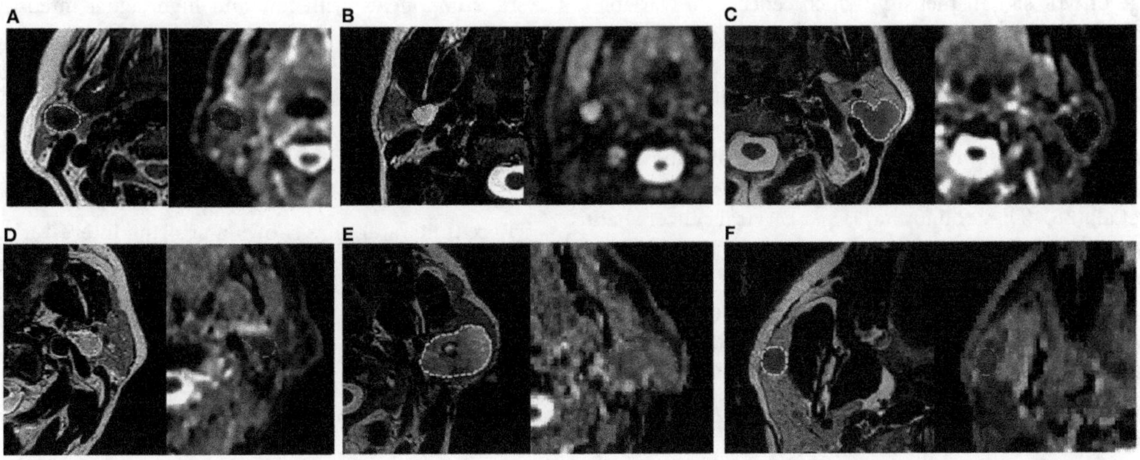

FIGURE 1 | On the top: three correctly classified lesions in the training dataset: **(A)** Warthin's tumor with low T2 intensity, ovoidal shape and decreased ADC value (P25 of ADC = 0.834 × 10^{-3} mm^2/s), **(B)** pleomorphic adenoma with typical T2 hyperintensity, sharp margins and high ADC value (P25 of ADC is 1.693 × 10^{-3} mm^2/s) **(C)** malignant tumor with irregular margins, T2 hypointensity and low ADC value, (P25 = 0.744 × 10^{-3} mm^2/s). At the bottom: three misdiagnosed cases in the validation set: **(D)** Warthin's tumor with high T2 hyperintensity and irregular shape (P25 of ADC = 0.930 × 10^{-3} mm^2/s); **(E)** pleomorphic adenoma with no typical T2 intensity and low ADC value (P25 of ADC = 1.109 × 10^{-3} mm^2/s); **(F)** malignant tumor with typical very low T2 intensity but regular and sharp margin and ovoidal shape (P25 of ADC = 0.836 × 10^{-3} mm^2/s). Each frame illustrates T2-weighted axial image with the user-defined lesion contour on the left and the corresponding ADC map on the right.

restrictive water molecule mobility. Thus, it is potentially related to a tumor region with a higher cell density. This finding suggests that instead of mean/median ADC values, it would be preferable to use a histogram-based approach to better address the tissue heterogeneity inside the tumor, which typically characterizes both benign and malignant parotid lesions (6, 8, 18). In this context, an interesting study of Khalek Abdel Razek et al. (31) evaluated the added value of Diffusion Tensor Imaging (DTI) to differentiate subtypes of parotid tumors, on the basis of fractional anisotropy (FA) and mean diffusivity, reporting very high accuracies. Even though DTI cannot be considered part of routine head and neck oncologic protocols, it showed a great potential to accurately separate Warthin's tumors from malignant tumors, as well as Warthin's tumours among all the other benign tumors. In particular, FA appeared to be associated to the complexity and heterogeneity of tissue microstructure and it may provide deeper insights into the parotid tumor cytoarchitecture, compared to conventional ADC.

The volume density AEE derived from T2-w images showed discriminatory potential for separating Warthin's tumors from other parotid tumors. This feature is directly related to the volume sphericity and showed increased values for Warthins' tumors, indicating that this kind of lesion has a more spherical shape than both malignant and benign tumors ($p = 0.025$ and $p = 0.04$ respectively, Mann-Whitney test). Concerning T2-w images, P10 was found to be relevant for differentiating benign and malignant lesions, with the latter showing significantly lower P10 values ($p = 0.007$, Mann-Whitney test) according to previous studies (5, 19, 23, 32, 33). In fact, it was demonstrated that high, intermediate, and low signal intensity can be associated with benign lesions (pleomorphic adenoma), intermediate, and highly malignant tumors, respectively (5, 32). Therefore, the use of heavily T2-w sequences is strongly suggested (33).

Recently, Sarioglu et al. (12) reported a texture-based study of T2-w images and contrast-enhanced T1-w images to discriminate the most common parotid tumors, in addition to several qualitative scores, as we similarly proposed. Due to the small number of malignant parotid tumors included and to differences in MR sequences considered for the analysis, a direct comparison with our findings is not possible. However, the authors showed that both skewness and kurtosis were significantly different between pleomorphic adenoma, Warthin's tumors, and mucoepidermoid carcinoma. In the present study, the skewness was also found to be discriminative for the separation of benign and malignant/ Warthin's lesions, even though it was not included in the final model. The role of the minimum histogram gradient from T2-w images in the model is less obvious for differentiating benign and Warthin's tumors. This feature was strongly associated with several GLCM-based features, such as the dissimilarity, contrast, and inverse difference (Spearman's coefficient Rho = 0.894, 0.870, and -0.906 with $p < 0.0001$), with the latter being a measure of homogeneity (16). Therefore, an increased value of the minimum histogram gradient in the group of benign lesions should suggest higher contrast and inhomogeneity compared to the group of Warthin's tumors.

The explanation for this phenomenon is not straightforward, considering that Warthin's lesions typically show high tissue heterogeneity (22, 27). In fact, the tissue contrast of this kind of lesion can be affected by degenerative alterations in the interstitial tissue and may depend on the degree of differentiation of tumor cells, as well as the presence or absence of necrosis and cystic components (27, 34). This causes a broad range of MR signal intensity, which reflects the variable proportion of microcytic components and lymphoid stroma inside the lesion (34). On the other hand, benign lesions may also show tissue heterogeneity on T2-w images due to cystic, solid, or mixoid components. Moreover, it was recently reported that the volume of the lesion may impact the value of some T2-w radiomic features, such as dissimilarity and energy, as shown by Wormald et al. (35). They found that larger cervical cancers had lower dissimilarity and higher energy and thus higher homogeneity and uniformity than smaller ones. In our dataset, Warthin's tumors showed a tendency to be larger (median, 5.2 cm^3) than benign lesions (median, 2.7 cm^3), even though there was no statistically significant difference between these volumes ($p = 0.22$, Mann-Whitney test). This may partially explain our findings.

The macroscopic imaging signs involved in the models (i.e., the type of margins and CE) were previously found to be useful in differential diagnosis (12). In fact, an ill-defined tumor border and low-grade contrast enhancement were observed as independent risk factors for malignancy, while a well-defined tumor margin was reported as a good qualitative indicator of benignity (12, 23).

The potential role of contrast enhancement and perfusion in discriminating various subtypes of parotid tumors was specifically addressed by some previous studies, which proposed the use of arterial-spin labeling (ASL) (30), dynamic susceptibility contrast perfusion-weighted MRI or dynamic contrast enhanced MRI (2, 4, 36, 37). These investigations consistently indicated that Warthins's tumors are characterized by a higher tissue vascularity than pleomorphic adenomas, and generally by a lower vascularity than malignant tumors. Although further efforts should be made to improve the repeatability and reproducibility of perfusion-weighted techniques (38) before including them as part of routine head and neck oncologic protocols, they are very promising and merit future investigation.

Lastly, we tested the performance of the developed prediction models on an external validation dataset, which is strongly suggested for a complete radiomic analysis to verify the reproducibility and transportability in a clinical setting (10). The predictive performance on the validation cohort indicated comparable accuracies, even though the model discriminating between Warthin's and malignant tumors showed lower specificity and negative predictive power (they decreased from 86.6 to 57.1, and from 73.3 to 66.7%, respectively).

This is consistent with a recent study of Gabelloni et al. (25), who also proposed a radiomic analysis of parotid tumors on T2-w MR images and obtained the best classification performance when comparing benign tumors with Warthin's tumors, while a lower accuracy was found in differentiating Warthin's and malignant tumors. Radiologists have particular difficulties in differentiating this type of lesion, the reason is that it may present a solid component with low signal intensity in T2-w images, which is also found in malignant lesions. Furthermore, they may have cystic components with low and high signal intensity in T1-w images, which indicate the presence of cystic fluid or high protein fluid, respectively (2, 27, 39). As mentioned, DWI has the potential to appreciably improve this misclassification, as Warthin's tumors typically show lower ADC values than both benign and low grade malignant tumors (22, 27).

Recent literature has shown a growing interest in the clinical applicability of radiomics for the parotid tumor characterization (12, 25, 26), thanks to significant improvements in diagnostic accuracy obtained with a multiparametric approach to quantitative MRI (2, 4, 6, 30, 31, 36, 37). However, no consensus exists regarding the most appropriate sequences to consider for the extraction of radiomics features and only a few studies used standardized software, previously validated according to the updated IBSI guidelines (16). Moreover, the lack of an external validation set in most of current papers makes impossible to verify the transportability of the proposed models. In general, further efforts are needed for a standardization of the entire workflow, from image acquisition and processing to feature extraction, statistical analysis and clinical validation (40). This could facilitate a direct comparison between findings from single centers, helping to clarify the added role of MRI-based radiomics in oncologic applications.

The present study has some limitations. First, its retrospective nature may have introduced bias and confounding factors. Secondly, our findings should be confirmed in a larger patient population as only a small number of benign and malignant tumors were included in the training cohort. Another limitation is the lack of differentiation between low and high-grade lesions in the context of malignant neoplasms due to the low number of patients, which could allow us to develop specific predictive models as a function of tumor grade.

CONCLUSIONS

Radiomic analysis of ADC and T2-w images in addition to qualitative scores evaluating margins and CE allowed us to obtain good to excellent diagnostic accuracies in differentiating parotid lesions, which was confirmed by testing on an external validation cohort.

ETHICS STATEMENT

The studies involving human participants were reviewed and approved by Institutional Review Board, Regina Elena National Cancer Institute (IRCCS), Rome, Italy. Written informed consent for participation was not required for this study in accordance with the national legislation and the institutional requirements.

AUTHOR CONTRIBUTIONS

FP and AV conceived of the study and drafted the manuscript. SM carried out the radiomic analysis and contributed to the draft. RP contributed to the patient enrollment and data gathering. RCo provided the histological data on surgical specimens. VF and FP carried out the image delineation and participated in the image analysis. MR, DF, and RCa provided the external validation dataset and contributed to the design of the study. IT performed the statistical analysis. All authors contributed to the article and approved the submitted version.

REFERENCES

1. Gao M, Hao Y, Huang MX, Ma DQ, Chen Y, Luo HY, et al. Salivary Gland Tumours in a Northern Chinese Population: A 50-Year Retrospective Study of 7190 Cases. *Int J Oral Maxillofac Surg* (2017) 46:343–9. doi: 10.1016/j.ijom.2016.09.021
2. Espinoza S, Felter A, Malinvaud D, Badoual C, Chatellier G, Siauve N, et al. Warthin's Tumor of Parotid Gland: Surgery or Follow-Up? Diagnostic Value of a Decisional Algorithm With Functional MR. *Diagn Interventional Imaging* (2016) 97:37–43. doi: 10.1016/j.diii.2014.11.024
3. Monsour N, Hofauer B. Knopf AJ Ultrasound Elastography in Diffuse and Focal Parotid Gland Lesions. *Otorhinolaryngol Relat Spec* (2017) 79:54–64. doi: 10.1159/000455727
4. Yuan Y, Tang W, Tao X. Parotid Gland Lesions: Separate and Combined Diagnostic Value of Conventional MRI, Diffusion-Weighted Imaging and Dynamic Contrast-Enhanced MRI. *Br J Radiol* (2016) 89(1060):20150912. doi: 10.1259/bjr.20150912
5. Christe A, Waldherr C, Hallett R, Zbaeren P, Thoeny H. MR Imaging of Parotid Tumors: Typical Lesion Characteristics in MR Imaging Improve Discrimination Between Benign and Malignant Disease. *AJNR Am J Neuroradiol* (2011) 32:1202–7. doi: 10.3174/ajnr.A2520
6. Gökçe E. Multiparametric Magnetic Resonance Imaging for the Diagnosis and Differential Diagnosis of Parotid Gland Tumors. *J Magn Reson Imaging* (2020) 52:11–32. doi: 10.1002/jmri.27061
7. Teresi LM, Lufkin RB, Wortham DC, Abemayor E, Hanafee WN. Parotid Masses: MR Imaging. *Radiology* (1989) 163:405–9. doi: 10.1148/radiology.163.2.3562818
8. Kessler AT, Bhatt AA. Review of the Major and Minor Salivary Glands, Part 2: Neoplasms and Tumor-like Lesions. *J Clin Imaging Sci* (2018) 8:48. doi: 10.4103/jcis.JCIS_46_18
9. Habermann CR, Arndt C, Graessner J, Diestel L, Petersen KU, Reitmeier F. Diffusion-Weighted Echo-Planar MR Imaging of Primary Parotid Gland Tumors: Is a Prediction of Different Histologic Subtypes Possible? *AJNR Am J Neuroradiol* (2009) 30:591–6. doi: 10.3174/ajnr.A1412
10. Lambin P, Leijenaar RTH, Deist TM, Peerlings J, de Jong EEC, van Timmeren J, et al. Radiomics: The Bridge Between Medical Imaging and Personalized Medicine. *Nat Rev Clin Oncol* (2017) 14:749–62. doi: 10.1038/nrclinonc.2017.141
11. Song J, Yin Y, Wang H, Zhihui Chang Z, Zhaoyu Liu Z, Cui L. A Review of Original Articles Published in the Emerging Field of Radiomic. *Eur J Radiol* (2020) 127:108991. doi: 10.1016/j.ejrad.2020.108991
12. Sarioglu O, Sarioglu FC, Akdogan AI, Kucuk U, Arslan IB, Cukurova I, et al. MRI-Based Texture Analysis to Differentiate the Most Common Parotid Tumours. *Clin Radiol* (2020) 75:877.e15–e23. doi: 10.1016/j.crad.2020.06.018
13. Kassner A, Thornhill RE. Texture Analysis: A Review of Neurologic MRI Applications. *AJNR Am J Neuroradiol* (2010) 31:809–16. doi: 10.3174/ajnr.A2061
14. Bettinelli A, Branchini M, De Monte F, Scaggion A, Paiusco M. Technical Note: An IBEX Adaption Toward Image Biomarker Standardization. *Med Phys* (2020) 47(3):1167–73. doi: 10.1002/mp.13956
15. Zhang L, Fried DV, Fave XJ, Hunter LA, Yang J, Court LE. Ibex: An Open Infrastructure Software Platform to Facilitate Collaborative Work in Radiomics. *Med Phys* (2015) 42:1341–53. doi: 10.1118/1.4908210
16. Zwanenburg A, Leger S, Vallières M, Löck S. Image Biomarker Standardisation Initiative:Standardized Quantitative Radiomics for High-Throughput Image-based Phenotyping. *Radiology* (2020) 295:328–38. doi: 10.1148/radiol.2020191145
17. Haga A, Takahashi W, Aoki S, Nawa K, Yamashita H, Abe O, et al. Standardization of Imaging Features for Radiomics Analysis. *J Med Invest* (2019) 66:35–7. doi: 10.2152/jmi.66.35
18. Abdel Razek AAK, Mukherji SK. State-of-the-Art Imaging of Salivary Gland Tumors. *Neuroimaging Clin N Am* (2018) 28:303–17. doi: 10.1016/j.nic.2018.01.009
19. Mayerhoefera ME, Breitensehera M, Amannd G, Dominkuse M. Are Signal Intensity and Homogeneity Useful Parameters for Distinguishing Between Benign and Malignant Soft Tissue Masses on MR Images? Objective Evaluation by Means of Texture Analysis. *Magn Reson Imaging* (2008) 26:1316–22. doi: 10.1016/j.mri.2008.02.013
20. Wang H, Zhang J, Bao S, Liu J, Hou F, Huang Y, et al. Preoperative MRI-Based Radiomic Machine-Learning Nomogram May Accurately Distinguish Between Benign and Malignant Soft-Tissue Lesions: A Two-Center Study. *J Magn Reson Imaging* (2020) 52:873–82. doi: 10.1002/jmri.27111
21. Nogueira L, Nunes RG. Radiomics Based on Multimodal MRI for the Differential Diagnosis of Benign and Malignant Breast Lesions, Editorial. *J Magn Reson Imaging* (2020) 52:608–9. doi: 10.1002/jmri.27168
22. Fruehwald-Pallamar J, Czerny C, Holzer-Fruehwald L, Nemec SF, Mueller-Mang C, Weber M, et al. Texture-Based and Diffusion-Weighted Discrimination of Parotid Gland Lesions on MR Images At 3.0 Tesla. *NMR BioMed* (2013) 26:1372–9. doi: 10.1002/nbm.2962
23. Wu Q, Zhu LN, Jiang JS, Bu SS, Xu XQ, Wu FY. Characterization of Parotid Gland Tumors Using T2 Mapping Imaging: Initial Findings. *Acta Radiol* (2020) 61:629–35. doi: 10.1177/0284185119875646
24. Chang YJ, Huang TY, Liu YJ, Chung HW, Juan CJ. Classification of Parotid Gland Tumors by Using Multimodal MRI and Deep Learning. *NMR BioMed* (2020) 34:e4408. doi: 10.1002/nbm.4408
25. Gabelloni M, Faggioni L, Attanasio S, Vani V, Goddi A, Colantonio S, et al. Can Magnetic Resonance Radiomics Analysis Discriminate Parotid Gland Tumors? A Pilot Study. *Diagnostics (Basel)* (2020) 310(11):900. doi: 10.3390/diagnostics10110900
26. Zheng YM, Li J, Liu S, Cui JF, Zhan JF, Pang J, et al. Mri-Based Radiomics Nomogram for Differentiation of Benign and Malignant Lesions of the Parotid Gland. *Eur Radiol* (2020) 19:1–11. doi: 10.1007/s00330-020-07483-4
27. Wang CW, Chu YH, Chiu DY, Shin N, Hsu HH, Lee JC, et al. Journal CLUB: The Warthin Tumor Score: A Simple and Reliable Method to Distinguish Warthin Tumors From Pleomorphic Adenomas and Carcinomas. *AJR Am J Roentgenol* (2018) 210:1330–7. doi: 10.2214/AJR.17.18492
28. Zhang Z, Song C, Zhang Y, Wen B, Zhu J, Cheng J. Apparent Diffusion Coefficient (ADC) Histogram Analysis: Differentiation of Benign From Malignant Parotid Gland Tumors Using Readout-Segmented Diffusion-Weighted Imaging. *Dentomaxillofac Radiol* (2019) 48:20190100. doi: 10.1259/dmfr.20190100
29. Matsushima N, Maeda M, Takamura M. Takeda K.Apparent Diffusion Coefficients of Benign and Malignant Salivary Gland Tumors. Comparison to Histopathological Findings. *J Neuroradiol* (2017) 34:183–9. doi: 10.1016/j.neurad.2007.04.002

30. Razek AAKA. Multi-Parametric MR Imaging Using Pseudo-Continuous Arterial-Spin Labeling and Diffusion-Weighted MR Imaging in Differentiating Subtypes of Parotid Tumors. *Magn Reson Imaging* (2019) 63:55–9. doi: 10.1016/j.mri.2019.08.005
31. Khalek Abdel Razek AA. Characterization of Salivary Gland Tumours With Diffusion Tensor Imaging. *Dentomaxillofac Radiol* (2018) 47:20170343. doi: 10.1259/dmfr.20170343
32. Espinoza S, Halimi P. Interpretation Pearls For MR Imaging Of Parotid Gland Tumor. *Eur Ann Otorhinolaryngol Head Neck Dis* (2013) 130:30–5. doi: 10.1016/j.anorl.2011.12.006
33. Sakamoto M, Sasano T, Higano S, Takahashi S, Iikubo M, Kakehata S. Usefulness of Heavily T(2) Weighted Magnetic Resonance Images for the Differential Diagnosis of Parotid Tumours. *Dentomaxillofac Radiol* (2003) 32:295–9. doi: 10.1259/dmfr/32387150
34. Kato H, Fujimoto K, Matsuo M, Mizuta K. Aoki M. Usefulness of Diffusion-Weighted MR Imaging for Differentiating Between Warthin's Tumor and Oncocytoma of the Parotid Gland. *Jpn J Radiol* (2017) 35:78–85. doi: 10.1007/s11604-016-0608-5
35. Wormald BW, Doran SJ, Ind TE, D'Arcy J, Petts J, deSouza NM. Radiomic Features of Cervical Cancer on T2- and Diffusion-Weighted MRI: Prognostic Value in Low-Volume Tumors Suitable for Trachelectomy. *Gynecol Oncol* (2020) 156:107–14. doi: 10.1016/j.ygyno.2019.10.010
36. Razek AAKA. Multi-Parametric MR Imaging Using Pseudo-Continuous Arterial-Spin Labeling and Diffusion-Weighted MR Imaging in Differentiating Subtypes of Parotid Tumors. *Magn Reson Imaging* (2019) 63:55–9. doi: 10.1016/j.mri.2019.08.005
37. Xu Z, Zheng S, Pan A, Cheng X, Gao M. A Multiparametric Analysis Based on DCE-MRI to Improve the Accuracy of Parotid Tumor Discrimination. *Eur J Nucl Med Mol Imaging* (2019) 46:2228–34. doi: 10.1007/s00259-019-04447-9
38. Shukla-Dave A, Obuchowski NA, Chenevert TL, Jambawalikar S, Schwartz LH, Malyarenko D, et al. Quantitative Imaging Biomarkers Alliance (QIBA) Recommendations for Improved Precision of DWI and DCE-MRI Derived Biomarkers in Multicenter Oncology Trials. *J Magn Reson Imaging* (2019) 49: e101–21. doi: 10.1002/jmri.26518
39. Ikeda M, Motoori K, Hanazawa T, Nagai Y, Yamamoto S, Ueda T, et al. Warthin Tumor of the Parotid Gland: Diagnostic Value of MR Imaging With Histopathologic Correlation. *AJNR Am J Neuroradiol* (2004) 25:1256–62. doi: 10.1016/j.ijrobp.2018.08.032
40. Morin O, Vallières M, Jochems A, Woodruff HC, Valdes G, Braunstein SE, et al. A Deep Look Into the Future of Quantitative Imaging in Oncology: A Statement of Working Principles and Proposal for Change. *Int J Radiat Oncol Biol Phys* (2018) 102(4):1074–82. doi: 10.1016/j.ijrobp.2018.08.032

7

Lingual Lymph Node Metastasis in cT1-2N0 Tongue Squamous Cell Carcinoma: Is it an Indicator for Elective Neck Dissection

Wenli Yang*, Minglei Sun, Qiaoyan Jie, Haixia Zhou, Peng Zhang* and Juanfang Zhu*

Department of Stomatology, The First Affiliated Hospital of Zhengzhou University, Zhengzhou, China

***Correspondence:**
Wenli Yang
yangwenli7412540@163.com
Peng Zhang
sunqiangsqs456@163.com
Juanfang Zhu
zzyouzi@163.com

Objective: Accurate predictors for occult metastasis in cT1-2N0 tongue squamous cell carcinoma (SCC) remains scarce, the main goal in current study was to evaluate whether there is significant association between lingual lymph node (LLN) metastasis and occult lymph node metastasis as well as whether there is prognostic value of LLN metastasis in early stage tongue SCC.

Methods: Patients with surgically treated primary cT1-2N0 tongue SCC were prospectively enrolled from January 2010 to December 2018. LLNs were dissected independently for pathologic analysis. The main study endpoints were locoregional control survival (LRC) and disease-specific survival (DSS). The Chi-square test and multivariate regression analysis were used to assess the predictors for occult metastasis. The Kaplan-Meier approach and Cox model were used to analyze the potential prognostic factors.

Results: A total of 317 patients were enrolled for analysis. Eighty-eight patients had occult metastasis with a prevalence of 27.8%. LLNs presented in 89 patients, in which 43 patients had LLN metastasis. In the 43 patients with positive LLNs, 20 patients had occult metastasis, in 274 patients with negative LLNs or no LLNs, 68 patients had occult metastasis, the difference was significant ($p = 0.012$). Further multivariate regression analysis confirmed the independence of LLN metastasis in predicting the occult metastasis. In patients without LLNs, the 5-year LRC rate was 79%, in patients with negative LLNs, the 5-year LRC rate was 78%, in patients with positive LLNs, the 5-year LRC rate was 62%, the difference was significant ($p = 0.024$). In patients without LLNs, the 5-year DSS rate was 84%, in patients with negative LLNs, the 5-year DSS rate was 74%, in patients with positive LLNs, the 5-year DSS rate was 51%, the difference was significant ($p < 0.001$), further Cox model confirmed the independence of LLN metastasis in affecting the LRC and DSS.

Conclusions: LLN metastasis is significantly associated with occult neck lymph node metastasis, and decrease the LRC and DSS in early stage tongue SCC.

Keywords: lingual lymph node, occult metastasis, early stage tongue squamous cell carcinoma, squamous cell carcinoma, elective neck dissection

INTRODUCTION

Tongue squamous cell carcinoma (SCC) is the most common oral cavity malignancy (1, 2), its prognosis has not improved significantly despite advances in diagnosis and treatment, neck lymph node metastasis is one of the most important prognostic factors (3, 4), but unfortunately these positive lymph nodes are usually occult or subclinical at the initial treatment in early stage tongue SCC. Owing to a wide range of occult metastasis rate (5, 6), either elective neck dissection (END) or the watchful waiting policy has been the favored treatment for cT1-2N0 tongue SCC (7, 8). Investigators favoring for END comment that END allows more accurate disease stage and decision of the need for adjuvant therapies, and resection of metastatic lymph nodes could potentially reduce the recurrence risk (9, 10), however, the main concern according to the traditional watchful waiting policy is the associated surgical complication including shoulder dysfunction and over-treatment for those patients having no pathologic metastases (11). Considering there is no accurate diagnostic procedure for staging the neck preoperatively, the elective management of the neck in cT1-2N0 tongue SCC has been the subject of much debate during the past three decades and continues to be controversial.

Lingual lymph nodes (LLNs) were firstly introduced by Rouviere et al. (12). These authors have divided LLNs into two groups: the lateral lingual nodes are lateral to the genioglossus or the hyoglossus muscles, and the median lingual node resides between the medial side of the genioglossus muscle and the lingual septum (12, 13). A number of researchers have reported the phenomenon of LLN metastasis in primary or recurrent oral SCC by cases reports (14–22), but whether there is significant association between LLN metastasis and occult lymph node metastasis as well as whether there is prognostic value of LLN metastasis in early stage tongue SCC remain unknown. Therefore, the current study aimed to clarify these questions.

METHODS

The Zhengzhou University institutional research committee approved our study, and all participants provided written informed consent for medical research prior to enrollment in the study. All experiments were performed in accordance with relevant guidelines and regulations.

From January 2010 to December 2018, patients with primary cT1-2N0 tongue SCC according to the 7th AJCC classification were prospectively investigated. The only inclusion criteria was that patients underwent surgical treatment for primary cancer disease; patients who lost their visits were excluded for analysis. Information including age, sex, adverse pathologic characteristics, and follow-up of enrolled patients was collected and analyzed. All patients had underwent a neck dissection. Drinkers were defined as those who consumed at least one alcoholic drink per day for at least 1 year (2, 3), smokers were defined as those smoked on a daily basis or had quit smoking for less than 5 years (2, 3). cT1-2 was defined as a maximum diameter of tumors <2 cm or a diameter ranging from 2 to 4 cm, patients were considered to have cN0 disease if they had no evidence of nodal metastasis on clinical examination, ultrasound, or radiographic imaging (23, 24).

All pathologic sections were reviewed by at least two pathologists, and perineural invasion was considered to be present if tumor cells were identified within the perineural space and/or nerve bundle; lymphovascular infiltration was positive if tumor cells were noted within the lymphovascular channels (23). The pathologic depth of invasion (DOI) was measured from the level of the adjacent normal mucosa to the deepest point of tumor infiltration, regardless of the presence or absence of ulceration (24).

All patients underwent radical primary tumor excision with a minimum margin of 1 cm, the muscle of the mouth floor was preserved in highest measure, the adipose tissue in the mouth floor including the sublingual gland was separated from the primary tumor, and then dissected for any possible lymph nodes (**Figure 1**) for postoperative pathology analysis independently, END (levelI-III) was routinely performed for tongue SCC patients with the exception of very early-stage disease in our cancer center. Indication for adjuvant treatment included perineural invasion, lymphovascular invasion, positive margin, and cervical lymph node metastasis. All patients were regularly followed every 3 months within the first 2 years after

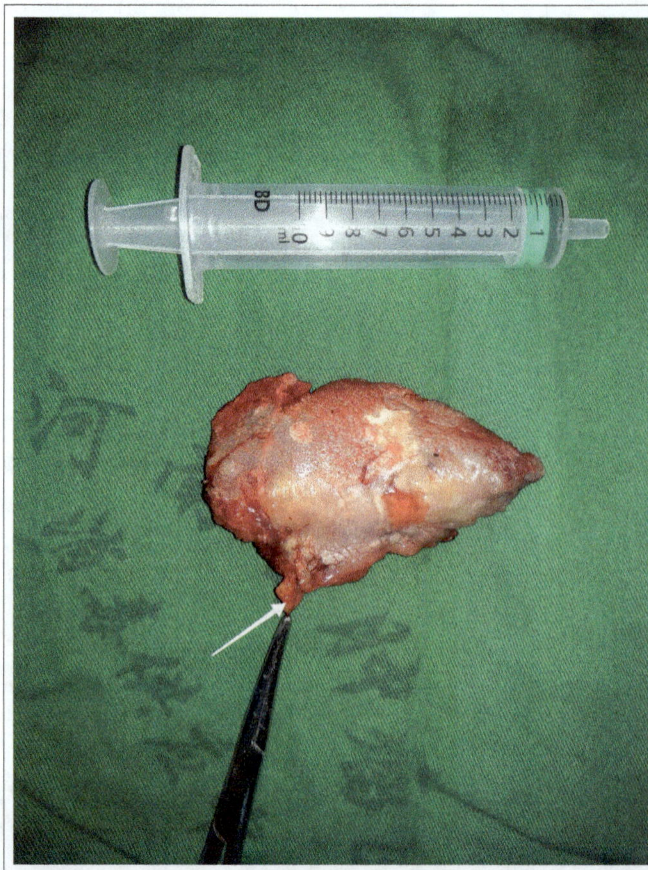

FIGURE 1 | Lingual lymph node (white row).

the operation and every 6 months within the third to fifth year after the operation. If there was any doubt regarding disease recurrence, active interference was performed. (25).

The association between neck occult metastasis and clinical pathologic variables was firstly evaluated by the Chi-square test, and then by multivariate regression analysis for detecting the independent predictor. The main study endpoints were locoregional control (LRC) and disease specific survival (DSS), and the survival time was calculated from date of surgery to the date of an event or latest follow-up. The Kaplan-Meier approach (log-rank test) was used to calculate the LRC and DSS rates. The factors which were significant in univariate analysis were then analyzed in the multivariate proportional hazard Cox model for determining the independent prognostic factors. All statistical analyses were performed on SPSS 20.0, and a $p < 0.05$ was considered significant.

RESULTS

There were 317 patients (227 male and 90 female) enrolled in total, the mean age was 58.3 (range: 28–78) years. Smoker and drinker were noted in 189 (59.6%) and 130 (41.0%) patients, respectively. Clinical tumor stages were distributed as T1 in 143 (45.1%) patients and T2 in 174 (54.9%) patients, respectively. Perineural invasion and lymphovascular invasion were noted in 46 (14.5%) and 33 (10.4%) patients, respectively. Pathologic tumor grade was distributed as well in 122 (38.4%) patients, moderate in 143 (45.1%) patients, and poor in 52 (16.4%) patients. The mean pathologic DOI was 6.9 (range: 3.0–15.8) mm. Negative margin was achieved in all patients (100%). There were 65 (20.5%) patients underwent flap reconstruction for tongue restoration including 25 platysma myocutaneous flaps, 17 submental island flaps, 15 radial forearm flaps, and eight anterolateral thigh flaps.

LLNs were reported in 89 (28.1%) patients, the mean number of LLNs was 1.4 (range: 1–3), 43 of the 89 patients had pathologic LLN metastasis, the mean number of positive LLNs was 1.3 (range: 1–3), the overall LLN metastasis rate was 13.6% (43/317). As described by **Table 1**, the LLN metastasis was significantly associated with cervical lymph node metastasis and tumor stage.

Occult neck lymph node metastasis occurred in 88 (27.8%) patients. There was no extracapsular spread. Seventy-eight patients had isolate level I metastasis, nine patients had simultaneous level I and II metastasis, and 1 patient had simultaneous level I, II, and III metastasis. In 43 patients with positive LLNs, 20 patients had occult metastasis, in 46 patients with negative LLNs, 12 patients had occult metastasis, in 228 patients with no LLNs, 56 patients had occult metastasis, the difference was significant ($p = 0.012$). The sensitivity of positive LLN to predict positive occult neck node metastasis was 22.7% (95% CI, 14.5–32.9%), and the positive test likelihood ratio was 2.3 (95% CI, 1.3–3.9). The Chi-square test also reported the significant association between occult metastasis and tumor stage, pathologic DOI, and pathologic tumor grade (all $p < 0.05$). Further multivariate regression described the factors of tumor stage ($p = 0.005$, 2.445[1.247–6.332]), pathologic DOI ($p = 0.033$, 2.118[1.684–5.226]), LLN status ($p = 0.041$, 1.984[1.247–3.222]), and pathologic tumor grade ($p = 0.008$, 3.221[1.647–7.669]) independently increased the risk of occult neck lymph node metastasis (**Table 2**).

TABLE 1 | Association between clinical pathologic variables and lingual lymph node metastasis.

Variables	Lingual lymph node status		*p*
	Positive (*n* = 43)	Negative or none (*n* = 274)	
Age			
<40	7	23	
≥40	36	251	0.101
Sex			
Male	33	194	
Female	10	80	0.422
Smoking			
Yes	23	166	
No	20	108	0.378
Drinking			
Yes	15	115	
No	28	159	0.380
Tumor stage			
T1	12	131	
T2	31	143	0.015
DOI*			
<5 mm	15	132	
≥5 mm	28	142	0.104
PI#			
Yes	8	38	
No	35	236	0.412
LVI%			
Yes	5	28	
No	38	246	0.779
Occult metastasis			
Negative	23	206	
Positive	20	68	0.003
Tumor grade			
Well	13	109	
Moderate	20	123	
Poor	10	42	0.313

**, depth of invasion; #, perineural invasion; %, lymphovascular invasion.*

Table 3 analyzed the cervical metastasis pattern according to the status of the LLNs, and it described that there might be a trending of more extensive metastasis if there was LLN metastasis.

After follow-up with mean time of 37.5 (range: 2–93) months, 100 patients received adjuvant radiotherapy, and 10 patients also received adjuvant chemotherapy, locoregional recurrence occurred in 58 patients, disease-specific death occurred in 43 patients.

The 5-year LRC rate was 77%. In patients without LLNs, the 5-year LRC rate was 79%, in patients with negative LLNs,

TABLE 2 | Association between clinical pathologic variables and occult neck lymph node metastasis.

Variables	Occult metastasis		X^2	Multivariate regression	
	+ (n = 88)	− (n = 229)	p	p	RR[95% CI]
Age					
<40	7	23			
≥40	81	206	0.569		
Sex					
Male	63	164			
Female	25	65	0.996		
Smoking					
Yes	53	136			
No	35	93	0.107		
Drinking					
Yes	35	95			
No	53	134	0.781		
Tumor stage					
T1	25	118			
T2	63	111	<0.001	0.005	2.445[1.247–6.332]
DOI*					
<5 mm	32	115			
≥5 mm	56	114	0.027	0.033	2.118[1.684–5.226]
PI#					
Yes	15	31			
No	73	198	0.427		
LVI%					
Yes	13	20			
No	75	209	0.115		
LLN&					
No	56	172			
Negative	12	34			
Positive	20	23	0.012	0.041	1.984[1.247–3.222]
Tumor grade					
Well	26	96			
Moderate	40	103			
Poor	22	30	0.018	0.008	3.221[1.647–7.669]

**, depth of invasion; #, perineural invasion; %, lymphovascular invasion; &, lingual lymph node.*

TABLE 3 | Cervical metastasis pattern according to the status of lingual lymph node (LLN) status.

Level metastasis	LLN status		
	Positive	Negative	None
I	20	12	56
II	2	2	6
III	1	0	0

the 5-year LRC rate was 78%, in patients with positive LLNs, the 5-year LRC rate was 62%, the difference was significant (p = 0.024, **Figure 2**). As described by **Table 4**, the factors of tumor stage, LLN status, neck lymph node metastasis, perineural invasion, lymphovascular invasion, and pathologic DOI were associated with the locoregional control, further Cox model confirmed the independence of LLN status, neck lymph node metastasis, perineural invasion, and pathologic DOI in predicting the LRC survival.

The 5-year DSS rate was 78%. In patients without LLNs, the 5-year DSS rate was 84%, in patients with negative LLNs, the 5-year DSS rate was 74%, in patients with positive LLNs, the 5-year DSS rate was 51%, the difference was significant (p < 0.001, **Figure 3**). As described by **Table 5**, the factors

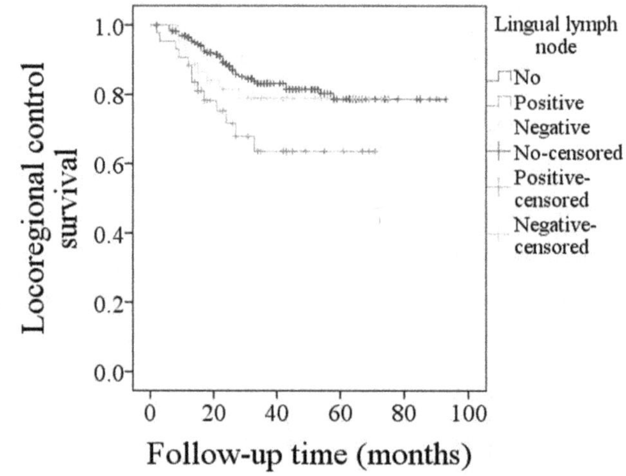

FIGURE 2 | Comparison of locoregional control survival in patients with different lingual lymph node status (p = 0.024).

TABLE 4 | Prognostic factors for the locoregional control in patients with cT1-2N0 tongue squamous cell carcinoma.

Variables	Univariate analysis	Cox model	
	p	P	HR[95%CI]
Age (<40 vs. ≥40)	0.547		
Sex	0.336		
Smoking	0.147		
Drinking	0.225		
Tumor stage (T1 vs. T2)	0.005	0.174	3.664[0.786–12.004]
Neck node stage (N0 vs. N+)	0.001	<0.001	4.222[1.782–9.664]
DOI* (<5 vs. ≥5 mm)	0.026	0.013	2.643[1.844–6.449]
Perineural invasion	0.014	0.008	2.847[1.471–7.552]
Lymphovascular invasion	0.008	0.085	3.412[0.925–9.227]
Pathologic tumor grade	0.111		
Well			
Moderate			
Poor			
LLN status	0.024		
No			
Negative		0.845	1.235[0.158–2.111]
Positive		0.015	1.999[1.325–4.668]
Adjuvant treatment	0.521		

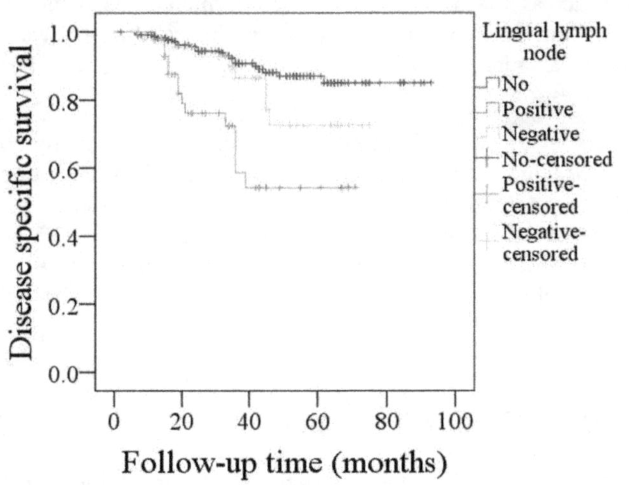

FIGURE 3 | Comparison of disease specific survival in patients with different lingual lymph node status ($p < 0.001$).

TABLE 5 | Prognostic factors for the disease specific survival in patients with cT1-2N0 tongue squamous cell carcinoma.

Variables	Univariate analysis	Cox model	
	p	P	HR[95%CI]
Age (<40 vs. ≥40)	0.254		
Sex	0.631		
Smoking	0.215		
Drinking	0.334		
Tumor stage (T1 vs. T2)	0.088		
Neck node stage (N0 vs. N+)	0.002	<0.001	2.222[1.258–5.331]
DOI* (<5 vs. ≥5 mm)	0.015	0.003	3.524[1.631–8.552]
Perineural invasion	0.263		
Lymphovascular invasion	0.014	0.005	2.338[1.726–5.434]
Pathologic tumor grade	0.021		
Well			
Moderate		0.015	2.114[1.235–4.002]
Poor		<0.001	4.669[1.978–9.224]
LLN status	<0.001		
No			
Negative		0.098	1.735[0.896–3.425]
Positive		<0.001	1.845[1.137–3.987]
Adjuvant treatment	0.521		

of LLN status, lymphovascular invasion, neck lymph node metastasis, pathologic tumor grade, and pathologic DOI were associated with the DSS, further Cox model confirmed the independence of LLN status, neck lymph node metastasis, pathologic tumor grade, and pathologic DOI in predicting the DSS.

DISCUSSION

The most important finding in current study was that the LLN metastasis was significantly associated with the risk of occult metastasis as well as the prognosis in early stage tongue SCC. It could provide benefit in decision making regarding neck management in cT1-2N0 tongue SCC, and also it suggested more advanced treatment would be required in despite of the neck lymph node status.

The presence of neck lymph node metastasis was an important prognostic factor for head and neck SCC (1–3). END was usually an important part in primary operation, but owing to the wide range of occult metastasis rate in cT1-2N0 tongue SCC (10), the neck management of cT1-2N0 tongue SCC has been debated over the years remaining its controversy. Although there was high quality literature including D'Cruz et al. (26) and Ren et al. (27) showed the benefit associated with routine neck dissection, the ideal treatment for patients with cT1-2N0 tongue SCC must be balanced between and the possible surgical morbidity and optimal oncological outcomes. The common principle was that N0 necks should be treated electively when the occult metastatic rate was more than 20% (28). In current study, the overall occult metastasis rate was 27.8%, but the occult metastasis rate was just 17.5% for T1 disease, all patients underwent END. Therefore, there was a number of patients were over-treated, there were at least three aspects for explaining this phenomenon: firstly, the high requirement of routine follow-up of wait-and-see policy was usually out of our patients' ability, as described by our previous studies (13, 25), patients in our cancer hospital usually came from low income family and remote districts; secondly, there was abundant evidence indicating that there was often a low salvage rate on disease recurrence in patients who do not have prophylactic therapy of the clinically N0 neck (1–5), thirdly, also the most important one, there were no reliable predictors for occult neck lymph node metastasis from previous studies.

A number of researchers had aimed to explore the potential predictors for the occult neck lymph node metastasis. Tumor budding was defined as the presence of small clusters of cancer cells or isolated single cancer cell, it suggested a more aggressive biologic behavior and carried more possibility of migrating to the adjacent stroma. Xie et al. (29) described the tumor budding intensity was significantly associated with occult lymph node metastasis. Systemic inflammatory response could promote tumor cell proliferation, microvascular regeneration, and tumor metastasis, further, the peripheral neutrophil-to-lymphocyte ratio (NLR) was an accurate and reliable inflammatory marker. High NLR is thought to be significantly associated with worse survival in solid cancers (28). Abbate et al. (30) firstly presented there was higher risk for occult neck lymph node metastasis when pre-treatment NLR was greater than 2.93. Loganathan et al. (31) recently reported END should be considered when the tumor thickness exceeds 5 mm based on the significant relationship between tumor thickness and occult neck lymph node metastasis. Other analyzed variables included perineural invasion, lymphovascular invasion, and pathologic DOI (32, 33). However, data regarding the these pathologic factors usually could not be obtained preoperatively or during operation, and pretreatment NLR were nonspecific parameters because they could be influenced by concomitant conditions, such as infections or inflammation. Therefore, more accurate indicators were needed. In current study it was noted that LLN metastasis was related to additional nearly 2-fold risk of occult metastasis, and might promote more extensive metastasis. The status of LLNs was easily obtained by frozen section, it might act as a useful indicator for END in early stage tongue SCC. LLNs were not included in any N groups in TNM stage system, the lymph pathway draining to the LLNs passes through the medial side of the submandibular gland parahyoid area and connects to the middle internal jugular lymph nodes (13, 19). Saito et al. (19) firstly described the feasibility of LLN acting as the sentinel lymph node in tongue SCC by imaging methods, current study would support this comment. However, we must considered the fact that the sensitivity and positive test likelihood ratio of positive LLN to predict occult metastasis was a little poor, it was insufficient for deciding neck management, we should not rely solely on the LLN positivity to justify the neck lymph node dissection, more other parameters were needed to increase its reliability.

Prognostic factors for tongue SCC were extensively analyzed, common predictors for worse prognosis included high tumor stage, poor pathologic tumor grade, perineural invasion, lymphovascular invasion, high pathologic DOI, neck lymph node metastasis, high NLR, and so on (2, 3, 13, 14). But the significance of LLN metastasis was rarely assessed. Jia et al. (14) recently reported all the patients with LLN metastases had an advanced neck lymph node classification in their 111 patients, the incidence and metastasis of the LLNs were associated with pathological classifications of SCC of the tongue and the floor of the mouth. Similar finding was also noted in a prospective study by Fang et al. (13), the authors also described LLN metastasis was uncommon, but it could decreased the LRC in advanced tongue SCC. But whether there was similar phenomenon in early stage tongue SCC remained unclear. We were the first to present LLN metastasis significantly decreased the LRC and DSS. In a letter to the editors, Calabrese et al. (34) stated that LLN metastasis could worsen the prognosis and may act as the same way as level I lymph node metastasis. Our findings may support this hypothesis; however, we do not have such data, more studies were needed to clarify this question.

There are some limitations in current study: firstly, the statistical power was reduced by our relatively small sample size. Secondly, there might be more interesting findings found in the future if the follow-up time was longer. Thirdly, lingual lymph nodes were partially dissected by surgeons, and because of our subjective knowledge, there might be bias for detecting the LLNs (35).

CONCLUSIONS

In summary, LLN metastasis is relatively uncommon in early stage tongue SCC, but it is significant associated with the occurrence of occult neck lymph node metastasis, and it apparently decrease the LRC and DSS.

ETHICS STATEMENT

The studies involving human participants were reviewed and approved by Zhengzhou University. The patients/participants provided their written informed consent to participate in this study.

AUTHOR CONTRIBUTIONS

WY, QJ, and PZ: study design and manuscript writing. QJ and PZ: studies selecting and data analysis. WY, MS, HZ, QJ, and JZ: study quality evaluating. WY, JZ, MS, HZ, QJ, and PZ: manuscript revising. All authors have read and approved the final manuscript.

REFERENCES

1. Farhood Z, Simpson M, Ward GM, Walker RJ, Osazuwa-Peters N. Does anatomic subsite influence oral cavity cancer mortality? A SEER database analysis. *Laryngoscope.* (2019) 129:1400–6. doi: 10.1002/lary.27490
2. Fang QG, Shi S, Liu FY, Sun CF. Tongue squamous cell carcinoma as a possible distinct entity in patients under 40 years old. *Oncol Lett.* (2014) 7:2099–102. doi: 10.3892/ol.2014.2054
3. Fang QG, Shi S, Liu FY, Sun CF. Squamous cell carcinoma of the oral cavity in ever smokers: a matched-pair analysis of survival. *J Craniofac Surg.* (2014) 25:934–7. doi: 10.1097/SCS.0000000000000710
4. Afzali P, Ward BB. Management of the neck in oral squamous cell carcinoma: background, classification, and current philosophy. *Oral Maxillofac Surg Clin North Am.* (2019) 31:69–84. doi: 10.1016/j.coms.2018.09.004
5. Yuen AP, Wei WI, Wong YM, Tang KC. Elective neck dissection versus observation in the treatment of early oral tongue carcinoma. *Head Neck.* (1997) 19:583–8. doi: 10.1002/(SICI)1097-0347(199710)19:7<583::AID-HED4>3.0.CO;2-3
6. Mücke T, Mitchell DA, Wagenpfeil S, Ritschl LM, Wolff K-D, Kanatas A. Incidence and outcome for patients with occult lymph node involvement in T1 and T2 oral squamous cell carcinoma: a prospective study. *BMC Cancer.* (2014) 14:346. doi: 10.1186/1471-2407-14-346
7. Feng Z, Li JN, Li CZ, Guo CB. Elective neck dissection versus observation in the management of early tongue carcinoma with clinically node-negative neck: a retrospective study of 229 cases. *J Craniomaxillofac Surg.* (2014) 42:806–10. doi: 10.1016/j.jcms.2013.11.016
8. Cao Y, Wang T, Yu C, Guo X, Li C, Li L. Elective neck dissection versus wait-and-watch policy for oral cavity squamous cell carcinoma in early stage: a systematic review and meta-analysis based on survival data. *J Oral Maxillofac Surg.* (2019) 77:2154–67. doi: 10.1016/j.joms.2019.03.015
9. Lim YC, Lee JS, Koo BS, Kim SH, Kim YH, Choi EC. Treatment of contralateral N0 neck in early squamous cell carcinoma of the oral tongue: elective neck dissection versus observation. *Laryngoscope.* (2006) 116:461–5. doi: 10.1097/01.mlg.0000195366.91395.9b
10. Abu-Ghanem S, Yehuda M, Carmel NN, Leshno M, Abergel A, Gutfeld O, et al. Elective neck dissection vs observation in early-stage squamous cell carcinoma of the oral tongue with no clinically apparent lymph node metastasis in the neck: a systematic review and

meta-analysis. *JAMA Otolaryngol Head Neck Surg.* (2016) 142:857–65. doi: 10.1001/jamaoto.2016.1281

11. Fakih AR, Rao RS, Borges AM, Patel AR. Elective versus therapeutic neck dissection in early carcinoma of the oral tongue. *Am J Surg.* (1989) 158:309–13. doi: 10.1016/0002-9610(89)90122-0
12. Rouviere H. *Anatomy of the Human Lymphatic System.* Ann Arbor, MI: Edward Brothers (1938).
13. Fang Q, Li P, Qi J, Luo R, Chen D, Zhang X. Value of lingual lymph node metastasis in patients with squamous cell carcinoma of the tongue. *Laryngoscope.* (2019) 129:2527–30. doi: 10.1002/lary.27927
14. Jia J, Jia MQ, Zou HX. Lingual lymph nodes in patients with squamous cell carcinoma of the tongue and the floor of the mouth. *Head Neck.* (2018) 40:2383–8. doi: 10.1002/hed.25340
15. Ando M, Asai M, Ono T, Nakanishi Y, Asakage T, Yamasoba T. Metastases to the lingual nodes in tongue cancer: a pitfall in a conventional neck dissection. *Auris Nasus Larynx.* (2010) 37:386–9. doi: 10.1016/j.anl.2009.10.001
16. Dutton JM, Graham SM, Hoffman HT. Metastatic cancer to the floor of mouth: the lingual lymph nodes. *Head Neck.* (2002) 24:401–5. doi: 10.1002/hed.10026
17. Han W, Yang X, Huang X, Hu Q, Wang Z. Metastases to lingual lymph nodes from squamous cell carcinoma of the tongue. *Br J Oral Maxillofac Surg.* (2008) 46:376–8, doi: 10.1016/j.bjoms.2007.12.002
18. Zhang T, Ord RA, Wei WI, Zhao J. Sublingual lymph node metastasis of early tongue cancer: report of two cases and review of the literature. *Int J Oral Maxillofac Surg.* (2011) 40:597–600. doi: 10.1016/j.ijom.2010.12.009
19. Saito M, Nishiyama H, Oda Y, Shingaki S, Hayashi T. The lingual lymph node identified as a sentinel node on CT lymphography in a patient with cN0 squamous cell carcinoma of the tongue. *Dentomaxillofac Radiol.* (2012) 41:254–8. doi: 10.1259/dmfr/61883763
20. Woolgar JA. Histological distribution of cervical lymph node metastases from intraoral/oropharyngeal squamous cell carcinomas. *Br J Oral Maxillofac Surg.* (1999) 37:175–80. doi: 10.1054/bjom.1999.0036
21. Umeda M, Minamikawa T, Shigeta T, Oguni A, Kataoka T, Takahashi H, et al. Metastasis to the lingual lymph node in patients with squamous cell carcinoma of the floor of the mouth: a report of two cases. *Kobe J Med Sci.* (2010) 55:E67–72.
22. Ozeki S, Tashiro H, Okamoto M, Matsushima T. Metastasis to the lingual lymph node in carcinoma of the tongue. *J Maxillofac Surg.* (1985) 13:277–81. doi: 10.1016/S0301-0503(85)80064-3
23. Skulsky SL, O'Sullivan B, McArdle O, Leader M, Roche M, Conlon PJ, et al. Review of high-risk features of cutaneous squamous cell carcinoma and discrepancies between the American Joint Committee on Cancer and NCCN Clinical Practice Guidelines In Oncology. *Head Neck.* (2017) 39:578–94. doi: 10.1002/hed.24580
24. Lydiatt WM, Patel SG, O'Sullivan B, Brandwein MS, Ridge JA, Migliacci JC, et al. Head and Neck cancers-major changes in the American Joint Committee on cancer eighth edition cancer staging manual. *CA Cancer J Clin.* (2017) 67:122–37. doi: 10.3322/caac.21389
25. Dai L, Fang Q, Li P, Wu J, Zhang X. Secondary squamous cell carcinoma of the oral cavity after nasopharyngeal carcinoma. *Cancer Res Treat.* (2020) 52:109–16. doi: 10.4143/crt.2019.202
26. D'Cruz AK, Vaish R, Kapre N, Dandekar M, Gupta S, Hawaldar R, et al. Elective versus therapeutic neck dissection in node-negative oral cancer. *N Engl J Med.* (2015) 373:521–9. doi: 10.1056/NEJMoa1506007
27. Ren ZH, Xu JL, Li B, Fan TF, Ji T, Zhang CP. Elective versus therapeutic neck dissection in node-negative oral cancer: evidence from five randomized controlled trials. *Oral Oncol.* (2015) 51:976–81. doi: 10.1016/j.oraloncology.2015.08.009
28. Weiss MH, Harrison LB, Isaacs RS. Use of decision analysis in planning a management strategy for the stage N0 neck. *Arch Otolaryngol Head Neck Surg.* (1994) 120:699–702. doi: 10.1001/archotol.1994.01880310005001
29. Xie N, Wang C, Liu X, Li R, Hou J, Chen X, et al. Tumor budding correlates with occult cervical lymph node metastasis and poor prognosis in clinical early-stage tongue squamous cell carcinoma. *J Oral Pathol Med.* (2015) 44:266–72. doi: 10.1111/jop.12242
30. Abbate V, Dell'Aversana Orabona G, Salzano G, Bonavolontà P, Maglitto F, Romano A, et al. Pre-treatment neutrophil-to-lymphocyte ratio as a predictor for occult cervical metastasis in early stage (T1-T2 cN0) squamous cell carcinoma of the oral tongue. *Surg Oncol.* (2018) 27:503–7. doi: 10.1016/j.suronc.2018.06.002
31. Loganathan P, Sayan A, Hsu DWK, Paraneetharan S, Ilankovan V. Squamous cell carcinoma of the anterior tongue: is tumour thickness an indicator for cervical metastasis? *Int J Oral Maxillofac Surg.* (2017) 46:407–12. doi: 10.1016/j.ijom.2016.11.003
32. Lim SC, Zhang S, Ishii G, Endoh Y, Kodama K, Miyamoto S, et al. Predictive markers for late cervical metastasis in stage I and II invasive squamous cell carcinoma of the oral tongue. *Clin Cancer Res.* (2004) 10(1 Pt 1):166–72. doi: 10.1158/1078-0432.CCR-0533-3
33. Sparano A, Weinstein G, Chalian A, Yodul M, Weber R. Multivariate predictors of occult neck metastasis in early oral tongue cancer. *Otolaryngol Head Neck Surg.* (2004) 131:472–6. doi: 10.1016/j.otohns.2004.04.008
34. Calabrese L, Renne G, De Cicco C, Chiesa F. Metastatic cancer to the floor of mouth: the lingual lymph nodes. *Head Neck.* (2003) 25:341–2. doi: 10.1002/hed.10259
35. Fang Q, Liu F, Seng D. Oncologic outcome of parotid mucoepidermoid carcinoma in pediatric patients. *Cancer Manag Res.* (2019) 11:1081–5. doi: 10.2147/CMAR.S192788

8

Amplification of 3q26.2, 5q14.3, 8q24.3, 8q22.3 and 14q32.33 are Possible Common Genetic Alterations in Oral Cancer Patients

Melvin A. Ambele[1,2*], *Andre van Zyl*[3], *Michael S. Pepper*[2], *Marlene B. van Heerden*[1] and *Willie F. P. van Heerden*[1]

[1] *Department of Oral Pathology and Oral Biology, Faculty of Health Sciences, School of Dentistry, University of Pretoria, Pretoria, South Africa,* [2] *Department of Immunology, and SAMRC Extramural Unit for Stem Cell Research and Therapy, Faculty of Health Sciences, Institute for Cellular and Molecular Medicine, University of Pretoria, Pretoria, South Africa,* [3] *Specialist in Oral Medicine and Periodontics, Private Practice, Stellenbosch, South Africa*

Correspondence:
Melvin A. Ambele
melvin.ambele@up.ac.za

The lack of clinical biomarkers for head and neck cancer subtypes limits early diagnosis and monitoring of disease progression. This study investigates genetic alterations in clinically identical tumor, tumor-adjacent dysplastic epithelium (TADE) and normal epithelium (NE) in five oral cancer patients to identify differences and commonalities between oral cancer, TADE and NE. A VELscope®Vx device was used to identify TADE and NE surrounding a clinical tumor for analysis of genetic alterations using the OncoScan® assay. One of the tumor samples examined was an "M" class tumor with a high confidence *BRAF*:p.G469A:c.1406G>C somatic mutation, which is the first to be reported in oral cancer. Another tumor showed mosaicism in genetic alterations, indicating the presence of multiple clones. Overall, each patient's tumor, TADE and NE showed a distinct genetic profile which indicates intertumoral clonal/genetic diversity. Interestingly, four tumors showed gain of 3q26.2, 5q14.3, 8q24.3, 8q22.3, 14q32.33 and loss/LOH in 9p21.3 while all TADE had LOH on 22q11.23. In addition, some genetic alterations progressed from NE through TADE into tumor in individual patients. Furthermore, no molecular event was identified that is common to all NE and/or TADE that progressed into tumor. This pilot study demonstrates the presence of genetic heterogeneity in oral tumorigenesis, and suggests that there might exist some common genetic alterations between tumors and TADE. However, this observation would need to be further investigated and validated in a larger cohort of oral cancer patients for its potential role in oral tumorigenesis.

Keywords: oral squamous cell carcinomas, head and neck cancer, genomic heterogeneity, intratumor clonal heterogeneity, intertumoral clonal diversity, OncoScan® FFPE assay, VELscope®Vx device

INTRODUCTION

The Globocan 2018 statistics reported 887,659 new cases of head and neck cancer (lip & oral cavity; 354,864, salivary gland; 52,799, oropharynx; 92,887, nasopharynx; 129,079, hypopharynx; 80,608 and larynx; 177,422 cases) with 453,307 deaths worldwide (http://gco.iarc.fr/today/fact-sheets-cancers). Significant genomic instability and resultant clonal diversity are hallmark characteristics of head and neck squamous cell carcinoma (HNSCC). Heterogeneity in phenotype, etiology, biology and clinical presentation are common features of HNSCC, and this may account for the dismal 5-year survival rates which are as low as 50% in all patients, despite treatment. Except for tumor human papilloma virus (HPV) status, the molecular risk factors investigated in HNSCC have yielded limited clinical utility. Risk stratification for HNSCC is based largely on the tumor anatomical site, stage and histological characteristics (1). Of interest is oral squamous cell carcinoma (OSCC) that develops through a multistep process involving the accumulation of multiple genetic mutations. This process is influenced both by genetic predisposition and environmental risk factors such as tobacco, alcohol, and HPV infection (2). Differences in tumor evolution and progression as well as resistance to therapy in oral cancer can be attributed to intratumoral clonal heterogeneity and intertumoralal clonal diversity, which are seen in clinical cases of oral cancer and other cancers of the head and neck region (1, 3–6). Understanding the molecular mechanisms of clonal heterogeneity within a tumor and clonal diversity between tumors may lead to better treatment outcomes in affected patients.

Field cancerization is to date the most acceptable molecular progression model for OSCC development. The model was proposed by Slaughter et al. and linked the presence of dysplastic changes in tumor-adjacent epithelium of oral cancer specimens with local recurrence and multifocal areas of cancer development process in many cells as a result of exposure to a carcinogen such as tobacco (7). A previous study in our group has also demonstrated this concept of field cancerization in OSCC with heterozygosity in p16 expression (8). Genetic alterations, mainly loss of heterozygosity (LOH) or deletion in chromosomal regions 9p (*CDKN2A*) (2, 9), 3p (*FHIT* & *RSSFIA*) (10, 11), and 17p (*TP53*) (2) have been observed in relatively high proportions of dysplastic lesions and are considered early events in oral carcinogenesis. Losses at 13q and 8p are observed more frequently in carcinomas than in dysplasia, and are associated with late stages of oral carcinogenesis (2, 12).

Inactivation of tumor suppressor genes (TSGs) by loss of heterozygosity (LOH) or deletion and/or the activation of oncogenes by gene amplification are the two major types of genetic alterations most often associated with OSCC tumorigenesis (1, 12, 13). In this study, a VELscope®Vx Handpiece (LED Dental Inc, Canada) was used to identify tumor-adjacent dysplastic epithelium (TADE) and normal epithelium (NE) surrounding a clinically detected cancer. The Affymetrix OncoScan® FFPE assay was then used to investigate the genetic alterations in these specimens with the aim of identifying common molecular events in all tumor, TADE and NE samples. Significant findings could be further explored in a larger cohort of oral cancer patients for their potential role in early to late stages of oral tumorigenesis.

MATERIALS AND METHODS

Clinical Diagnosis of Oral Cancer Patients

Patients with OSSC were referred to the Pretoria Oral and Dental Hospital. Each patient was seen in a specialist clinic where the primary lesion was identified, and a scalpel biopsy was done for histological confirmation of the OSSC. Written informed consent was obtained from all five patients and the study was approved by the Faculty of Health Sciences Research Ethics Committee (Reference number 44/2010).

VELscope® Screening of Oral Cancer Patients and Tissue Collection

The VELscope®Vx Handpiece (LED Dental Inc, Canada) is a portable device with a 40–460 nm light source that has been shown to be effective at identifying lesions at risk of developing cancer in clinically normal mucosa (14). This device has a sensitivity of 98% and a specificity of 100% for identification of oral dysplasia and cancer (15). VELscope® is a diagnostic aid that when applied, results in pale green autofluorescence of normal mucosa and shows loss of fluorescence with abnormal tissue. This fluorescence is viewed through the narrow-band filter built into the eyepiece (16). It has also been shown to be effective at identifying lesions at risk of developing cancer in clinically normal mucosa as seen under normal light (14). One study showed that VELscope® is able to identify LOH at 3p and 9p in mucosa surrounding a clinically detected cancer, with margins as wide as 25 mm (17). Hence, each patient received a comprehensive intra-oral clinical examination with the use of the VELscope® to identify TADE and NE sites (**Figure 1**) for tissue sampling.

DNA Extraction, Quantification, and OncoScan® FFPE Assay

Formalin fixed paraffin embedded (FFPE) specimens of tumor, TADE and NE were prepared from hemi-glossectomy specimens (**Figure 2**) with different histological classification (**Figure 3**). Genomic DNA (gDNA) was extracted from each FFPE sample (tumor, TADE and NE) using the QIAamp DNA FFPE Tissue kit (QIAGEN GmbH, Hilden, Germany) according to the manufacturer's protocol. DNA was quantified using a Quant-iT™ PicoGreen® dsDNA Assay Kit (Life Technologies) following the manufacturer's recommended protocol. Eighty nanogram gDNA was prepared for each sample and run on the Affymetrix OncoScan® FFPE assay kit (Affymetrix; Thermo Fisher Scientific company) according to the manufacturers' instructions (18). The Affymetrix OncoScan® FFPE assay is a molecular analytical tool that works efficiently on formalin-fixed paraffin-embedded (FFPE) samples. It provides a comprehensive coverage of whole genome copy number alterations, LOH and somatic mutations of genes that have been implicated in cancer and tumor progression by utilizing the molecular inversion Probe (MIP) technology (18). Briefly, to each 80 ng of gDNA sample, copy number variation and somatic mutations MIP mixes was added followed by denaturation for 5 min at 95°C and an overnight annealing for 17 h at 58°C. The product of each sample was split into two wells to which dATP (A) and dTTP (T) (A/T) was added into one well while dGTP (G) and dCTP (C) (G/C) was added to the other well to perform a gap fill reaction according to the manufacture's manual. A cocktail of exonucleases supplied with the OncoScan® kit was used to digest gDNA and uncircularized MIP. Cleavage enzymes supplied with the OncoScan® kit

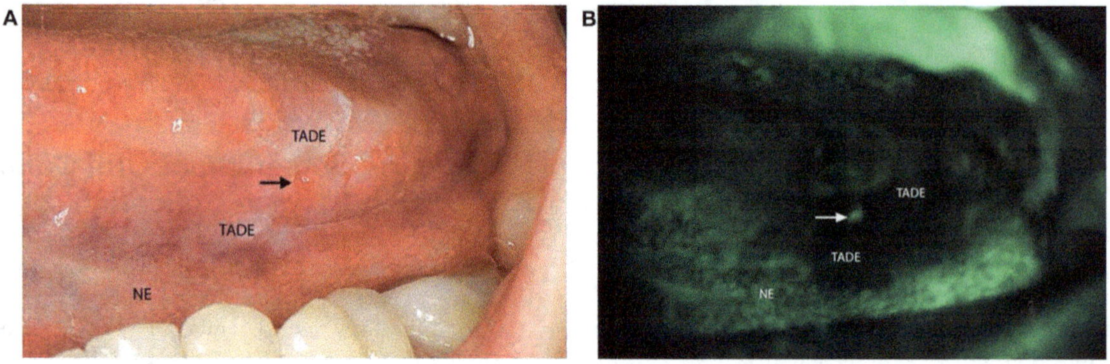

FIGURE 1 | Clinical photo of VELscope® oral cancer screening of a patient. **(A)** Image of a patient with a squamous cell carcinoma on the left side of the tongue presenting as an ulcer (arrow). The tumor adjacent dysplastic epithelium (TADE) that showed loss of fluorescence with the VELscope® is present around the ulcer with the distant clinical normal epithelium (NE) that did not show loss of fluorescence. **(B)** Photograph of the VELscope® analysis showing the ulcer (arrow) with surrounding TADE with loss of autofluorescence and NE showing normal autofluorescence. (Number of patients screened = 5).

were then used to linearize the circular MIP that had been gap filled by A/T or G/C nucleotides followed by a PCR amplification. A second round of PCR amplification was then performed using Haeii enzyme supplied with the OncoScan® kit to cleave amplicons from the previous PCR reaction. The cleaved fragments were then hybridized onto the OncoScan® assay array overnight for 17 h according the manufacturer's protocol. The arrays were then washed and stained using the Affymetrix GeneChip® Fluidics Station 450 and scanned on the Affymetrix GeneChip® Scanner 3000 7G. Each scanned array generates array images known as a DAT file that were automatically converted into fluorescence intensity (CEL) files by the Affymetrix® GeneChip® Command Console® (AGCC) software version 4. CEL files were imported onto the Affymetrix OncoScan™ Console software version 1.3 and processed to generate OSCHP files which were analyzed using Chromosome Analysis Suite (ChAS) for copy number alterations (CNAs) and LOH in approximately 900 cancer genes as well as for 74 clinically actionable somatic mutations in nine cancer genes (*BRAF, EGFR, IDH1, IDH2, KRAS, NRAS, PIK3CA, PTEN,* and *TP53*) (18).

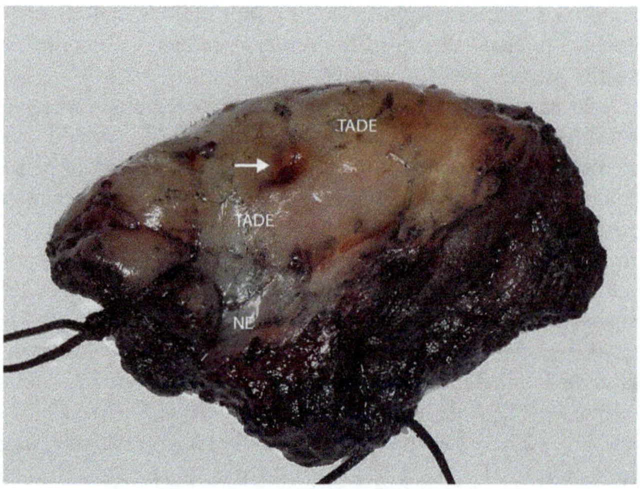

FIGURE 2 | Photograph of hemi-glossectomy specimen. Image showing the carcinoma (arrow) as well as the TADE and NE areas (as determined previously using the VELscope®, number of patients screened = 5).

RESULTS

Sample Size and Classification

Fifteen clinical specimens consisting of 5 tumors, 5 TADE and 5 distant NE from five oral cancer patients were examined in this pilot study for genetic changes such as copy number alterations (CNAs), loss of heterozygosity (LOH) and other somatic mutations (SMs). Of the five tumor samples, four were characterized by high CNAs (referred to as C class tumors) and showed a progressive development of genomic instability characterized by LOH and CNAs from NE through TADE to tumor. One patient's tumor was characterized by a high confidence somatic mutation with few CNAs (referred to as an M class tumor) (19) when compared to the TADE and NE in the same patient.

Genetic Alterations Reveal Both Intratumoral Clonal Heterogeneity and Intertumoral Clonal Diversity

Tumor 1 showed a characteristic HNSCC mutation profile including the amplification of 3q26/28 (*TP63, SOX2, PIK3CA*), *FGFR1*, 11q13 (*CCND1, FADD, CTTN*), *E2F1, PTK2*, loss of *NSD1* and LOH in *CDKN2A* and *TP53* (20). The TADE and NE showed mutations in certain chromosomal regions that do not contain any of the well described HNSCC associated gene mutations. However, some observed molecular events such as the size of a Cn-LOH on 5q14.3 in NE, increased in TADE and changed to a CNL-LOH in the tumor. Also, Cn-LOH on 16q21 in NE and TADE changed to a CNL-LOH in the tumor. Extensive functional studies would be important to validate the significance of these two events in the development and progression of this tumor.

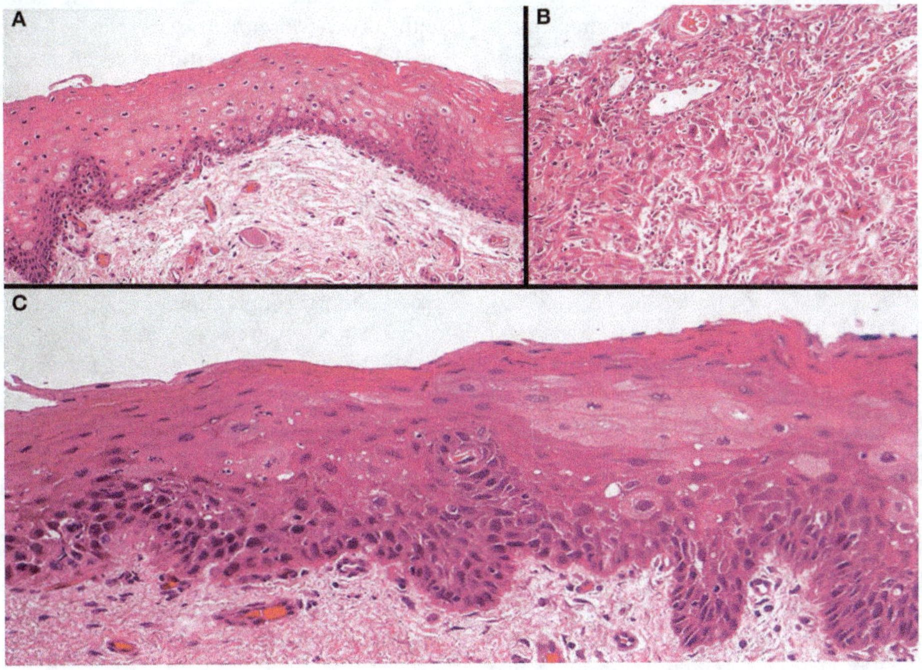

FIGURE 3 | Photomicrograph of the three different areas. Histology of the normal epithelium showing basal cell hyperplasia with no atypia **(A)**. The base of the tumor ulcer consisted of a poorly differentiated squamous cell carcinoma **(B)**. The tumor adjacent dysplastic epithelium (TADE) that showed loss of fluorescence with the VELscope® showed the presence of moderate epithelial dysplasia **(C)**. Original magnification X200.

Tumor 2 is an "M" class tumor (tumor driven by mutation rather than CNAs) typified by a high confidence *BRAF*:p.G469A:c.1406G>C somatic mutation with less genomic instability compared to the TADE and NE. This somatic mutation resulted from the substitution of glycine (G) by alanine (A) at position 469 in *BRAF*. This mutation has been reported in non-small-cell lung cancer (21–23) and in colorectal cancer (24) but not in oral cancer. Loss in *FHIT* and *RB1* were the only well described HNSCC associated mutations (25) detected in TADE and which were absent from both the tumor and NE, suggesting this TADE is an independent clone and not related to the tumor. Interestingly, the size of a loss on 3p26.3 in NE that increased in this TADE would be important to investigate further for possible role in early genetic event in the NE, since a loss in this region has been suggested to be an independent prognostic factor in OSCC patients (26, 27).

Tumor 3 showed mosaicism in CNAs which is indicative of a highly heterogenous tumor with multiple clones. This tumor showed mosaicism in the amplification of *TP63*, *PIK3CA*, *SOX2*, *FADD*, *CTTN*, *CCND1*, *NOTCH1*, *E2F1*, *HRAS*, *BIRC2*, *EGFR*, *MYC*, *PTK2*, loss in *FHIT* and *CDKN2A*, and LOH in *NSD1*, *FAT1* and *APC*. All these mutations constitute a combination of distinct mutation profiles for various molecular sub-types of HNSCC of different etiology (1, 13, 25). Genetic alterations in TADE and NE did not involve any well described HNSCC associated mutations.

Tumor 4 showed amplification of *PIKC3A*, *SOX2*, *TP63*, *EGFR*, *PTK2*, *NOTCH 1, 2 & 3*, *AJUBA*, *TRAF3*, *ERBB2*, *MYC*, and *KMT2D*, loss of *CDKN2A*, *FAT1*, *APC*, *RB1*, *KLK12*, *SMAD4*, and *PTEN*, and LOH of *FHIT*, *CDKN2A*, *CASP8*, *TP53* and *NFE2L2*, which have all been reported in HNSCC (1, 13). TADE and NE had no detectable HNSCC associated mutations. However, the size of a LOH at 3p21.31 in NE and TADE increased in the tumor. In addition, the size of a homozygous deletion of 19p13.2 in NE and TADE that increased in the tumor; this warrants further investigation as it may have played a role in oral cancer development and progression in this patient.

Tumor 5 had a high confidence *PIK3CA*:p.H1047R:c.3140A>G somatic mutation resulting from the substitution of histidine (H) by arginine (R) at position 1047 of the *PIK3CA* gene. This somatic mutation has previously been detected in HNSCC patients (28). This tumor also showed additional mutations such as amplification of *TP63*, *SOX2*, *PIK3CA*, *FADD*, *CTTN*, *CCND1*, *EGFR*, *FGFR1*, *CASP8*, *SMAD4*, *TP53*, *NFE2L2*, *NOTCH1, 2,& 3*, *MYC*, *PTK2*, *AJUBA*, *TRAF3*, *ERBB2*, *NRAS*, *KRAS*, *HRAS*, *FAT1*, *KEAP1*, *E2F1*, and *SMAD2*, loss of *RASSF1*, *FHIT*, *CDKN2A*, *KMT2D*, *RB1*, *APC*, *CSMD1*, *PTPRD*, *MET*, *CUL3*, and *NSD1* and a LOH of *TP53*, *NOTCH1*, *APC*, *RB1*, *CSMD1*, *PTPRD*, *CUL3*, *NSD1*, *CDKN2A*, *FHIT*, and *RASSF1*, which have been reported in HNCSS (1, 13, 25). Mutations detected in TADE and NE were not those that have been well described to be associated with HNSCC.

Identification of Molecular Events Common to Histologically Identical Samples From all Patients

We examined the mutation profile of the three groups of histologically identical sample types (tumor, TADE, and NE) from all five patients in an attempt to identify genetic alterations that are unique to each sample in the different groups (inter-patient heterogeneity) as well as those that are common to all samples in each group, which could potentially be explored in a larger cohort study of oral cancer patients for their clinical significance.

Tumor

With the exception of tumor 2, all tumor samples showed characteristic mutations of HNSCC including amplification of 3q26.2 (*TP63*, *SOX2*, *PIK3CA*) (1), 5q14.3 (*APC*) (13, 29, 30), 8q24.3 (*PTK2*) (25), 8q22.3 (*LRP12*) (27) as well as loss and/or LOH of 9p21.3 (*CDKN2A*) (1, 31). Other characteristic HNSCC mutations such as loss of 4q35.1 (*FAT1*) (1, 31), 5q35.2 (*NSD1*) (1, 31), LOH of 17p13.2 (*TP53*) (1, 31), and amplification of 7p11.2 (*EGFR*) (1, 31), 8q24.21 (*MYC*) (1, 25, 32) and 11q13.3 (*CCND1*, *FADD*, *CTTN*) (1) were detected in three tumors. Interestingly, we also found genetic alterations not previously described in HNSCC such as amplification of 14q32.33 (*LINC00221*) and 20q11.22 in 4 tumors, and loss and/or LOH of 5q23.2, 5q35.1 and loss of 3p24.1 (*NEK10*) in three tumors. There were many other undescribed detectable genetic alterations present in at least 3 tumor samples (**Table S1**). Despite some common molecular features of HNSCC detected in all tumor samples, the type of alteration (gain, loss or LOH) detected in some of the affected chromosomal locations and in certain HNSCC associated genes, differ from one tumor to another, thereby making each tumor genetically distinct (**Table 1**).

Tumor-Adjacent Dysplastic Epithelium (TADE)

Except for TADE 2, all TADE showed fewer CNAs compared to their respective tumor samples. The number of genetic alterations that were common to at least 3 TADE were fewer and different from those found among tumor samples (**Table 2**). Interestingly, a LOH event on 22q11.23 (*GSTTP1*, *LOC391322*, *GSTT1*, *GSTTP2*) was present in all 5 TADE. Other alterations detected in at least 3 TADE includes amplification of 1p13.3 (*GSTM2*, *GSTM1*, *GSTM5*), 14q32.33 (*LINC00221*) and LOH of 3p21.1 (*NEK4*) and 3p21.31. *NEK4* has not been reported in HNSCC tumorigenesis and this gene is known to regulate cell entry into replicative senescence as well as the response to double strand DNA damage (33). Thus, LOH of *NEK4* in OSCC should be functionally investigated further as it could be suggestive of a putative TSG in the development of dysplastic lesions in the oral mucosal. Genetic alterations of a specific type (gain, loss or LOH) in affected chromosomal locations/genes were consistent among TADE unlike in tumor samples. Notwithstanding the limited number of mutations found to be common among TADE, there were alterations that were present and/or absent in a subset of TADE thereby resulting in each patient's TADE having a unique genetic profile (**Table 2**).

Normal Epithelium (NE)

In all patients, NE had fewer CNAs compared to their respective TADE. Only two genetic alterations were common to at least two out of the five NE (**Table 3**). Surprisingly, one of the genetic events—loss and/or LOH of 3p21.3—was common in all the five NE. Inactivating mutations in this region have been a consistent finding in cancers, especially HNSCC, and have been associated with early development of dysplastic lesions in HNSCC (13, 27, 34–43). The clinical significance of this genetic event in NE is unknown and warrants further investigation.

Is There a Marker for Progression in Oral Cancer Tumorigenesis?

We examined genetic alterations present in NE and/or TADE that were also found in tumor and as such could denote progression through clonal expansion from a single progenitor clone. Such progressive genetic alterations from NE and/or TADE to tumor could be suggestive of an early marker for oral cancer development and/or progression. We could not find a single genetic event that was common to all five NE and/or TADE which progressed to tumor. This demonstrates a high level of genetic diversity among all five patients' samples. Nevertheless, the activating mutation of the novel putative oncogene *LINC00221* (14q32.33) and the inactivating mutation of the novel putative TSG *NEK4* (3p21.1) that were detected in TADE1 & 5, were retained as they progressed into their respective tumors.

DISCUSSION

Genetic heterogeneity in HNSCC has been described in tumors from various anatomical sites analyzed using different techniques (3, 5, 44). This pilot study reports analysis of the genome of tumor, TADE and NE from five patients with OSCC with the aim of identifying molecular events in tumor, TADE and NE samples, which could be explored further in a larger cohort study of oral cancer patients for their significance in oral tumorigenesis. Tumor from each patient showed a unique interpatient mutation profile. Differences in the types of genetic alterations (gain, loss and/or LOH) at the same chromosomal location and in some HNSCC associated genes observed in tumor samples are indicative of intertumoral genetic diversity. Tumor 2 showed a high confidence *BRAF*:p.G469A:c.1406G>C somatic mutation (classified as "M" class tumor), which is the first to be reported in oral cancer. This tumor sample showed less genomic instability compared to TADE and NE. "M" class tumors have previously been observed in oral cancer (1, 19). Except for tumor 2, all tumors were characterized by high CNAs classified as "C" class tumors. Tumor 3 showed mosaicism in CNAs, which is indicative of intratumoral clonal heterogeneity. Lack of uniformity in the mutational landscape of all 5 tumors suggests intertumoral clonal/genetic diversity. Except for tumor 2, all tumors showed focal deletion of 3p and amplification of 5p and 8q which contain genes not previously described to be associated with HNSCC. Furthermore, amplification of 14q32.33 (*LINC00221*) and 20q11.22 in all 4 tumors and a loss and/or LOH of 5q23.2, 5q35.1 and 3p24.1 (*NEK10*) in three tumors are interesting findings which would require more detailed functional studies to evaluate their possible role as putative oncogenes and TSGs, respectively, in these regions. *NEK10*, not previously described in HNSCC tumorigenesis, has been reported to mediate G2/M cell cycle arrest (45) and could be a potential TSG in oral cancer.

TABLE 1 | Genetic alterations on the same chromosomal location common to at least three tumors.

Chromosome cytoband start location	Types of alteration in tumor				
	Tumor 1	Tumor 2	Tumor 3	Tumor 4	Tumor 5
1q31.1	–	LOH	–	Gain	Gain
3p26.3 (26, 27)	–	–	Loss	Loss	Loss
4q31.2	–	–	Loss	Gain	Gain
4q35.1 (*FAT1*) (1, 31)	–	–	Loss	Loss	Gain
5q11.2	Loss	–	–	Loss	Loss
6p25.2	LOH	–	Gain	Gain	LOH
7p11.2 (*EGFR*) (1, 31)	–	–	Gain	Gain	Gain
9p23	LOH	Gain	Gain	Loss	LOH
11q13.3 (*CCND1*, *FADD*, *CTTN*) (1)	Gain	–	Gain	–	Gain
12q24.12 (*ALDH2*)	LOH	LOH	–	Gain	–
13q13.1	Loss	–	–	LOH	Loss
15q11.2	Gain	–	Loss	Loss	Gain
16p13.3	LOH	–	Loss	Gain	Gain
17p13.2 (*TP53*) (1, 31)	LOH	–	–	LOH	Gain + LOH
20q11.21	Gain	–	Gain	–	Gain
22q11.23 (*GSTT1*)	–	–	Gain	Gain	Gain

The same chromosomal location revealed intertumoral genetic diversity of all five tumors based on either (a) a discrepancy in the genetic alterations (gain, loss, or LOH) or (b) the presence/absence of a genetic alteration only in certain tumors.

TABLE 2 | Genetic alterations on the same chromosomal location common to at least two TADE.

Chromosome cytoband start location	Types of alteration in TADE				
	TADE 1	TADE 2	TADE 3	TADE 4	TADE 5
1p13.3 (*GSTM1*) (46)	–	Gain	–	Gain	Gain
3p21.1 (*NEK4*)	LOH	LOH	–	–	LOH
3p21.31 (*RASSF1*)	LOH	Loss	–	LOH	–
14q32.33 (*LINC00221*)	Gain	Gain	–	–	Gain
22q11.23 (*GSTT1*) (47)	LOH	LOH	Gain + LOH	LOH	Gain +LOH

All 5 TADE showed differences in genetic alteration (LOH, gain, gain + LOH, or none) at the same loci.

TABLE 3 | Genetic alterations common to at least two NE.

Chromosome cytoband start location	Types of alteration in NE				
	NE 1	NE 2	NE 3	NE 4	NE 5
3p21.3	LOH	Loss + LOH	LOH	Loss + LOH	LOH
5q23.3	–	LOH	LOH	–	–
11p11.12	LOH	–	–	–	Gain

Genetic alterations detected were mostly loss and LOH on chromosomes 3p, 5q, and 11p which could be used to distinguish between individual patient's NE.

Interestingly, TADE from all 5 patients showed inactivating mutations of 22q11.23 (*GSTTP1*, *LOC391322*, *GSTT1*, *GSTTP2*). The clinical significance of this genetic alteration in all five patients is unknown. However, given the presence of a traditional risk factor (tobacco consumption) in all patients, further studies are warranted.

Surprisingly, all five NE showed inactivating mutations of 3p21.3, known to contain TSGs or resident cancer genes. Alterations in this region are one of the most consistent genetic events reported not only in HNSCC but also in other cancer types (13, 27, 34–43). The presence of this genetic alteration in NE of all patients is therefore very surprising; could it possibly be that this particular region of the human genome is naturally very unstable? Further investigation of NE in both healthy individuals and oral cancer patients would be beneficial in understanding this genomic region and its associated genetic alterations.

CONCLUSION

Amplification of 3q26.2, 5q14.3, 8q24.3, 8q22.3, 14q32.33, 20q11.22 together with a loss/LOH on 9p21.3 was detected in four out of the five oral cancer samples, and a LOH on 22q11.23 detected in all five TADE. Furthermore, no molecular event was identified that is common to all NE and/or TADE that progressed into tumor. The small sample size limits the clinical significance of these findings. We therefore recommend further studies in a larger cohort of oral cancer patients to determine their significance in oral cancer biology.

ETHICS STATEMENT

The studies involving human participants were reviewed and approved by University of Pretoria Faculty of Health Sciences Research Ethics Committee (Reference number 44/2010). The patients/participants provided their written informed consent to participate in this study.

AUTHOR CONTRIBUTIONS

MA performed the OncoScan® assay, data analysis, interpretation, and wrote the first draft of the manuscript. AZ conceptualized the study, performed clinical examination of patients, the Velscope® screening, data interpretation, and edited the manuscript, MP contributed to the study design, data interpretation, edited the manuscript, and provided funding for the study. MH prepared FFPE specimen of all tissues, performed DNA isolation, and edited the manuscript. WH conceptualized the study, performed clinical examination of patients, data interpretation, edited the manuscript, and provided funding for the study.

ACKNOWLEDGMENTS

The authors would like to thank the five oral cancer subjects that consented and participated in this study and Izak Storm at BIOCOM Africa and Jo Mcbride at the Centre for Proteomic & Genomic Research, Cape Town for their technical support with the OncoScan® assay.

REFERENCES

1. The Cancer Genome Atlas N, Lawrence MS, Sougnez C, Lichtenstein L, Cibulskis K, Lander E, et al. Comprehensive genomic characterization of head and neck squamous cell carcinomas. *Nature.* (2015) 517:576. doi: 10.1038/nature14129
2. Califano J, van der Riet P, Westra W, Nawroz H, Clayman G, Piantadosi S, et al. Genetic progression model for head and neck cancer: implications for field cancerization. *Cancer Res.* (1996) 56:2488–92. doi: 10.1016/S0194-5998(96)80631-0
3. Mroz EA, Rocco JW. Intra-tumor heterogeneity in head and neck cancer and its clinical implications. *World J Otorhinolaryngol Head Neck Surg.* (2016) 2:60–7. doi: 10.1016/j.wjorl.2016.05.007
4. Zhang XC, Xu C, Mitchell RM, Zhang B, Zhao D, Li Y, et al. Tumor evolution and intratumor heterogeneity of an oropharyngeal squamous cell carcinoma revealed by whole-genome sequencing. *Neoplasia.* (2013) 15:1371–8. doi: 10.1593/neo.131400
5. Sarode G, Sarode SC, Tupkari J, Patil S. Is oral squamous cell carcinoma unique in terms of intra- and inter-tumoral heterogeneity? *Transl Res Oral Oncol.* (2017) 2:2057178X17703578. doi: 10.1177/2057178X17703578
6. Klussmann JP. Head and neck cancer - new insights into a heterogeneous disease. *Oncol Res Treat.* (2017) 40:318–9. doi: 10.1159/000477255
7. Slaughter DP, Southwick HW, Smejkal W. Field cancerization in oral stratified squamous epithelium; clinical implications of multicentric origin. *Cancer.* (1953) 6:963–8. doi: 10.1002/1097-0142(195309)6:5<963::AID-CNCR2820060515>3.0.CO;2-Q
8. Ambele MA, Pepper MS, van Heerden MB, van Heerden WFP. Heterozygosity of p16 expression in an oral squamous cell carcinoma with associated loss of heterozygosity and copy number alterations. *Head Neck.* (2019) 41:E62–5. doi: 10.1002/hed.25566
9. Mao L, Lee JS, Fan YH, Ro JY, Batsakis JG, Lippman S, et al. Frequent microsatellite alterations at chromosomes 9p21 and 3p14 in oral premalignant lesions and their value in cancer risk assessment. *Nat Med.* (1996) 2:682–5. doi: 10.1038/nm0696-682
10. Masayesva BG, Ha P, Garrett-Mayer E, Pilkington T, Mao R, Pevsner J, et al. Gene expression alterations over large chromosomal regions in cancers include multiple genes unrelated to malignant progression. *Proc Natl Acad Sci USA.* (2004) 101:8715–20. doi: 10.1073/pnas.0400027101
11. Garnis C, Baldwin C, Zhang L, Rosin MP, Lam WL. Use of complete coverage array comparative genomic hybridization to define copy number alterations on chromosome 3p in oral squamous cell carcinomas. *Cancer Res.* (2003) 63:8582–5.
12. Choi S, Myers JN. Molecular pathogenesis of oral squamous cell carcinoma: implications for therapy. *J Dental Res.* (2008) 87:14–32. doi: 10.1177/154405910808700104
13. Kasamatsu A, Uzawa K, Usukura K, Koike K, Nakashima D, Ishigami T, et al. Loss of heterozygosity in oral cancer. *Oral Sci Int.* (2011) 8:37–43. doi: 10.1016/S1348-8643(11)00027-9
14. Poh CF, Ng SP, Williams PM, Zhang L, Laronde DM, Lane P, et al. Direct fluorescence visualization of clinically occult high-risk oral premalignant disease using a simple hand-held device. *Head Neck.* (2007) 29:71–6. doi: 10.1002/hed.20468
15. Lane PM, Gilhuly T, Whitehead P, Zeng H, Poh CF, Ng S, et al. Simple device for the direct visualization of oral-cavity tissue fluorescence. *J Biomed Opt.* (2006) 11:024006. doi: 10.1117/1.2193157
16. Lingen MW, Kalmar JR, Karrison T, Speight PM. Critical evaluation of diagnostic aids for the detection of oral cancer. *Oral Oncol.* (2008) 44:10–22. doi: 10.1016/j.oraloncology.2007.06.011
17. Poh CF, Zhang L, Anderson DW, Durham JS, Williams PM, Priddy RW, et al. Fluorescence visualization detection of field alterations in tumor

margins of oral cancer patients. *Clin Cancer Res.* (2006) 12:6716–22. doi: 10.1158/1078-0432.CCR-06-1317

18. Foster JM, Oumie A, Togneri FS, Vasques FR, Hau D, Taylor M, et al. Cross-laboratory validation of the OncoScan(R) FFPE Assay, a multiplex tool for whole genome tumour profiling. *BMC Med Genom.* (2015) 8:5. doi: 10.1186/s12920-015-0079-z
19. Ciriello G, Miller ML, Aksoy BA, Senbabaoglu Y, Schultz N, Sander C. Emerging landscape of oncogenic signatures across human cancers. *Nat Genet.* (2013) 45:1127–33. doi: 10.1038/ng.2762
20. Hanahan D, Weinberg RA. Hallmarks of cancer: the next generation. *Cell.* (2011) 144:646–74. doi: 10.1016/j.cell.2011.02.013
21. Cardarella S, Ogino A, Nishino M, Butaney M, Shen J, Lydon C, et al. Clinical, pathologic, and biologic features associated with BRAF mutations in non-small cell lung cancer. *Clin Cancer Res.* (2013) 19:4532–40. doi: 10.1158/1078-0432.CCR-13-0657
22. Davies H, Bignell GR, Cox C, Stephens P, Edkins S, Clegg S, et al. Mutations of the BRAF gene in human cancer. *Nature.* (2002) 417:949–54. doi: 10.1038/nature00766
23. Paik PK, Arcila ME, Fara M, Sima CS, Miller VA, Kris MG, et al. Clinical characteristics of patients with lung adenocarcinomas harboring BRAF mutations. *J Clin Oncol.* (2011) 29:2046–51. doi: 10.1200/JCO.2010.33.1280
24. Rizzo S, Bronte G, Fanale D, Corsini L, Silvestris N, Santini D, et al. Prognostic vs predictive molecular biomarkers in colorectal cancer: is KRAS and BRAF wild type status required for anti-EGFR therapy? *Cancer Treat Rev.* (2010) 36 (Suppl. 3):S56–61. doi: 10.1016/S0305-7372(10)70021-9
25. Leemans CR, Braakhuis BJ, Brakenhoff RH. The molecular biology of head and neck cancer. *Nat Rev Cancer.* (2011) 11:9–22. doi: 10.1038/nrc2982
26. Uchida K, Oga A, Nakao M, Mano T, Mihara M, Kawauchi S, et al. Loss of 3p26.3 is an independent prognostic factor in patients with oral squamous cell carcinoma. *Oncol Rep.* (2011) 26:463–9. doi: 10.3892/or.2011.1327
27. Vincent-Chong VK, Salahshourifar I, Woo KM, Anwar A, Razali R, Gudimella R, et al. Genome wide profiling in oral squamous cell carcinoma identifies a four genetic marker signature of prognostic significance. *PLoS ONE.* (2017) 12:e0174865. doi: 10.1371/journal.pone.0174865
28. Janku F, Wheler JJ, Naing A, Falchook GS, Hong DS, Stepanek VM, et al. PIK3CA mutation H1047R is associated with response to PI3K/AKT/mTOR signaling pathway inhibitors in early-phase clinical trials. *Cancer Res.* (2013) 73:276–84. doi: 10.1158/0008-5472.CAN-12-1726
29. Largey JS, Meltzer SJ, Sauk JJ, Hebert CA, Archibald DW. Loss of heterozygosity involving the APC gene in oral squamous cell carcinomas. *Oral Surg Oral Med Oral Pathol.* (1994) 77:260–3. doi: 10.1016/0030-4220(94)90295-X
30. Rivero ER, Horta MC, Silva Guerra EN, Ferraz AR, Nunes FD. Loss of heterozygosity of the APC gene in oral squamous cell carcinoma. *Pathol Res Pract.* (2008) 204:793–7. doi: 10.1016/j.prp.2008.05.003
31. Leemans CR, Snijders PJF, Brakenhoff RH. The molecular landscape of head and neck cancer. *Nat Rev Cancer.* (2018) 18:269–82. doi: 10.1038/nrc.2018.11
32. Rodrigo JP, Lazo PS, Ramos S, Alvarez I, Suarez C. MYC amplification in squamous cell carcinomas of the head and neck. *Arch Otolaryngol Head Neck Surg.* (1996) 122:504–7. doi: 10.1001/archotol.1996.01890170038008
33. Nguyen CL, Possemato R, Bauerlein EL, Xie A, Scully R, Hahn WC. Nek4 regulates entry into replicative senescence and the response to DNA damage in human fibroblasts. *Mol Cell Biol.* (2012) 32:3963–77. doi: 10.1128/MCB.00436-12
34. Ghosh S, Ghosh A, Maiti GP, Alam N, Roy A, Roy B, et al. Alterations of 3p21.31 tumor suppressor genes in head and neck squamous cell carcinoma: Correlation with progression and prognosis. *Int J Cancer.* (2008) 123:2594–604. doi: 10.1002/ijc.23834
35. Angeloni D. Molecular analysis of deletions in human chromosome 3p21 and the role of resident cancer genes in disease. *Brief Funct Genom Proteom.* (2007) 6:19–39. doi: 10.1093/bfgp/elm007
36. Marsit CJ, Hasegawa M, Hirao T, Kim DH, Aldape K, Hinds PW, et al. Loss of heterozygosity of chromosome 3p21 is associated with mutant TP53 and better patient survival in non-small-cell lung cancer. *Cancer Res.* (2004) 64:8702–7. doi: 10.1158/0008-5472.CAN-0 4-2558
37. Wang K, Ling T, Wu H, Zhang J. Screening of candidate tumor-suppressor genes in 3p21.3 and investigation of the methylation of gene promoters in oral squamous cell carcinoma. *Oncol Rep.* (2013) 29:1175–82. doi: 10.3892/or.2012.2213
38. Dasgupta S, Chakraborty SB, Roy A, Roychowdhury S, Panda CK. Differential deletions of chromosome 3p are associated with the development of uterine cervical carcinoma in Indian patients. *Mol Pathol.* (2003) 56:263–9. doi: 10.1136/mp.56.5.263
39. Martin CL, Reshmi SC, Ried T, Gottberg W, Wilson JW, Reddy JK, et al. Chromosomal imbalances in oral squamous cell carcinoma: examination of 31 cell lines and review of the literature. *Oral Oncol.* (2008) 44:369–82. doi: 10.1016/j.oraloncology.2007.05.003
40. Hogg RP, Honorio S, Martinez A, Agathanggelou A, Dallol A, Fullwood P, et al. Frequent 3p allele loss and epigenetic inactivation of the RASSF1A tumour suppressor gene from region 3p21.3 in head and neck squamous cell carcinoma. *Eur J Cancer.* (2002) 38:1585–92. doi: 10.1016/S0959-8049(01) 00422-1
41. Maestro R, Gasparotto D, Vukosavljevic T, Barzan L, Sulfaro S, Boiocchi M. Three discrete regions of deletion at 3p in head and neck cancers. *Cancer Res.* (1993) 53:5775–9.
42. Chakraborty SB, Sabbir MG, Roy A, Sengupta A, Panda CK. Multiple deletions in chromosome 3p are associated with the development of head and neck squamous cell carcinoma. *Int J Human Genet.* (2003) 3:79–87. doi: 10.1080/09723757.2003.11885832
43. Chakraborty SB, Dasgupta S, Roy A, Sengupta A, Ray B, Roychoudhury S, et al. Differential deletions in 3p are associated with the development of head and neck squamous cell carcinoma in Indian patients. *Cancer Genet Cytogenet.* (2003) 146:130–8. doi: 10.1016/S0165-4608(03)00127-4
44. Mroz EA, Tward AD, Hammon RJ, Ren Y, Rocco JW. Intra-tumor genetic heterogeneity and mortality in head and neck cancer: analysis of data from the Cancer Genome Atlas. *PLoS Med.* (2015) 12:e1001786. doi: 10.1371/journal.pmed.1001786
45. Moniz LS, Stambolic V. Nek10 mediates G2/M cell cycle arrest and MEK autoactivation in response to UV irradiation. *Mol Cell Biol.* (2011) 31:30–42. doi: 10.1128/MCB.00648-10
46. Zhang X, Huang M, Wu X, Kadlubar S, Lin J, Yu X, et al. GSTM1 copy number and promoter haplotype as predictors for risk of recurrence and/or second primary tumor in patients with head and neck cancer. *Pharmacogenom Personal Med.* (2013) 6:9–17. doi: 10.2147/PGPM.S 35949
47. Singh M, Shah PP, Singh AP, Ruwali M, Mathur N, Pant MC, et al. Association of genetic polymorphisms in glutathione S-transferases and susceptibility to head and neck cancer. *Mutat Res.* (2008) 638:184–94. doi: 10.1016/j.mrfmmm.2007.10.003

9

"Fistula Zero" Project After Total Laryngectomy: The Candiolo Cancer Institute Experience

Erika Crosetti [1], Giulia Arrigoni [1], Andrea Elio Sprio [2] and Giovanni Succo [1,3]*

[1] Head and Neck Oncology Unit, Candiolo Cancer Institute, Fondazione del Piemonte per l'Oncologia - IRCCS (FPO-IRCCS), Candiolo, Italy, [2] Department of Biomedical and Clinic Sciences, University of Turin, Orbassano, Italy, [3] Department of Oncology, University of Turin, Orbassano, Italy

***Correspondence:**
Erika Crosetti
erika.crosetti@ircc.it*

Objectives: Pharyngocutaneous fistula (PCF) is a troublesome complication after total laryngectomy. The "Fistula zero" project aims to reduce the number of PCF by following a detailed protocol based on three fundamental key points.

Materials and Methods: The Fistula zero project included 77 patients who underwent total laryngectomy in the period from January 2019 to December 2020. The protocol consisted of three main aspects: the systematic placement of a Har-El salivary bypass tube, the continuous horizontal watertight pharyngeal suture using a barbed suture, onlay insetting of a pedicled flap in pre-treated patients.

Results: One case of PCF (1.3%) and three small blind fistulas (3.9%) were observed in this series. The mean length of hospitalization was 18 days.

Conclusion: Pharyngocutaneous fistula (PCF) prolongs hospitalization and delays adjuvant treatments. Thanks to a strict adherence to the protocol, it was possible to reduce PCF rates, avoiding lengthy hospitalization and additional surgical procedures.

Keywords: laryngeal cancer, total laryngectomy, pharyngocutaneous fistula, complications, Montgomery tube, bypass tube, pedicled flap, head and neck cancer

INTRODUCTION

Total laryngectomy (TL) is considered the gold standard surgical treatment for advanced laryngeal cancer. Surgery can be performed as primary treatment or as salvage treatment after failure of previous surgical or non-surgical protocols.

Pharyngocutaneous fistula (PCF) is a common complication after TL, with an incidence ranging from 3% to 65% (1–4) [9–25% after primary surgery, 30–70% after salvage laryngectomy (5)]. When PCFs occur after total laryngectomy, several challenging consequences have to be expected: delays for adjuvant treatments, frequent need for revision surgery, an increase in the length of hospitalization, delays in the rehabilitation process leading up to oral food intake, reduction in quality of life, and higher costs (both social and economic).

Abbreviations: COPD, chronic obstructive pulmonary disease; PCF, pharyngocutaneous fistula; TL, total laryngectomy; NGT, naso-gastric tube; ND, neck dissection; TLM, transoral laser microsurgery; OPHL, open partial horizontal laryngectomy.

Many studies have focused on the risk factors associated with PCF (6, 7) and many surgical strategies have been proposed to reduce its incidence (3, 5, 8, 9). Of these, one is represented by the routine placement of a salivary bypass tube. Even though some interesting results related to this strategy are reported in the literature, robust evidence is still lacking (10, 11).

The main aim of this study is to present the results of the project, titled "Fistula zero after total laryngectomy."

MATERIALS AND METHODS

In total, 77 consecutive patients underwent primary/salvage TL at the Head and Neck Oncological Unit of the FPO IRCCS, Candiolo Cancer Institute, in the period from January 2019 to December 2020 and were included in this study.

All of the procedures performed were considered to be conventional in terms of technique and indications, according to the current guidelines, to the ethical standards of the Institutional and/or National Research Committee and to the 1964 Helsinki Declaration and its later amendments. Ethical review and approval were not required for this study in accordance with the national and institutional requirements. Before surgery, every patient signed a consent form for the disclosure of appropriate personal data for scientific purposes. Written informed consent was obtained from all of the patients. They all underwent the same clinical assessment during the 3 weeks before surgery, including clinical examination, nutritional status evaluation (body mass index [BMI]), biopsy/pathological examination, maxillofacial and neck MRI/CT scan, and total body PET scan. Two surgeons (GS and EC) carried out all of the procedures. Demographic data for the study population are summarized in **Table 1**.

The "fistula zero protocol" was adopted for the whole series. Following the protocol, a Har-El salivary bypass tube (Boston Medical™, Westborough, MA, USA) was placed in the neopharynx with a naso-gastric tube (NGT) positioned inside it before performing the pharyngeal closure; the bypass tube was secured by a stitch passing through the base of the tongue toward the skin, where it was knotted to prevent pressure ulcers (**Figures 1A–E**). The Har-El pharyngeal tube was chosen because of its particular funnel shape, designed to be easily anchored at the tongue base. The posterior aspect of the tube is higher while the anterior wall has a lower, flattened profile: this feature prevents it from being displaced upward into the oropharynx.

A watertight pharyngeal suture was performed using a continuous barbed suture (V-lock suture; Covidien™, Mansfield, VA, USA). Two resorbable stitches were placed at each end of the neopharynx to keep the mucosa stretched; two V-lock sutures were used to suture each hemipharynx as far as the midline. A second layer of reinforcement was then made with a third barbed suture. In pre-treated patients [radiotherapy (RT) with or without concomitant chemotherapy (CRT)], a pedicled flap (pectoralis major myofascial flap) was harvested and placed upon the pharyngeal suture.

Patients who had undergone earlier laryngeal surgical procedures [transoral laser microsurgery (TLM)/open partial horizontal laryngectomy (OPHL)] were not included in this group. This study focused on patients pre-treated with chemoradiotherapy, since such treatments may represent one of the main risk factors for postoperative fistula formation.

In every patient, a barium dynamic swallowing test with liquid and semi-liquid bolus was performed in both antero-posterior and lateral projections before commencing oral intake. The exam was performed on the 9th postoperative day in the group of patients where no reconstructive surgery was carried out, and on the 12th postoperative day in the group of patients who underwent reconstructive surgery by pectoralis major myofascial flap. In the case of absence of PCF, oral food intake started on the 10th postoperative day for patients who underwent only total laryngectomy without reconstruction, and on the 13th postoperative day for those who underwent reconstructive surgery. Oral feeding began with the salivary bypass tube in place and after 2 days, the patient was discharged. The NGT was removed on the same day as commencement of oral feeding and the salivary bypass tube was removed 1 week after the barium swallowing test (if it showed no fistulas).

When the barium swallowing test indicated the presence of a PCF/blind fistula, a compressive cervical dressing was put in place and oral feeding was delayed.

RESULTS

The fistula zero protocol was applied in 77 patients (70 men, 7 women) who underwent primary/salvage TL for laryngeal cancer; the median age was 67 years (range, 47–90 years).

In total, 27 patients (35.1%) were pre-treated [RT: 7 patients (9.1%), CRT: 20 patients (26.0%)]. Comorbidities were scored by applying the Adult Comorbidity Evaluation-27 Index (12). This score is composed of 12 organ system related categories and 27 subcategories; it aims to quantify a specific disease. The Overall Comorbidity Score was defined according to the highest ranked single disorder (0 = none, 1 = mild, 2 = moderate, and 3 = severe). More than two grade 2 scores gave an overall score of 3.

Nineteen patients (25%) were staged pT3: they were not amenable to OPHL or organ-sparing protocols due to important comorbidities (ACE-27 grade 2). Moreover, some of them had undergone previous chemoradiotherapeutic treatments for oropharyngeal squamous cell carcinoma/non-Hodgkin lymphoma. Four patients (5%) were very old (>80 years) and had severe comorbidities (ACE-27 grade 3): in these cases, we preferred to carry out a total laryngectomy.

The median intraoperative time for the surgical procedure was 210 min.

The salivary bypass tube demonstrated good patient-tolerability with no complications (bypass tube dislocation, migration, granulation tissue formation). The average length of hospitalization was 18 days (range, 12–40 days): 21 days for patients who underwent reconstruction and 16 days for those who did not.

TABLE 1 | Demographic data for the 77 patients in this study.

Characteristic	No. of patients (%)
Age, years	
Mean	67 ± 10
Range	47–90
Sex	
Male	70 (90.9)
Female	7 (9.1)
Comorbidities	
No	15 (19.5)
1 comorbidity	18 (23.4)
2 comorbidities	30 (38.9)
≥3 comorbidities	14 (18.2)
ACE-27 Grade 1	39 (50)
ACE-27 Grade 2	19 (24)
ACE-27 Grade 3	4 (5)
BMI	
Mean	24
Range	17–31
Pre-treatment	
Yes	27 (35.1)
No	50 (64.9)
Pathological status	
pT4a	27 (35.1)
pT3	19 (24.7)
pT2	4 (5.2)
ypT4	16 (20.8)
ypT3	6 (7.8)
ypT2	5 (6.5)
Neck dissection	
Ipsilateral	30 (39)
Pre-treated	12 (17)
Primary	18 (23)
Bilateral	40 (51.9)
Pre-treated	8 (10)
Primary	32 (41)
None	
Pre-treated	7 (9.1)
Thyroidectomy	
Hemi-thyroidectomy	20 (26)
Total thyroidectomy	27 (35.1)
Hystmectomy	30 (38.9)
Complications	
PCF	1 (1.3) [not-pre treated]
Minimum extraluminal spill of barium	3 (3.9) [2 pre-treated (2.5%), 1 primary patient (1%)]

PCF occurred in only one patient who had not been pre-treated (1.3%), who experienced more than three comorbidities (cardiopathy, diabetes, kidney failure, chronic obstructive pulmonary disease, ACE-27 grade 3) and who was treated by revision surgery (a pectoralis major myofascial flap was harvested and placed to cover the PCF). Three patients (3.9%), two pre-treated and one not pre-treated, developed a minimum extraluminal spill of barium (blind fistula), successfully managed with a compression dressing. In these cases, oral feeding was postponed. Donor-site complication (seroma) occurred in four pre-treated patients (5%) and was managed with a compression dressing.

DISCUSSION

Complications after TL are always associated with delayed adjuvant treatment, a longer hospitalization due to the delayed rehabilitation, and the need for additional postoperative surgical procedures. However, a trend toward a reduction in postoperative complications has recently been reported. In a systematic review of 522 studies (2177 patients), Sayles and Grant reported an incidence of 14.3% for pharyngocutaneous fistula in patients treated by primary laryngectomy with an increased incidence of 27.6% after salvage laryngectomy (3).

There are several risk factors related to PCF, which can be summarized as patient-related, disease-related and treatment-related. Concerning patient-related risk factors, age > 60 years, presence of > 1 comorbidity (lung disease, cardiopathy, diabetes), smoking status, nutritional status, low albumin level, and low hemoglobin level (7, 13–16) have to be considered. Disease-related risk factors are represented by advanced T stage and tumor site (supraglottic region) (17). Regarding treatment-related risk factors, previous treatments, such as RT/CRT, causing tissue fibrosis and skin necrosis, can lead to delayed mucosa healing, resulting in PCF. Neck dissection, requiring a longer operating time, could lead to an increased risk of wound infection and PCF formation. In addition, the skill of the surgeon, especially with regard to watertight closure of the pharyngeal wall, could represent a risk factor for PCF formation.

The "fistula zero protocol" was introduced to minimize the rate of PCF formation after TL, based on information from literature data. Many studies have analyzed the usefulness of the salivary bypass tube in preventing PCF formation, but the heterogeneity of patients included in those studies did not allow a meaningful meta-analysis to support strong evidence in clinical practice (11). The salivary bypass tube, placed for the first time in 1978 by Montgomery (18) to bridge the gap between the pharyngostome and esophagostome after laryngoesophagectomy, is recommended in high-risk patients to prevent PCF formation after total laryngectomy and to prevent stenosis of the cervical esophagus and tracheoesophageal fistula (11, 19).

More recently, Gilardi et al. precisely described how to manage the positioning of a salivary bypass tube with the help of a Cuffed-Reinforced Oral/Nasal Tracheal Tube, to prevent or treat some complications of laryngeal and hypopharyngeal surgery (20). Moreover, many authors have previously endorsed the application of a salivary pharyngeal tube, often in association with reconstructive surgery, to help wound healing in patients who developed PCF after laryngeal surgery (21–24).

Concerning the present study, the calyx-shaped Har-El pharyngeal tube allows better adaptability to the pharynx, allowing an efficient collection of saliva inside the tube, therefore reducing its spread over the pharyngeal suture.

On the other hand, based on literature data, closure of the pharyngeal wall could represent a risk factor for PCF formation. Several studies have demonstrated that a mechanical pharyngeal suture could represent an advantage in patients undergoing total laryngectomy, mainly for the reduction in PCF formation (8.7% with an absolute risk reduction of 15%). Nevertheless, the benefits offered by stapler-assisted closure could not be

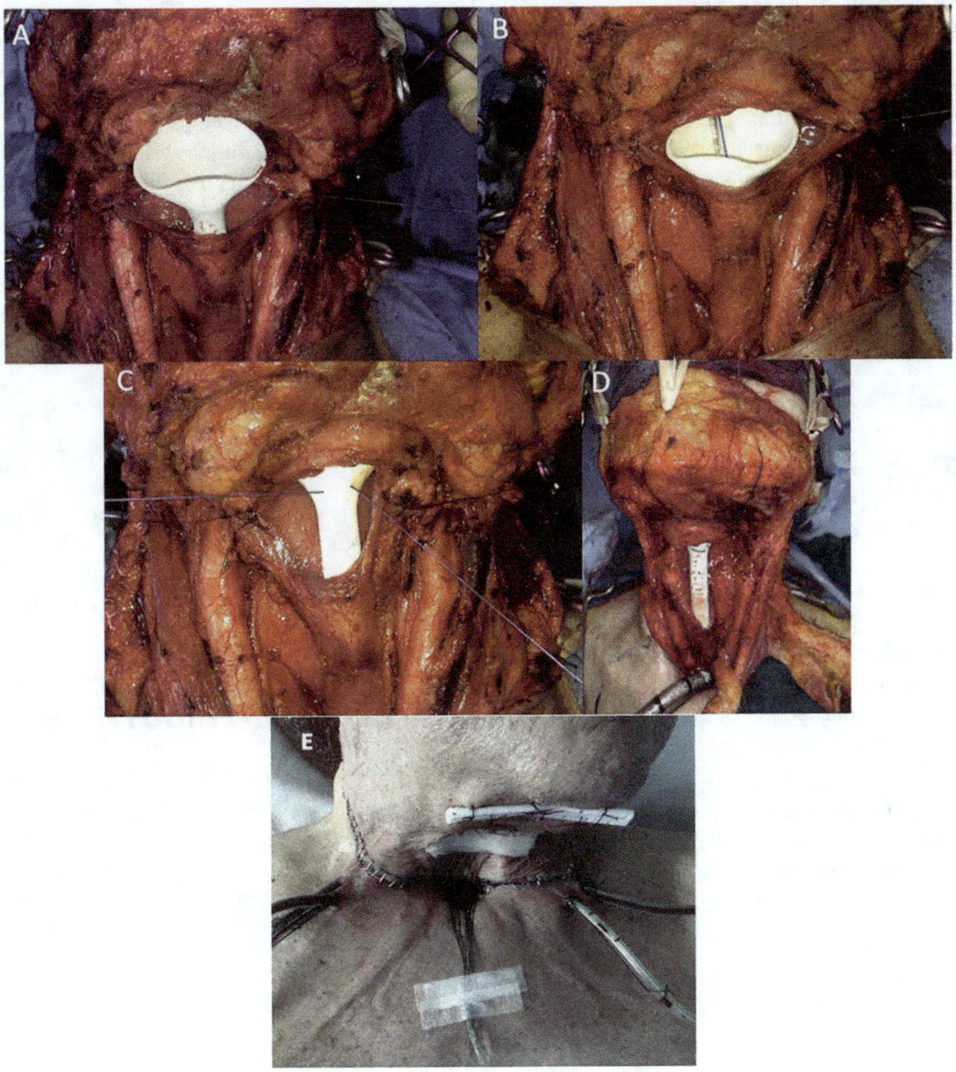

FIGURE 1 | **(A)** Intraoperative positioning of salivary bypass tube. **(B)** Naso-gastric tube (NGT) insertion inside salivary tube. **(C, D)** Transcutaneous securing of salivary tube. **(E)** Salivary stent fixation on the skin.

definitively identified among patients who had previously undergone organ-sparing protocols (25).

In the fistula zero protocol, the pharyngeal suture is performed horizontally using a barbed suture. Currently, three types of barbed suture are commercially available: the Quill Self-Retaining System (SRS) (B. Braun Medical Ltd, Sheffield, UK), the bidirectional barbed suture (Angiotech, Vancouver, BC, Canada) and the V-Loc unidirectional barbed suture (V-lock suture; Covidien^{TM}, Mansfield, VA, USA) (26–28). The barbed stitches allow for a continuous suture, without tension, reducing the possibility of knots slipping, secondary dehiscence to knot breakage, extrusion or suture splitting and necrosis caused by knot compression on tissues. Furthermore, a continuous suture without knots gives a better seal against liquids, reducing the potential infiltration of saliva between tissues of different thickness and consistency. Three stitches are normally used to complete the tension-free suture.

The third key point of our project is using a pedicled flap to reinforce the pharyngeal suture in pre-treated patients (radiotherapy with or without concomitant chemotherapy). The onlay of a pedicled/free flap in pre-treated patients is now widely supported in the literature, because of the radiation-induced microvascular injury that leads to hypovascular, hypocellular, and hypoxic tissue. Many authors suggest that reinforcing the pharyngeal suture with well-vascularized tissue will help to reduce the incidence of PCF formation in these patients (5, 29, 30). The pectoralis major myofascial flap is one of the most reliable flaps, but many other reconstructive options are described (supraclavicular artery island flap, fasciocutaneous free flaps, mammary artery perforator propeller flap, latissimus dorsi flaps, and facial artery-based cutaneous island flap) (21, 22, 31–34).

In our practice, a pectoralis major myofascial flap was sutured over the pharyngeal suture, without compressing it. The systematic and rigorous adoption of our protocol allowed us to observe excellent results in terms of minimal complications (1.3%), especially when comparing pre-treated (1.3%) and untreated (3.9%) patients, showing similar low rates of complications, also stratifying the patients on the basis of patient- and disease-related risk factors.

The management of PCF has a huge economic impact. Parikh et al. estimated that 57% of patients who develop a fistula require surgical revision. They reported postoperative complications in 22% of patients, with a final cost, which included hospitalization and surgical procedures, of about $58 000 for each fistula (35).

The results of this study seem to be encouraging from both a clinical and economic perspective. In our cohort, the mean hospitalization time was 18 days (range 12–40 days). Hospitalization was longer (21 days) in pre-treated patients (reconstruction; donor-site seroma occurred in four patients and was managed with compression dressing) and shorter (16 days) for patients who did not undergo reconstruction. Higher surgery-related costs (mean € 550 for each procedure) are balanced by a reduction in the length of hospitalization and the absence of delayed adjuvant therapy and oral feeding.

The strengths of this study are represented by the relatively large series and uniformity of surgical procedures. The main limitation of the study is the lack of a control group of patients not treated with this protocol. The preliminary results obtained in this study encourage us to propose a multi-institutional perspective study to validate the usefulness of the Har-El salivary bypass tube in preventing PCF after TL.

CONCLUSION

Sustainability of medical care, especially in oncology, is a delicate and debated topic, especially in a world where comorbidities increase with increasing age of the population. More standardized procedures are required, and total laryngectomy represents an excellent model from this point of view.

"Fistula zero" is undoubtedly an ambitious project (there is no surgery without complications) but not an unapproachable strategy. Thanks to a careful attitude and a meticulous approach, the project achieved very low rates of pharyngocutaneous fistula and small blind fistula formation.

The results of this study were obtained by rigid adherence to the protocol and uniformity of surgical procedure and suggest that, with a small increase in surgical costs, it is possible to reduce overall costs for PCF management.

ETHICS STATEMENT

Ethical review and approval was not required for the study on human participants in accordance with the local legislation and institutional requirements. The patients/participants provided their written informed consent to participate in this study.

AUTHOR CONTRIBUTIONS

EC, conception and design of the study, surgeon, writing and editing the manuscript. GA, data collection. AS, medical statistician who performed statistical analysis. GS, conception and design of the study, surgeon, editing the manuscript. All authors contributed to the article and approved the submitted version.

REFERENCES

1. Thawley SE. Complications of Combined Radiation Therapy and Surgery for Carcinoma of the Larynx and Inferior Hypopharynx. *Laryngoscope* (1981) 91 (5):677–700. doi: 10.1288/00005537-198105000-00001
2. Bresson K, Rasmussen H, Rasmussen PA. Pharyngo-Cutaneous Fistulae in Totally Laryngectomized Patients. *J Laryngol Otol* (1974) 88(9):835–42. doi: 10.1017/s0022215100079433
3. Sayles M, Grant DG. Preventing Pharyngo-Cutaneous Fistula in Total Laryngectomy: A Systematic Review and Meta-Analysis. *Laryngoscope* (2014) 124(5):1150–63. doi: 10.1002/lary.24448
4. Süslü N, Senirli RT, Günaydın RÖ, Özer S, Karakaya J, Hoşal AŞ. Pharyngocutaneous Fistula After Salvage Laryngectomy. *Acta Otolaryngol* (2015) 135(6):615–21. doi: 10.3109/00016489.2015.1009639
5. Sittitrai P, Srivanitchapoom C, Reunmakkaew D. Prevention of Pharyngocutaneous Fistula in Salvage Total Laryngectomy: Role of the Pectoralis Major Flap and Peri-Operative Management. *J Laryngol Otol* (2018) 132(3):246–51. doi: 10.1017/S0022215118000178
6. Lemaire E, Schultz P, Vergez S, Debry C, Sarini J, Vairel B, et al. Risk Factors for Pharyngocutaneous Fistula After Total Pharyngolaryngectomy [Published Online Ahead of Print, 2020 Feb 25]. *Ear Nose Throat J* (2020) 1–7. doi: 10.1177/0145561319901035 145561319901035.
7. Wang M, Xun Y, Wang K, Lu L, Yu A, Guan B, et al. Risk Factors of Pharyngocutaneous Fistula After Total Laryngectomy: A Systematic Review and Meta-Analysis. *Eur Arch Otorhinolaryngol* (2020) 277(2):585–99. doi: 10.1007/s00405-019-05718-9
8. Minni A, Ralli M, Di Cianni S, Cialente F, Candelori F, Colizza A, et al. Montgomery Salivary Bypass Tube in Head and Neck Cancer: The Experience

of Our Otolaryngology Clinic. *Ear Nose Throat J* (2020) 12:1–5. doi: 10.1177/0145561320961754 145561320961754.

9. Piazza C, Paderno A, Del Bon F, Grammatica A, Montalto N, Bresciani L, et al. Fascio-Cutaneous-Free Flaps As Primary Reconstruction in Salvage Total Laryngectomy. *Eur Arch Otorhinolaryngol* (2021) 278(1):219–26. doi: 10.1007/s00405-020-06137-x
10. Hone RWA, Rahman E, Wong G, Annan Y, Alexander V, Al-Lami A, et al. Do Salivary Bypass Tubes Lower the Incidence of Pharyngocutaneous Fistula Following Total Laryngectomy? A Retrospective Analysis of Predictive Factors Using Multivariate Analysis. *Eur Arch Otorhinolaryngol* (2017) 274(4):1983–91. doi: 10.1007/s00405-016-4391-9
11. Kamhieh Y, Fox H, Hallett E, Berry S. Routine Use of Salivary Bypass Tubes in Laryngectomy Patients: Systematic Review. *J Laryngol Otol* (2018) 132 (5):380–4. doi: 10.1017/S0022215118000154
12. Bang D, Piccirillo JF, Littenberg B, Johnston A. The Adult Comorbidity Evaluation-27 (Ace-27) Test: A New Comorbidity Index for Patients With Cancer, in: *36th Annual Meeting of American Society of Clinical Oncology*, May 20, 2000. New Orleans, LA.
13. Redaelli de Zinis LO, Ferrari L, Tomenzoli D, Premoli G, Parrinello G, Nicolai P. Postlaryngectomy Pharyngocutaneous Fistula: Incidence, Predisposing Factors, and Therapy. *Head Neck* (1999) 21(2):131–8. doi: 10.1002/(sici)1097-0347(199903)21:2<131::aid-hed6>3.0.co;2-f
14. Paydarfar JA, Birkmeyer NJ. Complications in Head and Neck Surgery: A Meta-Analysis of Postlaryngectomy Pharyngocutaneous Fistula. *Arch Otolaryngol Head Neck Surg* (2006) 132(1):67–72. doi: 10.1001/archotol.132.1.67
15. Wulff NB, Kristensen CA, Andersen E, Charabi B, Sørensen CH, Homøe P. Risk Factors for Postoperative Complications After Total Laryngectomy Following Radiotherapy or Chemoradiation: A 10-Year Retrospective Longitudinal Study in Eastern Denmark. *Clin Otolaryngol* (2015) 40(6):662–71. doi: 10.1111/coa.12443
16. Busoni M, Deganello A, Gallo O. Pharyngocutaneous Fistula Following Total Laryngectomy: Analysis of Risk Factors, Prognosis and Treatment Modalities. *Acta Otorhinolaryngol Ital* (2015) 35(6):400–5. doi: 10.14639/0392-100X-626
17. Lebo NL, Caulley L, Alsaffar H, Corsten MJ, Johnson-Obaseki S. Peri-Operative Factors Predisposing to Pharyngocutaneous Fistula After Total Laryngectomy: Analysis of a Large Multi-Institutional Patient Cohort. *J Otolaryngol Head Neck Surg* (2017) 46(1):54. doi: 10.1186/s40463-017-0233-z
18. Montgomery WW. Salivary Bypass Tube. *Ann Otol Rhinol Laryngol* (1978) 87 (2 Pt 1):159–62. doi: 10.1177/000348947808700202
19. Bondi S, Giordano L, Limardo P, Bussi M. Role of Montgomery Salivary Stent Placement During Pharyngolaryngectomy, to Prevent Pharyngocutaneous Fistula in High-Risk Patients. *J Laryngol Otol* (2013) 127(1):54–7. doi: 10.1017/S0022215112002502
20. Gilardi A, Colizza A, Minni A, de Vincentiis M. A New Montgomery® Salivary Bypass Tube Placement Technique: Report of Procedures Performed on Patients With Tracheoesophageal Fistula or Pharyngoesophageal Stenosis. *Ear Nose Throat J* (2021) 25:1–3. doi: 10.1177/01455613211006002 1455613211006002.
21. Piazza C, Bon FD, Paderno A, Grammatica A, Montalto N, Taglietti V, et al. Fasciocutaneous Free Flaps for Reconstruction of Hypopharyngeal Defects. *Laryngoscope* (2017) 127(12):2731–7. doi: 10.1002/lary.26705
22. López F, Obeso S, Camporro D, Fueyo A, Suárez C, Llorente JL. Outcomes Following Pharyngolaryngectomy With Fasciocutaneous Free Flap Reconstruction and Salivary Bypass Tube. *Laryngoscope* (2013) 123(3):591–6. doi: 10.1002/lary.23695
23. Murray DJ, Gilbert RW, Vesely MJ, Novak CB, Zaitlin-Gencher S, Clark JR, et al. Functional Outcomes and Donor Site Morbidity Following Circumferential Pharyngoesophageal Reconstruction Using an Anterolateral Thigh Flap and Salivary Bypass Tube. *Head Neck* (2007) 29(2):147–54. doi: 10.1002/hed.20489
24. Varvares MA, Cheney ML, Gliklich RE, Boyd JM, Goldsmith T, Lazor J, et al. Use of the Radial Forearm Fasciocutaneous Free Flap and Montgomery Salivary Bypass Tube for Pharyngoesophageal Reconstruction. *Head Neck* (2000) 22:463–8. doi: 10.1002/1097-0347(200008)22:5<463::aid-hed4>3.0.co;2-s
25. Aires FT, Dedivitis RA, Castro MAF, Bernardo WM, Cernea CR, Brandão LG. Efficacy of Stapler Pharyngeal Closure After Total Laryngectomy: A Systematic Review. *Head Neck* (2014) 36(5):739–42. doi: 10.1002/hed.23326
26. Crosetti E, Caracciolo A, Arrigoni G, Delmastro E, Succo G. Barbed Suture in Oral Cavity Reconstruction: Preliminary Results. *Acta Otorhinolaryngol Ital* (2019) 39(5):308–15. doi: 10.14639/0392-100X-2130
27. Villa MT, White LE, Alam M, Yoo SS, Walton RL. Barbed Sutures: A Review of the Literature. *Plast Reconstr Surg* (2008) 121(3):102e–8e. doi: 10.1097/01.prs.0000299452.24743.65
28. Moya AP. Barbed Sutures in Body Surgery. *Aesthet Surg J* (2013) 33(3 Suppl):57S–71S. doi: 10.1177/1090820X13499577
29. Oosthuizen JC, Leonard DS, Kinsella JB. The Role of Pectoralis Major Myofascial Flap in Salvage Laryngectomy: A Single Surgeon Experience. *Acta Otolaryngol* (2012) 132(9):1002–5. doi: 10.3109/00016489.2012.672768
30. Patel UA, Keni SP. Pectoralis Myofascial Flap During Salvage Laryngectomy Prevents Pharyngocutaneous Fistula. *Otolaryngol Head Neck Surg* (2009) 141 (2):190–5. doi: 10.1016/j.otohns.2009.03.024
31. Emerick KS, Herr MA, Deschler DG. Supraclavicular Flap Reconstruction Following Total Laryngectomy. *Laryngoscope* (2014) 124(8):1777–82. doi: 10.1002/lary.24530
32. Pabiszczak M, Banaszewski J, Pastusiak T, Szyfter W. Supraclavicular Artery Pedicled Flap in Reconstruction of Pharyngocutaneous Fistulas After Total Laryngectomy. *Otolaryngol Pol* (2015) 69(2):9–13. doi: 10.5604/00306657.1147032
33. lmadori G, De Corso E, Visconti G, Almadori A, Di Cintio G, Mele DA, et al. Impact of Internal Mammary Artery Perforator Propeller Flap in Neck Resurfacing and Fistula Closure After Salvage Larynx Cancer Surgery: Our Experience. *Head Neck* (2019) 41(11):3788–97. doi: 10.1002/hed.25903
34. Gupta DK, Chugh R, Singh SK, Pati S. Use of the Facial Artery-Based Cutaneous Island Flap (Melo-Labial Flap) for Reconstruction of the Neopharynx Following Total Laryngectomy: A Novel Technique. *BMJ Case Rep* (2019) 12(8):e230712. doi: 10.1136/bcr-2019-230712
35. Parikh SR, Irish JC, Curran AJ, Gullane PJ, Brown DH, Rotstein LE. Pharyngocutaneous Fistulae in Laryngectomy Patients: The Toronto Hospital Experience. *J Otolaryngol* (1998) 27(3):136–40.

10

Integrated Analysis Reveals *ENDOU* as a Biomarker in Head and Neck Squamous Cell Carcinoma Progression

Chengzhi Xu[1†], Yunbin Zhang[2,3†], Yupeng Shen[4], Yong Shi[1], Ming Zhang[1] and Liang Zhou[1]*

[1] Department of Otolaryngology—Head and Neck Surgery, Eye Ear Nose and Throat Hospital, Fudan University, Shanghai, China, [2] Shanghai Institute of Biochemistry and Cell Biology, Chinese Academy of Sciences, University of Chinese Academy of Sciences, Shanghai, China, [3] Department of Respirology, Shanghai Public Health Clinical Center, Fudan University, Shanghai, China, [4] Department of Otolaryngology—Head and Neck Surgery, Bethune International Peace Hospital, Shijiazhuang, China

***Correspondence:**
Liang Zhou
Zl76856@126.com

[†]These authors have contributed equally to this work

Background: Head and neck squamous cell carcinoma (HNSCC) is a leading cancer with high morbidity and mortality worldwide. The aim is to identify genes with clinical significance by integrated bioinformatics analysis and investigate their function in HNSCC.

Methods: We downloaded and analyzed two gene expression datasets of GSE6631 and GSE107591 to screen differentially expressed genes (DEGs) in HNSCC. Common DEGs were functionally analyzed by Gene ontology and KEGG pathway enrichment analysis. Protein-protein interaction (PPI) network was constructed with STRING database and Cytoscape. *ENDOU* was overexpressed in FaDu and Cal-27 cell lines, and cell proliferation and migration capability were evaluated with MTT, scratch and transwell assay. The prognostic performance of ENDOU and expression correlation with tumor infiltrates in HNSCC were validated with TCGA HNSCC datasets.

Results: Ninety-eight genes shared common differential expression in both datasets, with core functions like extracellular matrix organization significantly enriched. 15 genes showed prognostic significance, and *COBL* and *ENDOU* serve as independent survival markers in HNSCC. In-vitro *ENDOU* overexpression inhibited FaDu and Cal-27 cells proliferation and migration, indicating its tumor-suppressing role in HNSCC progression. GSEA analysis indicated *ENDOU* down-stream pathways like DNA replication, mismatch repair, cell cycle and IL-17 signaling pathway. *ENDOU* showed relative lower expression in HNSCC, especially HPV-positive HNSCC samples. At last, *ENDOU showed* negative correlation with tumor purity and tumor infiltrating macrophages, especially M2 macrophages.

Conclusion: This study identified *ENDOU* as a biomarker with prognostic significance in HNSCC progression.

Keywords: head and neck squamous cell carcinoma, *ENDOU*, prognosis, tumor suppressor, bioinformatics

INTRODUCTION

HNSCC is a leading cancer with high morbidity and mortality worldwide (1, 2). It can be categorized by the area of the head or neck in which they begin, like oral cavity, pharynx, oropharynx, larynx, paranasal sinuses and nasal cavity and salivary glands. The most important pathogenic risk factors of HNSCC are tobacco and alcohol consumption and at least 75% of head and neck cancers are attributed to them (3). Molecular pathogenesis is still a comprehensive but largely not understood problem in HNSCC. Due to the phenotypic heterogeneity of each individual patient, it is hard to match suitable and effective treatments. Over the past decades, the development of high-throughput sequencing, increasing researchers have focused on the biological genetic functions of genes involved in the tumor-genesis of HNSCC (4–12).They have illustrated a lot of large-scale gene-expression profiles of HNSCC samples. The first successful therapeutic strategy for HNSCC was to inhibit the epidermal growth factor receptor (EGFR). In-depth understanding of the molecular carcinogenesis of HNSCC could help to develop novel and accurate treatment strategies for individual HNSCC patient.

The Cancer Genome Atlas (TCGA) network group of NIH generated comprehensive genomic characterization of HNSCC in 2015 (5). It profiled 279 HNSCC samples and provided a large-scale landscape of genetic and epigenetic characterizations of HNSCC, pointing the pivotal roles of *PIK3CA*, *TRAF3*, *E2F1*, *TP53*, *NOTCH* and other regulators in Wnt signaling pathways in tumor-genesis of HNSCC. Before that, Chen and his colleagues also compared 22-paired samples of HNSCC and normal tissues in 2004 (13). They found critically altered genes in the pathogenic processes of HNSCC through combinatorial analysis of microarray data. However, HNSCC is a cancer with complicated pathogenesis as well as diverse tissue origins. At present, most researches of HNSCC focus on star pathways or molecules, like PI3K signaling pathway or *TP53* protein. Therefore, it's necessary and urgent to dig out more potential targets for HNSCC treatment.

In this study, we downloaded two published and well-generated profiling datasets about HNSCC tumor and normal tissues from the Gene Expression Omnibus (GEO). Then novel potential prognostic markers were dig out to find more avenues to effective clinical treatments of HNSCC *via* multiple bioinformatics analysis, including biological process functional annotation and pathway enrichment analysis, protein-protein interaction network analysis as well as gene expression profiling interactive survival analysis. Gene *ENDOU* showed differential expression, correlation with tumor infiltrates and prognostic significance, and were functionally investigated.

MATERIALS AND METHODS

Data Collection

The expression profiles of RNAs were screened from the National Center of Biotechnology Information Gene Expression Omnibus (http://www.ncbi.nlm.nih.gov/gds/). The GSE6631 dataset is composed of 22 paired HNSCC tumor and normal samples. The platform is GPL8300 [HG_U95Av2] Affymetrix Human Genome U95 Version 2 Array. The GSE107591 dataset contains 23 normal and 24 tumor tissues. The platform is GPL6244 [HuGene-1_0-st] Affymetrix Human Gene 1.0 ST Array.

Identification of Differentially Expressed Genes (DEGs)

We utilized quartile normalization algorithm to subtract and correct background of these downloaded datasets firstly (14). Then we filtered probes without corresponding gene symbols and calculated the average value of gene symbols with multiple probes. We further used *R* software *Limma* package to screen DEGs by filtering *p.adj* value of student's t-test and fold change (FC) (15). Finally, with a threshold of p.adj-value <0.05 and absolute value of FC >2 (16, 17), volcano plot was performed by using R software ggplot2 package to identify the DEGs with statistical significance between two groups. Hierarchical clustering and combined analyses were performed for the DEGs.

Functional Analysis of DEGs in HNSCC Pathogenesis

GO enrichment analyses of differentially expressed mRNAs were implemented with annotation, visualization and integrated discovery (DAVID) (http://david.abcc.ncifcrf.gov/). GO terms (including Molecular Function, Biological Processes and Cellular Components) with p-value less than 0.05 were considered significantly enriched by DEGs. KEGG is a database resource for understanding high-level functions and effects of the biological systems (http://www.genome.jp/kegg/). DAVID was also used to test the significantly statistical enrichment of DEGs in KEGG pathways. Cytoscape (version 3.40) was used to visualize the relationships between biological processes terms and DEGs.

Protein-Protein Interaction (PPI) Network Analysis

Protein-protein interaction analysis was further conducted in STRING database (https://string-db.org/). The higher or larger score protein-protein interaction pairs were selected to construct PPI networks. Then, the regulatory relationships between genes were visualized *via* Cytoscape (version 3.4.0) (18). The sub-networks were extracted from the whole PPI network by using MCODE app.

Survival Analysis and Tumor Filtrating Immune Cells Analysis

To conduct survival analysis, clinical data and RNA expression data from TCGA dataset were downloaded. Univariate and Multivariate Cox analysis was conducted with SPSS, and forest plot was conducted with R. Then Kaplan-Meier survival plot and LogRank analysis was done. The correlation of *ENDOU* expression with tumor infiltrating cells were conducted with TIMER (https://cistrome.shinyapps.io/timer/) (19). For macrophage markers, *CCL2*, *CD68*, and *IL10* were used for tumor associated macrophages (TAM), *NOS2*, *IRF5*, and *PTGS2* for M1 macrophages and *CD163*, *VSIG4*, and *MS4A4A* for M2 macrophages, referring to previous study (20).

Cells Culture

The FaDu and Cal-27 human carcinoma cell lines were propagated and carefully maintained in our laboratory. FaDu and Cal-27 cells were cultured in Dulbecco's modified Eagle's medium supplemented with 10% fetal bovine serum at 37°C in a humid atmosphere containing 5% CO2.

Lentivirus Mediated *ENDOU* Overexpression

CDS of *ENDOU* (NM_001172440) was inserted into a recombinant lentiviral expression vector (pGSIL) containing green fluorescent proteins (GFP) tag. To generate lentiviral particles, the recombinant expression plasmid was co-transfected with a packaging plasmid system (psPAX2 and pMD2G) into FaDu and Cal-27 cells, and viral particles were collected after 48 h. FaDu and Cal-27 cells were infected with *ENDOU* lentiviral vector or with a negative control (NC) for 24 h. The infection efficiency was preliminarily assessed in each experiment under a fluorescence microscope and then measured by sorting GFP-positive cells by flow cytometry (Beckman Coulter, USA). The stably infected cells were expanded and harvested for further experiments. The overexpression of *ENDOU* was examined with western blotting, using monoclonal antibody (Abcam, Cambridge, MA, USA). GAPDH was used as the house-keeping gene.

MTT Assay

The cell proliferation activity of FaDu and Cal-27 cells was examined with MTT Cell Proliferation and Cytotoxicity Assay Kit (Dojindo Laboratories, Tokyo, Japan). The cells were incubated for 24, 48, 72, and 96 h. After incubation, the MTT solution was removed and replaced with dimethyl sulfoxide (DMSO; 150 µl, 4%; Sigma). A microplate reader (Bio-Tek, Instruments, Neufahrn, Germany) was used to measure the absorbance at 570 nm.

Transwell Assay

Cells in logarithmic growth phase were seeded at the upper transwell chamber insert (Corning, USA) at a density of 2 × 104 cells per well. The chamber was placed in a 24- well plate in which the upper chamber contained serum-free cell culture medium and the lower chamber contained 10% FBS complete medium. The culture was continued for 24 h. The medium was discarded, and stained with a crystal violet solution to observe the number of migrated cells.

Scratch Wound Healing Assay

FaDu and Cal-27 cells were grown in complete growth medium until 90% confluence after transfection. A 3 mm wound was introduced across the diameter of each plate. Cell migration was observed by microscopy at 24 h.

Statistical Analysis

Student's t-test or ANOVA were performed to analyze the differential expression. Kaplan-Meier analysis was used to estimate overall survival rate or time; the differences between the survival curves were analyzed using the log-rank test. In all analyses, $P<0.05$ was considered to indicate a statistically significant result. Continuous data are presented as the mean ± standard deviation.

RESULTS

DEGs Identification in Two HNSCC Datasets

Two GEO datasets of HNSCC, GSE6631 and GSE107591 were first normalized (**Figure S1**) and analyzed to acquire significantly differential expressed genes (DEGs), respectively. Both datasets contains more than twenty tumor and normal samples, and with the same microarray platform of Affymetrix gene expression microarray. The GSE107591 dataset contains 23 normal and 24 tumor tissues. As GSE6631 comprises 22 paired HNSCC tumor and normal samples, we conducted paired comparison. With a threshold of p.adj-value <0.05 and absolute value of FC >2, the expression of DEGs in HNSCC tumor and normal tissues were shown in **Figure 1**. We found 91 genes significantly up-regulated and 121 genes down-regulated in GSE6631 dataset (**Figures 1A, C**). For GSE107591, we found 194 up-regulated and 278 down-regulated genes in HNSCC tumor samples compared with normal tissues (**Figures 1B, D**).

Functional Analysis of 98 Common DEGs Enriched Hub Pathways in HNSCC

To further figure out the roles of these DEGs in HNSCC, we searched the common DEGs both altered in these two datasets. A total of 98 DEGs (37 up-regulated and 61 down-regulated DEGs) showed dysregulation in both datasets (**Figure 2A**). To further detailed unravel the function of these common DEGs in HNSCC, we constructed protein-protein interaction (PPI) network *via* STRING database (https://string-db.org/). The genes with larger scores were selected to construct PPI networks (**Figure 2B**), and their function was uploaded to DAVID database for KEGG pathway and GO enrichment analysis. As shown in **Figure 2C**, biological processes with the largest number of common DEGs and smallest p-value includes extracellular matrix disassemble, collagen catabolic process, extracellular matrix organization, cell adhesion, aging and angiogenesis. As for the KEGG enrichment analysis in **Figure 2C**, not surprisingly, items like Pathways in cancer, ECM-receptor interaction, Focal adhesion and PI3K-Akt signaling pathways are significantly enriched and showed the largest number of common DEGs. The PI3K-Akt signaling was inappropriately activated in many cancers, including head and neck cancer (21). Somatic mutations of *PIK3CA* had been also described before and are found in about 15% of HNSCC (22–24). These findings might help us find more new therapy targets for HNSCC.

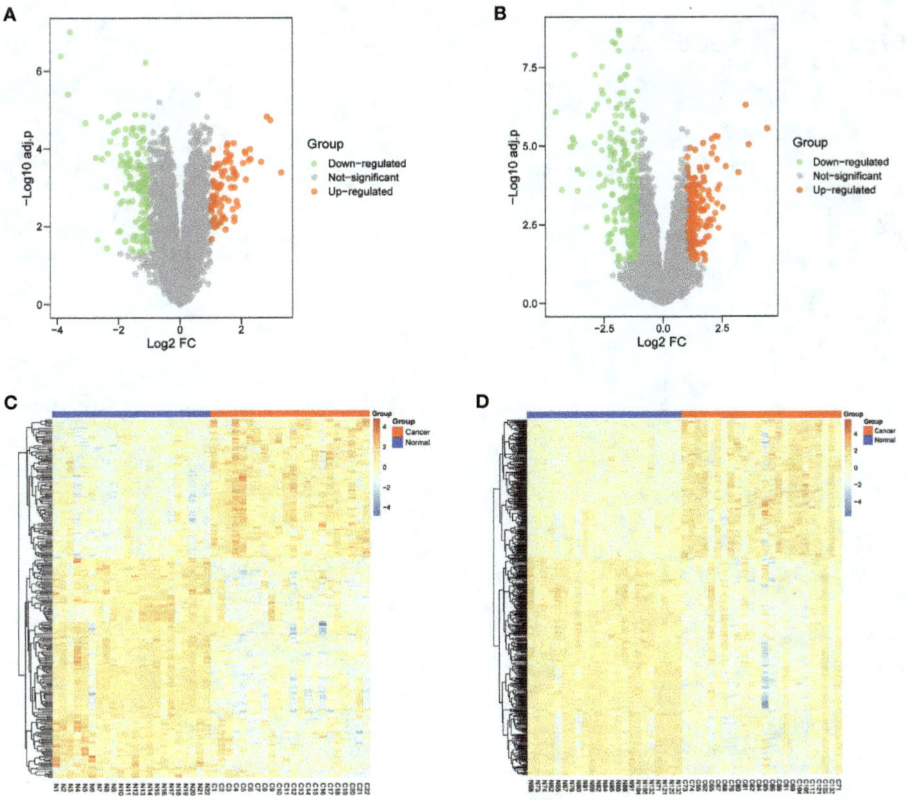

FIGURE 1 | Differentially expressed genes (DEGs) of normal and Head and neck squamous cell carcinoma (HNSCC) tissue from GSE6631 and GSE107591. **(A)** Volcano plot showing significantly deregulated genes in GSE6631; **(B)** Volcano plot showing significantly deregulated genes in GSE107591; **(C)** Heatmap clustering of all DEGs in normal and HNSCC tissue from GSE6631; **(D)** Heatmap clustering of all DEGs in normal and HNSCC tissue from GSE107591; UP, genes with significant increased expression in HNSCC group were labeled in red. DW, genes with significant decreased expression in HNSCC group were labeled in green, genes with no different were in HNSCC group were labelled in grey.

Clinical Significance of 15 Genes Were Analyzed With TCGA HNSCC Datasets

To further explore the clinical significance of DEGs in HNSCC, we first validated the expression of 98 common DEGs with TCGA HNSCC dataset. A total of 2230 DEGs were acquired in HNSCC datasets and 92 genes (in 98 common DEGs, **Table S1**) showed significant dysregulation in all datasets (**Figures 3A, B**). Then the prognostic significance of the 92 DEGs were analyzed with univariate analysis. As shown in **Figure 3C**, 15 genes showed promising performance with HNSCC overall survival. Nine genes of *LAMC2* (HR=1.5, P=0.00319), *SEMA3C* (HR=1.35, P=0.029), *FAP* (HR=1.42, P=0.0112), *COBL* (HR=1.38, P=0.0184), *SERPINE1* (HR=1.61, P=0.000616), *PLAU* (HR=1.49, P=0.00373), *MYO1B* (HR=1.35, P=0.028), *DUSP5* (HR=1.31, P=0.0498), *LAMB3* (HR=1.49, P=0.00407) were hazardous, and 6 genes of *CEACAM1* (HR=0.709, P=0.00049), *CEACAM6* (HR=0.751, P=0.0362), *ALDH3A1* (HR=0.763, P=0.0478), *ENDOU* (HR=0.711, P=0.0135), *SPINK5* (HR=0.736, P=0.0249) and *METTL7A* (HR=0.765, P=0.0494) were potential protective markers. At last, the multivariate analysis was conducted and only *COBL* and *ENDOU* showed significance (**Figure 3D**), indicating *COBL* (HR=1.55, P=0.00233) and *ENDOU* (HR=0.712, P=0.0361) as independent prognostic overall markers in HNSCC, and the Kaplan-Meier overall survival plot of *COBL* and *ENDOU* was shown in **Figures 3E, F**, and other 13 genes were shown in **Figure S2**.

Cordon-Bleu WH2 Repeat Protein (*COBL*) contains WH2 domains (WASP, Wiskott-Aldrich syndrome protein, homology domain-2) and has been reported to play an important role in the reorganization of the actin cytoskeleton (25–27). In acute lymphoblastic leukemia, *COBL* is a hotspot for *IKZF1* deletions (28), and we will study the function of *COBL* in HNSCC in the future. *ENDOU*, also known as *PP11* (Placental Protein 11), encodes uridylate-specific endoribonuclease expressed in the placenta. *ENDOU was reported to* displays RNA binding capability and cleaves single stranded RNA in a Mn (2+)-dependent manner at uridylates (29). Studies of *ENDOU* in cancer dates back to 1980s (30, 31). *ENDOU* was annotated with the function of in proteolysis (Gene Ontology term GO:0006508), and members like matrix metalloproteinases (MMPs) play an important function in cancer progression, by depredating extracellular matrix. Considering the significant enrichment of functional items of extracellular matrix in **Figures 2C, D**, we chose *ENDOU* for the following study.

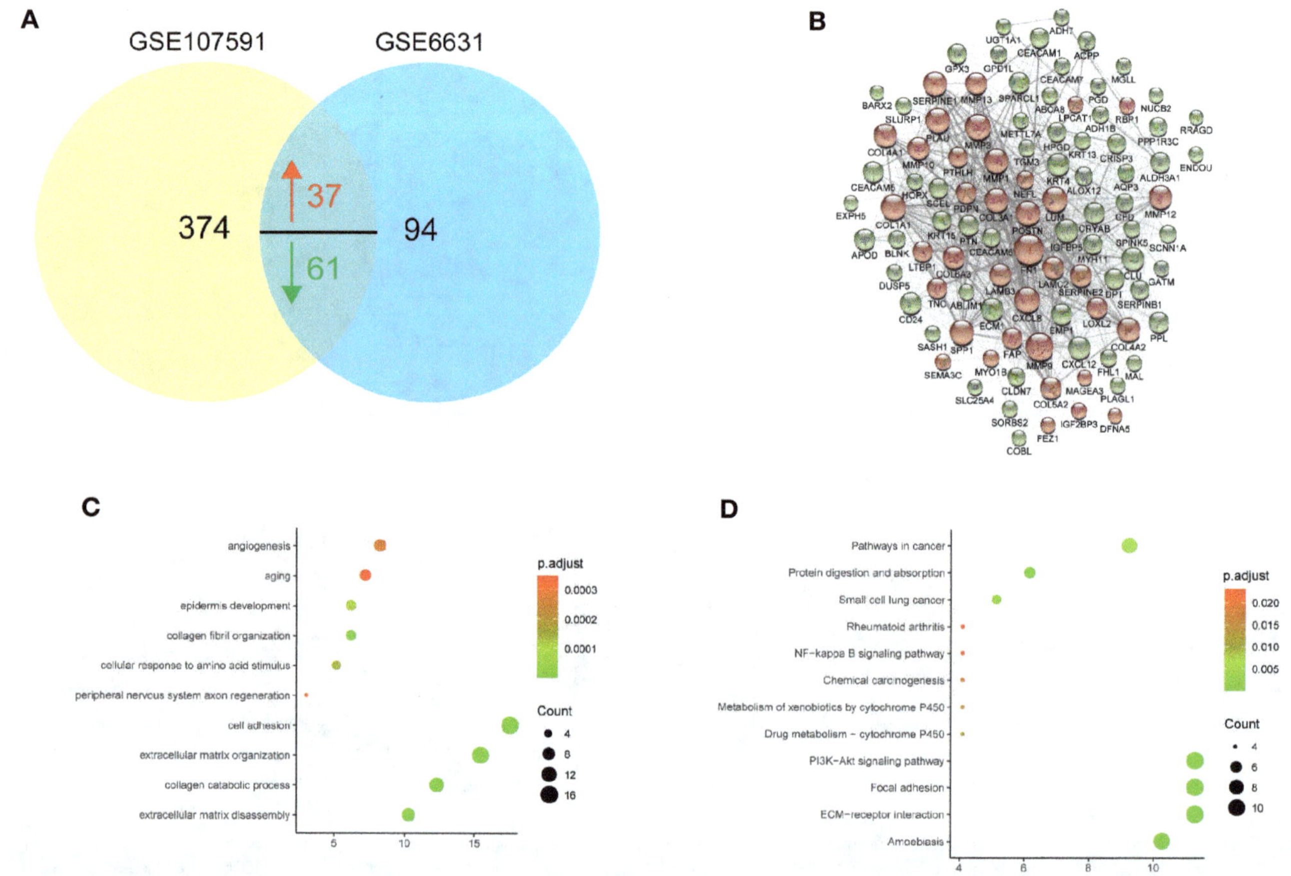

FIGURE 2 | Gene Ontology (GO) and KEGG pathway analysis of 98 commonly deregulated genes in GSE6631 and GSE107591. P value, count and ratio of top 10 enriched functional items were shown. **(A)** Venn plot of 98 commonly deregulated genes in GSE6631 and GSE107591; **(B)** Protein-protein interaction (PPI) network of 98 commonly deregulated genes; **(C)** Top 10 enriched Gene Ontology biological processes, including extracellular matrix disassembly were significantly identified; **(D)** Top 10 enriched KEGG pathways including ECM-receptor interaction were shown.

At last, the clinical association between ENDOU expression and clinicopathological variables in TCGA HNSCC patients was analyzed. As shown in **Table 1**, ENDOU expression showed significant correlation with survival status (P=0.03), gender (P=0.011), alcohol history (P=0.017), clinical N stage (P=0.001), lymphovascular invasion status (P=0.001), neoplasm histologic grade (P<0.001) and pathologic N stage (P<0.001). In sum, *ENDOU* may serve as an independent prognostic marker in HNSCC.

ENDOU Inhibits HNSCC Cancer Cell Proliferation and Migration *In Vitro*

As *ENDOU* shows consistent lower expression and hazardous prognostic significance in HNSCC, to explore the function of *ENDOU* in HNSCC, we conducted in-vitro over-expression (OE) studies in two cell lines of Fadu and Cal-27. The proliferation and migration capability was examined. As shown in **Figure 4A**, the proliferation capability of Fadu and Cal-27cells in *ENDOU* overexpression group was significantly decreased. Then wound healing assay and transwell assay was applied to study the effect of *ENDOU* overexpression on cell migration and invasion. In **Figures 4B, C**, the migration distance of *ENDOU* overexpression group was significantly larger than vector groups, and cells numbers was significantly decreased, implying that *ENDOU* may serve as a tumor suppressor in HNSCC.

To explore the potential mechanism of *ENDOU* as a tumor suppressor in HNSCC, we applied Gene Set Enrichment Analysis (GSEA) analysis to enrich *ENDOU* related KEGG pathways and biological processes. As shown in **Figure 5**, DNA replication, mismatch repair, cell cycle and IL-17 showed significant enrichment, which supported the cellular phenotype of *ENDOU* in HNSCC.

ENDOU Expression Showed Significant Correlation With Macrophages in HNSCC

In addition to HNSCC, we analyzed the expression of *ENDOU* in other cancer types, as shown in **Figure 6A**, decreased expression was also observed in bladder cancer (BLCA), breast cancer (BRCA), liver cancer (LIHC) and other cancer samples, indicating a universal role of *ENDOU in cancer. For HNSCC,* Human papillomavirus (HPV) positive HNSCC has a far better prognosis than HPV negative HNSCC, and HPV infection has

TABLE 1 | Clinical association between ENDOU expression and clinicopathological variables in HNSCC patients.

Characteristics	n	No. of Patients (%)	ENDOU		
			Low	High	*p*
Status	500				0.03
Alive		282(56.4)	129	163	
Death		218(43.6)	121	97	
Gender	500				0.011
Female		133(26.6)	54	79	
Male		367(73.4)	196	171	
Age	499				0.616
<60		220(44.1)	107	113	
≥60		279(55.9)	142	137	
Alcohol_history	489				0.017
No		157(32.1)	66	91	
Yes		332(67.9)	178	154	
Clinical_N	478				0.001
N0		239(50)	101	138	
N1-3		239(50)	139	100	
Clinical_T	485				0.731
T1-2		176(36.3)	86	90	
T3-4		309(63.7)	156	153	
Clinical_stage	486				0.096
I-II		114(23.5)	49	65	
III-IV		372(76.5)	193	179	
Lymph_node_count	407				0.52
Low		203(49.9)	102	101	
High		204(50.1)	96	108	
Lymphovascular_invasion_present	339				0.001
No		219(64.6)	95	124	
Yes		120(35.4)	74	46	
Neoplasm_histologic_grade	481				0
G1-2		360(74.8)	151	209	
G3-4		121(25.2)	88	33	
Recurrence	442				0.39
No		317(71.7)	153	164	
Yes		125(28.3)	66	59	
Pathologic_N	407				0
N0		171(42.0)	63	108	
N1-3		236(58.0)	132	104	
Pathologic_T	444				0.799
T1-2		177(39.9)	84	93	
T3-4		267(60.1)	130	137	
Pathologic_stage	435				0.133
I-II		98(22.5)	41	57	
III-IV		337(77.5)	170	167	
Perineural_invasion	351				0.311
No		186(53.0)	88	98	
Yes		165(47.0)	87	78	
Smoker	490				0.914
No		111(22.7)	56	55	
Yes		379(77.3)	189	190	

been linked with intratumoral immune cell infiltrates (e.g. IL-17 +CD8+T lymphocytes) in HNSCC (32, 33). Then we compared the expression of *ENDOU* in HPV-negative and HPV-positive HNSCC samples, and *ENDOU* showed significant lower expression in HPV-positive HNSCC samples (**Figure 6A**). At last, we analyzed the expression of *ENDOU* with tumor immune infiltrates, in HPV-negative and HPV-positive HNSCC samples. As shown in **Figure 6B**, *ENDOU* showed significant negative correlation with neutrophils, dendritic cells and especially macrophages. As the correlation was most significant in tumor infiltrating macrophages, correlation of TAMs, M1 and M2 macrophages markers with *ENDOU* expression were analyzed. As shown in **Figure 6C**, the markers of M2 macrophages (*CD163*, *VSIG4*, and *MS4A4A*) all showed significant negative correlation coefficient with *ENDOU*, implicating potential role of *ENDOU* in tumor infiltrating M2 macrophages.

DISCUSSION

At present, head and neck cancer is the sixth most common cancer with a poor prognosis and high mortality over the world

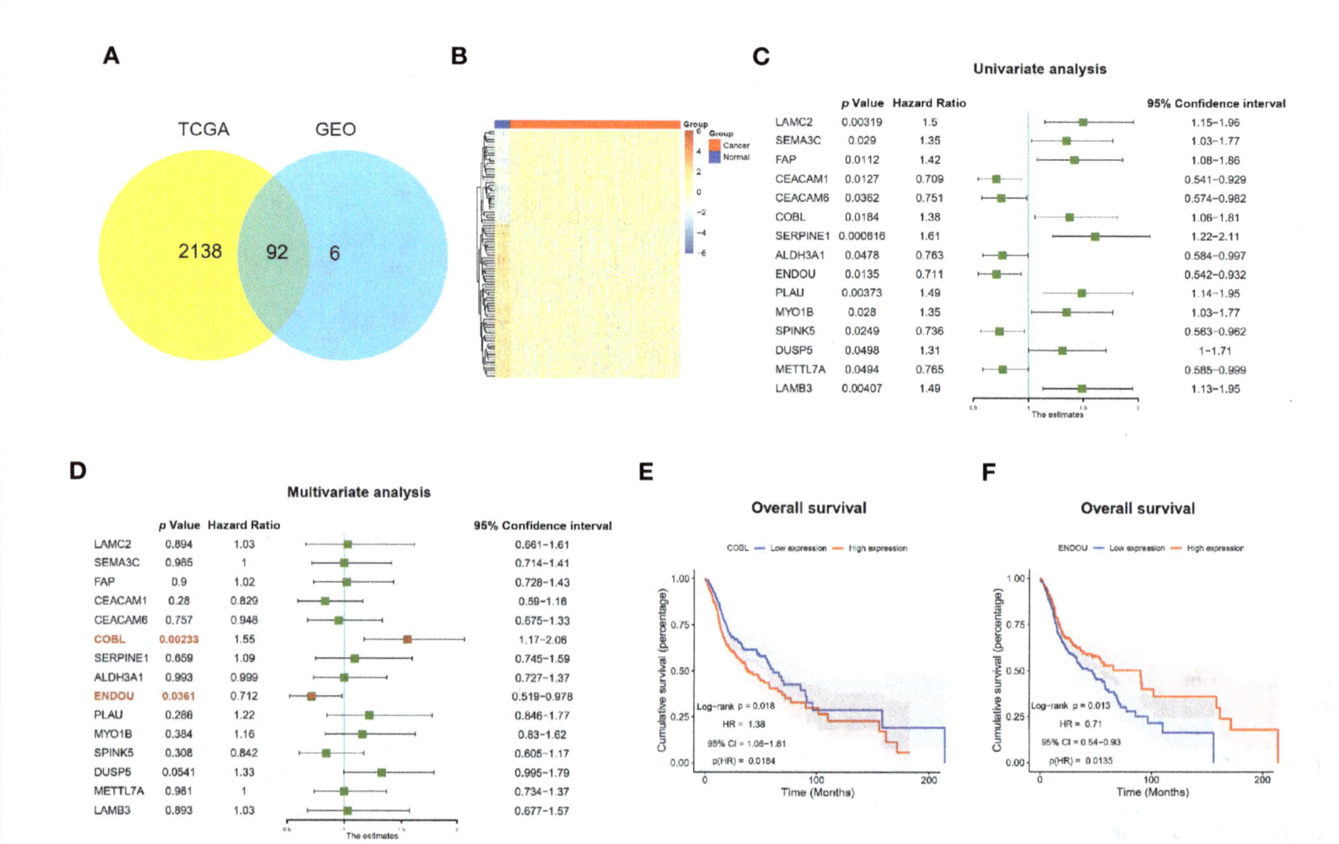

FIGURE 3 | Prognostic significance of genes in The Cancer Genome Atlas (TCGA) HNSCC dataset. **(A)** Ninety-two genes showed consistent dysregulation in TCGA dataset, and were shown with Venn plot; **(B)** Heatmap of the dysregulated 92 genes in TCGA HNSCC cancer and normal samples; **(C)** Univariate analysis identified 15 genes with prognostic significance in TCGA HNSCC datasets; **(D)** Multivariate analysis further identified COBL and ENDOU as independent prognostic markers in HNSCC; **(E, F)** Kaplan-Meier overall survival plot of COBL **(E)** and ENDOU **(F)** in HNSCC.

accounting for approximately 4% of all cancers in the United States (34). HNSCC is a kind of highly heterogeneous malignancy and appropriate clinical treatments remain a major challenge for HNSCC because of heterogeneity. Hence, personalized care for HNSCC patients requires a better understanding of the molecular mechanism of HNSCC. Though some biomarkers in head and neck squamous cell carcinoma progression have been reported yet (35, 36), accepted biomarkers for HNSCC prognosis in the clinic is still raw. Effective prognostic care for HNSCC patients requires a better understanding of the molecular mechanism. With the recent development of next generation sequencing and other "omics" profiling methods, we began to focus on genomic analysis of HNSCC to illustrate the detailed or new causes of HNSCC pathogenesis and to try to develop new markers for treatments of this cancer.

In the present study, gene expression data of HNSCC were downloaded from GEO, which revealed significant differences between survival status and clinical treatments of HNSCC patients. Hence, we reanalyzed two published microarray datasets, GSE6631 and GSE107591 in this study. Finally, we found 98 common DEGs between 45 normal and 46 HNSCC tumor samples. Gene functional annotation and pathway enrichment analysis of these DEGs showed that extracellular matrix disassemble collagen catabolic process, extracellular matrix organization, cell adhesion, aging and angiogenesis were enriched in HNSCC. These results revealed that our bioinformatics analysis may help a better understanding of the regulation of these genes in HNSCC. There are also many researchers focusing on extracellular matrix organization play an important role in HNSCC (37, 38). They pointed out that extracellular matrix organization was one of the most frequently altered pathways in HNSCC, consistent with our results.

By integrating the clinical information in TCGA, we screened 9 hazardous and 6 protective prognostic markers. Of the 15 genes, *LAMC2* (39–41), *SERPINE1* (41–43), *PLAU* (44), *MYO1B* (45), *LAMB3* (46), *CEACAM1* (41, 47), *CEACAM6* (48, 49), *ALDH3A1* (50) and *SPINK5* (51) has been reported as HNSCC prognostic markers, and in this study, we first uncovered the clinical significance of *SEMA3C*, *FAP*, *COBL*, *DUSP5*, *ENDOU* and *METTL7A* with HNSCC survival. Semaphorin 3C (*SEMA3C*) has been reported to play a pivotal role in tumor microenvironment driven neuroblastoma metastasis and progression (52). Fibroblast Activation Protein Alpha (*FAP*) was proven to serve as a marker in metastatic prostate cancer (53), pancreatic cancer (54) and ovarian cancer (55). Cordon-Bleu WH2 Repeat Protein (*COBL*) has been reported to play an

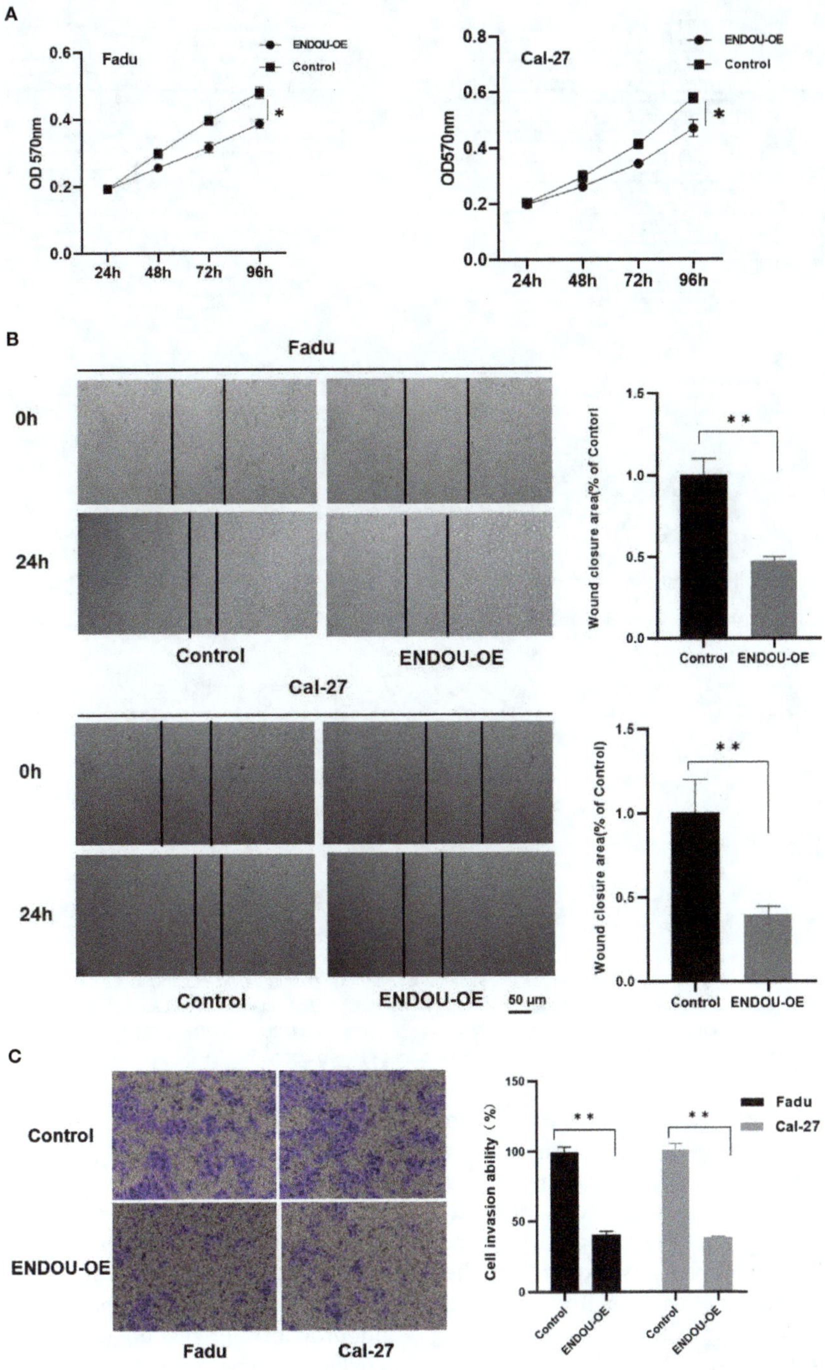

FIGURE 4 | ENDOU overexpression inhibits Fadu and Cal-27 cells proliferation and migration *in vitro*. **(A)** MTT assay results indicated *ENDOU* overexpression (OE) inhibited Fadu and Cal-27 cells proliferation. Each assay was replicated three times. *P < 0.05. **(B)** Scratch healing assay showed decreased migration capability in *ENDOU* overexpressing Fadu and Cal-27 cells. Each assay was replicated three times. *P < 0.05. **(C)** Transwell assay showed that *ENDOU* overexpression (OE) attenuated the invasion capability of Fadu and Cal-27 cells. Each assay was replicated three times. *P < 0.05, **P < 0.01.

important role in the reorganization of the actin cytoskeleton (25–27), and as a hotspot for *IKZF1* deletions (28) in acute lymphoblastic leukemia. Dual Specificity Phosphatase 5 (*DUSP5*) is tumor suppressor in ovarian cancer (56). Methyltransferase Like 7A (*METTL7A*) promoted cell viability and reduced apoptosis following methotrexate in choriocarcinoma (57). Further functional and mechanism studies of *SEMA3C*, *FAP*, *COBL*, *DUSP5*, *ENDOU*, and *METTL7A* may provide more detailed information to reveal their potential role as therapeutic targets in HNSCC.

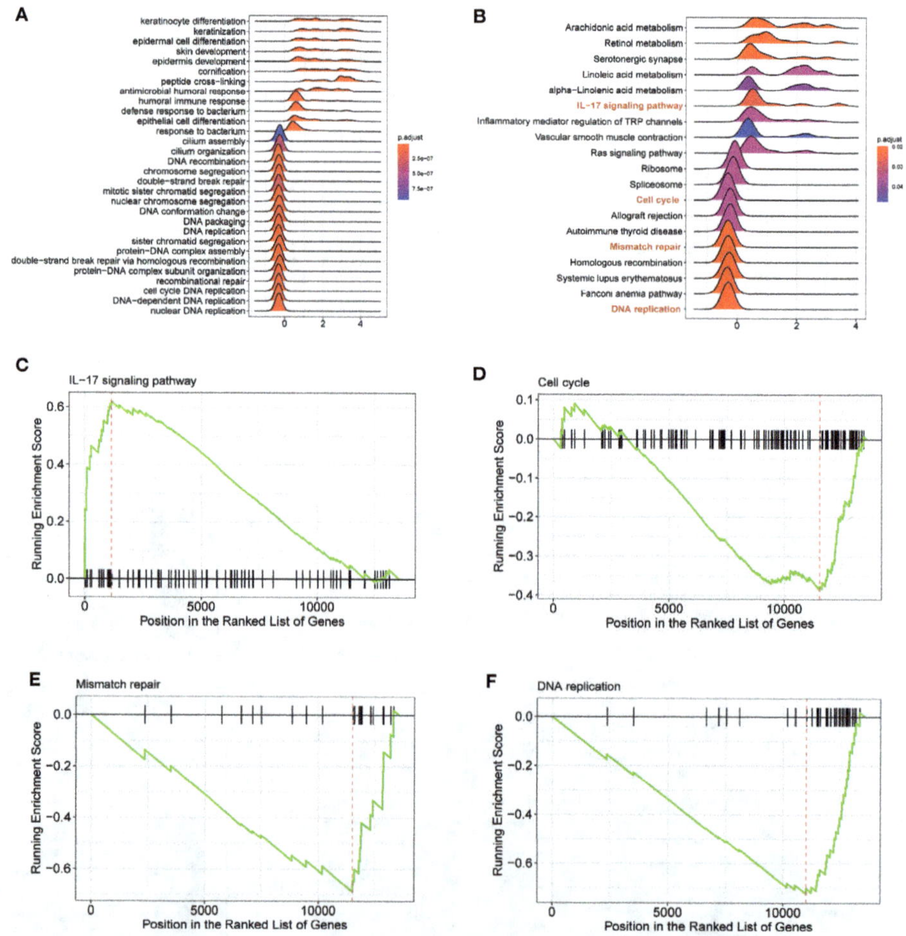

FIGURE 5 | Gene Set Enrichment Analysis (GSEA) analysis reveals DNA replication, Mismatch repair, Cell cycle and IL-17 signaling pathway as potential ENDOU functional mechanism. **(A)** GSEA analysis of Gene ontology enrichment items of ENDOU; **(B)** GSEA analysis of KEGG pathway enrichment items of ENDOU; **(C)** GSEA Enrichment plot of IL-17 signaling pathway in head and neck squamous cell carcinoma (HNSCC); **(D)** GSEA Enrichment plot of Cell cycle in HNSCC; **(E)** GSEA Enrichment plot of Mismatch repair in HNSCC; **(F)** GSEA Enrichment plot of DNA replication in HNSCC.

Then, *ENDOU* not only showed significant lower expression in HNSCC cancer samples (compared with normal samples), but also decreased level in higher stage cancer samples, implicating its tumor suppressing function in HNSCC occurrence and progression. *ENDOU*, also known as *PP11* (Placental Protein 11), encodes uridylate-specific endoribonuclease expressed in the placenta. *ENDOU was reported to* displays RNA binding capability and cleaves single stranded RNA in a Mn (2 +)-dependent manner at uridylates (29). Studies of *ENDOU* in cancer dates back to 1980s (30, 31), and this is the first time investigating the role of *ENDOU* in HNSCC. In this study, *ENDOU* was negatively correlated with tumor purity and then were functionally investigated in cancer cell lines. MTT, scratch healing and transwell assay demonstrated that *ENDOU* indeed inhibited the proliferation and migration capability, supporting it tumor suppressing role in HNSCC cancer cells. Meanwhile, there are several limits in this part. First, the effect of *ENDOU* overexpression can be validated in other HNSCC cell lines, and if possible, the impact of *ENDOU* silencing or mutation on HNSCC cell lines to support the conclusion. Secondly, an *in vivo* study of *ENDOU* would provide more solid evidence, as the function of genes *in vitro* and *in vivo* are not always consistent. Lastly, the underlying mechanism of *ENDOU* inhibiting FaDu cells proliferation and migration may be explored.

At last, tumor infiltrating immune cells in tumor microenvironment plays a pivotal role in HNSCC progression and prognosis prediction (58, 59). In this study, we found *ENDOU* negative correlates with tumor infiltrating neutrophils, dendritic cells and macrophages, especially M2 macrophages. Macrophages were reported to be involved in HNSCC metastasis (60–62), chemotherapy (63) and prognosis (64). Macrophages were polarized into M1 and M2 subtypes depending on their environment (65), and were reported to be functionally distinct in cancer (66). M2 polarized macrophages were found to be correlated with poor prognosis in nasopharyngeal carcinoma patients (67). HNSCC cancer cells were found to contribute to M2 polarization in several ways, like secreting microRNA-21 abundant exosomes (68) and lactic acid (69). Based on the

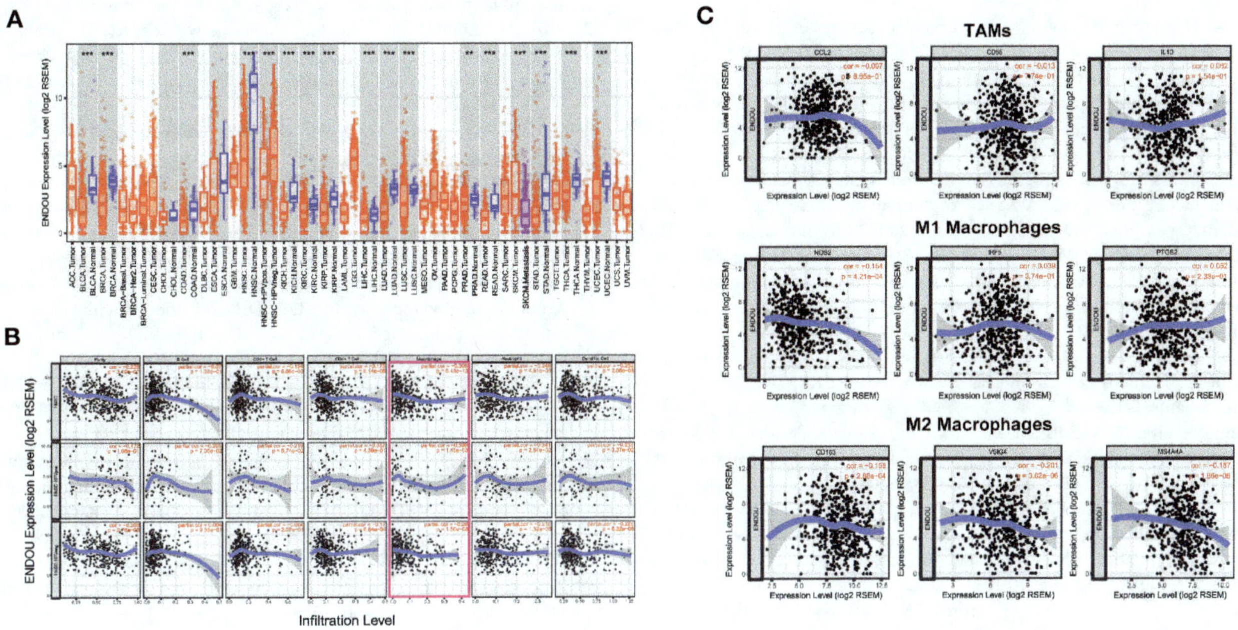

FIGURE 6 | *ENDOU* showed significant down-regulation in head and neck squamous cell carcinoma (HNSCC) development and correlates with tumor infiltrating immune cells. **(A)** *ENDOU* was significantly downregulated in HNSCC samples, compared with normal tissue. *ENDOU* showed significant lower expression in HPV-positive HNSCC samples. Decreased expression was also observed in bladder cancer (BLCA), breast cancer (BRCA), liver cancer (LIHC) and other cancer samples. **P < 0.01; ***P < 0.001; **(B)** The correlation of *ENDOU* expression with tumor infiltrates were analyzed, and *ENDOU* expression showed significant negative correlation with tumor purity, macrophages, neutrophils and dendritic cells; **(C)** *ENDOU* expression showed negative correlation with M2 macrophages markers, including *CD163*, *VSIG4*, and *MS4A4A*.

founding that tumor suppressor gene *ENDOU* was negatively correlated with M2 markers of *CD163*, *VSIG4*, and *MS4A4A*, we speculated that *ENDOU* may also inhibit macrophages M2 polarization in tumor microenvironment.

In sum, our multiple bioinformatics analysis identified 98 genes with core functions like extracellular matrix organization significantly enriched. 15 genes showed prognostic significance, and *COBL* and *ENDOU* serve as independent survival markers in HNSCC. In-vitro *ENDOU* overexpression inhibited FaDu and Cal-27 cells proliferation and migration, indicating its tumor-suppressing role in HNSCC progression. GSEA analysis indicated *ENDOU* down-stream pathways like DNA replication, mismatch repair, cell cycle and IL-17 signaling pathway. *ENDOU* showed relative lower expression in HNSCC, especially HPV-positive HNSCC samples. At last, *ENDOU showed* negative correlation with tumor purity and tumor infiltrating macrophages, especially M2 macrophages. It was the first time that *ENDOU* was identified as a tumor suppressor, with prognostic significance and negative correlation with tumor infiltrating M2 macrophages. However, further biological and basic studies are needed to validate our findings.

ETHICS STATEMENT

The experiment was approved the Ethics Committee of Eye Nose and Throat Hospital, Fudan University.

AUTHOR CONTRIBUTIONS

CX, YZ, and LZ conceived and designed the study. YZ analyzed the data. YPS, YS, and MZ performed the experiments. YZ and LZ wrote the paper. CX and YPS reviewed and edited the manuscript. All authors contributed to the article and approved the submitted version.

Supplementary Figure 1 | Normalization and MDS plot of GSE6631 and GSE107591; **A, B**) Normalization boxplot of GSE6631 and GSE107591; **C, D**) MDS plot of GSE6631 and GSE107591.

Supplementary Figure 2 | Kaplan-Meier survival plot of **(A)** PLAU; **(B)** ALDH3A1; **(C)** SERPINE1; **(D)** CEACAM6; **(E)** CEACAM61; **(F)** LAMB3; **(G)** METTL7A; **(H)** DUSP5; **(I)** SPINK5; **(J)** MYO1B; **(K)** FAP; **(L)** SEMA3C; **(M)** LAMC2 in HNSCC.

REFERENCES

1. Jou A, Hess J. Epidemiology and Molecular Biology of Head and Neck Cancer. *Oncol Res Treat* (2017) 40(6):328–32. doi: 10.1159/000477127
2. Kamangar F, Dores GM, Anderson WF. Patterns of cancer incidence, mortality, and prevalence across five continents: defining priorities to reduce cancer disparities in different geographic regions of the world. *J Clin Oncol* (2006) 24(14):2137–50. doi: 10.1200/JCO.2005.05.2308
3. Moskovitz JM, Moy J, Seiwert TY, Ferris RL. Immunotherapy for Head and Neck Squamous Cell Carcinoma: A Review of Current and Emerging Therapeutic Options. *Oncologist* (2017) 22(6):680–93. doi: 10.1634/theoncologist.2016-0318
4. Agrawal N, Frederick MJ, Pickering CR, Bettegowda C, Chang K, Li RJ. Exome sequencing of head and neck squamous cell carcinoma reveals inactivating mutations in NOTCH1. *Science* (2011) 333(6046):1154–7. doi: 10.1126/science.1206923
5. Cancer Genome Atlas N. Comprehensive genomic characterization of head and neck squamous cell carcinomas. *Nature* (2015) 517(7536):576–82. doi: 10.1038/nature14129
6. Diehn M, Eisen MB, Botstein D, Brown PO. Large-scale identification of secreted and membrane-associated gene products using DNA microarrays. *Nat Genet* (2000) 25(1):58–62. doi: 10.1038/75603
7. El-Naggar AK, Kim HW, Clayman GL, Coombes MM, Le B, Lai S. Differential expression profiling of head and neck squamous carcinoma: significance in their phenotypic and biological classification. *Oncogene* (2002) 21(53):8206–19. doi: 10.1038/sj.onc.1206021
8. Lemaire F, Millon R, Young J, Cromer A, Wasylyk C, Schultz I, et al. Differential expression profiling of head and neck squamous cell carcinoma (HNSCC). *Br J Cancer* (2003) 89(10):1940–9. doi: 10.1038/sj.bjc.6601373
9. Stransky N, Egloff AM, Tward AD, Kostic AD, Cibulskis K, Sivachenko A, et al. The mutational landscape of head and neck squamous cell carcinoma. *Science* (2011) 333(6046):1157–60. doi: 10.1126/science.1208130
10. Emmert-Buck MR, Strausberg RL, Krizman DB, Bonaldo MF, Bonner RF, Bostwick DG, et al. Molecular profiling of clinical tissues specimens: feasibility and applications. *J Mol Diagn* (2000) 2(2):60–6. doi: 10.1016/s1525-1578(10) 60617-4
11. Pollack JR, Perou CM, Alizadeh AA, Eisen MB, Pergamenschikov A, Williams CF, et al. Genome-wide analysis of DNA copy-number changes using cDNA microarrays. *Nat Genet* (1999) 23(1):41–6. doi: 10.1038/12640
12. Zhang L, Zhou W, Velculescu VE, Kern SE, Hruban RH, Hamilton SR, et al. Gene expression profiles in normal and cancer cells. *Science* (1997) 276 (5316):1268–72. doi: 10.1126/science.276.5316.1268
13. Kuriakose MA, Chen WT, He ZM, Sikora AG, Zhang P, Zhang ZY, et al. Selection and validation of differentially expressed genes in head and neck cancer. *Cell Mol Life Sci* (2004) 61(11):1372–83. doi: 10.1007/s00018-004-4069-0
14. Irizarry RA, Bolstad BM, Collin F, Cope LM, Hobbs B, Speed TP. Summaries of Affymetrix GeneChip probe level data. *Nucleic Acids Res* (2003) 31(4):e15. doi: 10.1093/nar/gng015
15. Diboun I, Wernisch L, Orengo CA, Koltzenburg M. Microarray analysis after RNA amplification can detect pronounced differences in gene expression using limma. *BMC Genomics* (2006) 7:252. doi: 10.1186/1471-2164-7-252
16. Zou Y, Zhang M, Zeng D, Ruan Y, Shen L, Mu Z, et al. Periplaneta americana Extracts Accelerate Liver Regeneration a Complex Network of Pathways. *Front Pharmacol* (2020) 11:1174. doi: 10.3389/fphar.2020.01174
17. Babačić H, Lehtiö J, Pico de Coaña Y, Pernemalm M, Eriksson H. In-depth plasma proteomics reveals increase in circulating PD-1 during anti-PD-1 immunotherapy in patients with metastatic cutaneous melanoma. *J Immunother Cancer* (2020) 8(1). doi: 10.1136/jitc-2019-000204
18. Scardoni G, Petterlini M, Laudanna C. Analyzing biological network parameters with CentiScaPe. *Bioinformatics* (2009) 25(21):2857–9. doi: 10.1093/bioinformatics/btp517
19. Li T, Fan J, Wang B, Traugh N, Chen Q, Liu JS, et al. TIMER: A Web Server for Comprehensive Analysis of Tumor-Infiltrating Immune Cells. *Cancer Res* (2017) 77(21):e108–10. doi: 10.1158/0008-5472.CAN-17-0307
20. Pan JH, Zhou H, Cooper L, Huang JL, Zhu SB, Zhao XX, et al. LAYN Is a Prognostic Biomarker and Correlated With Immune Infiltrates in Gastric and Colon Cancers. *Front Immunol* (2019) 10:6. doi: 10.3389/fimmu.2019. 00006
21. Engelman JA. Targeting PI3K signalling in cancer: opportunities, challenges and limitations. *Nat Rev Cancer* (2009) 9(8):550–62. doi: 10.1038/nrc2664
22. Kozaki K, Imoto I, Pimkhaokham A, Hasegawa S, Tsuda H, Omura K, et al. PIK3CA mutation is an oncogenic aberration at advanced stages of oral squamous cell carcinoma. *Cancer Sci* (2006) 97(12):1351–8. doi: 10.1111/ j.1349-7006.2006.00343.x
23. Qiu W, Schonleben F, Li X, Ho DJ, Close LG, Manolidis S, et al. PIK3CA mutations in head and neck squamous cell carcinoma. *Clin Cancer Res* (2006) 12(5):1441–6. doi: 10.1158/1078-0432.CCR-05-2173
24. Murugan AK, Hong NT, Fukui Y, Munirajan AK, Tsuchida N. Oncogenic mutations of the PIK3CA gene in head and neck squamous cell carcinomas. *Int J Oncol* (2008) 32(1):101–11. doi: 10.3892/ijo.32.1.101
25. Hou W, Nemitz S, Schopper S, Nielsen ML, Kessels MM, Qualmann B. Arginine Methylation by PRMT2 Controls the Functions of the Actin Nucleator Cobl. *Dev Cell* (2018) 45(2):262–275 e8. doi: 10.1016/ j.devcel.2018.03.007
26. Hou W, Izadi M, Nemitz S, Haag N, Kessels MM, Qualmann B. The Actin Nucleator Cobl Is Controlled by Calcium and Calmodulin. *PloS Biol* (2015) 13 (9):e1002233. doi: 10.1371/journal.pbio.1002233
27. Schwintzer L, Koch N, Ahuja R, Grimm J, Kessels MM, Qualmann B. The functions of the actin nucleator Cobl in cellular morphogenesis critically depend on syndapin I. *EMBO J* (2011) 30(15):3147–59. doi: 10.1038/emboj.2011.207
28. Lopes BA, Meyer C, Barbosa TC, Poubel CP, Mansur MB, Duployez N, et al. IKZF1 Deletions with COBL Breakpoints Are Not Driven by RAG-Mediated Recombination Events in Acute Lymphoblastic Leukemia. *Transl Oncol* (2019) 12(5):726–32. doi: 10.1016/j.tranon.2019.02.002
29. Laneve P, Gioia U, Ragno R, Altieri F, Di Franco C, Santini T, et al. The tumor marker human placental protein 11 is an endoribonuclease. *J Biol Chem* (2008) 283(50):34712–9. doi: 10.1074/jbc.M805759200
30. Inaba N, Renk T, Daume E, Bohn H. Ectopic production of placenta-"specific" tissue proteins (PP5 and PP11) by malignant breast tumors. *Arch Gynecol* (1981) 231(1):87–90. doi: 10.1007/BF02110028
31. Inaba N, Renk T, Wurster K, Rapp W, Bohn H. Ectopic synthesis of pregnancy specific beta 1-glycoprotein (SP1) and placental specific tissue proteins (PP5, PP10, PP11, PP12) in nontrophoblastic malignant tumours. Possible markers in oncology. *Klin Wochenschr* (1980) 58(15):789–91. doi: 10.1007/BF01478287
32. Song L, Xie H, Tong F, Yan B, Zhang S, Fu E, et al. Association of lnc-IL17RA-11 with increased radiation sensitivity and improved prognosis of HPV-positive HNSCC. *J Cell Biochem* (2019) 120(10):17438–48. doi: 10.1002/jcb.29008
33. Partlova S, Boucek J, Kloudova K, Lukesova E, Zabrodsky M, Grega M, et al. Distinct patterns of intratumoral immune cell infiltrates in patients with HPV-associated compared to non-virally induced head and neck squamous cell carcinoma. *Oncoimmunology* (2015) 4(1):e965570. doi: 10.4161/ 21624011.2014.965570
34. Siegel RL, Miller KD, Jemal A. Cancer Statistics, 2017. *CA Cancer J Clin* (2017) 67(1):7–30. doi: 10.3322/caac.21387
35. Wicker C, Takiar V, Suganya R, Arnold S, Brill Y, Chen L, et al. Evaluation of antioxidant network proteins as novel prognostic biomarkers for head and neck cancer patients. *Oral Oncol* (2020) 111:104949. doi: 10.1016/ j.oraloncology.2020.104949
36. Li W, Chen Y, Nie X. Regulatory Mechanisms of lncRNAs and Their Target Gene Signaling Pathways in Laryngeal Squamous Cell Carcinoma. *Front Pharmacol* (2020) 11:1140. doi: 10.3389/fphar.2020.01140
37. Koontongkaew S, Amornphimoltham P, Monthanpisut P, Saensuk T, Leelakriangsak M. Fibroblasts and extracellular matrix differently modulate MMP activation by primary and metastatic head and neck cancer cells. *Med Oncol* (2012) 29(2):690–703. doi: 10.1007/s12032-011- 9871-6
38. Taitz A, Petruzzelli GJ, Lozano Y, Shankar R, Young MR. Bi-directional stimulation of adherence to extracellular matrix components by human head and neck squamous carcinoma cells and endothelial cells. *Cancer Lett* (1995) 96(2):253–60. doi: 10.1016/0304-3835(95)03939-T
39. Ge Y, Li W, Ni Q, He Y, Chu J, Wei P. Weighted Gene Co-Expression Network Analysis Identifies Hub Genes Associated with Occurrence and Prognosis of Oral Squamous Cell Carcinoma. *Med Sci Monit* (2019) 25:7272– 88. doi: 10.12659/MSM.916025

40. Mendez E, Houck JR, Doody DR, Fan W, Lohavanichbutr P, Rue TC, et al. A genetic expression profile associated with oral cancer identifies a group of patients at high risk of poor survival. *Clin Cancer Res* (2009) 15(4):1353–61. doi: 10.1158/1078-0432.CCR-08-1816
41. Zhao L, Chi W, Cao H, Cui W, Meng W, Guo W, et al. Screening and clinical significance of tumor markers in head and neck squamous cell carcinoma through bioinformatics analysis. *Mol Med Rep* (2019) 19(1):143–54. doi: 10.3892/mmr.2018.9639
42. Arroyo-Solera I, Pavon MA, Leon X, Lopez M, Gallardo A, Cespedes MV, et al. Effect of serpinE1 overexpression on the primary tumor and lymph node, and lung metastases in head and neck squamous cell carcinoma. *Head Neck* (2019) 41(2):429–39. doi: 10.1002/hed.25437
43. Saleh AD, Cheng H, Martin SE, Si H, Ormanoglu P, Carlson S, et al. Integrated Genomic and Functional microRNA Analysis Identifies miR-30-5p as a Tumor Suppressor and Potential Therapeutic Nanomedicine in Head and Neck Cancer. *Clin Cancer Res* (2019) 25(9):2860–73. doi: 10.1158/1078-0432.CCR-18-0716
44. Yang K, Zhang S, Zhang D, Tao Q, Zhang T, Liu G, et al. Identification of SERPINE1, PLAU and ACTA1 as biomarkers of head and neck squamous cell carcinoma based on integrated bioinformatics analysis. *Int J Clin Oncol* (2019) 24(9):1030–41. doi: 10.1007/s10147-019-01435-9
45. Yamada Y, Koshizuka K, Hanazawa T, Kikkawa N, Okato A, Idichi T, et al. Passenger strand of miR-145-3p acts as a tumor-suppressor by targeting MYO1B in head and neck squamous cell carcinoma. *Int J Oncol* (2018) 52 (1):166–78. doi: 10.3892/ijo.2017.4190
46. Liu L, Jung SN, Oh C, Lee K, Won HR, Chang JW, et al. LAMB3 is associated with disease progression and cisplatin cytotoxic sensitivity in head and neck squamous cell carcinoma. *Eur J Surg Oncol* (2019) 45(3):359–65. doi: 10.1016/j.ejso.2018.10.543
47. Tam K, Schoppy DW, Shin JH, Tay JK, Moreno-Nieves U, Mundy DC, et al. Assessing the Impact of Targeting CEACAM1 in Head and Neck Squamous Cell Carcinoma. *Otolaryngol Head Neck Surg* (2018) 159(1):76–84. doi: 10.1177/0194599818756627
48. Bednarek K, Kostrzewska-Poczekaj M, Szaumkessel M, Kiwerska K, Paczkowska J, Byzia E, et al. Downregulation of CEACAM6 gene expression in laryngeal squamous cell carcinoma is an effect of DNA hypermethylation and correlates with disease progression. *Am J Cancer Res* (2018) 8(7):1249–61.
49. Cameron S, de Long LM, Hazar-Rethinam M, Topkas E, Endo-Munoz L, Cumming A, et al. Focal overexpression of CEACAM6 contributes to enhanced tumourigenesis in head and neck cancer via suppression of apoptosis. *Mol Cancer* (2012) 11:74. doi: 10.1186/1476-4598-11-74
50. Okazaki S, Shintani S, Hirata Y, Suina K, Semba T, Yamasaki J, et al. Synthetic lethality of the ALDH3A1 inhibitor dyclonine and xCT inhibitors in glutathione deficiency-resistant cancer cells. *Oncotarget* (2018) 9(73):33832–43. doi: 10.18632/oncotarget.26112
51. Lv Z, Wu K, Qin X, Yuan J, Yan M, Zhang J, et al. A Novel Tumor Suppressor SPINK5 Serves as an Independent Prognostic Predictor for Patients with Head and Neck Squamous Cell Carcinoma. *Cancer Manag Res* (2020) 12:4855–69. doi: 10.2147/CMAR.S236266
52. Delloye-Bourgeois C, Bertin L, Thoinet K, Jarrosson L, Kindbeiter K, Buffet T, et al. Microenvironment-Driven Shift of Cohesion/Detachment Balance within Tumors Induces a Switch toward Metastasis in Neuroblastoma. *Cancer Cell* (2017) 32(4):427–443 e8. doi: 10.1016/j.ccell.2017.09.006
53. Hintz HM, Gallant JP, Vander Griend DJ, Coleman IM, Nelson PS, LeBeau AM. Imaging Fibroblast Activation Protein Alpha Improves Diagnosis of Metastatic Prostate Cancer with Positron Emission Tomography. *Clin Cancer Res* (2020) 26(18):4882–91. doi: 10.1158/1078-0432.CCR-20-1358
54. Ogawa Y, Masugi Y, Abe T, Yamazaki K, Ueno A, Fujii-Nishimura Y, et al. Three distinct stroma types in human pancreatic cancer identified by image analysis of fibroblast subpopulations and collagen. *Clin Cancer Res* (2020). doi: 10.1158/1078-0432.CCR-20-2298
55. Hussain A, Voisin V, Poon S, Karamboulas C, Bui NHB, Meens J, et al. Distinct fibroblast functional states drive clinical outcomes in ovarian cancer and are regulated by TCF21. *J Exp Med* (2020) 217(8). doi: 10.1084/jem.20191094
56. Hua KT, Wang MY, Chen MW, Wei LH, Chen CK, Ko CH, et al. The H3K9 methyltransferase G9a is a marker of aggressive ovarian cancer that promotes peritoneal metastasis. *Mol Cancer* (2014) 13:189. doi: 10.1186/1476-4598-13-189
57. Jun F, Peng Z, Zhang Y, Shi D. Quantitative proteomic analysis identifies novel regulators of methotrexate resistance in choriocarcinoma. *Gynecol Oncol* (2020) 157(1):268–79. doi: 10.1016/j.ygyno.2020.01.013
58. Badr M, Johrens K, Allgauer M, Boxberg M, Weichert W, Tinhofer I, et al. Morphomolecular analysis of the immune tumor microenvironment in human head and neck cancer. *Cancer Immunol Immunother* (2019) 68 (9):1443–54. doi: 10.1007/s00262-019-02378-w
59. Chimote AA, Hajdu P, Sfyris AM, Gleich BN, Wise-Draper T, Casper KA, et al. Kv1.3 Channels Mark Functionally Competent CD8+ Tumor-Infiltrating Lymphocytes in Head and Neck Cancer. *Cancer Res* (2017) 77 (1):53–61. doi: 10.1158/0008-5472.CAN-16-2372
60. Tsujikawa T, Yaguchi T, Ohmura G, Ohta S, Kobayashi A, Kawamura N, et al. Autocrine and paracrine loops between cancer cells and macrophages promote lymph node metastasis via CCR4/CCL22 in head and neck squamous cell carcinoma. *Int J Cancer* (2013) 132(12):2755–66. doi: 10.1002/ijc.27966
61. Topf MC, Harshyne L, Tuluc M, Mardekian S, Vimawala S, Cognetti DM, et al. Loss of CD169(+) Subcapsular Macrophages during Metastatic Spread of Head and Neck Squamous Cell Carcinoma. *Otolaryngol Head Neck Surg* (2019) 161(1):67–73. doi: 10.1177/0194599819829741
62. She L, Qin Y, Wang J, Liu C, Zhu G, Li G, et al. Tumor-associated macrophages derived CCL18 promotes metastasis in squamous cell carcinoma of the head and neck. *Cancer Cell Int* (2018) 18:120. doi: 10.1186/s12935-018-0620-1
63. Balermpas P, Rodel F, Liberz R, Oppermann J, Wagenblast J, Ghanaati S, et al. Head and neck cancer relapse after chemoradiotherapy correlates with CD163 + macrophages in primary tumour and CD11b+ myeloid cells in recurrences. *Br J Cancer* (2014) 111(8):1509–18. doi: 10.1038/bjc.2014.446
64. Ooft ML, van Ipenburg JA, Sanders ME, Kranendonk M, Hofland I, de Bree R, et al. Prognostic role of tumour-associated macrophages and regulatory T cells in EBV-positive and EBV-negative nasopharyngeal carcinoma. *J Clin Pathol* (2018) 71(3):267–74. doi: 10.1136/jclinpath-2017-204664
65. Wang Y, Smith W, Hao D, He B, Kong L. M1 and M2 macrophage polarization and potentially therapeutic naturally occurring compounds. *Int Immunopharmacol* (2019) 70:459–66. doi: 10.1016/j.intimp.2019.02.050
66. Yuan A, Hsiao YJ, Chen HY, Chen HW, Ho CC, Chen YY, et al. Opposite Effects of M1 and M2 Macrophage Subtypes on Lung Cancer Progression. *Sci Rep* (2015) 5:14273. doi: 10.1038/srep14273
67. Huang H, Liu X, Zhao F, Lu J, Zhang B, Peng X, et al. M2-polarized tumour-associated macrophages in stroma correlate with poor prognosis and Epstein-Barr viral infection in nasopharyngeal carcinoma. *Acta Otolaryngol* (2017) 137(8):888–94. doi: 10.1080/00016489.2017.1296585
68. Hsieh CH, Tai SK, Yang MH. Snail-overexpressing Cancer Cells Promote M2-Like Polarization of Tumor-Associated Macrophages by Delivering MiR-21-Abundant Exosomes. *Neoplasia* (2018) 20(8):775–88. doi: 10.1016/j.neo.2018.06.004
69. Ohashi T, Aoki M, Tomita H, Akazawa T, Sato K, Kuze B, et al. M2-like macrophage polarization in high lactic acid-producing head and neck cancer. *Cancer Sci* (2017) 108(6):1128–34. doi: 10.1111/cas.13244

11

Regulatory Role of Hexokinase 2 in Modulating Head and Neck Tumorigenesis

Wan-Chun Li [1,2,3], Chien-Hsiang Huang [1], Yi-Ta Hsieh [1], Tsai-Ying Chen [1], Li-Hao Cheng [1], Chang-Yi Chen [1], Chung-Ji Liu [1,2,4,5], Hsin-Ming Chen [6], Chien-Ling Huang [7], Jeng-Fan Lo [1,2,3,8] and Kuo-Wei Chang [1,2,3,8]*

[1] Institute of Oral Biology, School of Dentistry, National Yang-Ming University, Taipei, Taiwan, [2] Department of Dentistry, School of Dentistry, National Yang-Ming University, Taipei, Taiwan, [3] Cancer Progression Research Center, National Yang-Ming University, Taipei, Taiwan, [4] Department of Oral and Maxillofacial Surgery, MacKay Memorial Hospital, Taipei, Taiwan, [5] Department of Medical Research, MacKay Memorial Hospital, Taipei, Taiwan, [6] School of Dentistry and Department of Dentistry, National Taiwan University Medical College and National Taiwan University Hospital, Taipei, Taiwan, [7] Department of Health Technology and Informatics (HTI), The Hong Kong Polytechnic University (PolyU), Kowloon, Hong Kong, [8] Department of Stomatology, Taipei Veterans General Hospital, Taipei, Taiwan

***Correspondence:**
Wan-Chun Li
wcli@ym.edu.tw

To support great demand of cell growth, cancer cells preferentially obtain energy and biomacromolecules by glycolysis over mitochondrial oxidative phosphorylation (OxPhos). Among all glycolytic enzymes, hexokinase (HK), a rate-limiting enzyme at the first step of glycolysis to catalyze cellular glucose into glucose-6-phosphate, is herein emphasized. Four HK isoforms, HK1-HK4, were discovered in nature. It was shown that HK2 expression is enriched in many tumor cells and correlated with poorer survival rates in most neoplastic cells. HK2-mediated regulations for cell malignancy and mechanistic cues in regulating head and neck tumorigenesis, however, are not fully elucidated. Cellular malignancy index, such as cell growth, cellular motility, and treatment sensitivity, and molecular alterations were determined in HK2-deficient head and neck squamous cell carcinoma (HNSCC) cells. By using various cancer databases, HK2, but not HK1, positively correlates with HNSCC progression in a stage-dependent manner. A high HK2 expression was detected in head and neck cancerous tissues compared with their normal counterparts, both in mouse and human subjects. Loss of HK2 in HNSCC cells resulted in reduced cell (*in vitro*) and tumor (*in vivo*) growth, as well as decreased epithelial-mesenchymal transition–mediated cell movement; in contrast, HK2-deficient HNSCC cells exhibited greater sensitivity to chemotherapeutic drugs cisplatin and 5-fluorouracil but are more resistant to photodynamic therapy, indicating that HK2 expression could selectively define treatment sensitivity in HNSCC cells. At the molecular level, it was found that HK2 alteration drove metabolic reprogramming toward OxPhos and modulated oncogenic Akt and mutant TP53-mediated signals in HNSCC cells. In summary, the present study showed that HK2 suppression could lessen HNSCC oncogenicity and modulate therapeutic sensitivity, thereby being an ideal therapeutic target for HNSCCs.

Keywords: head and neck cancer, hexokinase 2, cellular malignancy, metabolic shift, therapeutic efficacy

INTRODUCTION

Most cancers have acquired the same set of functional capabilities during tumorigenesis including sustained proliferative signal, evaded growth suppressors, resisted cell death, sustained angiogenesis, and deregulated cellular energetics (1). In the aspect of energy production, glucose is a major source of bioenergetics and biomolecules used to maintain cellular homeostasis. Glucose molecules could be metabolized by glycolysis to generate pyruvate in cells; the pyruvate could be either oxidatively metabolized to generate up to 38 ATPs through the process of oxidative phosphorylation (OxPhos) or be reductively converted into organic acids or alcohols by fermentation producing only 2 ATP (2). In general, normal cells in non-malignant tissues developed an evolutionary choice of "Pasteur effect" to allow a system to fine tune cell metabolism in unfavorable environment (3, 4). On the contrary, cancer cells exhibited a unique metabolic system by taking advantage of aerobic glycolysis for demands of energy and biomolecules regardless of oxygen status; in this way, cancer cells preferentially drive their metabolism away from OxPhos toward glycolysis, so-called Warburg effect (5).

Previous studies have sought to target different cancer-specific metabolic pathways, in particular glycolysis, for development of antitumor treatments (6–9). There are three irreversible reactions in glycolysis. It is well-known that the glycolytic rate is limited by the phosphorylation state of glycolytic enzymes hexokinases (HKs), because at the first step of glycolysis, HKs catalyze the intake glucose into glucose-6-phosphate (G-6-P) (10). Hexokinase-mediated catalysis is ATP dependent and a key determinant for the direction and magnitude of glucose flux within cells; thus, it would more efficient to target glucose metabolism in cancer cells by cutting down this earliest step of glucose flux (11). Four HK isoforms including HK1, HK2, HK3, and HK4 encoded by different genes were found in nature. Among them, HK1 is ubiquitously expressed in most mammalian tissues, and HK2 is detected in adipose, skeletal, and cardiac muscles, whereas HK3 and HK4 show relatively low expression in mammalian tissues (12). In the aspect of protein structure, two catalytic domains, both in N- and C-terminal portions, are detected in HK2, resulting in greater glycolytic rate compared with HK1-mediated glycolysis, whereas only one catalytic domain was found at the carboxyl terminal part in HK1 protein (13). In clinic, HK2 is rarely expressed in normal tissues as a high level of HK2 expression was detected in many solid tumors (14) and is associated with elevated progression, poorer overall survival, and treatment resistance in breast cancer (both primary and metastatic kinds) (15–18), bladder cancer (19), cervical squamous cell carcinoma (20), colorectal cancer (21), epithelial ovarian tumors (22), glioblastoma multiforme (23), hepatocellular carcinoma (24), laryngeal squamous cell carcinoma (25), lung cancer (26), neuroblastoma (27), neuroendocrine tumor (28), pancreatic cancer (29), and prostate cancer (30), making it an excellent target for development of anticancer therapy. Moreover, given its selective expression in tumors, HK2 has drawn increasing attention on its clinical implications forming the basis of fluorodeoxyglucose F-18 positron emission tomography imaging, a widely used clinical procedure to detect tumors. Indeed, a recent meta-analysis provides evidence that HK2 could be a marker to predict the risk of all-cause mortality and cancer progression in patients with tumors of the digestive system (31).

Numbers of molecular cues including signal transducer and activator of transcription 3 (32–35), protein kinase B (PKB), also known as Akt (19, 36–38), mammalian target of rapamycin (38–40), and PH domain leucine-rich repeat protein phosphatase (41), as well as autophagy (42, 43), have been found to control HK2-mediated metabolic alterations, thereby regulating tumor identity. Moreover, HK2 contains an N-terminal hydrophobic domain allowing it to bind to outer mitochondrial membrane voltage-dependent anion channel (VDAC) protein, thereby resulting in Bax-mediated apoptosis. HK2–VDAC interaction could also provide kinetic benefits in HK2 exhibiting greater affinity to ATP over G-6-P, suggesting that HK2 could regulate oncogenicity via modulation of mitochondrial physiology (44–47). More recent studies further discovered that p53-inducible protein TIGAR (Tp53-induced Glycolysis and Apoptosis Regulator), Akt, and ER stress sensor kinase could regulate mitochondrial HK2 localization (48–51). Interestingly, mitochondrial TIGAR–HK2 complex upregulated HK2 and hypoxia-inducible factor 1 activity limiting reactive oxygen species production and protecting from tumor cell death under hypoxic condition implying that p53 could be an essential key regulator for HK2-mediated oncogenesis (26, 30, 48). In addition to signaling factors, HK2 regulated by epigenetic mediators including microRNAs (32, 52–55), long non-coding RNAs (56–58), and histone/DNA methylation (59) are also important to modulate HK2-mediated tumorigenicity. Taken together, HK2 seems to be a master promoting factor in controlling carcinogenesis in different cancers; to date, however, the role of HK2 in controlling head and neck squamous cell carcinoma (HNSCC) development was rarely focused. The present study was therefore conceived to determine cellular, molecular, and physiological alterations of HNSCC cells in response to HK2 silencing.

MATERIALS AND METHODS

Basic Reagents, Cells, and Animal and Human Protocols

All experimental reagents including 4-nitroquinoline 1-oxide (4-NQO), 3-(4,5-Dimethylthiazol-2-yl)-2,5-diphenyltetrazolium bromide (MTT), cisplatin (CDDP), and 5-fluorouracil (5-FU) were purchased from Sigma. The HNSCC cell lines, clinical human HNSCC tissues, and animal procedure were obtained and described elsewhere (60, 61).

Establishment of HK2 Silencing HNSCC Cells

Three plasmids encoding small hairpin RNAs (shRNAs) targeting HK2 gene were purchased from the National RNAi Core Facility (NRCF), Academia Sinica, Taipei, Taiwan. The targeting sequences were as listed: 5-GCCTGGCTAACTTCATGGATA-3 (A), 5-CCGTAACATTCTCATCGATTT-3 (B), and 5-GCTTGA AGATTAGGTACTATC-3 (C) (NRCF). The control nucleotide sequence of shRNA was 5-GCGGTTGCCAAGAGGTTCCAT-3, which was the random sequence that targets luciferase (shLuc) mRNA. Lentiviral vectors containing shHK2/shLuc were generated in 293T cells.

Cellular and Molecular Assays

Cell growth (MTT and trypan blue exclusion assays), cell cycle, annexin V–fluorescein isothiocyanate–based cell apoptosis, Transwell-based cell migration/invasion, drug resistance (IC50 determination), quantitative real-time polymerase chain reaction (qRT-PCR), Western blot, aldehyde dehydrogenase (ALDH) activity, immunostaining analysis, human phospho-antibody array, and XF Metabolic Assay analyses were performed as previously described at Instrumentation Resource Center, National Yang Ming University (61, 62). Primers for qRT-PCR analysis (**Supplementary Table 1**) and antibodies used for protein assays (**Supplementary Table 2**) are listed. ImageJ (National Institute of Health, Bethesda, Maryland, United States) was used for quantification.

Aminolevulinic Acid–Photodynamic Therapy Treatment

5-Aminolevulinic acid (ALA) 1 mM was made by diluting 1 M ALA stock with serum-free medium and neutralized to pH 7.2 with NaOH immediately before use. The total number of 5×10^5 cells were incubated with 1 mM ALA for 3 h, and the medium was replaced with 100 μL phosphate-buffered saline to prevent thermal injury by the light. The cells were then exposed to various doses of light source (30.33 mW/cm^2) with a 635-nm wavelength emission of red light. After exposure, cells are replaced with culture medium and cultured for 24 h. Relative viable cells were determined by the MTT method.

Measurement of Lactate, ATP, and PDH Activity

Extracellular lactate, intracellular ATP level, and pyruvate dehydrogenase (PDH) activity were determined previously (62). Cell number or genomic DNA content was used to normalize detections.

Xenografic Model

The HNSCC cells 1×10^6 to 4×10^6 and 1 μL of each medium were mixed and subcutaneously injected into the back of nude mice. Tumor volume and size were recorded.

Statistical Analysis

All analyses were statistically determined using Microsoft Excel 2013 (Microsoft, Redmond, WA, United States)/Prism 5 (GraphPad, San Diego, CA, United States). All quantifications are presented as mean ± SEM. A significant difference was defined as $p < 0.05$.

RESULTS

HK2 Expression Defines HNSCC Progression in Clinic

By taking advantage of The Cancer Genomic Atlas–based UALCAN, Firebrowse, and The Human Protein Atlas (www.proteinatlas.org) databases (63–65), it was found that HK2 transcript, in comparison with HK1, is enriched in most primary tumor tissues compared with their normal counterparts (**Figures 1A,B**). Further analysis for HK1 and HK2 expression in HNSCCs indicated that (i) HK2 expression, but not HK1, is positively correlated with tumor stages and grades (**Figures 1C,D**); (ii) HK2 level, but not HK1, is upregulated in HPV$^-$ HNSCC tissues (**Figure 1E**); and (iii) HK2 expression, but not HK1, is increased in early metastatic HNSCCs [with one to three axillary lymph nodes (N1)] (**Figure 1F**). Furthermore, immunohistochemical analysis showed that HK2 is strongly detected in 4-NQO–induced mouse tongue neoplastic lesions compared with normal oral epithelium (**Figure 1G**), as well as human oral squamous cell carcinoma (**Figure 1H**). Surprisingly, differential HK1 level could better stratify cancer-specific survival rates than HK2 in HNSCC patients (**Supplementary Figure 1**), suggesting that HK1 and HK2 might play differential roles during HNSCC tumorigenesis. Taken together, these analyses suggest that HK2 serves as a rather early prognostic indicator in the majority of HNSCC population.

HK2 Loss Modulates HNSCC Cell Growth and Motility

In consistent with former findings in other cancer tissues, HK2, both in mRNA and protein level, is highly expressed in tested HNSCC cell lines (**Supplementary Table 3**) compared to normal human oral keratinocytes (NHOKs) (**Figure 2A** and **Supplementary Figure 2**). A wide spectrum of cellular alterations and their potential underlying regulatory cues in response to HK2 loss were next focused on. As shRNA-mediated HK2-deficient HNSCC cells were successfully established without apparent morphological change (**Figures 2B,C** and **Supplementary Figure 3**), it was demonstrated that, by using both trypan blue exclusion (**Figure 2D**) and MTT (**Figure 2E**) assays, HK2-silencing resulted in decreased cell growth in HNSCC cells. Further analysis found no significant cell cycling change and cell apoptosis (data now shown) in HK2-silencing HNSCC cells compared with control cells, suggesting that HK2 could possibly control cell growth via self-protective machinery, such as autophagy (42, 43). *In vivo* growth for HK2-silencing tumors was also analyzed, and it was shown that HK2 loss resulted in significantly smaller xenografic tumors compared with control tumors (**Figure 2F**).

Potential impact of HK2 loss in regulating cell motility was also analyzed by using Transwell-based assays (62). The results indicated that HK2 deficiency led to significant decrease of cell migration and invasion in OECM-1 and HSC3 clones (**Figures 3A,B**). At cellular and molecular levels, lactate level, cytoskeletal organization and epithelial–mesenchymal transition (EMT) could modulate cell motility (66–68). While a slight, but not significant, increase in extracellular lactate production was detected in HK2-silencing HNSCC cells (**Supplementary Figure 4**), immunofluorescence staining analysis implied that lamellipodia-like F-actin (dot-lined in **Figure 3C**) was predominantly found in HK2-deficient

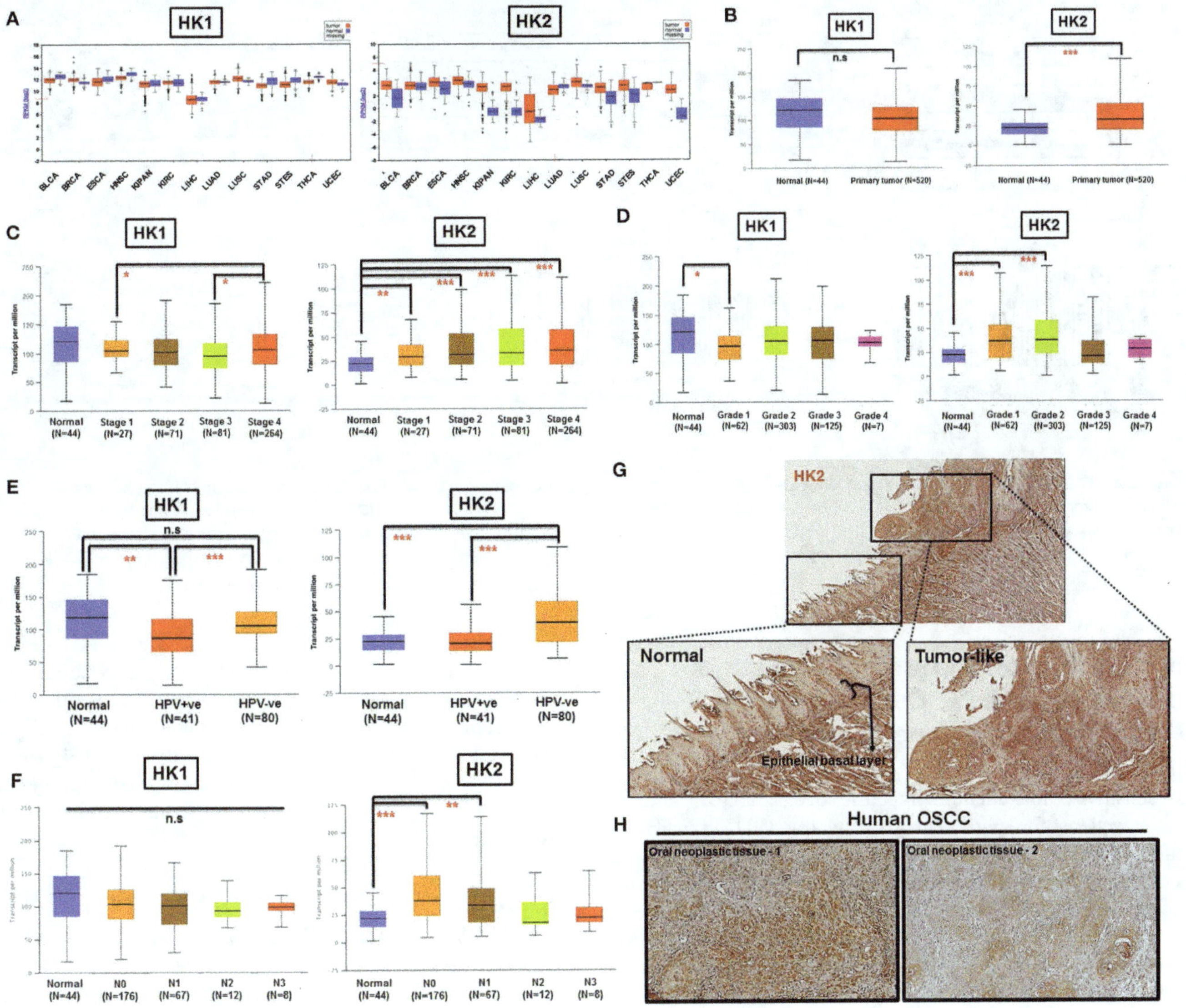

FIGURE 1 | HK2 level positively correlates with HNSCC progression in clinic. **(A)** HK1, but not HK2, mRNA expression is enriched in most human tumors by using Firebrowser database. BCLA, bladder urothelial carcinoma; BRCA, breast invasive carcinoma; ESCA, esophageal carcinoma; HNSCC, head and neck squamous cell carcinoma; KIPAN, Pan-kidney cohort (KICH+KIRC+KIRP); KIRC, kidney renal clear cell carcinoma; LIHC, liver hepatocellular carcinoma; LUAD, lung adenocarcinoma; LUSC, lung squamous cell carcinoma; STAD, stomach adenocarcinoma; STES, stomach and esophageal carcinoma; THCA, Thyroid carcinoma; UCEC, uterine corpus endometrial carcinoma. **(B)** Statistical analysis for HK1 and HK2 mRNA levels in normal and primary HNSCC tissues as well as tumor tissues, classified by clinical **(C)** stages, **(D)** grade, **(E)** HPV infection status, and **(F)** nodal metastasis status from UALCAN database. Immunohistochemical analysis for HK2 in **(G)** in 12-week 4-NQO–treated mouse tongue and **(H)** human oral squamous cell carcinoma (hOSCC) tissues. Data are shown as mean ± SEM. ***$p < 0.001$, **$p < 0.01$, *$p < 0.05$, and n.s., non-significant.

HNSCC cells in comparison with control cells those contain more evident filopodia-like protrusions. Interestingly, as shRNA-mediated HK2 manipulation seems to heterogeneously silence HK2 protein, HNSCC cells with greater HK2 loss (white arrows in **Figure 3C**) showed more and compacted F-actin staining signals compared with cells with less HK2 expression (yellow arrows in **Figure 3C**), revealing that HK2 loss potentially reduces F-actin level in a single-cell basis. Moreover, increased epithelial marker E-cadherin accompanied with decreased mesenchymal markers N-cadherin, Snail, and Twist was detected in mRNA level (**Figure 3D**), further supporting the important role of EMT in HK2-mediated cell motility alteration. The role of HK2 in regulating tumor metastasis *in vivo* was further defined in a previously established primary and metastatic xenografic tumor model (60). By using microarray analysis, it was found that HK2, but not HK1 and HK3, is enriched in highly migrating cells in this model (**Figure 3E**). In brief, multiple molecular factors play key roles in regulating cell movement upon HK2 loss.

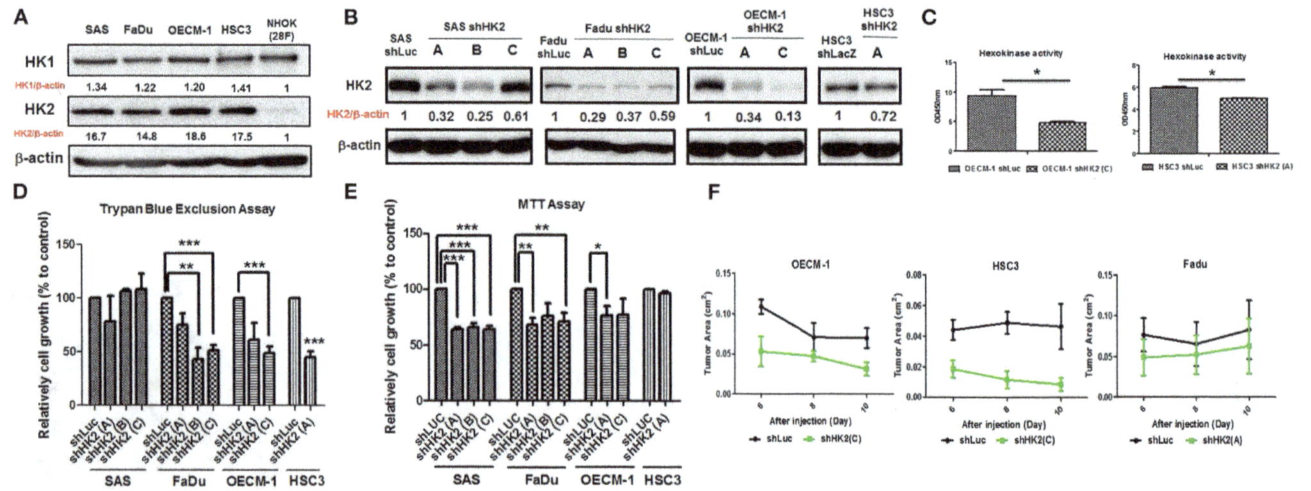

FIGURE 2 | Differential HNSCC cell growth and HNSCC-bearing xenografic tumor growth in response to HK2 loss. Respective Western blot analysis for HK1 and HK2 protein expression in **(A)** HNSCC and NHOK cells and **(B)** shRNA-mediated HK2-silencing HNSCCC cells. **(C)** Colorimetric hexokinase activity assay showed functional deficient in HK2-silencing OECM-1 and HSC3 cells. Cell growth was examined in HK2-silencing HNSCC cells using **(D)** trypan exclusion and **(E)** MTT assays. **(F)** HK2 loss downregulated HNSCC-bearing xenografic tumor growth. shLuc vector is used as a control plasmid. Data are shown as mean ± SEM ($N \geq 3$). ***$p < 0.001$, **$p < 0.01$, and *$p < 0.05$.

HK2 Expression Determines Treatment Resistance in HNSCCs Through Regulations of Stemness and Differentiation

The sensitivity for chemotherapeutic drugs, CDDP and 5-FU, as well as for photodynamic therapy (PDT), in HK2-silencing HNSCC cells was next examined. The results showed a common pattern of decreased half maximal inhibitory concentration (IC50) level for CDDP and 5-FU in HK2-deficient HNSCC cells compared with control cells (**Figure 4A**). Photodynamic therapy is an approved adjuvant treatment to lessen the disease mass of various premalignant and malignant lesions, including HNSCCs (69, 70). Photodynamic therapy–mediated cell apoptosis could be induced under numbers of physiological and pathological conditions, and one of the main advantages of PDT treatment is the higher selectivity to target transformed cells over normal cells (71). As HK2 loss could potentially reduce cell malignancy in HNSCC cells, it is expected that HK2-silencing HNSCC cells are less sensitive to PDT treatment (**Figure 4B**). At molecular level, previous study has shown that HK2 is essential for tumor initiation and survival in Kras-driven mouse lung cancer and ErbB2-driven mouse breast cancer, indicating that HK2 could be important to regulate cancer stemness (24). Moreover, it was also shown that elevated stemness could be a key factor underlying chemoresistance in HNSCCs (72). Consistent with this notion, stemness indicators Nanog and Oct4 mRNA (**Figure 4C**) and ALDH activity (**Figure 4D**) were downregulated in HK2-silencing HNSCC cells. Further analysis showed that HK2 protein is enriched in stem-like/high-grade sphere cells (**Figure 4E**), and strikingly, HK2 loss resulted in significantly less sphere number in selective medium used to culture head and neck cancer–initiating cells (**Figure 4F**). On the other hand, epithelial differentiation marker involucrin in OECM-1 cells with greater HK2 loss (clone C) was highly detected (**Figure 4G**), further supporting that HK2 change could regulate stemness and differentiation status, which modulate treatment sensitivity in HNSCC cells.

Molecular Alterations and Metabolic Shift in HK2-Silencing HNSCC Cells

HK2-mediated metabolic and molecular regulators for HNSCC malignancy were next examined. Metabolic reprogramming was recently proposed, suggesting that cancer cells could adapt to unfavorable metabolic stresses (73). Numbers of investigations have been reported showing metabolic shift upon HK2 changes in non-HNSCC cells (32, 40, 50, 54); in agreement with these findings, Seahorse analysis showed that HK2 loss led to increased basal and maximal mitochondrial respiration (**Figures 5A,B**), implying HK2-silencing HNSCC cells were metabolically programmed, being more dependent on mitochondrial metabolism. This statement could be further supported by the results showing a greater extracellular acidification rate (ECAR) upon addition of ATPase inhibitor oligomycin (**Figure 5C**) and increased PDH activity (**Figure 5D**) in HK2-silencing HNSCC cells. Unexpectedly, HK2 deficiency–mediated decreased cell growth did not result from reduction of cellular ATP level (**Figure 5E**), suggesting that bioenergetics could be dispensable for metabolism-mediated cell growth. Using a high-throughput human protein array, it was discovered that Akt (S473), TP53 (S15, S46, and S392), and p27 (T198) proteins were downregulated in HK2-silencing OECM-1 cells

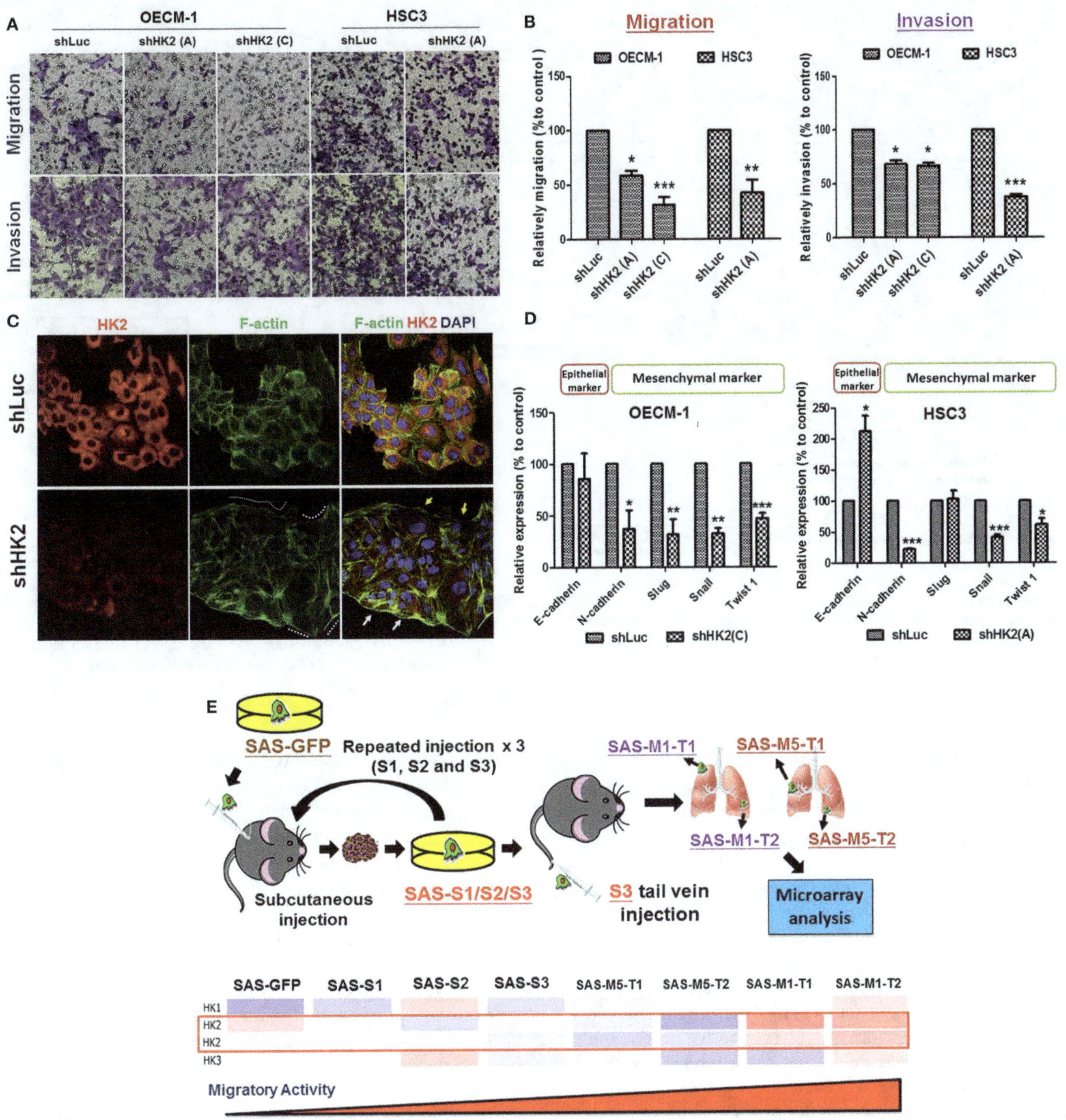

FIGURE 3 | Cell motility changes in HK2-silencing HNSCC Cells. **(A,B)** Transwell cell migration and invasion assays were performed in HK2-silencing HNSCC cells. HK2 knockdown led to significantly less migration and invasion in HNSCC cells. The changes of cell motility could result from **(C)** rearrangement of lamellipodia-like (dot-lined) and filopodia-like F-actin structures. HK2-silencing OECM-1 cells showed heterogeneous population, whereas cells with higher HK2 expression exhibited more condense F-actin structure (white arrows), while cells with less HK2 expression displayed little F-actin staining; and **(D)** altered EMT-associated mRNA expression. **(E)** Microarray analysis showed an increasing HK2, but not HK1 and HK3, mRNA expression in *in situ* injected (S1/2/3) and distant metastatic (M1/M5) HNSCC derived tumors. Data are presented as mean ± SEM ($N \geq 3$). $^{***}p < 0.001$, $^{**}p < 0.01$, and $^{*}p < 0.05$.

(**Figure 5F**). Western blot analysis further confirmed that Akt activity, but not another common oncogenic signaling factor Erk1/2, was deceased in HK2-deficient OECM-1 and HSC3 cells (**Figure 5G**).

DISCUSSION

In the present study, it was shown that HK2 loss downregulated cell growth, EMT-mediated cell movement,

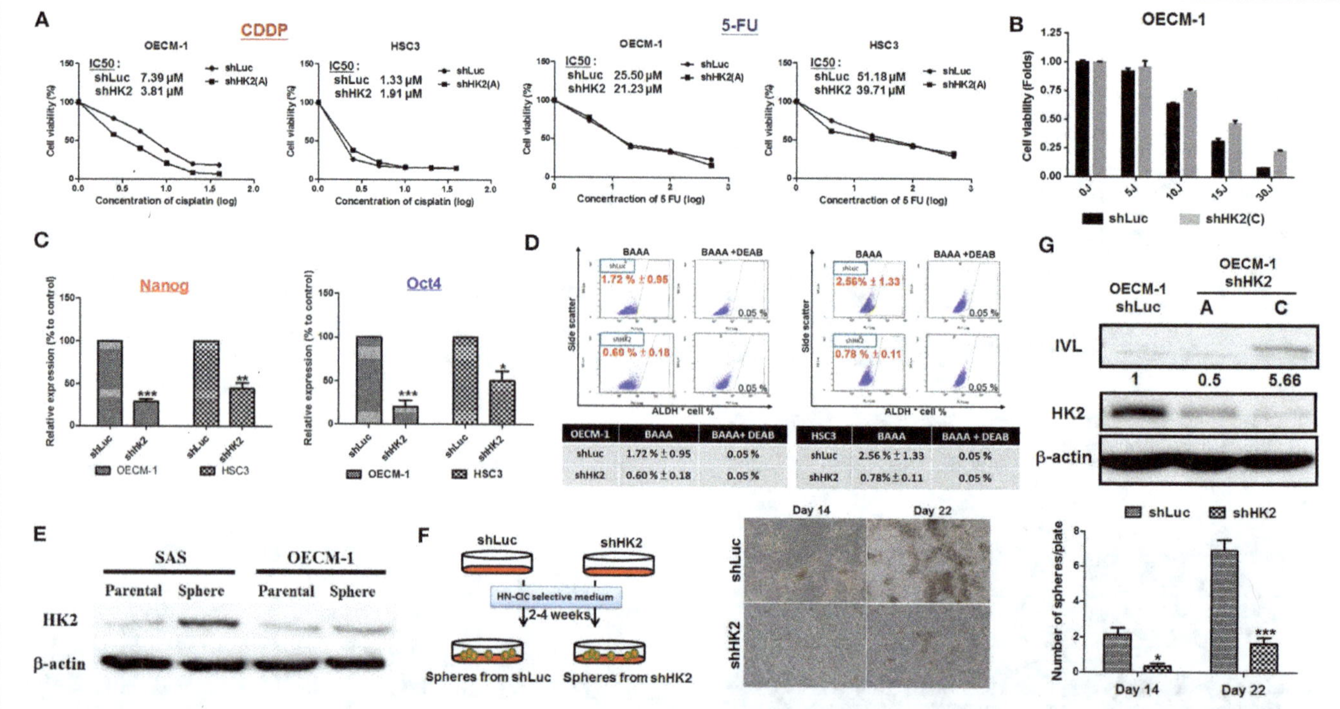

FIGURE 4 | HK2 loss modulated therapeutic sensitivity in HNSCC Cells. **(A)** Decreased IC50 for clinical chemotherapeutic agent CDDP and 5-FU, whereas **(B)** greater resistance in response to photodynamic therapy was detected in HK2-deficient HNSCC cells. This effect is probably regulated via decreased **(C)** Nanog/Oct4 mRNA expression and/or **(D)** ALDH activity. While **(E)** HK2 is highly expressed in SAS and OECM-1 derived sphere cells compared with parental cells, **(F)** HK2 loss resulted in decease of sphere formation. **(G)** Upregulation for cellular differentiation marker involucrin (IVL) protein was detected by Western blot analysis in HK2-silencing HNSCC cells. Data are presented as mean ± SEM ($N \geq 3$). ***$p < 0.001$, **$p < 0.01$, and *$p < 0.05$.

and stemness/differentiation-related treatment sensitivity; in addition, altered bioenergetics and modulation of oncogenic signaling molecules including Akt and phosphorylated TP53 could underlie HK2-mediated regulations in HNSCC cells (**Figure 5H**). Overall findings concluded that targeting HK2 could be an ideal therapeutic strategy in treating HNSCCs. One interesting discovery from the current study is that in HNSCC cells HK2-mediated malignant suppression is likely through glycolytic manipulation based on the following data: (i) HK2 is highly expressed in HNSCC cells implying that HNSCCs are "glycolytic" tumor; (ii) HK2 inhibition triggers metabolic shift away from glycolysis toward mitochondrial metabolism and (iii) it is found that mitochondria are swelling and lack cristae in HNSCC cells compared with human oral fibroblasts (**Supplementary Figure 5**). This finding agreed with previous investigations showing that HK2-mediated metabolic modulation is a key machinery to control cancerous characteristics (41, 54, 74, 75), even though it is required to further define the potential impact of mitochondrial HK2 (49, 51) in controlling tumorigenesis in HNSCC cells in the current experimental setting.

Another interesting finding is the potential involvement of phosphorylated TP53 and p27 proteins in HK2-mediated regulations for HNSCC oncogenicity. Based on protein array analysis, HK2 loss resulted in decreased phosphorylated TP53 at transactivation domain (S15 and S46) and C-terminal domain (S392) in OECM-1 cells. While previous sequencing analysis for TP53 gene in OECM-1 cells showed that OECM-1 cells carry mutant TP53 (P139R/V239L) (62), phosphorylation on S15, S46, and S392 of TP53 could be oncogenic in OECM-1 cells. This statement could be supported by previous studies showing that S15 phosphorylation of TP53 contributed mutant TP53 stability, thereby prolonging cell viability in ovarian cancer cells (76), and S392 phosphorylation in mutant TP53 could lead to tumor progression in esophageal squamous cell carcinoma (77). While it was reported that T198 phosphorylation of cell cycle regulator p27 promotes cyclin D1–CDK4–p27 complex assembly (78), as well as increases p27-RhoA–mediated cell motility (79), HK2 silencing–mediated T198 p27 loss could be a potential underlying cue in controlling HNSCC cell growth and migration. Further elucidation for roles of different TP53 phosphorylation sites in both wild-type and mutant HNSCC cells in regulating tumorigenicity is expected.

With extensive studies, including the present investigation, showing that HK2 is a master promoting factor in different stages of carcinogenesis (**Supplementary Table 4**), much efforts were put in exploring HK-mediated tumor inhibitors, despite that no potent drugs targeting HK2 are yet available in clinic (80–84). Taking the most promising HK2-targeting drug, 3-bromopyruvate (3-BP), as an example, although single treatment of 3-BP, at the appropriate dose and formulation, could effectively destroy glycolytic tumors and seems to be

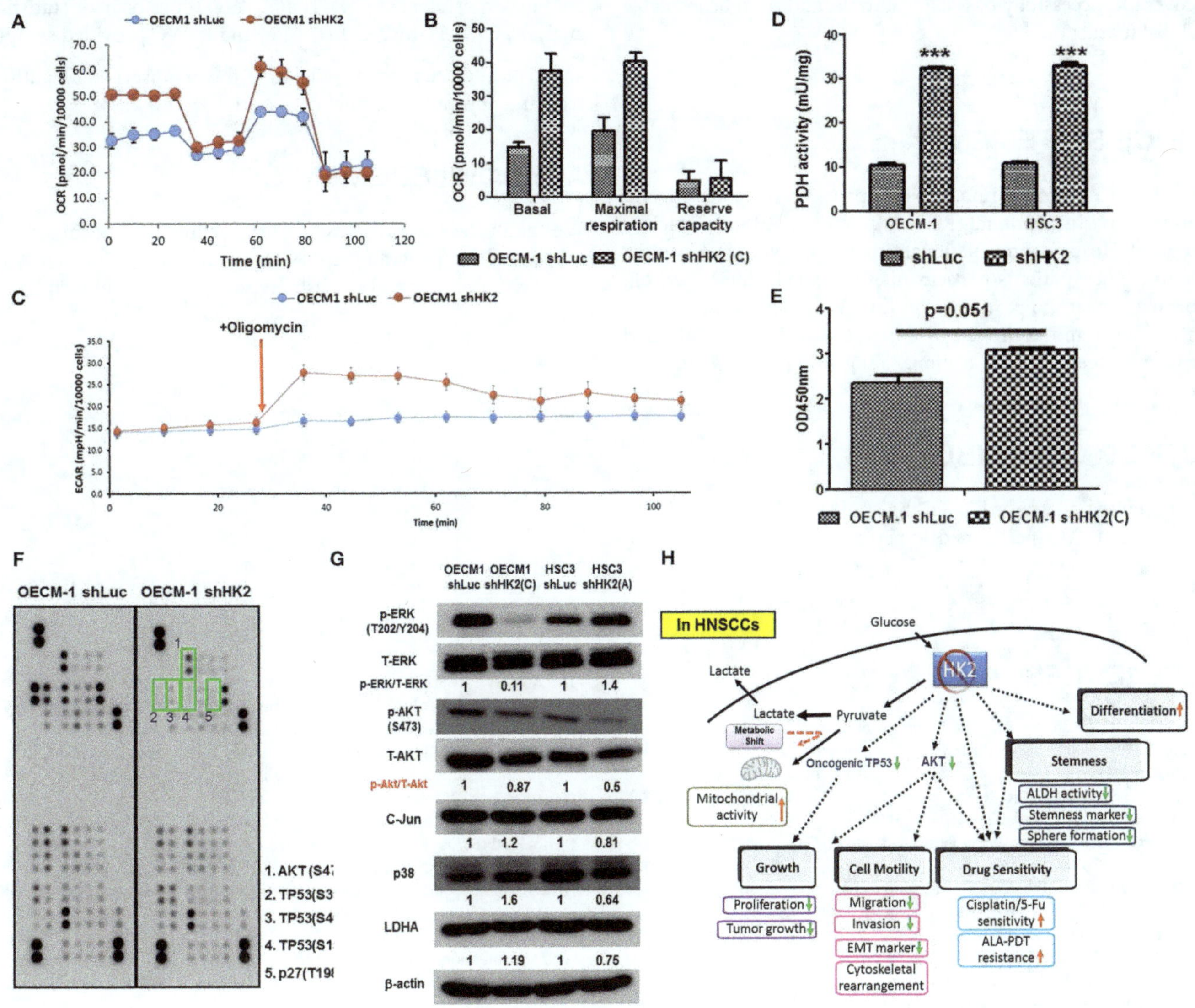

FIGURE 5 | Metabolic and molecular changes in HK2-silencing HNSCC cells. **(A,B)** Seahorse metabolic analysis showed an elevated basal respiration and maximal respiration in HK2 deficient OECM-1 cells. **(C)** Sharp increase of ECAR upon addition of ATPase inhibitor oligomycin and **(D)** increased pyruvate dehydrogenase activity reflected that HK2 loss triggers HNSCC cells toward mitochondrial metabolism. **(E)** ATP level was slightly increased in HK2-silencing OECM-1 cells. **(F)** Human protein array analysis for phosphorylated proteins differentially expressed in HK2-silencing OECM-1 cells was performed. Green boxes indicated oncogenic phosphorylated molecules: (1) Akt (S473), (2) TP53 (S392), (3) TP53 (S46), (4) TP53 (S15), and (5) p27 (T198). **(G)** Western blot analysis confirmed that phosphorylated PKB/Akt proteins is downregulated in HK2-silencing HNSCC cells. p38, P38 mitogen-activated protein kinase; LDHA, lactate dehydrogenase A. **(H)** Graphic summary of HK2-mediated regulations in HNSCC cells. Data are presented as mean ± SEM ($N > 3$). ***$P < 0.001$.

non-toxic to all sorts of vertebrates, certain failure cases were still reported in clinical test (83). It is noteworthy that 3-BP administration also resulted in great pain and inflammation in an HNSCC patient enrolled in a 3-BP trial at the Dayspring Cancer Clinic (http://www.dayspringcancerclinic.com). In addition to a demand of a larger clinical cohort, to achieve better outcomes by using 3-BP or other HK2 inhibitors, as stated in **Supplementary Table 4**, to cure cancer in clinic, a very recent article suggested that simultaneous or sequential treatment of 3-BP and other conventional therapeutic agents needs to be tested for optimal tumor-killing ability, and/or localized delivery of 3-BP directly into tumor tissues should be considered without affecting normal cells (85). Based on current findings, a more systemic study to test synergic antiproliferative effects of different HK2 inhibitors, not only for 3-BP but also for other known small molecules (listed in **Supplementary Table 4**), and their underlying molecular mechanisms in combination of treatments of chemotherapeutic drugs, radiotherapy, and targeted therapy (such as EGFR antagonist cetuximab), needs to be conducted, both *in vitro* and *in vivo*. In addition to BP-3, it is hoped that other inexpensive and safe anticancer HK2 inhibitors could also be discovered, successfully pass clinical trials, and soon be available in global market.

ETHICS STATEMENT

The studies involving human participants were reviewed and approved by Institutional Review Boards (IRB) of MacKay Memorial Hospital and National Taiwan University Hospital, Taiwan. The patients/participants provided their written informed consent to participate in this study. This animal study was reviewed and approved by Institutional Animal Care and Use Committee (IACUC), National Yang-Ming University.

AUTHOR CONTRIBUTIONS

W-CL devised and coordinated the study. C-HH, Y-TH, T-YC, L-HC, and C-YC performed experiments. C-HH conducted animal experiments. C-HH and Y-TH performed statistical analysis. C-JL, H-MC, C-LH, J-FL, and K-WC provided samples and critical discussion. W-CL wrote the manuscript. All authors read and approved the final manuscript.

ACKNOWLEDGMENTS

We thank the National RNAi Core Facility at Academia Sinica in Taiwan for providing shRNA reagents. We thank Dr. Jude Clapper for review and English revision for the manuscript.

REFERENCES

1. Hanahan D, Weinberg RA. The hallmarks of cancer. *Cell.* (2000) 100:57–70. doi: 10.1016/S0092-8674(00)81683-9
2. Nijsten MW, van Dam GM. Hypothesis: using the Warburg effect against cancer by reducing glucose and providing lactate. *Med Hypotheses.* (2009) 73:48–51. doi: 10.1016/j.mehy.2009.01.041
3. Dang CV. Links between metabolism and cancer. *Genes Dev.* (2012) 26:877–90. doi: 10.1101/gad.189365.112
4. Racker E. History of the Pasteur effect and its pathobiology. *Mol Cell Biochem.* (1974) 5:17–23. doi: 10.1007/BF01874168
5. Warburg O. On the origin of cancer cells. *Science.* (1956) 123:309–14. doi: 10.1126/science.123.3191.309
6. Hsieh YT, Chen YF, Lin SC, Chang KW, Li WC. Targeting Cellular Metabolism Modulates Head and Neck Oncogenesis. *Int J Mol Sci.* (2019) 20:E3960. doi: 10.3390/ijms20163960
7. Vander Heiden MG Targeting cancer metabolism: a therapeutic window opens. *Nat Rev Drug Discov.* (2011) 10:671–84. doi: 10.1038/nrd3504
8. Vander Heiden MG, De Berardinis RJ. Understanding the Intersections between Metabolism and Cancer Biology. *Cell.* (2017) 168:657–669. doi: 10.1016/j.cell.2016.12.039
9. Hamanaka RB, Chandel NS. Targeting glucose metabolism for cancer therapy. *J Exp Med.* (2012) 209:211–5. doi: 10.1084/jem.20120162
10. Gatenby RA, Gillies RJ. Why do cancers have high aerobic glycolysis? *Nat Rev Cancer.* (2004) 4:891–9. doi: 10.1038/nrc1478
11. Lunt SY, Vander Heiden MG. Aerobic glycolysis: meeting the metabolic requirements of cell proliferation. *Annu Rev Cell Dev Biol.* (2011) 27:441–64. doi: 10.1146/annurev-cellbio-092910-154237
12. Wilson JE. Isozymes of mammalian hexokinase: structure, subcellular localization and metabolic function. *J Exp Biol.* (2003) 206, 2049–57. doi: 10.1242/jeb.00241
13. Roberts DJ and Miyamoto S. Hexokinase II integrates energy metabolism and cellular protection: akting on mitochondria and TORCing to autophagy. *Cell Death Differ.* (2015) 22:248–57. doi: 10.1038/cdd.2014.173
14. Liu Y, Wu K, Shi L, Xiang F, Tao K, Wang G. Prognostic significance of the metabolic marker hexokinase-2 in various solid tumors: a meta-analysis. *PLoS ONE.* (2016) 11:e0166230. doi: 10.1371/journal.pone.0166230
15. Bacci M, Giannoni E, Fearns A, Ribas R, Gao Q, Taddei ML, et al. Morandi: miR-155 drives metabolic reprogramming of ER+ breast cancer cells following long-term estrogen deprivation and predicts clinical response to aromatase inhibitors. *Cancer Res.* (2016) 76:1615–26. doi: 10.1158/0008-5472.CAN-15-2038
16. van't LJ Veer, Dai H, van de Vijver MJ, He YD, Hart AA, Mao M, et al. Gene expression profiling predicts clinical outcome of breast cancer. *Nature.* (2002) 415:530–6. doi: 10.1038/415530a
17. Liu X, Miao W, Huang M, Li L, Dai X, Wang Y. Elevated hexokinase II expression confers acquired resistance to 4-hydroxytamoxifen in breast cancer cells. *Mol Cell Proteomics.* (2019) 18:2273–2284. doi: 10.1074/mcp.RA119.001576
18. Palmieri D, Fitzgerald D, Shreeve SM, Hua E, Bronder JL, Weil RJ, et al. Analyses of resected human brain metastases of breast cancer reveal the association between up-regulation of hexokinase 2 and poor prognosis. *Mol Cancer Res.* (2009) 7:1438–45. doi: 10.1158/1541-7786.MCR-09-0234
19. Yang X, Cheng Y, Li P, Tao J, Deng X, Zhang X, et al. A lentiviral sponge for miRNA-21 diminishes aerobic glycolysis in bladder cancer T24 cells via the PTEN/PI3K/AKT/mTOR axis. *Tumour Biol.* (2015) 36:383–91. doi: 10.1007/s13277-014-2617-2
20. Huang X, Liu M, Sun H, Wang F, Xie X, Chen X, et al. HK2 is a radiation resistant and independent negative prognostic factor for patients with locally advanced cervical squamous cell carcinoma. *Int J Clin Exp Pathol.* (2015) 8:4054–63.
21. Iwamoto M, Kawada K, Nakamoto Y, Itatani Y, Inamoto S, Toda K, et al. Regulation of 18F-FDG accumulation in colorectal cancer cells with mutated KRAS. *J Nucl Med.* (2014) 55:2038–44. doi: 10.2967/jnumed.114.142927
22. Jin Z, Gu J, Xin X, Li Y, Wang H. Expression of hexokinase 2 in epithelial ovarian tumors and its clinical significance in serous ovarian cancer. *Eur J Gynaecol Oncol.* (2014) 35:519–24.
23. Wolf A, Agnihotri S, Micallef J, Mukherjee J, Sabha N, Cairns R, et al. Hexokinase 2 is a key mediator of aerobic glycolysis and promotes tumor

growth in human glioblastoma multiforme. *J Exp Med.* (2011) 208:313–26. doi: 10.1084/jem.20101470

24. Kwee SA, Hernandez B, Chan O, Wong L. Choline kinase alpha and hexokinase-2 protein expression in hepatocellular carcinoma: association with survival. *PLoS ONE.* (2012) 7:e46591. doi: 10.1371/journal.pone.0046591
25. Chen J, Zhang S, Li Y, Tang Z, Kong W. Hexokinase 2 overexpression promotes the proliferation and survival of laryngeal squamous cell carcinoma. *Tumour Biol.* (2014) 35:3743–53. doi: 10.1007/s13277-013-1496-2
26. Wang H, Wang L, Zhang Y, Wang J, Deng Y, Lin D. Inhibition of glycolytic enzyme hexokinase II (HK2) suppresses lung tumor growth. *Cancer Cell Int.* (2016) 16: 38. doi: 10.1186/s12935-016-0313-6
27. Botzer LE, Maman S, Sagi-Assif O, Meshel T, Nevo I, Yron I. Hexokinase 2 is a determinant of neuroblastoma metastasis. *Br J Cancer.* (2016) 114:759–66. doi: 10.1038/bjc.2016.26
28. Binderup T, Knigge UP, Federspiel B, Sommer P, Hasselby JP, Loft A. Gene expression of glucose transporter 1 (GLUT1), hexokinase 1 and hexokinase 2 in gastroenteropancreatic neuroendocrine tumors: correlation with F-18-fluorodeoxyglucose positron emission tomography and cellular proliferation. *Diagnostics.* (2013) 3:372–84. doi: 10.3390/diagnostics3040372
29. Ogawa H, Nagano H, Konno M, Eguchi H, Koseki J, Kawamoto K, et al. The combination of the expression of hexokinase 2 and pyruvate kinase M2 is a prognostic marker in patients with pancreatic cancer. *Mol Clin Oncol.* (2015) 3:563–571. doi: 10.3892/mco.2015.490
30. Wang L, Xiong H, Wu F, Zhang Y, Wang J, Zhao L, et al. Hexokinase 2-mediated Warburg effect is required for PTEN- and p53-deficiency-driven prostate cancer growth. *Cell Rep.* (2014) 8:1461–74. doi: 10.1016/j.celrep.2014.07.053
31. Wu J, Hu L, Wu F, Zou L, He T. Poor prognosis of hexokinase 2 overexpression in solid tumors of digestive system: a meta-analysis. *Oncotarget.* (2017) 8:32332–44. doi: 10.18632/oncotarget.15974
32. Jiang S, Zhang LF, Zhang HW, Hu S, Lu MH, Liang S, et al. A novel miR-155/miR-143 cascade controls glycolysis by regulating hexokinase 2 in breast cancer cells. *EMBO J.* (2012) 31:1985–98. doi: 10.1038/emboj.2012.45
33. Li M, Jin R, Wang W, Zhang T, Sang J, Li N, et al. STAT3 regulates glycolysis via targeting hexokinase 2 in hepatocellular carcinoma cells. *Oncotarget.* (2017) 8:24777–84. doi: 10.18632/oncotarget.15801
34. Li J, Liu T, Zhao L, Chen W, Hou H, Ye Z, et al. Ginsenoside 20(S)Rg3 inhibits the Warburg effect through STAT3 pathways in ovarian cancer cells. *Int J Oncol.* (2015) 46:775–81. doi: 10.3892/ijo.2014.2767
35. Li Z, Li X, Wu S, Xue M, Chen W. Long non-coding RNA UCA1 promotes glycolysis by upregulating hexokinase 2 through the mTOR-STAT3/microRNA143 pathway. *Cancer Sci.* (2014) 105:951–5. doi: 10.1111/cas.12461
36. Li W, Ma X, Li N, Liu H, Dong Q, Zhang J, et al. Resveratrol inhibits hexokinases II mediated glycolysis in non-small cell lung cancer via targeting Akt signaling pathway. *Exp Cell Res.* (2016) 349:320–327. doi: 10.1016/j.yexcr.2016.11.002
37. Liu CC, Chou KT, Hsu JW, Lin JH, Hsu TW, Yen DH, et al. High metabolic rate and stem cell characteristics of esophageal cancer stem-like cells depend on the Hsp27-AKT-HK2 pathway. *Int J Cancer.* (2019) 145:2144–2156. doi: 10.1002/ijc.32301
38. Gao X, Han H. Jolkinolide B inhibits glycolysis by downregulating hexokinase 2 expression through inactivating the Akt/mTOR pathway in non-small cell lung cancer cells. *J Cell Biochem.* (2018) 119:4967–4974. doi: 10.1002/jcb.26742
39. Kim JE, He Q, Chen Y, Shi C, Yu K. mTOR-targeted therapy: differential perturbation to mitochondrial membrane potential and permeability transition pore plays a role in therapeutic response. *Biochem Biophys Res Commun.* (2014) 447:184–91. doi: 10.1016/j.bbrc.2014.03.124
40. deWaal D, Nogueira V, Terry AR, Patra KC, Jeon SM, Guzman G, et al. Hexokinase-2 depletion inhibits glycolysis and induces oxidative phosphorylation in hepatocellular carcinoma and sensitizes to metformin. *Nat Commun.* (2018) 9:446. doi: 10.1038/s41467-017-02733-4
41. Xiong X, Wen YA, Mitov MI, CO M, Miyamoto S, Gao T. PHLPP regulates hexokinase 2-dependent glucose metabolism in colon cancer cells. *Cell Death Discov.* (2017) 3:16103. doi: 10.1038/cddiscovery.2016.103
42. Jiao L, Zhang HL, Li DD, Yang KL, Tang J, Li X, et al. Regulation of glycolytic metabolism by autophagy in liver cancer involves selective autophagic degradation of HK2 (hexokinase 2). *Autophagy.* (2018) 14:671–684. doi: 10.1080/15548627.2017.1381804
43. Zhang XY, Zhang M, Cong Q, Zhang MX, Zhang MY, Lu YY, et al. Hexokinase 2 confers resistance to cisplatin in ovarian cancer cells by enhancing cisplatin-induced autophagy. *Int J Biochem Cell Biol.* (2018) 95:9–16. doi: 10.1016/j.biocel.2017.12.010
44. Arora KK, Pedersen PL. Functional significance of mitochondrial bound hexokinase in tumor cell metabolism. Evidence for preferential phosphorylation of glucose by intramitochondrially generated ATP. *J Biol Chem.* (1988) 263:17422–8.
45. Mathupala SP, Ko YH, Pedersen PL. Hexokinase II: cancer's double-edged sword acting as both facilitator and gatekeeper of malignancy when bound to mitochondria. *Oncogene.* (2006) 25:4777–86. doi: 10.1038/sj.onc.1209603
46. Zhang D, Yip YM and Li L. *In silico* construction of HK2-VDAC1 complex and investigating the HK2 binding-induced molecular gating mechanism of VDAC1. *Mitochondrion.* (2016) 30:222–8. doi: 10.1016/j.mito.2016.08.009
47. Nagdas S, Kashatus JA, Nascimento A, Hussain SS, Trainor RE, Pollock SR, et al. Drp1 promotes KRas-driven metabolic changes to drive pancreatic tumor growth. *Cell Rep.* (2019) 28:45–59.e5. doi: 10.1016/j.celrep.2019.07.031
48. Cheung EC, Ludwig RL, Vousden KH. Mitochondrial localization of TIGAR under hypoxia stimulates HK2 and lowers ROS and cell death. *Proc Natl Acad Sci USA.* (2012) 109:20491–6. doi: 10.1073/pnas.1206530109
49. Neary CL, Pastorino JG. Akt inhibition promotes hexokinase 2 redistribution and glucose uptake in cancer cells. *J Cell Physiol.* (2013) 228:1943–8. doi: 10.1002/jcp.24361
50. Gao F, Li M, Liu WB, Zhou ZS, Zhang R, Li JL, et al. Epigallocatechin gallate inhibits human tongue carcinoma cells via HK2mediated glycolysis. *Oncol Rep.* (2015) 33:1533–9. doi: 10.3892/or.2015.3727
51. Hou X, Liu Y, Liu H, Chen X, Liu M, Che H, et al. PERK silence inhibits glioma cell growth under low glucose stress by blockage of p-AKT and subsequent HK2's mitochondria translocation. *Sci Rep.* (2015) 5:9065. doi: 10.1038/srep09065
52. Gregersen LH, Jacobsen A, Frankel LB, Wen J, Krogh A, Lund AH. MicroRNA-143 down-regulates Hexokinase 2 in colon cancer cells. *BMC Cancer.* (2012) 12:232. doi: 10.1186/1471-2407-12-232
53. Yoshino H, Enokida H, Itesako T, Kojima S, Kinoshita T, Tatarano S, et al. Tumor-suppressive microRNA-143/145 cluster targets hexokinase-2 in renal cell carcinoma. *Cancer Sci.* (2013) 104:1567–74. doi: 10.1111/cas.12280
54. Guo W, Qiu Z, Wang Z, Wang Q, Tan N, Chen T, et al. MiR-199a-5p is negatively associated with malignancies and regulates glycolysis and lactate production by targeting hexokinase 2 in liver cancer. *Hepatology.* (2015) 62:1132–44. doi: 10.1002/hep.27929
55. Qin Y, Cheng C, Lu H, Wang Y. MiR-4458 suppresses glycolysis and lactate production by directly targeting hexokinase2 in colon cancer cells. *Biochem Biophys Res Commun.* (2016) 469:37–43. doi: 10.1016/j.bbrc.2015.11.066
56. Song J, Wu X, Liu F, Li M, Sun Y, Wang Y, et al. Long non-coding RNA PVT1 promotes glycolysis and tumor progression by regulating miR-497/HK2 axis in osteosarcoma. *Biochem Biophys Res Commun.* (2017) 490:217–224. doi: 10.1016/j.bbrc.2017.06.024
57. Fan L, Huang C, Li J, Gao T, Lin Z, Yao T. Long noncoding RNA urothelial cancer associated 1 regulates radioresistance via the hexokinase 2/glycolytic pathway in cervical cancer. *Int J Mol Med.* (2018) 42:2247–59. doi: 10.3892/ijmm.2018.3778
58. Ma Y, Hu M, Zhou L, Ling S, Li Y, Kong B. Long non-coding RNA HOTAIR promotes cancer cell energy metabolism in pancreatic adenocarcinoma by upregulating hexokinase-2. *Oncol Lett.* (2019) 18:2212–9. doi: 10.3892/ol.2019.10551
59. Lee HG, Kim H, Son T, Jeong Y, Kim SU, Dong SM, et al. Regulation of HK2 expression through alterations in CpG methylation of the HK2 promoter during progression of hepatocellular carcinoma. *Oncotarget.* (2016) 7:41798–810. doi: 10.18632/oncotarget.9723
60. Chen YS, Huang WL, Chang SH, Chang KW, Kao SY, Lo JF, et al. Enhanced filopodium formation and stem-like phenotypes in a novel metastatic head and neck cancer cell model. *Oncol Rep.* (2013) 30:2829–37. doi: 10.3892/or.2013.2772
61. Liu CJ, Chang WJ, Chen CY, Sun FJ, Cheng HW, Chen TY, et al. Dynamic cellular and molecular modulations of diabetes mediated head

and neck carcinogenesis. *Oncotarget*. (2015) 6:29268–84. doi: 10.18632/oncotarget.4922
62. Chen TY, Hsieh YT, Huang JM, Liu CJ, Chuang LT, Huang PC, et al. Determination of pyruvate metabolic fates modulates head and neck tumorigenesis. *Neoplasia*. (2019) 21:641–52. doi: 10.1016/j.neo.2019.04.007
63. Deng M, Bragelmann J, Kryukov I, Saraiva-Agostinho N, Perner S. FirebrowseR: an R client to the broad institute's firehose pipeline. *Database*. (2017) 2017:160. doi: 10.1093/database/baw160
64. Chandrashekar DS, Bashel B, Balasubramanya SAH, Creighton CJ, Ponce-Rodriguez I, Chakravarthi B, et al. UALCAN: a portal for facilitating tumor subgroup gene expression and survival analyses. *Neoplasia*. (2017) 19:649–58. doi: 10.1016/j.neo.2017.05.002
65. Uhlen M, Zhang C, Lee S, Sjostedt E, Fagerberg L, Bidkhori G, et al. A pathology atlas of the human cancer transcriptome. *Science*. (2017) 357:eaan2507. doi: 10.1126/science.aan2507
66. San-Millan, Brooks GA. Reexamining cancer metabolism: lactate production for carcinogenesis could be the purpose and explanation of the Warburg Effect. *Carcinogenesis*. (2017) 38:119–33. doi: 10.1093/carcin/bgw127
67. Fife CM, McCarroll JA, Kavallaris M. Movers and shakers: cell cytoskeleton in cancer metastasis. *Br J Pharmacol*. (2014) 171:5507–23. doi: 10.1111/bph.12704
68. Brabletz T, Kalluri R, Nieto MA, Weinberg RA. EMT in cancer. *Nat Rev Cancer*. (2018) 18:128–134. doi: 10.1038/nrc.2017.118
69. Seshadri M, Spernyak JA, Mazurchuk R, Camacho SH, Oseroff AR, Cheney RT, et al. Tumor vascular response to photodynamic therapy and the antivascular agent 5,6-dimethylxanthenone-4-acetic acid: implications for combination therapy. *Clin Cancer Res*. (2005) 11:4241–50. doi: 10.1158/1078-0432.CCR-04-2703
70. Nokes B, Apel M, Jones C, Brown G, Lang JE. Aminolevulinic acid (ALA): photodynamic detection and potential therapeutic applications. *J Surg Res*. (2013) 181:262–71. doi: 10.1016/j.jss.2013.02.002
71. Fayter D, Corbett M, Heirs M, Fox D, Eastwood A. A systematic review of photodynamic therapy in the treatment of pre-cancerous skin conditions, barrett's oesophagus and cancers of the biliary tract, brain, head and neck, lung, oesophagus and skin. *Health Technol Assess*. (2010) 14:1–288. doi: 10.3310/hta14370
72. Kulsum S, Sudheendra HV, Pandian R, Ravindra DR, Siddappa G, R N, et al. Cancer stem cell mediated acquired chemoresistance in head and neck cancer can be abrogated by aldehyde dehydrogenase 1 A1 inhibition. *Mol Carcinog*. (2017) 56:694–711. doi: 10.1002/mc.22526
73. Keibler MA, Wasylenko TM, Kelleher JK, Iliopoulos O, Vander Heiden MG, Stephanopoulos G. Metabolic requirements for cancer cell proliferation. *Cancer Metab*. (2016) 4:16. doi: 10.1186/s40170-016-0156-6
74. Gershon TR, Crowther AJ, Liu H, Miller CR, Deshmukh M. Cerebellar granule neuron progenitors are the source of Hk2 in the postnatal cerebellum. *Cancer Metab*. (2013) 1:15. doi: 10.1186/2049-3002-1-15
75. Li LQ, Yang Y, Chen H, Zhang L, Pan D, Xie WJ. MicroRNA-181b inhibits glycolysis in gastric cancer cells via targeting hexokinase 2 gene. *Cancer Biomark*. (2016) 17:75–81. doi: 10.3233/CBM-160619
76. Sonego M, Schiappacassi M, Lovisa S, Dall'Acqua A, Bagnoli M, Lovat F, et al. Stathmin regulates mutant p53 stability and transcriptional activity in ovarian cancer. *EMBO Mol Med*. (2013) 5:707–22. doi: 10.1002/emmm.201201504
77. Matsumoto M, Furihata M, Kurabayashi A, Sasaguri S, Araki K, Hayashi H, et al. Prognostic significance of serine 392 phosphorylation in overexpressed p53 protein in human esophageal squamous cell carcinoma. *Oncology*. (2004) 67:143–50. doi: 10.1159/000081001
78. Larrea MD, Liang J, Da Silva T, Hong F, Shao SH, Han K, et al. Phosphorylation of p27Kip1 regulates assembly and activation of cyclin D1-Cdk4. *Mol Cell Biol*. (2008) 28:6462–72. doi: 10.1128/MCB.02300-07
79. Larrea MD, Hong F, Wander SA, da Silva TG, Helfman D, Lannigan D, et al. RSK1 drives p27Kip1 phosphorylation at T198 to promote RhoA inhibition and increase cell motility. *Proc Natl Acad Sci USA*. (2009) 106:9268–73. doi: 10.1073/pnas.0805057106
80. Dai W, Wang F, Lu J, Xia Y, He L, Chen K, et al. By reducing hexokinase 2, resveratrol induces apoptosis in HCC cells addicted to aerobic glycolysis and inhibits tumor growth in mice. *Oncotarget*. (2015) 6:13703–17. doi: 10.18632/oncotarget.3800
81. Geng C, Li J, Ding F, Wu G, Yang Q, Sun Y, et al. Curcumin suppresses 4-hydroxytamoxifen resistance in breast cancer cells by targeting SLUG/Hexokinase 2 pathway. *Biochem Biophys Res Commun*. (2016) 473:147–53. doi: 10.1016/j.bbrc.2016.03.067
82. Li W, Zheng M, Wu S, Gao S, Yang M, Li Z, et al. Benserazide, a dopadecarboxylase inhibitor, suppresses tumor growth by targeting hexokinase 2. *J Exp Clin Cancer Res*. (2017) 36:58. doi: 10.1186/s13046-017-0530-4
83. Lis P, Dylag M, Niedzwiecka K, Ko YH, Pedersen PL, Goffeau A. The HK2 Dependent "Warburg effect" and mitochondrial oxidative phosphorylation in Cancer: targets for effective therapy with 3-Bromopyruvate. *Molecules*. (2016) 21:E1730. doi: 10.3390/molecules21121730
84. Lin H, Zeng J, Xie R, Schulz MJ, Tedesco R, Qu J, et al. Discovery of a Novel 2,6-disubstituted glucosamine series of potent and selective hexokinase 2 inhibitors. *ACS Med Chem Lett*. (2016) 7:217–22. doi: 10.1021/acsmedchemlett.5b00214
85. Abdel-Wahab F, Mahmoud W, Al-Harizy RM. Targeting glucose metabolism to suppress cancer progression: prospective of anti-glycolytic cancer therapy. *Pharmacol Res*. (2019) 150:104511. doi: 10.1016/j.phrs.2019.104511

12

Dual Inhibition of PARP and the Intra-S/G2 Cell Cycle Checkpoints Results in Highly Effective Radiosensitization of HPV-Positive HNSCC Cells

Katharina Hintelmann[1,2†], Thomas Berenz[1,2†], Malte Kriegs[2], Sabrina Christiansen[1,2], Fruzsina Gatzemeier[1,2], Nina Struve[2,3], Cordula Petersen[2], Christian Betz[1], Kai Rothkamm[2], Agnes Oetting[1,2‡] and Thorsten Rieckmann[1,2‡]*

[1] Department of Otorhinolaryngology, University Medical Center Hamburg-Eppendorf, Hamburg, Germany, [2] Department of Radiotherapy, University Medical Center Hamburg-Eppendorf, Hamburg, Germany, [3] Mildred-Scheel Cancer Career Center HATRICs4, University Medical Center Hamburg-Eppendorf, Hamburg, Germany

***Correspondence:**
Thorsten Rieckmann
t.rieckmann@uke.de

†These authors share first authorship

‡These authors share last authorship

In head and neck squamous cell carcinoma (HNSCC), tumors positive for human papillomavirus (HPV) represent a distinct biological entity with favorable prognosis. An enhanced radiation sensitivity of these tumors is evident in the clinic and on the cellular level when comparing HPV-positive and HPV-negative HNSCC cell lines. We could show that the underlying mechanism is a defect in DNA double-strand break repair associated with a profound and sustained G2 arrest. This defect can be exploited by molecular targeting approaches additionally compromising the DNA damage response to further enhance their radiation sensitivity, which may offer new opportunities in the setting of future de-intensified regimes. Against this background, we tested combined targeting of PARP and the DNA damage-induced intra-S/G2 cell cycle checkpoints to achieve effective radiosensitization. Enhancing CDK1/2 activity through the Wee1 inhibitor adavosertib or a combination of Wee1 and Chk1 inhibition resulted in an abrogation of the radiation-induced G2 cell cycle arrest and induction of replication stress as assessed by γH2AX and chromatin-bound RPA levels in S phase cells. Addition of the PARP inhibitor olaparib had little influence on these endpoints, irrespective of checkpoint inhibition. Combined PARP/Wee1 targeting did not result in an enhancement in the absolute number of residual, radiation induced 53BP1 foci as markers of DNA double-strand breaks but it induced a shift in foci numbers from S/G2 to G1 phase cells. Most importantly, while sole checkpoint or PARP inhibition induced moderate radiosensitization, their combination was clearly more effective, while exerting little effect in p53/G1 arrest proficient normal human fibroblasts, thus indicating tumor specificity. We conclude that the combined inhibition of PARP and the intra-S/G2 checkpoint is a highly effective approach for the radiosensitization of HPV-positive HNSCC cells and may represent a viable alternative for the current standard of concomitant cisplatin-based chemotherapy. *In vivo* studies to further evaluate the translational potential are highly warranted.

Keywords: head and neck cancer, human papillomavirus (HPV), molecular targeting, radiotherapy, radiosensitization, PARP, Wee1, Chk1

INTRODUCTION

In locally advanced squamous cell carcinoma of the head and neck (HNSCC), positivity for human papillomavirus (HPV) confers a favorable prognosis, especially for patients with tumors located in the oropharynx (OPSCC) (1, 2). Standard treatment of locally advanced disease is cisplatin-based chemoradiation, either in the primary setting or as adjuvant treatment after surgery. The combination of high cure rates but often dramatic toxicity under these regimes has resulted in the development of various clinical trials testing de-intensification approaches, and some early phase trials have reported promising results (3–7). Two phase 3 trials, however, which together recruited more than 1,000 patients, concordantly reported inferiority of the rather cautious de-intensification concept of exchanging cisplatin for the also approved anti-EGFR antibody cetuximab under maintenance of the full radiation dose (8, 9). In line with these negative clinical results, we had previously shown that cetuximab completely fails to radiosensitize HPV-positive HNSCC cells *in vitro* (10). This clearly urges caution and speaks in favor of careful preclinical evaluation of novel agents and concepts.

A way to very directly induce radiosensitization is the molecular targeting of proteins involved in the DNA damage response (DDR) and DNA repair. Poly(ADP-ribose) polymerase 1 (PARP1) is responsible for poly(ADP-ribose) polymerization at the sites of DNA damage, which marks the lesion and recruits further DNA repair factors. PARP1 is involved in single-strand break repair but also in double-strand break (DSB) repair *via* the alternative end-joining (alt-EJ) backup DSB repair pathway (11, 12). Sole PARP inhibition is especially effective in tumors with a severe deficiency in homologous recombination (HR). Following the well-known concept of synthetic lethality, PARP inhibition increases the need for effective HR by interfering with the repair of intrinsic single-strand lesions and PARP-trapping at the break sites. Upon collision with replication forks, these structures can lead to the formation of one-ended DSBs, the repair of which requires HR (13, 14). Ionizing radiation induces both single- and double-strand breaks, and PARP-inhibitors are well known radiosensitizers (15).

Cell cycle checkpoints constitute another important factor in the response towards irradiation, providing more time for DNA repair before entering S-phase or mitosis in order to avoid mutations and especially mitotic cell death (16). In HNSCC, the majority of HPV-positive and -negative tumors are functionally deficient for p53 and subsequently also for the G1-S cell cycle checkpoint, increasing the dependence on the G2-M checkpoint. Reduction of the radiation-induced G2 arrest can be achieved by inhibition of the ATR/Chk1/Wee1 axis, as the inhibition of any of these kinases finally counteracts Wee1-mediated inhibitory phosphorylation of cyclin dependent kinase 1 (CDK1), which, in its active state will continue to drive G2-M transition (16, 17). Premature mitotic entry and induction of severe replication stress are further therapeutic effects resulting from enhanced CDK1 and CDK2 activity upon inhibition of the ATR/Chk1/Wee1 axis also without irradiation (18–20).

We and others have demonstrated that PARP inhibition as well as inhibition of radiation induced cell cycle checkpoints *via* targeting of Chk1, ATR, or Wee1 can radiosensitize HPV-positive HNSCC cells (10, 21–25). Different mechanisms may account for the observed sensitization. HPV-positive HNSCC cells are described to rely on PARP-dependent alt-EJ (26, 27) and to be defective in homologous recombination (HR) (27–31). Due to an ineffective DSB repair, these cells further rely on an especially profound and long lasting radiation-induced G2 arrest for the repair of radiation-induced DSBs before the critical passage through mitosis (21, 22, 32, 33). Apart from interfering with G2 arrest, the inhibition of Wee1, Chk1, or ATR can directly compromise the ability to perform HR (34–36) and the induction of replication stress, which is to a large extent caused by nucleotide shortage due to unrestrained CDK activity and enhanced origin firing (18), that may create an unfavorable environment for DNA repair in S phase. Given these potential S/G2 phase-based mechanisms, it is easily imaginable that the combined inhibition of PARP and the S/G2 cell cycle checkpoints could be an especially effective treatment option for HPV-positive HNSCC cells, and its radiosensitizing effect has already been demonstrated in preclinical studies in a number of other cancer entities (37, 38). Against this background, we tested the combined inhibition of PARP and the S/G2 cell cycle checkpoint in intrinsically DSB repair-compromised HPV-positive HNSCC cells using clinically relevant inhibitors, all of which are already being tested in combination with radiotherapy in clinical trials in HNSCC.

MATERIAL AND METHODS

Cells and Cell Culture

All cell lines were grown in RPMI (Sigma-Aldrich, St. Louis, MO, USA) supplemented with 10% fetal bovine serum (FBS) (Biochrom AG, Berlin, Germany) at 37°C, 5% CO_2 and 100% humidification. HPV-positive HNSCC cells UD-SCC-2, UM-SCC-47 and UPCI-SCC-154, UPCI-SCC-90, 93VU-147T, UT-SCC-45, and normal human fibroblasts F184 were described previously (21, 33, 39). Tumor cell lines were identified by a short tandem repeat multiplex assay (Applied Biosystems, Waltham, MD, USA). PARP inhibition was performed using 1 µM olaparib (MyBiosource, San Diego, CA, USA). Wee1 inhibition was performed using 240 nM adavosertib (Selleckchem, Houston, TX, USA) and combined Wee1/Chk1 inhibition was performed at a dose of 60 nM adavosertib and 1 nM prexasertib (MedChemExpress, Monmouth Junction, NJ, USA) unless stated otherwise. Supplementation with nucleosides (EmbryoMax 100×, Sigma-Aldrich, St. Louis, MO, USA) was performed at a final dilution of 1/12.5.

Cell Proliferation

For cell proliferation analysis, cells were seeded into T25 cell culture flasks and after 4 h treated with inhibitors. The numbers of resulting cells were assessed after 5 days using a Coulter counter (Beckmann-Coulter, Brea, CA, USA).

Cell Cycle Assessment

Cells were harvested, fixed with 70% ethanol, briefly washed with PBS/0.2% Triton X-100, and subsequently incubated with PBS/

1% BSA/0.2% Triton X-100/DAPI (4′,6-Diamidin-2-phenylindol, 1 μg/ml) for 30 min at room temperature in the dark. Cells were washed once with PBS/0.2% Triton X-100, and flow cytometric analysis was performed using a MACSQuant10 with MACSQuantify Software (Miltenyi Biotec, Bergisch Gladbach, Germany). The proportion of cells in the respective cell cycle phases was calculated using ModFit LT™ software (Verity Software House, Topsham, ME, USA).

X-Irradiation

Cells were irradiated at room temperature with 200 kV X-rays (Gulmay RS225, Gulmay Medical Ltd., Suwanee, GA, USA; 200 kV, 15 mA, 0.8 mm Be + 0.5 mm Cu filtering; dose rate of 1.2 Gy/min).

DSB Reporter Gene Assay

Exponentially growing HNSCC cells containing stably integrated copies of the previously described GFP-based HR or NHEJ reporter plasmids pGC or pEJ (40) were transfected with an I-SceI expression vector for targeted DSB induction using Fugene HD (Promega, Fitchburg, WI, USA). Six hours post transfection, the medium was exchanged and supplemented with inhibitors or solvent (DMSO) as indicated, followed by another exchange plus supplementation 24 h post transfection. At 48 h post transfection, the cells were harvested and assessed for GFP expression by flow cytometry using a FACS Canto with FACS Diva software (Becton Dickinson, Franklin Lakes, NJ, USA). The gating of GFP-positive cells was set according to the negative control (Fugene HD + empty vector). Rates of DSB repair (% GFP-positive cells) were normalized to the respective transfection efficiency of the individual experiment as determined by parallel transfection with a GFP-expression vector (pEGFP-N1).

Immunofluorescence

Cells grown on glass cover slips were fixed with PBS/4% formaldehyde for 10 min, and permeabilized/blocked for 1 h or overnight with PBS/1% BSA/0.2%Triton X-100. The cells were subsequently incubated for 1 h at room temperature with the primary antibodies [mouse anti-53BP1 (clone BP13, Millipore, Billerica, MA, USA); rabbit anti-geminin (#10802-1-AP, Proteintech, Manchester, UK)] in blocking solution, washed four times with PBS/0.5% BSA/0.1% Triton X-100 before incubation with the secondary antibodies plus DAPI (1 μg/ml) and were then washed again four times before mounting with Vectashield mounting medium (Vector Laboratories, Burlingame, CA, USA). Cells were inspected using an AxioObserver Z1 fluorescence microscope with ApoTome and Axiovision Software (Zeiss, Oberkochen, Germany). 53BP1 foci per nucleus were manually counted using stack images in maximum intensity projection. Nuclei with ≥20 foci were scored as “20”.

Flow Cytometric Protein Quantification

Flow cytrometric measurement of relative protein staining intensity per cell in relation to the cell cycle phase was performed on either a FACS Canto with FACS Diva Software (Becton Dickinson, Franklin Lakes, NJ, USA) using FxCycle FarRed (Molecular Probes, Eugene, OR, USA) as nuclear counterstain or on a MACSQuant10 with MACSQuantify and Flowlogic Software (Miltenyi Biotec, Bergisch Gladbach, Germany & Inivai, Mentone Victoria, Australia) using DAPI as nuclear counter stain. In brief, cells were harvested, fixed with PBS/4% formaldehyde for 10 min, and then permeabilized and blocked with PBS/1% BSA/0.2% Triton X-100 for a minimum of 1 h. The cells were subsequently incubated (1 h; room temperature) with the primary antibody [rabbit anti-P-Histone3 (#06-570, Millipore, Billerica, MA, USA), mouse-anti-γ H2AX antibody (clone JBW301, Millipore, Billerica, MA, USA), and mouse anti-RPA32 (clone ME34, Santa Cruz, Santa Cruz, CA, USA)] in blocking solution, washed three times with PBS/0.5% BSA/0.1% Triton X-100 before incubation (1 h; room temperature) with the second antibody and were then washed again three times. DNA counterstaining was either performed with DAPI added to the secondary antibody or with FxCycle FarRed (Molecular Probes, Eugene, OR, USA) plus 300 ng/ml RNAse A and 0.2% Triton X-100 for 30 min at room temperature in the dark following the last washing step.

In case of RPA staining, the cells were pre-extracted after trypsinizaton by gentle resuspension (wide bore tips) of the harvested cell pellet in 500 μl ice cold PBS/0.1% Triton X-100/ 1 mM DTT followed by gentle shaking in horizontally placed reaction tubes on ice for 10 min. Afterwards, 1 ml cold PBS/1% BSA/1mM DTT was added, tubes were inverted several times, and the pre-extracted cells were collected in a pre-cooled centrifuge (5 min, 400 g). After discarding the supernatant, the pre-extracted cells were resuspended (wide bore tips) in PBS/4% formaldehyde and fixed for 10 min at room temperature before regular subsequent staining procedures as described above.

Colony Formation Assay

Radiosensitization was determined using delayed plating colony formation assay. Exponentially growing cells were treated with inhibitor and irradiated after 2 h of incubation. Twenty-four hours post irradiation the cells were seeded in defined numbers into T25 cell culture flasks without addition of inhibitors. Incubation time until colony formation varied between cell lines from 2 to 4 weeks; irradiated samples of HPV-positive cell lines were allowed to grow for an extended period of time, as colony formation was apparently delayed. The number of colonies containing more than 50 cells was assessed. In the case of UM-SCC-47, the cell number was adjusted to 5000 by addition of feeder cells (UM-SCC-47; 20 Gy) to support plating efficiency, and for UPCI-SCC-154 and F184 the medium was changed to a 1:1 mixture of RPMI/10% FBS and Amniomax C-100 medium/7.5% Amniomax Supplement (both Gibco, Thermo Fisher Scientific, Waltham, MA, USA)/7.5% FBS one (F184) or three (UPCI-SCC-154) weeks after seeding to facilitate colony formation.

Data Evaluation

Data analyses were performed using Excel (Microsoft, Redmond, WA, USA) and GraphPad Prism 6 (GraphPadSoftware, San Diego, CA, USA). All experiments were performed at least three times, and single experiments always contained the full set of substances and radiation doses as indicated. Values presented are mean ± SD unless indicated otherwise. Two-tailed Student's t-test was used to assess statistically significant differences using GraphPad Prism 6.

RESULTS

To assess whether the dual inhibition of PARP and Wee1 may exert some additive or synergistic effects in HPV-positive HNSCC cells, we tested a combination of the PARP inhibitor olaparib and the Wee1 inhibitor adavosertib (MK-1775/AZD-1775) with regard to cell proliferation and cell cycle distribution. To this end we used individual inhibitor doses that previously demonstrated moderate effects on their own with regard to the respective cell lines and endpoints or a maximum concentration of 1 µM olaparib in the cell cycle analyses, which was previously proven sufficient to completely suppress the poly(ADP)-ribosylation of HPV-positive HNSCC cells upon H_2O_2 treatment (10, 22). Regarding proliferation we observed several statistically significant differences and the generally strongest reduction under combined inhibition but without a clear hint for a meaningful synergistic effect (**Figure 1A**). Regarding cell cycle distribution, adavosertib induced an accumulation of cells in the S-phase, indicative of replication stress, while olaparib had little effect on its own or when added to Wee1 inhibition (**Figure 1B**).

Radiation-Induced Cell Cycle Arrest

While the previous results did not indicate prominent synergistic effects, we further tested dual PARP and S/G2 checkpoint inhibition combined with ionizing irradiation. To assess a direct effect on the radiation-induced G2 arrest, we quantified the amount of phospho-histone H3 positive mitotic cells 5 h after 6 Gy ± inhibitor treatment (**Figure 2A**). Sole adavosertib treatment (240 nM) increased the rate of mitotic cells in two cell lines, indicating unscheduled mitotic entry upon Wee1 inhibition as previously described (41). Irradiation largely blocked mitotic entry in all strains irrespective of olaparib treatment (1 µM). Adavosertib completely suppressed this G2 arrest, except for UD-SCC-2 cells, where it could only partially override checkpoint execution (**Figure 2B**). Additionally testing a later time point of 8 h post irradiation, adavosertib treatment ± olaparib further relieved UD-SCC-2 cells from the radiation-induced G2 checkpoint (**Figure 2C**). We had previously shown that Wee1 inhibition activates Chk1, which could in part compensate the reduction in Wee1 activity and, indeed, dual inhibition was effective at profoundly reduced doses (22). As low dose dual Wee1/Chk1 inhibition may potentially offer a clinical alternative to high dose single inhibitor treatment, we also included a combination using especially low concentrations of 60 nM adavosertib and 1 nM of the Chk1/2 inhibitor prexasertib, which showed limited effectiveness on their own (**Supplementary Figure S1**). This dual checkpoint inhibition resulted in checkpoint abrogation comparable to the higher dose (240 nm) of sole adavosertib treatment irrespective of the addition of olaparib in all strains (**Figure 2B**).

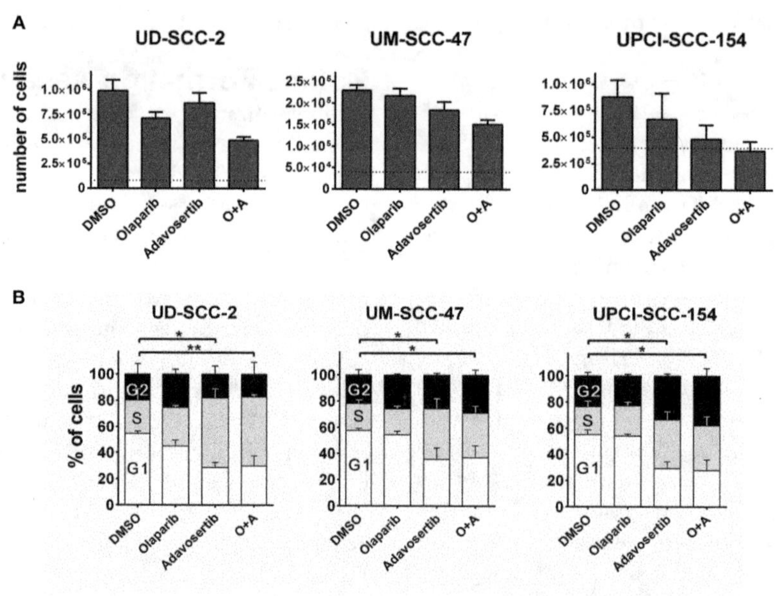

FIGURE 1 | Interactions of PARP and Wee1 inhibition. **(A)** Proliferation. Cells were seeded and after 4 h treatment with inhibitors as indicated. Five days later the respective numbers of cells were assessed. Dotted lines indicate the number of cells seeded. Adavosertib: UD-SCC-2 & UM-SCC-47, 120 nM; UPCI-SCC-154, 60 nM. Olaparib: all strains 500 nM. **(B)** Cell cycle. Cells were seeded and on the next day treated with the respective inhibitors. After 24 h, the cells were fixed and subjected to DAPI staining and flow cytometric assessment of cell cycle distribution. Adavosertib: UD-SCC-2 & UPCI-SCC-154, 480 nM; UM-SCC-47, 960 nM. Olaparib: all strains 1 µM. Statistical evaluation was performed for changes in the S-phase population; addition of olaparib did not induce any significant changes. Asterisks depict significant differences with * and ** indicating $p < 0.05$ and $p < 0.01$, respectively (two-tailed Student's t-test).

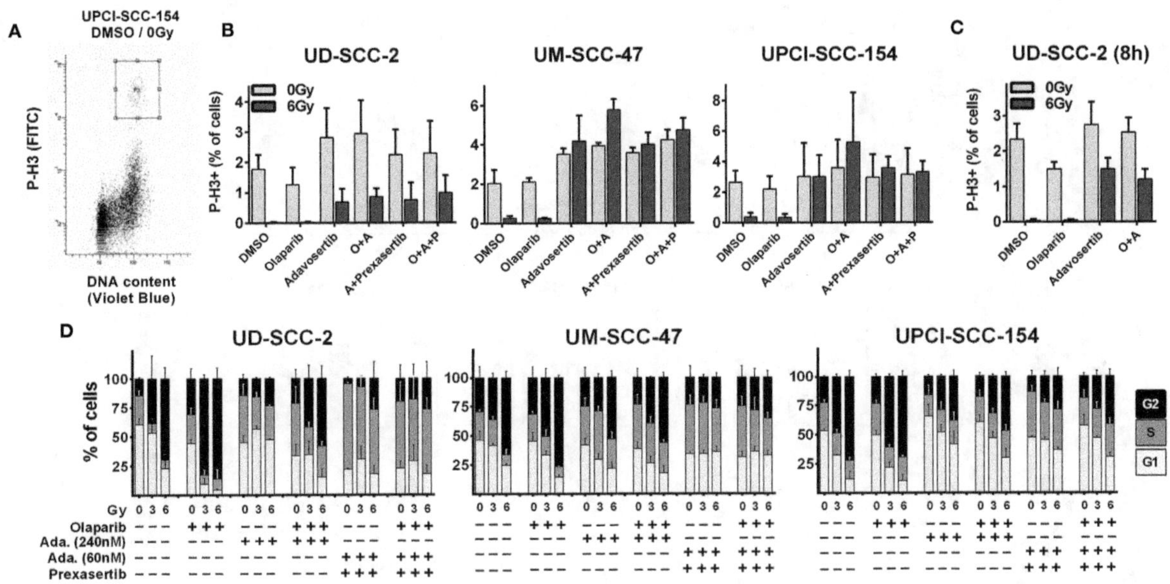

FIGURE 2 | Radiation-induced G2 arrest. **(A–C)** Fraction of mitotic cells. Exponentially growing cells were treated for 2 h with the inhibitors as indicated (olaparib: 1 µM; adavosertib: 240 nM; adavosertib + prexasertib: 60 nm + 1 nM, respectively), before irradiation with 0 or 6 Gy. Five or eight hours after irradiation cells were fixed and stained for phospho-histone H3 (P-H3+) to assess the number of mitotic cells. **(A)** Gating. **(B)** Quantification of the mitotic fraction at 5 h after irradiation. **(C)** Quantification at 8 h after irradiation. **(D)** Long term G2 arrest. Cells were treated and irradiated as in **(A–C)**. Twenty-four hours after irradiation the cells were fixed, and the cell cycle distribution was assessed by DAPI staining and flow cytometry.

As HPV-positive HNSCC cells show prolonged G2-checkpoint responses due to an inefficient DNA DSB repair (33), we further assessed cell cycle distribution at a later time point of 24 h after irradiation where all cell lines demonstrated profound radiation-induced G2 arrest (**Figure 2D**). In line with the short term experiments described above, adavosertib treatment reduced the amount of radiation-induced G2 arrest also at 24 h after irradiation but not to the full extent. The combination of adavosertib and prexasertib also reduced G2 arrest and partly increased the amount of S phase cells, suggesting severe replication stress. Addition of olaparib to adavosertib ± prexasertib did not induce any further accumulation in S-phase irrespective of radiation. In UD-SCC-2 cells, sole olaparib treatment resulted in a clear increase of cells in G2, especially after irradiation but also at baseline. In UM-SCC-47 and UPCI-SCC-154 the increase was subtle but highly reproducible, which is in line with enhanced DNA damage levels after PARP inhibition as frequently reported (**Supplementary Figure S2A**) (42–44). Enhanced damage levels are further supported by higher intensity of the DNA damage marker γH2AX in cells residing in radiation-induced G2-arrest after olaparib treatment in all three cell lines (**Supplementary Figure S2B**).

For all the following experiments, we continued with concentrations of 1 µM olaparib and 240 nM adavosertib or, alternatively, the reduced concentration of 60 nM adavosertib combined with 1 nM prexasertib, which demonstrated similar G2 checkpoint abrogation in these assays.

Replication Stress

Unscheduled activation of dormant origins and subsequent nucleotide depletion is described as a mechanism of antitumor activity through Weel and/or Chk1 inhibition (18, 20). This leads to replication stress and, if severe, S-phase arrest as partially observed for the combined Weel/Chk1 inhibition described above. Chk1 is further described as a replication fork protection factor (45) and PARP1, apart from its functions in DNA repair, was reported to be involved in the restart of stalled replication forks and Chk1-dependent S-phase checkpoint activation and fork protection (46–49).

In S-phase, cell stretches of single-strand DNA (ssDNA) upon replication fork stalling as well as DSBs upon replication fork collapse are recognized through the related ATR and ATM kinases, and such areas are subsequently decorated by γH2AX. In line with these mechanisms, the inhibition of Weel as well as the combined inhibition of Weel/Chk1 resulted in a strong increase in γH2AX signal intensity in S and partly G2 phase cells. However, neither olaparib alone nor the addition of olaparib to Weel or to Weel/Chk1 inhibition resulted in any substantial increase in γH2AX levels with the exception of sole addition in UD-SCC-2 cells. Here, a considerable number of cells demonstrated higher γH2AX levels, but the rise in signal intensity was very modest (**Figures 3A, B** and **Supplementary Figure S3A**). Although less uniform than the γH2AX staining, the results were in principle confirmed when assessing the amounts of chromatin-bound RPA, which, as the primary ssDNA binding and protection factor, represents a very direct and robust marker for replication stress (50) (**Figures 3C, D**). Notably here, in UD-SCC-2 and UPCI-SCC-154, sole Weel inhibition resulted in a more moderate induction of RPA signal intensity compared to combined Weel/Chk1 inhibition, in line with the stronger

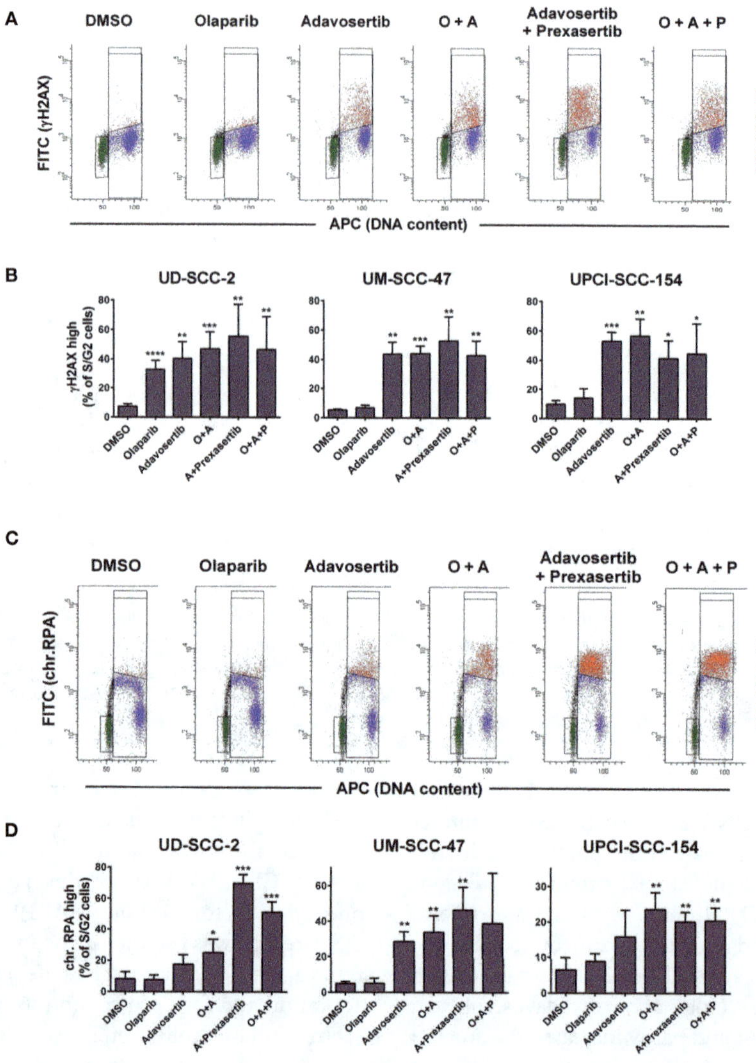

FIGURE 3 | Effect of PARP and intra-S/G2 checkpoint inhibition on γH2AX and chromatin-bound RPA staining intensity. Cells were treated with inhibitors as indicated for 24 h before fixation, staining, and flow cytometric measurements. In case of RPA staining the cells were pre-extracted before fixation. **(A)** Examples of the flow cytometric measurement of γH2AX. Gates are set to select cells in G1 (green), in S/G2 (red & blue) or cells in S/G2 with enhanced γH2AX levels (red). **(B)** Fraction of S/G2 phase cells that demonstrate enhanced γH2AX levels. **(C)** Examples of the flow cytometric measurement of chromatin-bound RPA, which is highest in the replicative S-phase. Gates are set to select cells in G1 (green), in S/G2 (red and blue) or cells in S with enhanced RPA levels (red). **(D)** Fraction of S/G2 phase cells that demonstrate enhanced RPA staining levels. Asterisks depict significant differences to solvent (DMSO) treatment with *, **, *** and **** indicating $p < 0.05$, $p < 0.01$, $p < 0.001$, and $p < 0.0001$, respectively (two-tailed Student's t-test).

accumulation in the S-phase described above (**Supplementary Figure S3B**). Adding the PARP inhibitor did not prominently change the amount of cells positive for γH2AX or chromatin-bound RPA.

Together these results demonstrate that under Weel and especially Weel/Chk1 inhibition S phase cells will have to repair radiation induced DNA damage under conditions of replication stress and with a severely reduced ability to halt the cell cycle in G2 and therefore without extra time for DNA repair before the critical passage through mitosis. Additional inhibition of PARP did not prominently impact on replication stress or inhibition of G2 arrest according to the endpoints measured.

DSB Repair

The reduced DNA DSB repair capacity of HPV-positive HNSCC cells has been frequently ascribed to a defect in the DNA repair pathway homologous recombination (HR) (28–31) and also a switch towards the error prone alt-EJ pathway has been reported (26, 27). As PARP1 is a key component of the latter (12) and Weel has been described as a relevant HR factor (35), we tested the influence of PARP- and Weel inhibition on NHEJ and HR using established GFP-based reporter gene constructs stably integrated in HPV-positive UD-SCC-2 and UPCI-SCC-154 cells (51) (**Supplementary Figures S4A, B**). Although the pEJ construct can interrogate classical NHEJ and alt-EJ repair (52),

PARP inhibition did not reduce the rate of measurable NHEJ in either cell line (**Supplementary Figure S4C**). Despite the reported HR defect of HPV-positive HNSCC cells, we had also been able to establish UD-SCC-2 and UPCI-SCC-154 HR reporter cells. Unexpectedly, Wee1 inhibition did not reduce the rate of HR repair as assessed through the pGC reporter construct and the combination with PARP inhibition even increased the rate of GFP-positive cells (**Supplementary Figure S4D**).

In line with the reporter gene assay results, we also did not observe an enhancement of residual 53BP1 nuclear foci as markers of unrepaired DSBs at 24 h after irradiation with 2 Gy under combined PARP/Wee1 inhibition in UD-SCC-2 and UPCI-SCC-154 and only a slight, non-significant increase in UM-SCC-47 (**Figure 4A** and **Supplementary Figure S5A**). We did, however, observe a common phenotype regarding the distribution of foci with respect to the cell cycle phase as determined by geminin co-staining, which marks cells in S and G2 phases (**Figure 4B**). In all cell lines, the average foci number in G1 increased significantly upon combined PARP/Wee1 inhibition, whereas foci in S/G2 phase cells decreased (**Figure 4C** and **Supplementary Figure S5B**). In line with the respective cell cycle data (**Figure 2**), this underscores that under combined inhibition cells with unrepaired DSBs exit G2 arrest and take the critical passage through mitosis despite the enhanced risk of acute and delayed mitotic cell death. In general, cells with low numbers of residual radiation-induced DSBs are the ones most likely to survive and the fraction of such potentially surviving cells after 2 Gy was decreased in all strains upon dual PARP/Wee1 inhibition, albeit in UD-SCC-2 slightly missing significance ($p = 0.0777$) (**Figure 4D**). Regarding cell cycle, this reduction was observed in the G1-phase in all strains, again underpinning premature mitotic passage (**Figure 4E**). Surprisingly, in UD-SCC-2 the fraction of cells with few residual foci was also significantly reduced in S/G2 phase cells upon dual inhibition, despite the overall decrease in average foci numbers in this fraction (**Figure 4C**).

Radiosensitization

So far while we did not observe clear hints pointing towards enhanced cytotoxicity when adding a PARP inhibitor to intra-S/G2 checkpoint inhibition, radiosensitization through PARP inhibition is clearly established owing to an enhanced induction of replication-induced one-ended DSBs, the inhibition of alt-EJ and further mechanisms (53). Moreover, we had previously observed highly effective radiosensitization in HPV-positive HNSCC cells when combining olaparib with the Chk1 inhibitor PF-00477736 (10). In line with these results, a significant reduction of colonies indicating radiosensitization was now observed upon combined PARP/Wee1 inhibition as

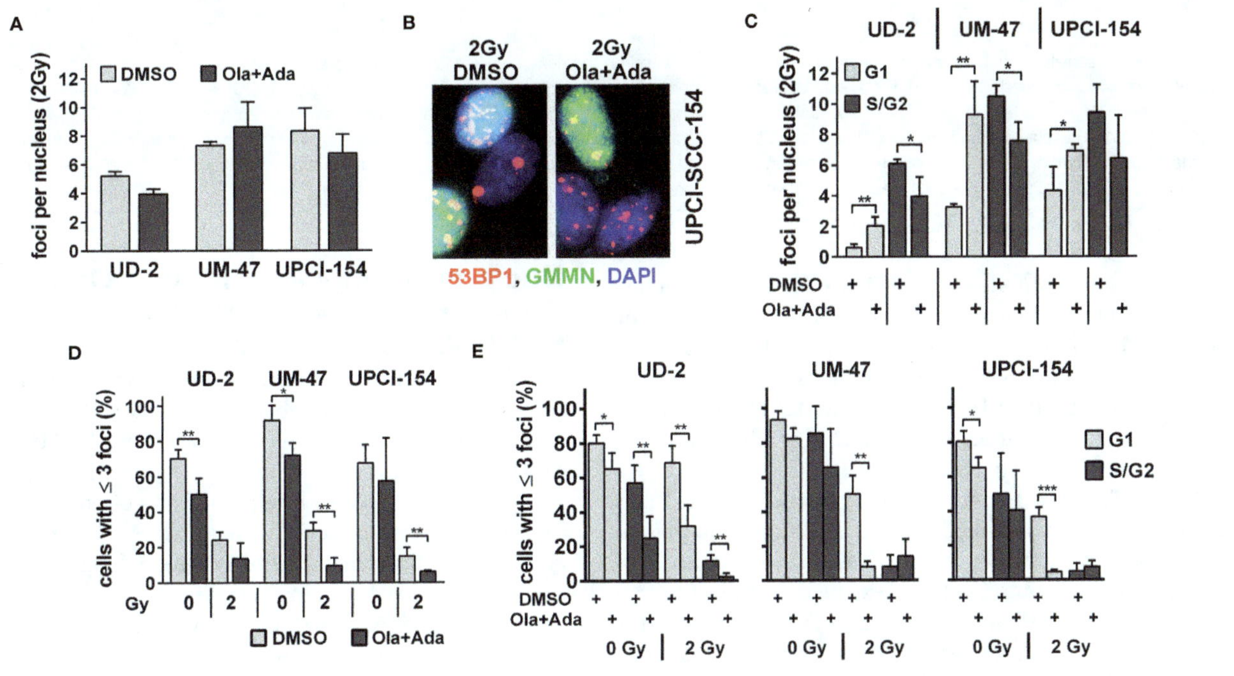

FIGURE 4 | Effect of PARP and Wee1 targeting on DSB repair. **(A)** Quantification of radiation-induced nuclear 53BP1 foci at 24 h after 2 Gy irradiation. Counts were normalized to the DNA content of the respective cell lines as assessed previously (33), foci numbers in non-irradiated controls were subtracted. **(B)** Example of immunofluorescence co-staining of 53BP1 and the S/G2 phase marker geminin (GMMN). **(C)** Quantification of radiation-induced nuclear 53BP1 foci with respect to the cell cycle phase as determined by geminin co-staining. Foci numbers in non-irradiated controls were subtracted. **(D)** Fraction of cells with ≤3 53BP1 nuclear foci. **(E)** Fraction of cells with ≤3 53BP1 nuclear foci with respect to cell cycle phase as determined by geminin co-staining. Significant changes are indicated with *, ** and *** indicating $p < 0.05$, $p < 0.01$, and $p < 0.001$, respectively (two-tailed Student's t-test).

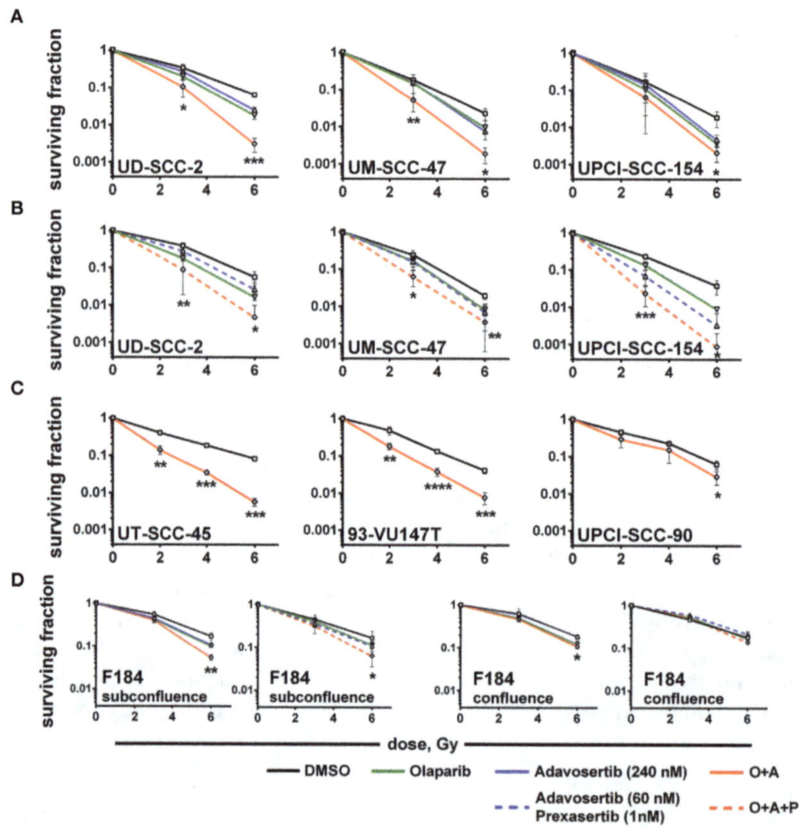

FIGURE 5 | Radiosensitization. Exponentially growing cells were seeded and on the next day treated with inhibitors as indicated and irradiated 2 h thereafter; 24 h later, irradiated cells were seeded in low, defined numbers for colony formation. **(A)** Radiosensitization of HPV-positive HNSCC cells using dual PARP/Wee1 inhibition or **(B)** combined PARP/Wee1/Chk1 inhibition. **(C)** Validation of radiosensitization through combined PARP/Wee1 inhibition using three additional HPV-positive HNSCC cell lines. **(D)** Effect on normal human fibroblasts as an example of normal tissue cells. Significance was assessed for solvent control *vs.* combined PARP + S/G2 checkpoint inhibition. In case of a statistically significant difference the respective dose points are marked with asterisks with *, **, *** and **** indicating p ≤ 0.05, p ≤ 0.01, p ≤ 0.001, and p ≤ 0.0001, respectively (two-tailed Student's t-test).

compared to single inhibitor usage (**Figure 5A**). Highly similar results were obtained when replacing the 240 nM adavosertib treatment with 60 nM adavosertib/1 nM prexasertib (**Figure 5B**). To further estimate whether radiosensitization occurs in a majority of HPV-positive HNSCC cells, we tested dual PARP/ Wee1 targeting in three additional strains, all of which were also sensitized, two very effectively and UPCI-SCC-90 to less extent (**Figure 5C**). To assess tumor specificity, we further tested dual targeting in p53/G1 arrest proficient normal human fibroblasts. In a proliferative state, fibroblasts were radiosensitized by combined inhibition but to a lesser extent than five of the six HPV-positive tumor cell lines. In confluent cultures, the effect of intra-S/G2 checkpoint targeting was completely lost, and radiosensitization was marginal or absent (**Figure 5D** and **Supplementary Table S1**). A comparison of the plating efficiency rates of the non-irradiated controls did not reveal a clear differential effect of the dual *vs.* the triple inhibition approach in HPV-positive HNSCC cells and virtually no reduction of survival in the normal fibroblasts (**Supplementary Figure S6**).

Nucleoside Supplementation Counteracts Radiosensitization Through Wee1 but Not PARP/Wee1 Inhibition

We finally wanted to estimate to what extent the induction of replication stress may contribute to the profound radiosensitization upon combined treatment. As a shortage in nucleotides contributes to replication stress upon intra-S/G2 checkpoint inhibition, it can partly be compensated by external addition of nucleosides (18, 54). To test the effect in our cells, we analyzed γH2AX levels in S-phase cells at 4 h after combined PARP/Wee1 inhibition, a time point corresponding to 2 h post irradiation in the colony formation assays when DSB repair would be highly active. We found γH2AX levels to be induced by combined inhibition in S phase cells and partly suppressed by nucleoside supplementation. A substantial degree of induction and normalization was observed in UD-SCC-2 and UPCI-SCC-154 cells (**Figures 6A, B**). Despite these similarities, nucleoside supplementation did not influence radiation sensitivity in UPCI-SCC-154 but in UD-SCC-2 induced a quite clear trend towards radioresistance in the PARP/Wee1-inhibited samples (6 Gy: p = 0.0862). Unexpectedly, resistance was induced in the

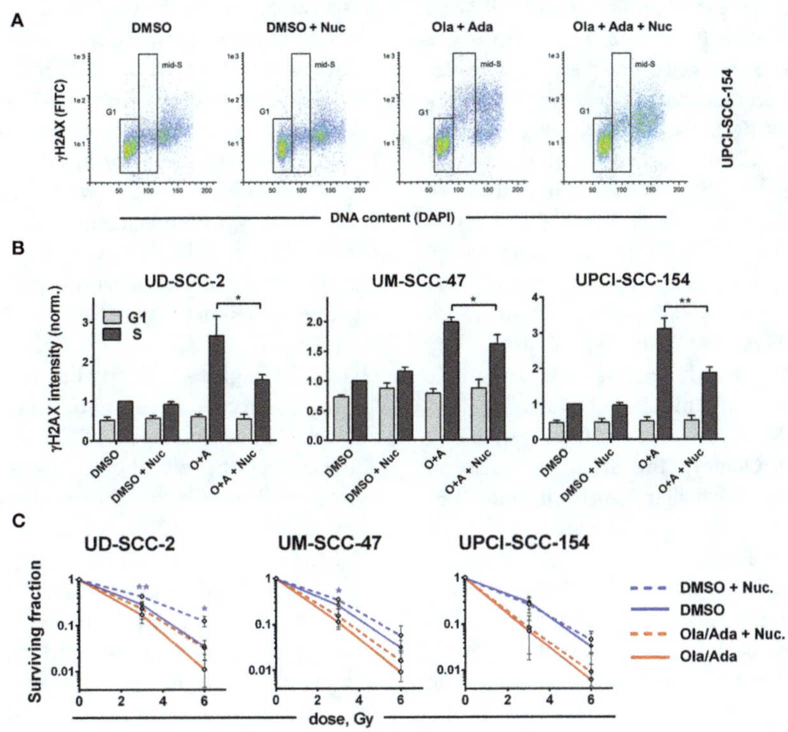

FIGURE 6 | Cell line-dependent induction of radioresistance through nucleoside supplementation. Exponentially growing cells were treated with or without the combination of olaparib and adavosertib and with or without external nucleosides as indicated. **(A)** Example of gating for γH2AX intensity measurement in G1 and mid-S phase cells as assessed by DAPI co-staining. The cells were fixed after 4 h of treatment and analyzed for γH2AX induction by flow cytometry. **(B)** Bars depict the average median γH2AX staining intensity of cells in G1 and mid-S phase. Values were normalized to the intensity of DMSO-treated mid-S phase cells of the respective experiments. Asterisks mark statistically significant differences upon nucleoside supplementation. **(C)** Two hours after addition of inhibitors ± nucleosides the cells were irradiated and after further 24 h seeded for colony formation without addition of inhibitors. Asterisks mark statistically significant differences in survival upon nucleoside supplementation, color indicates solvent controls or inhibitor treatment. Differences between DMSO treatment and dual inhibition without nucleoside supplementation (solid lines) were significant for all cell lines (not indicated). Significant changes are indicated with * and **indicating $p \leq 0.05$ and $p \leq 0.01$, respectively (two-tailed Student's t-test).

solvent-treated controls to a very similar extent reaching significance for the 6 Gy dose point (**Figure 6C**). In comparison, sole Wee1 inhibition induced a similar increase in γH2AX levels, and nucleoside supplementation resulted in a pertinent normalization. In contrast to the situation under combined targeting, nucleoside supplementation counteracted adavosertib-mediated radiosensitization in UM-SCC-47 and UPCI-SCC-154, with no or little effect in the respective solvent-treated controls. Solely in UD-SCC-2, nucleoside supplementation exerted a similar effect on adavosertib and control treated cells (**Supplementary Figure S7**). So while these data strongly suggest that replication stress caused by nucleotide shortage can play a prominent role in the radiosensitization under sole Wee1 inhibition, they question a meaningful role for the radiosensitization under combined PARP/Wee1 inhibition in our cells.

The cause for radioresistance under nucleoside supplementation in solvent treated UD-SCC-2 cells currently remains elusive. In a set of pilot experiments, nucleosides increased the fraction of G1 at the cost of S phase cells in UD-SCC-2 and reduced their proliferation speed (**Supplementary Figures S8A, B**). Also especially in UD-SCC-2, the radiation-induced G2 arrest was diminished upon nucleoside supplementation, suggesting that fewer residual DSBs were present to trigger the G2 cell cycle checkpoint (**Supplementary Figure S8A**). Finally, analyses of residual DSBs under nucleoside supplementation *via* 53BP1 nuclear foci in UD-SCC-2 cells demonstrated an increase in the fraction of cells with few (≤3) foci after irradiation, in line with radioresistance induction. The effect was present and significant in both cells that were or were not actively replicating at the time of irradiation (**Supplementary Figure S8C**). Further analyses will be necessary to clarify this intriguing finding of radioresistance through nucleoside supplementation in otherwise unperturbed cells.

DISCUSSION

Inhibition of Wee1 by adavosertib was recently described as a highly effective single-agent treatment for HPV-positive HNSCC dependent on FOXM1 activation (55) and single agent radio- and chemosensitization through PARP, as well as through intra-S/G2 checkpoint inhibition, which was repeatedly demonstrated in HPV-positive HNSCC models (10, 21–23, 25, 30, 31, 56, 57).

In this study we demonstrate a highly effective radiosensitization of HPV-positive HNSCC cells using dual inhibition of PARP and the S/G2 cell cycle checkpoint in five and moderate radiosensitization in one out of six cell lines tested. A similar result has recently been independently described for the HPV-positive strain UPCI-SCC-154 (24). Here it was suggested that the combination of PARP plus Chk1 inhibition is more effective in HPV-positive HNSCC cells, whereas the combination of PARP plus Wee1 inhibition is more effective in HPV-negative ones but the estimation was based on only one cell line per group. For this particular HPV-positive strain, we have indeed also observed an exceptionally strong radiosensitization when including a Chk1 inhibitor (**Figure 5**). The data are also in line with previous findings of strong radiosensitization using sole Chk1 and combined Chk1/Wee1 inhibition, but again the effect was only specific for UPCI-SCC-154 rather than for HPV-positive cells in general (22). Of note, this strain was also an outlier in the response to the particular Chk1 inhibitor PF-004776, but here demonstrated non-responsiveness for various endpoints, which further suggests irregularities (21). Effective radiosensitization through combined inhibition of PARP and the intra-S/G2 cell cycle checkpoint has also been described for other entities and for different approaches of checkpoint targeting, such as Chk1 or ATR inhibition (10, 58–60). The combination of PARP/Wee1 inhibition was previously tested in lung and pancreatic cancer cells with similarities but also some differences to our findings in HPV-positive HNSCC cells (61, 62). Contrasting these studies we did not observe inhibition of HR upon Wee1 inhibition in plasmid reconstruction assays and we neither observed a reduction of NHEJ upon PARP inhibition despite the reported enhanced usage of alt-EJ in HPV-positive HNSCC (26, 27). Furthermore, while replication stress was clearly evident upon intra-S/G2 checkpoint inhibition, we could not confirm an important role for the radiosensitization under combined inhibition, since for example in UD-SCC-2 targeting the intra-S/G2 checkpoint by combined Wee1/Chk1 inhibition induced replication stress more effectively than sole Wee1 inhibition but radiosensitization was highly similar (**Figures 2, 3, 5**). And while external nucleoside supplementation succeeded in partly relieving replication stress, it either failed to reduce radiosensitization (UPCI-SCC-154) or induced radioresistance in the solvent-treated controls to a similar extent as under combined PARP/Wee1 inhibition (UD-SCC-2) (**Figure 6**). In contrast, nucleoside supplementation demonstrated a pertinent reduction in replication stress and effectively counteracted radiosensitization upon sole Wee1 inhibition in two out of three cell lines tested (**Supplementary Figure S7**), suggesting additional mechanisms and a more robust radiosensitization upon combined inhibition. These findings are actually in line with previous reports, where the addition of nucleosides also counteracted radiosensitization under sole Wee1 (62, 63) but not under combined Wee1/PARP inhibition (62). Interestingly, nucleoside supplementation had also induced radioresistance in solvent treated samples in one of three (hepatocellular) carcinoma cell lines tested, while in NSCLC cells no results for the solvent treated controls were presented (62, 63). While clearly not the focus of this manuscript, our observation of profoundly enhanced radioresistance upon nucleoside supplementation in solvent-treated UD-SCC-2 cells is interesting and warrants future mechanistic investigations.

A puzzling finding of our study is the slight reduction in the overall number of 53BP1 foci upon combined treatment (**Figure 4**). In general, an enhancement in DNA damage in S/G2 phase upon PARP inhibition is very well established (13, 14, 64) and, accordingly, we observed an increase in G2 arrested cells and enhanced γH2AX levels in G2 phase cells upon PARP inhibition and moderate radiosensitization here and previously (**Figures 2, 5** and **Supplementary Figure S2**) (10). A possible explanation, in line with the cell cycle data and the shift in foci number from G2 to G1 phase cells (**Figures 2, 4**) may be that overriding the otherwise long lasting G2 checkpoint can result in immediate mitotic catastrophe and cell elimination, preferentially of those cells with high damage and foci levels that would otherwise reside long enough in G2 to be scored. In line with this theory, the proportion of irradiated G2 phase cells with ≥20 53BP1 foci decreased in UD-SCC-2 and UPCI-SCC-154 upon combined inhibition (data not shown). Importantly, the fraction of cells with very low foci numbers was reduced upon dual inhibition in all cell lines tested. Overall, our results point towards a mechanism for radiosensitization driven by the abrogation of the, in HPV-positive HNSCC cells extensive, G2 cell cycle arrest in combination with the induction of additional DNA damage in S/G2 through PARP inhibition. While differences may exist in detail, the described effectiveness in different entities and by application of various checkpoint inhibitors clearly point towards a very robust radiosensitization of proliferating tumor cells by this combinatorial approach (37, 38). In contrast, normal fibroblasts, representing p53-proficient normal tissue cells, were only modestly affected in our study (**Figure 5D**), which indicates a fair degree of tumor specificity, especially given that many normal tissues do not or only slowly proliferate.

From the translational view, HPV-positive HNSCC may represent an especially promising entity for radiosensitization through molecular targeting. Patients possess a favorable prognosis and therefore targeting agents may not be added to concomitant chemotherapy (CT) but could rather replace CT and this should reduce, instead of increase, the risk of severe systemic side effects. Safe de-intensification of treatment is already the common goal in clinical trials for HPV-positive HNSCC. A major drawback, however, was the reported inferiority of cetuximab compared to cisplatin despite maintaining full dose radiotherapy in two phase 3 trials (65). These studies clearly highlight the need for effectiveness and thorough preclinical evaluation of molecular targeting approaches despite the overall favorable prognosis. In the frame of recent clinical data on de-intensification, promising initial results were obtained for reducing radiation dose in definitive chemoradiation and after induction chemotherapy (ICT) (3, 5, 7). In the frame of the latter, effective targeting may also be an alternative to adjuvant chemotherapy after ICT in the frame of risk-adapted, de-intensified radiotherapy and may evade potential chemoresistance mechanisms selected for or acquired during ICT. All inhibitors used in this study are already being tested in clinical trials in combination with radiotherapy in HNSCC (66, 67) (NCT02555644, NCT01758731, NCT02308072, NCT02585973). Olaparib is clinically approved in other entities, and the combination of adavosertib and radiotherapy (plus gemcitabine) was recently reported to yield promising results in pancreatic cancer (68). Moreover, combined treatment with olaparib and adavosertib as well as with prexasertib is also being clinically tested in a number of entities (NCT02576444, NCT02511795, NCT03579316, NCT03330847), albeit so far not in combination with radiotherapy. From our point of view, the clinical stage of the inhibitors available and the preclinical evidence provided in this study clearly warrant subsequent *in vivo* experiments as a next step towards a possible clinical exploration of the described approaches in the frame of de-intensification trials in HPV-positive HNSCC.

AUTHOR CONTRIBUTIONS

KH, TB, AO, SC, and FG conducted experiments under the supervision of TR. KH, TB, AO, SC, FG, and TR analyzed the data. MK, KR, CP, CB, NS and TR contributed conception and design of the study; AO, NS, KR, and TR wrote the manuscript. All authors contributed to the article and approved the submitted version.

REFERENCES

1. Ang KK, Harris J, Wheeler R, Weber R, Rosenthal DI, Nguyen-Tân PF, et al. Human Papillomavirus and Survival of Patients With Oropharyngeal Cancer. *N Engl J Med* (2010) 363(1):24–35. doi: 10.1056/NEJMoa0912217
2. Sedghizadeh PP, Billington WD, Paxton D, Ebeed R, Mahabady S, Clark GT, et al. Is P16-Positive Oropharyngeal Squamous Cell Carcinoma Associated With Favorable Prognosis? A Systematic Review and Meta-Analysis. *Oral Oncol* (2016) 54:15–27. doi: 10.1016/j.oraloncology.2016.01.002
3. Chen AM, Felix C, Wang PC, Hsu S, Basehart V, Garst J, et al. Reduced-Dose Radiotherapy for Human Papillomavirus-Associated Squamous-Cell Carcinoma of the Oropharynx: A Single-Arm, Phase 2 Study. *Lancet Oncol* (2017) 18(6):803–11. doi: 10.1016/S1470-2045(17)30246-2
4. Chera BS, Amdur RJ, Tepper JE, Tan X, Weiss J, Grilley-Olson JE, et al. Mature Results of a Prospective Study of Deintensified Chemoradiotherapy for Low-Risk Human Papillomavirus-Associated Oropharyngeal Squamous Cell Carcinoma. *Cancer* (2018) 124(11):2347–54. doi: 10.1002/cncr.31338
5. Patel RR, Ludmir EB, Augustyn A, Zaorsky NG, Lehrer EJ, Ryali R, et al. De-Intensification of Therapy in Human Papillomavirus Associated Oropharyngeal Cancer: A Systematic Review of Prospective Trials. *Oral Oncol* (2020) 103:104608. doi: 10.1016/j.oraloncology.2020.104608
6. Takemoto N, Seo Y, Nakahara S, Yoshioka Y, Teshima T, Fujii T, et al. Radiation Therapy Alone for Human Papillomavirus-Related Squamous Cell Carcinoma of the Oropharynx: A Single-Arm, Phase 2 Study. *Int J Radiat Oncol Biol Phys* (2020) 110(2):403–11. doi: 10.1016/j.ijrobp.2020.12.025.
7. Yom SS, Torres-Saavedra P, Caudell JJ, Waldron JN, Gillison ML, Xia P, et al. Reduced-Dose Radiation Therapy for HPV-Associated Oropharyngeal Carcinoma (NRG Oncology Hn002). *J Clin Oncol* (2021) 39(9):956–65. doi: 10.1200/JCO.20.03128.
8. Gillison ML, Trotti AM, Harris J, Eisbruch A, Harari PM, Adelstein DJ, et al. Radiotherapy Plus Cetuximab or Cisplatin in Human Papillomavirus-Positive Oropharyngeal Cancer (NRG Oncology RTOG 1016): A Randomised, Multicentre, non-Inferiority Trial. *Lancet* (2019) 393(10166):40–50. doi: 10.1016/S0140-6736(18)32779-X
9. Mehanna H, Robinson M, Hartley A, Kong A, Foran B, Fulton-Lieuw T, et al. Radiotherapy Plus Cisplatin or Cetuximab in Low-Risk Human Papillomavirus-Positive Oropharyngeal Cancer (De-ESCALaTE HPV): An Open-Label Randomised Controlled Phase 3 Trial. *Lancet* (2019) 393 (10166):51 60. doi: 10.1016/S0140-6736(18)32752-1
10. Guster JD, Weissleder SV, Busch CJ, Kriegs M, Petersen C, Knecht R, et al. The Inhibition of PARP But Not EGFR Results in the Radiosensitization of HPV/p16-Positive HNSCC Cell Lines. *Radiother Oncol* (2014) 113(3):345–51. doi: 10.1016/j.radonc.2014.10.011
11. Satoh MS, Lindahl T. Role of Poly(ADP-Ribose) Formation in DNA Repair. *Nature* (1992) 356(6367):356–8. doi: 10.1038/356356a0
12. Wang M, Wu W, Wu W, Rosidi B, Zhang L, Wang H, et al. PARP-1 and Ku Compete for Repair of DNA Double Strand Breaks by Distinct NHEJ Pathways. *Nucleic Acids Res* (2006) 34(21):6170–82. doi: 10.1093/nar/gkl840
13. Bryant HE, Schultz N, Thomas HD, Parker KM, Flower D, Lopez E, et al. Specific Killing of BRCA2-Deficient Tumours With Inhibitors of Poly(ADP-Ribose) Polymerase. *Nature* (2005) 434(7035):913–7. doi: 10.1038/nature03443
14. Mateo J, Lord CJ, Serra V, Tutt A, Balmaña J, Castroviejo-Bermejo M, et al. A Decade of Clinical Development of PARP Inhibitors in Perspective. *Ann Oncol* (2019) 30(9):1437–47. doi: 10.1093/annonc/mdz192
15. Jannetti SA, Zeglis BM, Zalutsky MR, Reiner T. Poly(ADP-Ribose)Polymerase (PARP) Inhibitors and Radiation Therapy. *Front Pharmacol* (2020) 11:170. doi: 10.3389/fphar.2020.00170
16. Hauge S, Eek Mariampillai A, Rødland GE, Bay LTE, Landsverk HB, Syljuåsen RG. Expanding Roles of Cell Cycle Checkpoint Inhibitors in Radiation Oncology. *Int J Radiat Biol* (2021) p:1–10. doi: 10.1080/09553002.2021.1913529
17. Parker LL, Piwnica-Worms H. Inactivation of the P34cdc2-Cyclin B Complex by the Human WEE1 Tyrosine Kinase. *Science* (1992) 257(5078):1955–7. doi: 10.1126/science.1384126
18. Beck H, Nähse-Kumpf V, Larsen MS, O'Hanlon KA, Patzke S, Holmberg C, et al. Cyclin-Dependent Kinase Suppression by WEE1 Kinase Protects the Genome Through Control of Replication Initiation and Nucleotide Consumption. *Mol Cell Biol* (2012) 32(20):4226–36. doi: 10.1128/MCB.00412-12
19. Branigan TB, Kozono D, Schade AE, Deraska P, Rivas HG, Sambel L, et al. MMB-FOXM1-Driven Premature Mitosis is Required for CHK1 Inhibitor Sensitivity. *Cell Rep* (2021) 34(9):108808. doi: 10.1016/j.celrep.2021.108808
20. Sorensen CS, Syljuasen RG. Safeguarding Genome Integrity: The Checkpoint Kinases ATR, CHK1 and WEE1 Restrain CDK Activity During Normal DNA Replication. *Nucleic Acids Res* (2012) 40(2):477–86. doi: 10.1093/nar/gkr697

21. Busch CJ, Kriegs M, Laban S, Tribius S, Knecht R, Petersen C, et al. HPV-Positive HNSCC Cell Lines But Not Primary Human Fibroblasts are Radiosensitized by the Inhibition of Chk1. *Radiother Oncol* (2013) 108 (3):495–9. doi: 10.1016/j.radonc.2013.06.035
22. Busch CJ, Kröger MS, Jensen J, Kriegs M, Gatzemeier F, Petersen C, et al. G2-Checkpoint Targeting and Radiosensitization of HPV/p16-Positive HNSCC Cells Through the Inhibition of Chk1 and Wee1. *Radiother Oncol* (2016) 122 (2):260–6. doi: 10.1016/j.radonc.2016.11.017
23. Dok R, Glorieux M, Bamps M, Nuyts S. Effect of ATR Inhibition in RT Response of HPV-Negative and HPV-Positive Head and Neck Cancers. *Int J Mol Sci* (2021) 22(4). doi: 10.3390/ijms22041504
24. Molkentine JM, Molkentine DP, Bridges KA, Xie T, Yang L, Sheth A, et al. Targeting DNA Damage Response in Head and Neck Cancers Through Abrogation of Cell Cycle Checkpoints. *Int J Radiat Biol* (2020) p:1–8. doi: 10.1080/09553002.2020.1730014
25. Nickson CM, Moori P, Carter RJ, Rubbi CP, Parsons JL. Misregulation of DNA Damage Repair Pathways in HPV-Positive Head and Neck Squamous Cell Carcinoma Contributes to Cellular Radiosensitivity. *Oncotarget* (2017) 8 (18):29963–75. doi: 10.18632/oncotarget.16265
26. Leeman JE, Li Y, Bell A, Hussain SS, Majumdar R, Rong-Mullins X, et al. Human Papillomavirus 16 Promotes Microhomology-Mediated End-Joining. *Proc Natl Acad Sci USA* (2019) 116(43):21573–9. doi: 10.1073/pnas.1906120116
27. Liu Q, Ma L, Jones T, Palomero L, Pujana MA, Martinez-Ruiz H. Subjugation of TGFbeta Signaling by Human Papilloma Virus in Head and Neck Squamous Cell Carcinoma Shifts DNA Repair From Homologous Recombination to Alternative End Joining. *Clin Cancer Res* (2018) 24 (23):6001–14. doi: 10.1158/1078-0432.CCR-18-1346
28. Dok R, Kalev P, Van Limbergen EJ, Asbagh LA, Vázquez I, Hauben E, et al. P16ink4a Impairs Homologous Recombination-Mediated DNA Repair in Human Papillomavirus-Positive Head and Neck Tumors. *Cancer Res* (2014) 74(6):1739–51. doi: 10.1158/0008-5472.CAN-13-2479
29. Wang L, Zhang P, Molkentine DP, Chen C, Molkentine JM, Piao H, et al. TRIP12 as a Mediator of Human Papillomavirus/P16-Related Radiation Enhancement Effects. *Oncogene* (2016). doi: 10.1158/1538-7445.AM2016-1661
30. Weaver AN, Cooper TS, Rodriguez M, Trummell HQ, Bonner JA, Rosenthal EL, et al. DNA Double Strand Break Repair Defect and Sensitivity to Poly ADP-Ribose Polymerase (PARP) Inhibition in Human Papillomavirus 16-Positive Head and Neck Squamous Cell Carcinoma. *Oncotarget* (2015) 6 (29):26995–7007. doi: 10.18632/oncotarget.4863
31. Ziemann F, Seltzsam S, Dreffke K, Preising S, Arenz A, Subtil FSB, et al. Roscovitine Strongly Enhances the Effect of Olaparib on Radiosensitivity for HPV Neg. But Not for HPV Pos. HNSCC Cell Lines. *Oncotarget* (2017) 8 (62):105170–83. doi: 10.18632/oncotarget.22005
32. Kimple RJ, Smith MA, Blitzer GC, Torres AD, Martin JA, Yang RZ, et al. Enhanced Radiation Sensitivity in HPV-Positive Head and Neck Cancer. *Cancer Res* (2013) 73 (15):4791–800. doi: 10.1158/0008-5472.CAN-13-0587
33. Rieckmann T, Tribius S, Grob TJ, Meyer F, Busch CJ, Petersen C, et al. HNSCC Cell Lines Positive for HPV and P16 Possess Higher Cellular Radiosensitivity Due to an Impaired DSB Repair Capacity. *Radiother Oncol* (2013) 107(2):242–6. doi: 10.1016/j.radonc.2013.03.013
34. Buisson R, Niraj J, Rodrigue A, Ho CK, Kreuzer J, Foo TK, et al. Coupling of Homologous Recombination and the Checkpoint by ATR. *Mol Cell* (2017) 65 (2):336–46. doi: 10.1016/j.molcel.2016.12.007
35. Krajewska M, Heijink AM, Bisselink YJ, Seinstra RI, Silljé HH, de Vries EG, et al. Forced Activation of Cdk1 via Wee1 Inhibition Impairs Homologous Recombination. *Oncogene* (2013) 32(24):3001–8. doi: 10.1038/onc.2012.296
36. Sorensen CS, Hansen LT, Dziegielewski J, Syljuåsen RG, Lundin C, Bartek J, et al. The Cell-Cycle Checkpoint Kinase Chk1 is Required for Mammalian Homologous Recombination Repair. *Nat Cell Biol* (2005) 7(2):195–201. doi: 10.1038/ncb1212
37. Hintelmann K, Kriegs M, Rothkamm K, Rieckmann T. Improving the Efficacy of Tumor Radiosensitization Through Combined Molecular Targeting. *Front Oncol* (2020) 10:1260. doi: 10.3389/fonc.2020.01260
38. Parsels LA, Engelke CG, Parsels J, Flanagan SA, Zhang Q, Tanska D, et al. Combinatorial Efficacy of Olaparib With Radiation and ATR Inhibitor Requires PARP1 Protein in Homologous Recombination-Proficient Pancreatic Cancer. *Mol Cancer Ther* (2021) 20(2):263–73. doi: 10.1158/1535-7163.MCT-20-0365
39. Busch CJ, Becker B, Kriegs M, Gatzemeier F, Krüger K, Möckelmann N, et al. Similar Cisplatin Sensitivity of HPV-Positive and -Negative HNSCC Cell Lines. *Oncotarget* (2016) 7(24):35832–42. doi: 10.18632/oncotarget.9028
40. Mansour WY, Schumacher S, Rosskopf R, Rhein T, Schmidt-Petersen F, Gatzemeier F, et al. Hierarchy of Nonhomologous End-Joining, Single-Strand Annealing and Gene Conversion at Site-Directed DNA Double-Strand Breaks. *Nucleic Acids Res* (2008) 36(12):4088–98. doi: 10.1093/nar/gkn347
41. Tominaga Y, Li C, Wang RH, Deng CX. Murine Wee1 Plays a Critical Role in Cell Cycle Regulation and Pre-Implantation Stages of Embryonic Development. *Int J Biol Sci* (2006) 2(4):161–70. doi: 10.7150/ijbs.2.161
42. De Vos M, Schreiber V, Dantzer F. The Diverse Roles and Clinical Relevance of PARPs in DNA Damage Repair: Current State of the Art. *Biochem Pharmacol* (2012) 84(2):137–46. doi: 10.1016/j.bcp.2012.03.018
43. Murai J, Pommier Y. PARP Trapping Beyond Homologous Recombination and Platinum Sensitivity in Cancers. *Annu Rev Cancer Biol* (2019) 3:131–50. doi: 10.1146/annurev-cancerbio-030518-055914
44. Ray Chaudhuri A, Nussenzweig A. The Multifaceted Roles of PARP1 in DNA Repair and Chromatin Remodelling. *Nat Rev Mol Cell Biol* (2017) 18(10):610–21. doi: 10.1038/nrm.2017.53
45. Forment JV, Blasius M, Guerini I, Jackson SP. Structure-Specific DNA Endonuclease Mus81/Eme1 Generates DNA Damage Caused by Chk1 Inactivation. *PloS One* (2011) 6(8):e23517. doi: 10.1371/journal.pone.0023517
46. Bryant HE, Petermann E, Schultz N, Jemth AS, Loseva O, Issaeva N, et al. PARP is Activated at Stalled Forks to Mediate Mre11-Dependent Replication Restart and Recombination. *EMBO J* (2009) 28(17):2601–15. doi: 10.1038/emboj.2009.206
47. Ying S, Hamdy FC, Helleday T. Mre11-Dependent Degradation of Stalled DNA Replication Forks is Prevented by BRCA2 and PARP1. *Cancer Res* (2012) 72(11):2814–21. doi: 10.1158/0008-5472.CAN-11-3417
48. Haynes B, Murai J, Lee JM. Restored Replication Fork Stabilization, a Mechanism of PARP Inhibitor Resistance, can be Overcome by Cell Cycle Checkpoint Inhibition. *Cancer Treat Rev* (2018) 71:1–7. doi: 10.1016/j.ctrv.2018.09.003
49. Min W, Bruhn C, Grigaravicius P, Zhou ZW, Li F, Krüger A, et al. Poly(ADP-Ribose) Binding to Chk1 at Stalled Replication Forks is Required for S-Phase Checkpoint Activation. *Nat Commun* (2013) 4:2993. doi: 10.1038/ncomms3993
50. Toledo LI, Altmeyer M, Rask MB, Lukas C, Larsen DH, Povlsen LK, et al. ATR Prohibits Replication Catastrophe by Preventing Global Exhaustion of RPA. *Cell* (2013) 155(5):1088–103. doi: 10.1016/j.cell.2013.10.043
51. Schotz U, Balzer V, Brandt FW, Ziemann F, Subtil FSB, Rieckmann T, et al. Dual PI3K/mTOR Inhibitor NVP-BEZ235 Enhances Radiosensitivity of Head and Neck Squamous Cell Carcinoma (HNSCC) Cell Lines Due to Suppressed Double-Strand Break (DSB) Repair by Non-Homologous End Joining. *Cancers (Basel)* (2020) 12(2). doi: 10.3390/cancers12020467
52. Mansour WY, Rhein T, Dahm-Daphi J. The Alternative End-Joining Pathway for Repair of DNA Double-Strand Breaks Requires PARP1 But is Not Dependent Upon Microhomologies. *Nucleic Acids Res* (2010) 38(18):6065–77. doi: 10.1093/nar/gkq387
53. Lesueur P, Chevalier F, Austry JB, Waissi W, Burckel H, Noël G, et al. Poly-(ADP-Ribose)-Polymerase Inhibitors as Radiosensitizers: A Systematic Review of Pre-Clinical and Clinical Human Studies. *Oncotarget* (2017) 8 (40):69105–24. doi: 10.18632/oncotarget.19079
54. Parsels LA, Karnak D, Parsels JD, Zhang Q, Vélez-Padilla J, Reichert ZR, et al. PARP1 Trapping and DNA Replication Stress Enhance Radiosensitization With Combined WEE1 and PARP Inhibitors. *Mol Cancer Res* (2018) 16 (2):222–32. doi: 10.1158/1541-7786.MCR-17-0455
55. Diab A, Gem H, Swanger J, Kim HY, Smith K, Zou G, et al. FOXM1 Drives HPV+ HNSCC Sensitivity to WEE1 Inhibition. *Proc Natl Acad Sci USA* (2020) 117 (45):28287–96. doi: 10.1073/pnas.2013921117
56. Tanaka N, Patel AA, Wang J, Frederick MJ, Kalu NN, Zhao M, et al. Wee-1 Kinase Inhibition Sensitizes High-Risk HPV+ HNSCC to Apoptosis Accompanied by Downregulation of MCl-1 and XIAP Antiapoptotic Proteins. *Clin Cancer Res* (2015) 21(21):4831–44. doi: 10.1158/1078-0432.CCR-15-0279
57. Zeng L, Nikolaev A, Xing C, Della Manna DL, Yang ES. CHK1/2 Inhibitor Prexasertib Suppresses NOTCH Signaling and Enhances Cytotoxicity of Cisplatin and Radiation in Head and Neck Squamous Cell Carcinoma. *Mol Cancer Ther* (2020) 19(6):1279–88. doi: 10.1158/1535-7163.MCT-19-0946

58. Ahmed SU, Carruthers R, Gilmour L, Yildirim S, Watts C, Chalmers AJ. Selective Inhibition of Parallel DNA Damage Response Pathways Optimizes Radiosensitization of Glioblastoma Stem-Like Cells. *Cancer Res* (2015) 75 (20):4416–28. doi: 10.1158/0008-5472.CAN-14-3790
59. Carruthers RD, Ahmed SU, Ramachandran S, Strathdee K, Kurian KM, Hedley A, et al. Replication Stress Drives Constitutive Activation of the DNA Damage Response and Radioresistance in Glioblastoma Stem-Like Cells. *Cancer Res* (2018) 78(17):5060–71. doi: 10.1158/0008-5472.CAN-18-0569
60. Vance S, Liu E, Zhao L, Parsels JD, Parsels LA, Brown JL, et al. Selective Radiosensitization of P53 Mutant Pancreatic Cancer Cells by Combined Inhibition of Chk1 and PARP1. *Cell Cycle* (2011) 10(24):4321–9. doi: 10.4161/cc.10.24.18661
61. Karnak D, Engelke CG, Parsels LA, Kausar T, Wei D, Robertson JR, et al. Combined Inhibition of Wee1 and PARP1/2 for Radiosensitization in Pancreatic Cancer. *Clin Cancer Res* (2014) 20(19):5085–96. doi: 10.1158/1078-0432.CCR-14-1038
62. Parsels LA, Karnak D, Parsels JD, Zhang Q, Vélez-Padilla J, Reichert ZR, et al. The Contribution of DNA Replication Stress Marked by High-Intensity, Pan-Nuclear Gammah2ax Staining to Chemosensitization by CHK1 and WEE1 Inhibitors. *Cell Cycle* (2018) 17(9):1076–86. doi: 10.1080/15384101.2018.1475827
63. Cuneo KC, Morgan MA, Davis MA, Parcels LA, Parcels J, Karnak D, et al. Wee1 Kinase Inhibitor AZD1775 Radiosensitizes Hepatocellular Carcinoma Regardless of TP53 Mutational Status Through Induction of Replication Stress. *Int J Radiat Oncol Biol Phys* (2016) 95(2):782–90. doi: 10.1016/j.ijrobp.2016.01.028
64. Wu W, Wang M, Wu W, Singh SK, Mussfeldt T, Iliakis G. Repair of Radiation Induced DNA Double Strand Breaks by Backup NHEJ is Enhanced in G2. *DNA Repair (Amst)* (2008) 7(2):329–38. doi: 10.1016/j.dnarep.2007.11.008
65. Rieckmann T, Kriegs M. The Failure of Cetuximab-Based De-Intensified Regimes for HPV-Positive OPSCC: A Radiobiologists Perspective. *Clin Transl Radiat Oncol* (2019) 17:47–50. doi: 10.1016/j.ctro.2019.05.003
66. Kong A, Good J, Kirkham A, Savage J, Mant R, Llewellyn L, et al. Phase I Trial of WEE1 Inhibition With Chemotherapy and Radiotherapy as Adjuvant Treatment, and a Window of Opportunity Trial With Cisplatin in Patients With Head and Neck Cancer: The WISTERIA Trial Protocol. *BMJ Open* (2020) 10(3):e033009. doi: 10.1136/bmjopen-2019-033009
67. Yang ES, Deutsch E, Mehmet A, Fayette J, Tao Y, Nabell L, et al. A Phase 1b Trial of Prexasertib in Combination With Chemoradiation in Patients With Locally Advanced Head and Neck Squamous Cell Carcinoma. *Radiother Oncol* (2021) 157:203–9. doi: 10.1016/j.radonc.2021.01.032
68. Cuneo KC, Morgan MA, Sahai V, Schipper MJ, Parsels LA, Parsels JD, et al. Dose Escalation Trial of the Wee1 Inhibitor Adavosertib (AZD1775) in Combination With Gemcitabine and Radiation for Patients With Locally Advanced Pancreatic Cancer. *J Clin Oncol* (2019) 37(29):2643–50. doi: 10.1200/JCO.19.00730

13

Functional Genetic Variant of Long Pentraxin 3 Gene is Associated with Clinical Aspects of Oral Cancer in Male Patients

Chia-Ming Yeh [1,2,3], Chiao-Wen Lin [4,5], Chun-Yi Chuang [6,7], Yu-Fan Liu [8], Chia-Hsuan Chou [1], Shun-Fa Yang [1,9] and Mu-Kuan Chen [1,2,3]**

[1] Institute of Medicine, Chung Shan Medical University, Taichung, Taiwan, [2] Cancer Research Center, Changhua Christian Hospital, Changhua, Taiwan, [3] Department of Otorhinolaryngology-Head and Neck Surgery, Changhua Christian Hospital, Changhua, Taiwan, [4] Institute of Oral Sciences, Chung Shan Medical University, Taichung, Taiwan, [5] Department of Dentistry, Chung Shan Medical University Hospital, Taichung, Taiwan, [6] School of Medicine, Chung Shan Medical University, Taichung, Taiwan, [7] Department of Otolaryngology, Chung Shan Medical University Hospital, Taichung, Taiwan, [8] Department of Biomedical Sciences, College of Medicine Sciences and Technology, Chung Shan Medical University, Taichung, Taiwan, [9] Department of Medical Research, Chung Shan Medical University Hospital, Taichung, Taiwan

***Correspondence:**
Shun-Fa Yang
ysf@csmu.edu.tw
Mu-Kuan Chen
53780@cch.org.tw

Long pentraxin 3 (PTX3) is produced by various cell types and is correlated with tumor progression in various tumor types. However, the clinical significance of *PTX3* polymorphisms in oral cancer and their correlation with the risk of cancer are still unclear. In this study, we assessed the influence of *PTX3* gene polymorphisms and environmental factors on susceptibility to oral tumorigenesis. We recruited 865 cases with oral cancer and 1,189 controls. Four single-nucleotide variations of the *PTX3* gene (rs1840680, rs2305619, rs3816527, and rs2120243) were verified using a real-time polymerase chain reaction in control participants and cases with oral cancer. We found that rs3816527 in smokers was correlated with the development of late-stage cancer (odds ratio [OR], 2.328; 95% confidence interval [CI], 1.078–5.027) and increased lymph node metastasis (OR, 2.152; 95% CI, 1.047–4.422). Moreover, additional bioinformatics analysis results showed that the rs3816527 C allele variant to the A allele exhibited the strongest exonic splicing enhancer activity. In conclusion, our results suggested that *PTX3* rs3816527 plays a role in oral cancer development.

Keywords: long pentraxin 3, oral squamous cell carcinoma, single-nucleotide variation, metastasis, splicing, tumor progression

INTRODUCTION

The incidence of oral cancer in Asia and more particularly Taiwan increases annually. In addition to tobacco smoking and alcohol consumption, betel quid chewing is a major cause of oral cancer (1–4). Moreover, the annual number of deaths due to oral cancer among men is increasing rapidly (5). The global 5 year mortality rate of oral cancer is ~50%. Although considerable progress has been made in surgery, chemotherapy, and radiotherapy, no considerable improvements have been made in the preceding 50 years (6).

TABLE 1 | Information on *PTX3* SNPs.

Variable	rs2120243	rs2305619	rs3816527	rs1840680
Chromosome	3:157429779	3:157437072	3:157437525	3:157438240
Exon	–	–	2	–
Nucleotide change	A>C	A>G	C>A	A>G
mRNA position	–	–	286	–
Function	TFBS	Intron variant	Non-synonymous	Intron variant
dbSNP allele	–	–	GCC ⟹ GAC	–
Protein residue	–	–	A [Ala] ⟹ D [Asp]	–
Allele frequencies	0.6744	0.6358	0.7845	0.6738

Allele frequencies were obtained from population databases gnomAD (https://gnomad.broadinstitute.org/) for East Asian population.

Pentraxins (PTXs) are a superfamily of conserved proteins that contain the pentraxin domain. Proteins of the pentraxin family are multifunctional and participate in acute immunological responses (7). PTX3, also known as TGF14, is a transmembrane molecule expressed in a variety of human tissues (8, 9). PTX3 is secreted by natural immune cells in response to inflammatory cytokines, such as interleukin-1 β (IL-1β) and tumor necrosis factor α (TNFα), or selected pathogen-associated molecular patterns (9–11). Therefore, *PTX3* may play a vital role at the crossroads of inflammation increase (12, 13), innate immunity (14–16), tissue repair stimulation (17, 18), and cancer (19–21). *PTX3* promotes cell migration and invasion in several cancers, and the expression of *PTX3* correlates with tumor progression in various human tumor types (19, 22–24).

Genetic variations contribute to susceptibility to common diseases such as cardiovascular disease, diabetes, inflammatory disease, and cancer (25–29). Single-nucleotide variations (SNVs) may be a causative genetic variant that can affect the expression and structure of proteins, thereby directly contributing to disease (30). The *PTX3* gene is located on chromosome 3 and contains three exons and two introns. Previous studies have described that SNVs in *PTX3* (rs2305619 and rs1840680) have functional significance. Results indicated that the A allele of *PTX3* SNVs (rs2305619 and rs1840680) is associated with higher plasma levels of PTX3 (31, 32). In addition, the A alleles of rs2305619 and rs1840680 are associated with susceptibility to *Pseudomonas aeruginosa* and *Mycobacterium tuberculosis* infections (33, 34). Carmo et al. also revealed that genetic variations in *PTX3* (rs2305619 and rs1840680) and plasma levels were associated with hepatocellular carcinoma (35). Moreover, Hakelius et al. indicated that PTX3 played a major role in non-malignant and oral cancer malignant disease processes (36). However, few studies have investigated the association of *PTX3* polymorphisms in oral cancer. Therefore, we investigated the relationship between four *PTX3* gene polymorphisms (rs1840680, rs2305619, rs3816527, and rs2120243; **Table 1**) and clinicopathological characteristics of patients with oral cancer to identify those with an increased risk of oral cancer.

Abbreviations: PTX3, long pentraxin 3; OSCC, oral squamous cell carcinoma; OR, odds ratio; SNV, single-nucleotide variation.

TABLE 2 | Distribution of demographic characteristics in 1,189 controls and 865 male individuals with oral cancer.

Variable	Controls (*N* = 1,189)	Cases (*N* = 865)	*p*-value
AGE (YRS)			
≦55	607 (51.0%)	454 (52.5%)	$p = 0.521$
>55	582 (49.0%)	411 (47.5%)	
BETEL QUID CHEWING			
No	991 (83.4%)	188 (21.7%)	$p <0.001^*$
Yes	198 (16.6%)	677 (78.3%)	
CIGARETTE SMOKING			
No	558 (46.9%)	99 (11.5%)	$p <0.001^*$
Yes	631 (53.1%)	766 (88.5%)	
ALCOHOL DRINKING			
No	954 (80.2%)	414 (47.9%)	$p <0.001^*$
Yes	235 (19.8%)	451 (52.1%)	
STAGE			
I+II		431 (49.8%)	
III+IV		434 (50.2%)	
TUMOR T STATUS			
T1+T2		496 (57.3%)	
T3+T4		369 (42.7%)	
LYMPH NODE STATUS			
N0		583 (67.4%)	
N1+N2+N3		282 (32.6%)	
METASTASIS			
M0		856 (99.0%)	
M1		9 (1.0%)	
CELL DIFFERENTIATION			
Well-differentiated		119 (13.8%)	
Moderately or poorly differentiated		746 (86.2%)	

Mann–Whitney U-test or Fisher's exact test was used between healthy controls and individuals with oral cancer. $^*p < 0.05$ *was considered statistically significant.*

MATERIALS AND METHODS

Study Population

The participants of this case–control study were 865 male cases with oral cancer of squamous cell carcinoma recruited from Changhua Christian Hospital in Changhua and Chung Shan Medical University Hospital in Taichung, Taiwan, between 2007 and 2017, and 1,189 cancer-free male controls selected from the Taiwan Biobank. The oral cancers of squamous cell carcinoma in this study were pre-specified to include any cancers that originated from buccal mucosa (n = 314; 36.3%), tongue (n = 268; 31.0%), gingiva (n = 78; 9.0%), palate (n = 40; 4.6%), floor of the mouth (n = 25; 2.9%), and other areas (n = 140; 16.2%). The Institutional Review Board of Chung Shan Medical University approved this study (CSMUH No: CS13214-1). All participants provided written informed consent. Personal characteristics and information, including demographic characteristics; tobacco smoking, betel quid chewing, and alcohol consumption habits; and the medical histories of the participants, were investigated using interviewer-administered questionnaires.

Determination of Genotypes

Genomic DNA from peripheral blood leukocytes was extracted using a QIAamp DNA Blood Mini Kit (Qiagen, Valencia, CA, USA) following the manufacturer's protocol (37). DNA was dissolved in ethylenediaminetetraacetic acid (EDTA) buffer (10 mM Tris, 1 mM EDTA; pH 7.8) and then quantified by measuring absorbance at 260 nm. Finally, the preparation was stored in a −20°C refrigerator and later analyzed using a real-time polymerase chain reaction (PCR) system. Allelic discrimination for the PTX3 SNV was performed using a TaqMan assay (ID C_12069244_10 for rs1840680, C_22275654_10 for rs2305619, C_3035766_30 for rs3816527, and C_11796613_20 for rs2120243) with an ABI StepOne Real-Time PCR System (Applied Biosystems). The genotypic frequencies of *PTX3* were further evaluated using the SDS v3.0 software program.

Bioinformatics Analysis

Several bioinformatics tools were used to assess the putative functional relevance of the rs3816527 PTX3 polymorphism. SNPinfo was used to predict the function of the rs351855 polymorphism. Splicing enhancement activity was analyzed using ESEfinder. We used the National Center for Biotechnology Information (NCBI) database to determine splicing types of PTX3. Furthermore, protein structure homology modeling of PTX3 was performed using SWISS-MODEL.

Statistical Analysis

The Mann–Whitney *U*-test was used to compare differences in demographic characteristics between healthy controls and cases with oral cancer. Multiple logistic regression models were used to determine the association between genotypic frequencies and oral cancer risk after adjustment for age, betel quid chewing, cigarette smoking, and alcohol consumption. Data were analyzed using SAS 9.1 statistical software. A $p < 0.05$ was considered significant.

RESULTS

Demographic Characteristics of the Participants

Table 2 displays the results of the statistical analysis of the participants' demographic characteristics. A total of 2,054

TABLE 3 | Genotyping and allelic frequency of *PTX3* single-nucleotide variations (SNVs) in individuals with oral cancer and controls.

Variable	Controls (*N* = 1,189 (%))	Cases (*N* = 865 (%))	OR (95% CI)	AOR (95% CI)
rs1840680				
GG	531 (44.7%)	375 (43.4%)	1.000 (reference)	1.000 (reference)
GA	532 (44.7%)	407 (47.0%)	1.083 (0.901–1.303)	1.056 (0.832–1.341)
AA	126 (10.6%)	83 (9.6%)	0.933 (0.686–1.268)	0.876 (0.591–1.297)
GA+AA	658 (55.3%)	490 (56.6%)	1.054 (0.884–1.258)	1.020 (0.812–1.281)
G allele	1594 (67.0%)	1157 (66.9%)	1.000 (reference)	1.000 (reference)
A allele	784 (33.0%)	573 (33.1%)	1.007 (0.883–1.149)	0.978 (0.825–1.159)
rs2305619				
GG	493 (41.5%)	346 (40.0%)	1.000 (reference)	1.000 (reference)
GA	550 (46.3%)	428 (49.5%)	1.109 (0.920–1.336)	1.126 (0.885–1.433)
AA	146 (12.2%)	91 (10.5%)	0.888 (0.661–1.194)	0.786 (0.537–1.151)
GA + AA	696 (58.5%)	519 (60.0%)	1.062 (0.889–1.270)	1.050 (0.835–1.322)
G allele	1536 (64.6%)	1120 (64.7%)	1.000 (reference)	1.000 (reference)
A allele	842 (35.4%)	610 (35.3%)	0.994 (0.873–1.131)	0.960 (0.812–1.135)
rs3816527				
AA	734 (61.7%)	511 (59.1%)	1.000 (reference)	1.000 (reference)
AC	402 (33.8%)	317 (36.6%)	1.133 (0.941–1.364)	1.191 (0.937–1.515)
CC	53 (4.5%)	37 (4.3%)	1.003 (0.649–1.549)	1.110 (0.633–1.947)
AC + CC	455 (38.3%)	354 (40.9%)	1.118 (0.934–1.337)	1.182 (0.938–1.490)
A allele	1870 (78.6%)	1339 (77.4%)	1.000 (reference)	1.000 (reference)
C allele	508 (21.4%)	391 (22.6%)	1.075 (0.926–1.248)	1.130 (0.931–1.371)
rs2120243				
CC	530 (44.6%)	385 (44.5%)	1.000 (reference)	1.000 (reference)
CA	542 (45.6%)	401 (46.4%)	1.019 (0.847–1.224)	1.062 (0.837–1.347)
AA	117 (9.8%)	79 (9.1%)	0.930 (0.679–1.273)	1.129 (0.753–1.692)
CA + AA	659 (55.4%)	480 (55.5%)	1.003 (0.841–1.196)	1.073 (0.855–1.347)
C allele	1602 (67.4%)	1171 (67.7%)	1.000 (reference)	1.000 (reference)
A allele	776 (32.6%)	559 (32.3%)	0.986 (0.863–1.125)	1.059 (0.893–1.257)

Adjusted odds ratios (aORs) with their 95% confidence intervals (CIs) were estimated using multiple logistic regression models after controlling for betel quid chewing, cigarette smoking, and alcohol consumption.

TABLE 4 | Association of the combined effect of *PTX3* gene polymorphisms and betel quid chewing with susceptibility to oral cancer among 1,397 smokers.

Variable	Controls ($n = 631$) (%)	Cases ($n = 766$) (%)	OR (95% CI)	*p*-value	AOR (95% CI)	*p*-value
rs1840680						
GG genotype & non-betel quid chewing	208 (33.0%)	53 (6.9%)	1.00 (reference)		1.000 (reference)	
GA or AA genotype or betel quid chewing	312 (49.4%)	356 (46.5%)	**4.478 (3.195–6.277)**	$p < 0.001$	**4.230 (2.998–5.969)**	$p < 0.001$
GA or AA genotype with betel quid chewing	111 (17.6%)	357 (46.6%)	**12.622 (8.725–18.259)**	$p < 0.001$	**10.504 (7.198–15.327)**	$p < 0.001$
rs2305619						
GG genotype & non-betel quid chewing	188 (29.8%)	44 (5.7%)	1.00 (reference)		1.000 (reference)	
GA or AA genotype or betel quid chewing	322 (51.0%)	349 (45.6%)	**4.631 (3.226–6.647)**	$p < 0.001$	**4.455 (3.081–6.441)**	$p < 0.001$
GA or AA genotype with betel quid chewing	121 (19.2%)	373 (48.7%)	**13.171 (8.944–19.395)**	$p < 0.001$	**11.271 (7.586–16.745)**	$p < 0.001$
rs3816527						
AA genotype & non-betel quid chewing	283 (44.8%)	66 (8.6%)	1.00 (reference)		1.000 (reference)	
AC or CC genotype or betel quid chewing	270 (42.8%)	449 (58.6%)	**7.130 (5.243–9.697)**	$p < 0.001$	**6.652 (4.857–9.112)**	$p < 0.001$
AC or CC genotype with betel quid chewing	78 (12.4%)	251 (32.8%)	**13.798 (9.538–19.960)**	$p < 0.001$	**11.827 (8.099–17.271)**	$p < 0.001$
rs2120243						
CC genotype & non-betel quid chewing	194 (30.8%)	54 (7.1%)	1.00 (reference)		1.000 (reference)	
CA or AA genotype or betel quid chewing	339 (53.7%)	363 (47.4%)	**3.847 (2.749–5.383)**	$p < 0.001$	**3.664 (2.600–5.162)**	$p < 0.001$
CA or AA genotype with betel quid chewing	98 (15.5%)	349 (45.5%)	**12.794 (8.787–18.628)**	$p < 0.001$	**10.755 (7.330–15.779)**	$p < 0.001$

Adjusted odds ratios (aORs) with their 95% confidence intervals (CIs) were estimated using multiple logistic regression models after controlling for age and alcohol drinking.
P-values were adjusted for multiple comparisons by applying the Bonferroni correction.
Bold values were considered statistically significant.

participants were enrolled, namely 865 male cases with oral cancer and 1,189 male controls. Results revealed significant differences in cigarette smoking ($p < 0.001$), betel quid chewing ($p < 0.001$), and alcohol consumption ($p < 0.001$) between the cases with oral cancer and the controls.

PTX3 Gene Polymorphisms in Cases With Oral Cancer and Controls

To investigate the association between *PTX3* gene polymorphisms and oral cancer risk, the genotypic, and allelic frequencies of *PTX3* in the individuals with oral cancer and the controls were established in this investigation (**Table 3**). After adjustment for betel quid chewing, cigarette smoking, and alcohol consumption, no significant difference was observed between the participants with oral cancer who had rs1840680, rs2305619, rs3816527, and rs2120243 polymorphisms of the *PTX3* gene and those with wild-type (WT) genes.

Combined Effects of Environmental Factors and *PTX3* Gene Polymorphisms on Oral Cancer

To determine the combined effects of environmental factors and *PTX3* gene SNVs on oral cancer susceptibility, we conducted further analysis on 1,397 smokers (**Table 4**). As presented in **Table 4**, participants with at least one A allele of rs1840680, one A allele of rs2305619, one C allele of rs3816527, or one A allele of rs2120243 exhibited 12.622-fold (95% CI: 8.725–18.259), 13.171-fold (95% CI: 8.944–19.395), 13.798-fold (95% CI: 9.538–19.960), and 12.794-fold (95% CI: 8.787–18.628) higher risks of oral cancer, respectively, compared with individuals with WT homozygotes who did not chew betel quid.

Effects of Polymorphic Genotypes of *PTX3* on Clinical Status of Oral Cancer

We analyzed the relationship between the combined effect of cigarette smoking and PTX3 variants on oral cancer development. As depicted in **Table 5**, individuals who possessed the CC allele of rs3816527 and smoked cigarettes were more prone to developing late-stage tumors (stage III/IV: OR, 2.328; 95% CI, 1.078–5.027; $p = 0.0314$) and lymph node metastasis (OR, 2.152; 95% CI, 1.047–4.422; $p = 0.0371$) compared with individuals who were homozygous for the WT allele of rs3816527 (**Table 5**).

Functional Connotation of the *PTX3* rs3816527 Locus

We investigated the functional connotation of the rs3816527 SNV on the *PTX3* gene. The function of *PTX3* rs3816527 was

TABLE 5 | Genotyping frequency of the *PTX3* rs3816527 polymorphism on clinical status of oral cancer among 766 smokers.

	Clinical Stage		**OR (95% CI)**	**AOR (95% CI)[a]**
***PTX3* rs3816527**	**Stage I/II (n = 379) n (%)**	**Stage III/IV (n = 387) n (%)**		
AA	235 (62.0%)	222 (57.3%)	1.000 (reference)	1.000 (reference)
AC	134 (35.4%)	143 (37.0%)	1.130 (0.838–1.523)	1.111 (0.823–1.500)
CC	10 (2.6%)	22 (5.7%)	**2.328 (1.078–5.027)[b]**	**2.424 (1.114–5.273)[d]**
	Tumor size			
PTX3 rs3816527	<underline<>T2 (n = 436) n (%)	> T2 (n = 330) n (%)		
AA	262 (60.1%)	195 (59.1%)	1.000 (reference)	1.000 (reference)
AC	157 (36.0%)	120 (36.4%)	1.027 (0.760–1.388)	1.034 (0.764–1.400)
CC	17 (3.9%)	15 (4.5%)	1.186 (0.578–2.432)	1.202 (0.582–2.483)
	Lymph node metastasis			
PTX3 rs3816527	No (n = 519) n (%)	Yes (n = 247) n (%)		
AA	312 (60.1%)	145 (58.7%)	1.000 (reference)	1.000 (reference)
AC	191 (36.8%)	186 (34.8%)	0.969 (0.702–1.337)	0.950 (0.687–1.312)
CC	16 (3.1%)	16 (6.5%)	**2.152 (1.047–4.422)[c]**	**2.183 (1.053–4.528)[e]**
	Cell differentiation			
PTX3 rs3816527	Well (n = 111) n (%)	Moderate/poor (n = 655) n (%)		
AA	70 (63.1%)	387 (59.1%)	1.000 (reference)	1.000 (reference)
AC	38 (34.2%)	239 (36.5%)	1.138 (0.743–1.743)	1.117 (0.728–1.713)
CC	3 (2.7%)	29 (4.4%)	1.748 (0.518–5.897)	1.750 (0.515–5.939)

[a]*Adjustment for the effects of betel quid chewing and alcohol consumption.*
[b]*p = 0.0314.*
[c]*p = 0.0371.*
[d]*p = 0.0256.*
[e]*p = 0.0359.*
Bold values were considered statistically significant.

performed using several bioinformatics tools, namely SNPinfo, the NCBI database, ESEfinder, and SWISS-MODEL. Data indicated that *PTX3* rs3816527 was located on the exonic splice enhancer sequence of the *PTX3* gene (**Figure 1A**). The C allele had stronger enhancement activity than did the A allele and may be more likely to promote the splicing modification of the *PTX3* gene (**Figure 1B**). Two splicing forms of *PTX3* existed in the NCBI database (**Figure 1C**).

DISCUSSION

Head and neck cancers are common worldwide. Approximately 90% of head and neck cancers are squamous cell carcinomas, of which ~50% occur in the oral cavity (38, 39). In south Central Asia, oral cancer is the third most common type of cancer (40). Oral cancer is associated with the use of chronic stimuli such as tobacco smoking, alcohol consumption, and betel quid chewing in particular (3, 4, 41). PTX3 was recognized by proteomics as a critical candidate biomarker for liposarcoma (42), lung cancer (43), prostate cancer (44), and pancreatic cancer (22). For example, a high expression of PTX3 was found in pancreatic cancer cell lines and a direct relationship was found between tumor metastasis and PTX3 expression (22). Moreover, several studies have reported the role of *PTX3* in epithelial cancer progression due to EMT induction (45–48). A low expression of PTX3 has been associated with increased susceptibility to epithelial carcinogenesis (46). Previous studies have demonstrated that PTX3 mediated the induction of the EMT by reducing the expression of E-cadherin, increasing the expression of N-cadherin and vimentin, and promoting the migration of HK-2 cells (45). Moreover, results indicated that the expression of pentraxin family members was significantly associated with the poor prognosis of patients with pancreatic cancer (22). Furthermore, overexpression of PTX3 could promote the proliferation and invasion of cervical cancer *in vitro* and *in vivo* (24). However, few studies have discussed the role of PTX3 in oral cancer. In the present study, the combined effect of environmental factors and *PTX3* polymorphisms considerably increased the risk of oral cancer (**Table 4**). Moreover, patients with *PTX3* SNV rs3816527 with CC had the highest risk of tumors (**Table 5**).

The occurrence of cancer stems from the genetic and epigenetic alterations of the basic mechanisms of the normal cell cycle, such as replication control and cell death (49, 50). Most genes in the human genome consist of multiple introns and exons that are modified through splicing to form mature messenger ribonucleic acid and protein products (51, 52). Although alternative splicing (AS) provides cells with protein diversity, studies have found that pathological changes in splicing can contribute to the development of cancers. For instance, mutations and gene expression changes affect the splicing

A

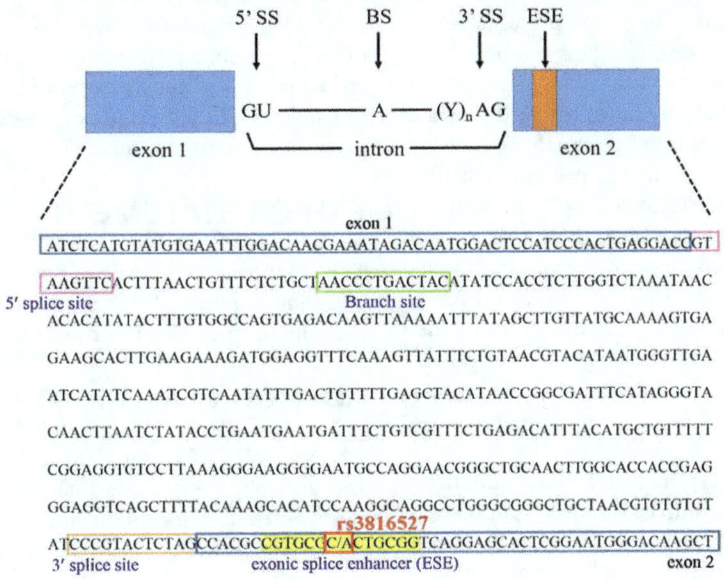

B

SNP	Allele	Position	Prediction Strand	Forward Sequence	Matrix	Method
rs3816527	C	3	+	CGCCTGC	SF2ASF2	ESEfind
rs3816527	A	3	+	CGACTGC	SF2ASF2	ESEfind

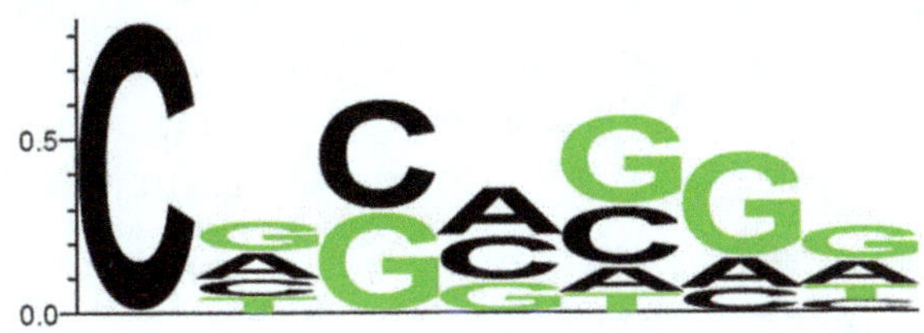

C

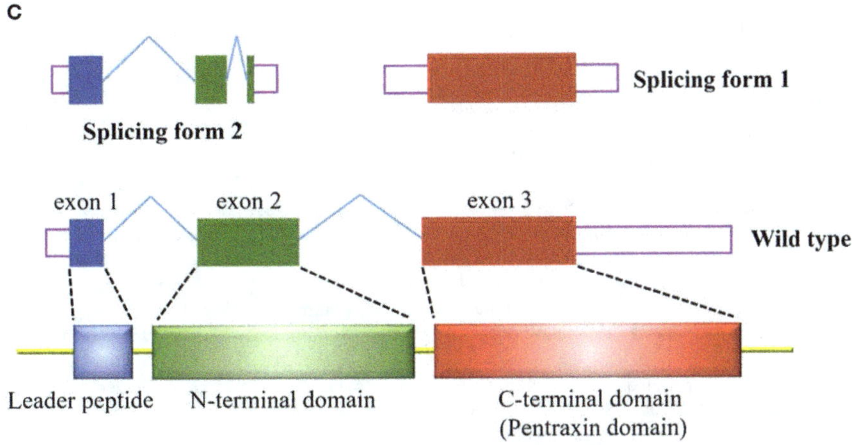

FIGURE 1 | Functional prediction profiling of *PTX3* SNV rs3816527. **(A)** The sequence of *PTX3* is from the NCBI reference sequences (RefSeq) (NM_002852.3). The cis-elements (5′ splice site, 3′ splice site, and branch site) and exonic splice enhancer (ESE) are indicated by various color squares. *PTX3* SNV rs3816527 is located on the ESE sequence. **(B)** The functional prediction of rs3816527 from SNPinfo web server is presented in this Figure. The relative frequency of the nucleotide for the ESE sequence is illustrated by the sequence logo. **(C)** *PTX3* gene consists of three exons. The first exon encodes the leader peptide, and the second and third exons encode N-terminal and C-terminal domains, respectively. Two common splicing forms of *PTX3* are accessed from the NCBI database.

regulatory sequences of key cancer-related genes (53) and the core or accessory components of spliceosome complexes (54–59).

PTX3 has two splice variants; one contains exon 1 or 2 (length of 453 bp) and the other contains exon 3 (length of 931 bp) (**Figure 1C**). ESEfinder analysis results revealed that the rs3816527 C allele had superior splicing enhancement activity for the A allele (**Figure 1B**). In addition, in the protein structure constructed by SWISS-MODEL, PTX3 was split into an N terminus and C terminus after splicing. Although the mechanism of action for this structure remains unclear, a molecular study indicated that the overexpression of PTX3 at the N terminus can considerably inhibit the oncogenic activity of transgenic adenocarcinoma mouse prostate-C2 transfectants, whereas C-terminal overexpression has only a minor effect on tumor growth (60).

We revealed an impact of *PTX3* gene variations on the development of oral cancer; however, there are some limitations in the study. As this study only included a discovery population and not a second independent study to replicate the findings, the associations between *PTX3* variations and oral cancer should be considered preliminary. The other concern is that we failed to exclude the possibility of potential selection bias and since the control group was enrolled among subjects without cancer on a hospital basis. In addition, determining the functional role of PTX3 in the development of oral cancer still requires further investigation.

In conclusion, our results suggest that the allelic effects of *PTX3* SNVs (rs1840680, rs2305619, rs3816527, and rs2120243) enhance the risk and progression of oral cancer in the presence of environmental factors such as tobacco smoking and betel quid chewing. This genetic association was observed most markedly in smokers. These results expose a novel genetic–environmental predisposition to oral cancer carcinogenesis.

ETHICS STATEMENT

The Institutional Review Board of Chung Shan Medical University approved this study (CSMUH No: CS13214-1). All participants provided informed consent.

AUTHOR CONTRIBUTIONS

C-MY, C-WL, S-FY, and M-KC contributed to conception, design and critically revised the manuscript. C-MY, S-FY, and M-KC contributed to conception and drafted the manuscript, C-YC, Y-FL, and C-HC contributed to performed experiments and analyzed data.

ACKNOWLEDGMENTS

This study was supported by grants from Ministry of Science and Technology, Taiwan (MOST-106-2314-B-371-005-MY3).

REFERENCES

1. Chiba I. Prevention of Betel Quid Chewers' Oral Cancer in the Asian-Pacific Area. *Asian Pac J Cancer Prev.* (2001) 2:263–9.
2. Jeng JH, Chang MC, Hahn LJ. Role of areca nut in betel quid-associated chemical carcinogenesis: current awareness and future perspectives. *Oral Oncol.* (2001) 37:477–92. doi: 10.1016/S1368-8375(01)00003-3
3. Su SC, Lin CW, Liu YF, Fan WL, Chen MK, Yu CP, et al. Exome sequencing of oral squamous cell carcinoma reveals molecular subgroups and novel therapeutic opportunities. *Theranostics.* (2017) 7:1088–99. doi: 10.7150/thno.18551
4. Yang SF, Huang HD, Fan WL, Jong YJ, Chen MK, Huang CN, et al. Compositional and functional variations of oral microbiota associated with the mutational changes in oral cancer. *Oral Oncol.* (2018) 77:1–8. doi: 10.1016/j.oraloncology.2017.12.005
5. Petti S, Scully C. How many individuals must be screened to reduce oral cancer mortality rate in the Western context? *Chall Oral Dis.* (2015) 21:949–54. doi: 10.1111/odi.12372
6. Miller C, Shay A, Tajudeen B, Sen N, Fidler M, Stenson K, et al. Clinical features and outcomes in young adults with oral tongue cancer. *Am J Otolaryngol.* (2019) 40:93–6. doi: 10.1016/j.amjoto.2018.09.022
7. Gewurz H, Zhang XH, Lint TF. Structure and function of the pentraxins. *Curr Opin Immunol.* (1995) 7:54–64. doi: 10.1016/0952-7915(95)80029-8
8. Garlanda C, Bottazzi B, Bastone A, Mantovani A. Pentraxins at the crossroads between innate immunity, inflammation, matrix deposition, and female fertility. *Ann Rev Immunol.* (2005) 23:337–66. doi: 10.1146/annurev.immunol.23.021704.115756
9. Lee GW, Lee TH, Vilcek J. TSG-14, a tumor necrosis factor- and IL-1-inducible protein, is a novel member of the pentaxin family of acute phase proteins. *J Immunol.* (1993) 150:1804–12.
10. Breviario F, d'Aniello EM, Golay J, Peri G, Bottazzi B, Bairoch A, et al. Interleukin-1-inducible genes in endothelial cells. Cloning of a new gene related to C-reactive protein and serum amyloid P component. *J Biol Chem.* (1992) 267:22190–7.
11. Vouret-Craviari V, Matteucci C, Peri G, Poli G, Introna M, Mantovani A. Expression of a long pentraxin, PTX3, by monocytes exposed to the mycobacterial cell wall component lipoarabinomannan. *Infect Immun.* (1997) 65:1345–50. doi: 10.1006/cyto.1997.0242
12. Bonavita E, Gentile S, Rubino M, Maina V, Papait R, Kunderfranco P, et al. PTX3 is an extrinsic oncosuppressor regulating complement-dependent inflammation in cancer. *Cell.* (2015) 160:700–14. doi: 10.1016/j.cell.2015.01.004
13. Daigo K, Mantovani A, Bottazzi B. The yin-yang of long pentraxin PTX3 in inflammation and immunity. *Immunol Lett.* (2014) 161:38–43. doi: 10.1016/j.imlet.2014.04.012
14. Jaillon S, Moalli F, Ragnarsdottir B, Bonavita E, Puthia M, Riva F, et al. The humoral pattern recognition molecule PTX3 is a key component of innate immunity against urinary tract infection. *Immunity.* (2014) 40:621–32. doi: 10.1016/j.immuni.2014.02.015
15. Kabbani D, Bhaskaran A, Singer LG, Bhimji A, Rotstein C, Keshavjee S, et al. Pentraxin 3 levels in bronchoalveolar lavage fluid of lung transplant recipients with invasive aspergillosis. *J Heart Lung Transpl.* (2017) 36:973–9. doi: 10.1016/j.healun.2017.04.007
16. Zhang J, Zhao GQ, Qu J, Lin J, Che CY, Yang XJ. Early expression of PTX3 in Aspergillus fumigatus infected rat cornea. *Inter J Ophthalmol.* (2018) 11:1084–9. doi: 10.18240/ijo.2018.07.02

17. Doni A, Garlanda C, Mantovani A. PTX3 orchestrates tissue repair. *Oncotarget.* (2015) 6:30435–6. doi: 10.18632/oncotarget.5453
18. Doni A, Musso T, Morone D, Bastone A, Zambelli V, Sironi M, et al. An acidic microenvironment sets the humoral pattern recognition molecule PTX3 in a tissue repair mode. *J Exp Med.* (2015) 212:905–25. doi: 10.1084/jem.20141268
19. Chang WC, Wu SL, Huang WC, Hsu JY, Chan SH, Wang JM, et al. PTX3 gene activation in EGF-induced head and neck cancer cell metastasis. *Oncotarget.* (2015) 6:7741–57. doi: 10.18632/oncotarget.3482
20. Garlanda C, Bottazzi B, Magrini E, Inforzato A, Mantovani A. PTX3, a humoral pattern recognition molecule in innate immunity, tissue repair, and cancer. *Physiol Rev.* (2018) 98:623–39. doi: 10.1152/physrev.00016.2017
21. Stallone G, Cormio L, Netti GS, Infante B, Selvaggio O, Fino GD, et al. Pentraxin 3: a novel biomarker for predicting progression from prostatic inflammation to prostate cancer. *Cancer Res.* (2014) 74:4230–8. doi: 10.1158/0008-5472.CAN-14-0369
22. Kondo S, Ueno H, Hosoi H, Hashimoto J, Morizane C, Koizumi F, et al. Clinical impact of pentraxin family expression on prognosis of pancreatic carcinoma. *Br J Cancer.* (2013) 109:739–46. doi: 10.1038/bjc.2013.348
23. Tung JN, Ko CP, Yang SF, Cheng CW, Chen PN, Chang CY, et al. Inhibition of pentraxin 3 in glioma cells impairs proliferation and invasion *in vitro* and *in vivo*. *J Neuro Oncol.* (2016) 129:201–9. doi: 10.1007/s11060-016-2168-z
24. Ying TH, Lee CH, Chiou HL, Yang SF, Lin CL, Hung CH, et al. Knockdown of Pentraxin 3 suppresses tumorigenicity and metastasis of human cervical cancer cells. *Sci Rep.* (2016) 6:29385. doi: 10.1038/srep29385
25. Eccles D, Tapper W. The influence of common polymorphisms on breast cancer. *Cancer Treat Res.* (2010) 155:15–32. doi: 10.1007/978-1-4419-6033-7_2
26. Hanahan D, Weinberg RA. The hallmarks of cancer. *Cell.* (2000) 100:57–70. doi: 10.1016/S0092-8674(00)81683-9
27. Hua KT, Liu YF, Hsu CL, Cheng TY, Yang CY, Chang JS, et al. 3'UTR polymorphisms of carbonic anhydrase IX determine the miR-34a targeting efficiency and prognosis of hepatocellular carcinoma. *Sci Rep.* (2017) 7:4466. doi: 10.1038/s41598-017-04732-3
28. Schmith VD, Campbell DA, Sehgal S, Anderson WH, Burns DK, Middleton LT, et al. Pharmacogenetics and disease genetics of complex diseases. *Cell Mol Life Sci.* (2003) 60:1636–46. doi: 10.1007/s00018-003-2369-4
29. Su SC, Hsieh MJ, Lin CW, Chuang CY, Liu YF, Yeh CM, et al. Impact of HOTAIR gene polymorphism and environmental risk on oral cancer. *J Dent Res.* (2018) 97:717–24. doi: 10.1177/0022034517749451
30. Sunyaev S, Ramensky V, Koch I, Lathe W 3rd, Kondrashov AS, Bork P. Prediction of deleterious human alleles. *Hum Mol Genet.* (2001) 10:591–7. doi: 10.1093/hmg/10.6.591
31. Barbati E, Specchia C, Villella M, Rossi ML, Barlera S, Bottazzi B, et al. Influence of pentraxin 3 (PTX3) genetic variants on myocardial infarction risk and PTX3 plasma levels. *PLoS ONE.* (2012) 7:e53030. doi: 10.1371/journal.pone.0053030
32. Diamond JM, Meyer NJ, Feng R, Rushefski M, Lederer DJ, Kawut SM, et al. Variation in PTX3 is associated with primary graft dysfunction after lung transplantation. *Am J Resp Crit Care Med.* (2012) 186:546–52. doi: 10.1164/rccm.201204-0692OC
33. Chiarini M, Sabelli C, Melotti P, Garlanda C, Savoldi G, Mazza C, et al. PTX3 genetic variations affect the risk of *Pseudomonas aeruginosa* airway colonization in cystic fibrosis patients. *Genes Immun.* (2010) 11:665–70. doi: 10.1038/gene.2010.41
34. Olesen R, Wejse C, Velez DR, Bisseye C, Sodemann M, Aaby P, et al. DC-SIGN (CD209), pentraxin 3 and vitamin D receptor gene variants associate with pulmonary tuberculosis risk in West Africans. *Genes Immun.* (2007) 8:456–67. doi: 10.1038/sj.gene.6364410
35. Carmo RF, Aroucha D, Vasconcelos LR, Pereira LM, Moura P, Cavalcanti MS. Genetic variation in PTX3 and plasma levels associated with hepatocellular carcinoma in patients with HCV. *J Viral Hepatit.* (2016) 23:116–22. doi: 10.1111/jvh.12472
36. Hakelius M, Reyhani V, Rubin K, Gerdin B, Nowinski D. Normal oral keratinocytes and head and neck squamous carcinoma cells induce an innate response of fibroblasts. *Anticanc Res.* (2016) 36:2131–7.
37. Su SC, Hsieh MJ, Liu YF, Chou YE, Lin CW, Yang SF. ADAMTS14 gene polymorphism and environmental risk in the development of oral cancer. *PLoS ONE.* (2016) 11:e0159585. doi: 10.1371/journal.pone.0159585
38. Boyle P, Levin B. *World Cancer Report 2008.* Lyon: IARC Press, International Agency for Research on Cancer (2008).
39. Jemal A, Siegel R, Ward E, Hao Y, Xu J, Thun MJ. Cancer statistics, 2009. *CA Cancer J Clin.* (2009) 59:225–49. doi: 10.3322/caac.20006
40. Petersen PE. The World Oral Health Report 2003: continuous improvement of oral health in the 21st century–the approach of the WHO Global Oral Health Programme. *Commun Dentist Oral Epidemiol. (2003)* 31(Suppl 1):3–23. doi: 10.1046/j..2003.com122.x
41. Su CW, Chien MH, Lin CW, Chen MK, Chow JM, Chuang CY, et al. Associations of genetic variations of the endothelial nitric oxide synthase gene and environmental carcinogens with oral cancer susceptibility and development. *Nitric Oxide Biol Chem.* (2018) 79:1–7. doi: 10.1016/j.niox.2018.06.005
42. Willeke F, Assad A, Findeisen P, Schromm E, Grobholz R, von Gerstenbergk B, et al. Overexpression of a member of the pentraxin family (PTX3) in human soft tissue liposarcoma. *Euro J Cancer.* (2006) 42:2639–46. doi: 10.1016/j.ejca.2006.05.035
43. Diamandis EP, Goodglick L, Planque C, Thornquist MD. Pentraxin-3 is a novel biomarker of lung carcinoma. *Clin Cancer Res.* (2011) 17:2395–9. doi: 10.1158/1078-0432.CCR-10-3024
44. Sardana G, Jung K, Stephan C, Diamandis EP. Proteomic analysis of conditioned media from the PC3, LNCaP, and 22Rv1 prostate cancer cell lines: discovery and validation of candidate prostate cancer biomarkers. *J Proteome Res.* (2008) 7:3329–38. doi: 10.1021/pr8003216
45. Hung TW, Tsai JP, Lin SH, Lee CH, Hsieh YH, Chang HR. Pentraxin 3 activates JNK signaling and regulates the epithelial-to-mesenchymal transition in renal fibrosis. *Cell Physiol Biochem.* (2016) 40:1029–38. doi: 10.1159/000453159
46. Ronca R, Di Salle E, Giacomini A, Leali D, Alessi P, Coltrini D, et al. Long pentraxin-3 inhibits epithelial-mesenchymal transition in melanoma cells. *Mol Cancer Therap.* (2013) 12:2760–71. doi: 10.1158/1535-7163.MCT-13-0487
47. Scimeca M, Antonacci C, Colombo D, Bonfiglio R, Buonomo OC, Bonanno E. Emerging prognostic markers related to mesenchymal characteristics of poorly differentiated breast cancers. *Tumour Biol.* (2016) 37:5427–35. doi: 10.1007/s13277-015-4361-7
48. Scimeca M, Antonacci C, Toschi N, Giannini E, Bonfiglio R, Buonomo CO, et al. Breast Osteoblast-like cells: a reliable early marker for bone metastases from breast cancer. *Clin Breast Cancer.* (2018) 18:e659–69. doi: 10.1016/j.clbc.2017.11.020
49. Feinberg AP, Koldobskiy MA, Gondor A. Epigenetic modulators, modifiers and mediators in cancer aetiology and progression. *Nat Rev Genet.* (2016) 17:284–99. doi: 10.1038/nrg.2016.13
50. Hanahan D, Weinberg RA. Hallmarks of cancer: the next generation. *Cell.* (2011) 144:646–74. doi: 10.1016/j.cell.2011.02.013
51. Pan Q, Shai O, Lee LJ, Frey BJ, Blencowe BJ. Deep surveying of alternative splicing complexity in the human transcriptome by high-throughput sequencing. *Nat Genet.* (2008) 40:1413–5. doi: 10.1038/ng.259
52. Wang ET, Sandberg R, Luo S, Khrebtukova I, Zhang L, Mayr C, et al. Alternative isoform regulation in human tissue transcriptomes. *Nature.* (2008) 456:470–6. doi: 10.1038/nature07509
53. Jung H, Lee D, Lee J, Park D, Kim YJ, Park WY, et al. Intron retention is a widespread mechanism of tumor-suppressor inactivation. *Nat Genet.* (2015) 47:1242–8. doi: 10.1038/ng.3414
54. Anczukow O, Rosenberg AZ, Akerman M, Das S, Zhan L, Karni R, et al. The splicing factor SRSF1 regulates apoptosis and proliferation to promote mammary epithelial cell transformation. *Nat Struct Mol Biol.* (2012) 19:220–8. doi: 10.1038/nsmb.2207
55. Jensen MA, Wilkinson JE, Krainer AR. Splicing factor SRSF6 promotes hyperplasia of sensitized skin. *Nat Struct Mol Biol.* (2014) 21:189–97. doi: 10.1038/nsmb.2756
56. Karni R, de Stanchina E, Lowe SW, Sinha R, Mu D, Krainer AR. The gene encoding the splicing factor SF2/ASF is a proto-oncogene. *Nat Struct Mol Biol.* (2007) 14:185–93. doi: 10.1038/nsmb1209
57. Quesada V, Conde L, Villamor N, Ordonez GR, Jares P, Bassaganyas L, et al. Exome sequencing identifies recurrent mutations of the splicing factor SF3B1 gene in chronic lymphocytic leukemia. *Nat Genet.* (2011) 44:47–52. doi: 10.1038/ng.1032

58. Wang L, Lawrence MS, Wan Y, Stojanov P, Sougnez C, Stevenson K, et al. SF3B1 and other novel cancer genes in chronic lymphocytic leukemia. *N Engl J Med.* (2011) 365:2497–506. doi: 10.1056/NEJMoa1109016
59. Yoshida K, Sanada M, Shiraishi Y, Nowak D, Nagata Y, Yamamoto R, et al. Frequent pathway mutations of splicing machinery in myelodysplasia. *Nature.* (2011) 478:64–9. doi: 10.1038/nature10496
60. Ronca R, Alessi P, Coltrini D, Di Salle E, Giacomini A, Leali D, et al. Long pentraxin-3 as an epithelial-stromal fibroblast growth factor-targeting inhibitor in prostate cancer. *J Pathol.* (2013) 230:228–38. doi: 10.1002/path.4181

14

BCL11A Promotes the Progression of Laryngeal Squamous Cell Carcinoma

Jian Zhou[1,2,3], Liang Zhou[2,3], Duo Zhang[2,3], Wei-Jing Tang[2,3], Di Tang[2,3], Xiao-Ling Shi[2,3], Yue Yang[2,3], Lin Zhou[1], Fei Liu[1], Yong Yu[4], Pentao Liu[4], Lei Tao[2,3] and Li-Ming Lu[1]**

[1] Shanghai Institute of Immunology, Shanghai Jiaotong University School of Medicine, Shanghai, China, [2] Department of Otolaryngology, Eye, Ear, Nose and Throat Hospital, Fudan University, Shanghai, China, [3] Shanghai Key Clinical Disciplines of Otorhinolaryngology, Shanghai, China, [4] Wellcome Trust Sanger Institute, Cambridge, United Kingdom

***Correspondence:**
Lei Tao
doctortaolei@163.com
Li-Ming Lu
lulunew2003@163.com

Background: We report functional and clinical data uncovering the significance of B-cell lymphoma/leukemia 11A (BCL11A) in laryngeal squamous cell carcinoma (LSCC).

Methods: We examined BCL11A expression in a cohort of LSCC patients and evaluated the association between BCL11A expression and clinicopathological features. We investigated the consequences of overexpressing BCL11A in the LSCC cell line on proliferation, migration, invasion, cell cycle, chemosensitivity, and growth *in vivo*. We explored the relationship between BCL11A and MDM2 in LSCC and tumorigenesis pathways by using the Human Cancer PathwayFinder Array.

Results: High levels of BCL11A were found in LSCC tissues and were more frequently associated with advanced lymphatic metastasis stages with poor prognoses. BCL11A overexpression enhanced LSCC proliferation *in vitro* and *vivo*. A positive correlation between MDM2 and BCL11A expression was identified.

Conclusions: These data uncover important functions of BCL11A in LSCC and identify BCL11A as a prognostic biomarker and potential therapeutic target in LSCC.

Keywords: BCL11A, LSCC, proto-oncogene, MDM2, prognosis

INTRODUCTION

Laryngeal squamous cell carcinoma (LSCC) is the eleventh most common tumor in males. The most deep-rooted risk factors for LSCC are alcohol abuse and tobacco use (1). The LSCC has a poor prognosis, with a 5 year survival rate <50%. The aforementioned is mostly attributed to regional and local recurrences, especially in patients with stage III or IV disease (2). Studies are needed to increase our understanding of the pathogenesis and prognosis of LSCC.

The *Bcl11a* gene encodes a C2H2 zinc finger transcription factor, which acts as a retroviral insertion site (Evi9) in myeloid leukemia in BXH-2 mice (3, 4). The gene was initially recognized in a rare $t_{(2;14)}$ (p16; q32.3) translocation in aggressive B-cell chronic lymphocytic leukemia, and it is usually co-amplified with the proto-oncogene REL in classical Hodgkin's lymphoma and non-Hodgkin's lymphoma (5, 6). The role of BCL11A in solid melanomas has not been widely studied. Khaled et al. studied the BCL11A oncogene in triple-negative breast tumors and reported that its overexpression promoted cancer development (7). Jiang et al. revealed that BCL11A protein expression levels were markedly upregulated in non-small-cell lung cancer (NSCLC) tissues, particularly in large cell cancer and squamous cell cancer (SCC). A multivariate analysis demonstrated that BCL11A was an independent prognostic factor for both overall survival and disease-free survival (8). To address these issues, we determined BCL11A expression in

LSCC and investigated its clinical significance by associating clinicopathologic parameters with BCL11A expression in LSCC patients. We further dissected the cellular and molecular mechanisms underlying BCL11A function in LSCC.

MATERIALS AND METHODS

Patient Population

Sixty-nine LSCC patients were recruited for this study. All of them had undergone total laryngectomy, with or without chemotherapy from November 2013 to September 2014 in the Otolaryngology Head and Neck Surgery Department of the Eye, Ear, Nose and Throat Hospital, Fudan University. Of 69 patients entered in this research, suitable tissues for Tissue Microarrays (TMA) were available for all 69 patients. All patients were categorized on the basis of UICC stage classification using specimens. All cases were collected according to study protocols permitted by the Ethics Committee of Fudan University, and all the participants offered written informed consent before the commencement of the research. The following data were recorded: patient's age, T stage, N stage, carcinoma stage, drinking status (non-drinker, drinker), smoking status (non-smoker, smoker), and tumor recurrence. Non-smokers were defined as those who smoked $\leq$10 packs/y, and smokers were defined as those who smoked >10 packs/y. All patients followed up for 2 years. Progression-free survival was defined as the time from registration to local or distant recurrence. Failure was recorded on the occasion of recurrent cancer or if the primary tumor was never wholly gone.

Cell Culture Conditions

Human laryngeal cancer cell line AMC-HN-8 cells were obtained from the Asian Medical Center, Ulsan University College of Medicine approximately 8 years ago. The cells were cultured in RPMI-1640 (Gibco, CA, U.S.A.), supplemented with streptomycin (100 μg/ml; Beyotime), penicillin (100 units/ml; Beyotime, China) and 10% fetal bovine serum (Gibco), in a 5% CO_2 incubator at 37°C.

Establishment of Stable Cell Lines With Overexpression of BCl11A

The lentiviral vectors expressing the Bcl11A-FLAG sequence (Bcl11A-OE) and the NCs were provided by Hanyin Co. (Shanghai). The primers were as follows:

Bcl11a-F: 5′ GACTAGTGCCACCATGTCTCGCCGCAAG CAAGG3′; Bcl11a-R: 5′ CGGGATCCTCACTTGTCGTCAT CGTCCTTGTAGTCGAACTTAAGGGCTCTCGAGCTT-3′.

Amplified flag-tagged Bcl11a was cloned into a pHY-LV-OE2.2 vector. Recombinant lentiviruses (Bcl11A-OE and NC) (Hanyin Co.) were then arranged and titered to 10^9 TU/ml. To establish stable cell lines, cells were plated in six-well plates and infected with the virus and polybrene the next day. Positive clones were then incubated with puromycin for 14 d. Bcl11A overexpression was verified by Western blot and qRT-PCR analyses.

Cell Proliferation Assays

The proliferation effects of AMC-HN-8-NC and AMC-HN-8-BCL11A cells were measured by CCK-8 assay. The cells were plated into 96-well plates, with 100 μl (1×10^4/ml) in each well in the exponential growth phase. The cells were then placed in an incubator at 37°C for 5 d, then 10 μl CCK-8 was added to every well then incubated for 1 h. The absorbance of every unit was assessed at 450 and 650 nm using a standard enzyme-linked immunosorbant assay. The absorbance values at A450 and A650 were calculated, and the results were measured in triplicate.

Colony Formation Assay

Cells were plated at 800 cells per well in six-well plates ($n = 2$). After 15 d of culture, the cells were stained with crystal violet, photographed and scored.

Transwell Migration Assays

In the transwell migration assays, 8.0 μm pore polyethylene terephthalate track-etched membrane cell culture inserts (FALCON) were used. A total volume of 600 μl of RPMI-1640 medium (Gibco), supplemented with 20% serum, was loaded into the lower chamber of a 24-well plate. Then, 1×10^5 cells in 100 μl of medium were added to the upper chamber, and the cells were allowed to migrate for 24 h at 37°C. Five random fields per insert were imaged at ×200 magnification. The migrated cells were calculated by ImageJ (NIH Image, NIH).

Invasion Assays

In the invasion assays, 8 μm transwells were coated with 1 mg/ml of Matrigel (BD Pharmingen). The medium (100 μl) containing the cells (2×10^5) was added to the higher unit, and the cells were allowed to migrate for 24 h in a 37°C incubator. All the experiments were performed in triplicate. The rest of the experimental methods were the same as those used in the migration assays.

Investigation of Cell Cycle Phase Using Flow Cytometry

The AMC-HN-8 cells were trypsinized, washed with PBS and then fixed by icy 70% ethanol for 24 h. The cells were stained with 1 ml of PI (0.1 mg/ml with 0.1% Triton X-100; Sangon Biotech) and cultured in the dark for half an hour. The cells were evaluated using a flow cytometer (FACSCalibur, Becton-Dickinson).

Immunochemistry

The tumor tissues were dissected, fixed and embedded in paraffin. The tissue microarray analysis (TMA) was completed with tumors by using multiple representative 1 mm cores from each tumor. Immunohistochemistry staining with haematoxylin/eosin (H&E) of 4–5 μm paraffin sections was performed. The primary antibodies were mouse monoclonal anti-human anti-BCL11A (Clone: EPR 14943-44, 1:100 dilution, Abcam, London, U.K.) and anti-MDM2 (Clone: SMP 14, 1:50 dilution, Abcam). Each tumor was assigned a score based on the staining intensity (no staining = 0, weak staining = 1, moderate staining = 2, and strong staining = 3). The extent of staining was classified as follows: 81–100% = 4, 51–80% = 3, 11–50% = 2, 1–10%

= 1, and 0% = 0 (9). The final score was determined by multiplying the intensity scores by the scores for the positively stained cells, with a maximum score of 12 and a minimum score of 0. Scores ≥ 6 were categorized as high expression, and scores lower than this were classified as low expression. The numbers of positively stained BCL11A and MDM2 cells were estimated by two independent researchers who were blinded to the clinical characteristics.

qRT-PCR Assays

Whole RNA was extracted by TRIzol (Invitrogen, CA, U.S.A.). The total RNA (1 μg) was used for cDNA synthesis by a reverse transcription kit (Takara, Japan) in a 20 μl reaction mixture containing 5 μM of random hexamers, 0.1 μM of a specific primer and 2.5 μM of an oligo (dT) primer. The assay was executed on an Applied Biosystems 7500 Fast System. The expression levels of the target gene RNAs were standardized to that of GAPDH. The BCL11A primer pair was as follow:F:ACAA ACGGAAACAATGCAATGG, R:TTTCATCTCGATTGGTGAA GGG.

Cancer PathwayFinder PCR Array

The RNA was extracted from the AMC-HN-8-BCL11A cells and AMC-HN-8-NC cells in the exponential growth phase using TRIzol (Invitrogen). The gene expression of 84 genes in nine biological tumorigenesis pathways was measured using the Human Cancer Pathway-Finder RT^2 Profiler PCR Array (SABiosciences) according to established guidelines and evaluated using the MX3005P Real-Time PCR System (Stratagene). Only genes with 1.5-fold variation or greater were selected for further research. The data were confirmed using a combination of qPCR and Western blot assays.

Western Blot Analysis

The total cell extracts were processed by denaturing proteins with SDS loading buffer (Beyotime, China). Equivalent amounts of protein were separated by 12% SDS-polyacrylamide gel electrophoresis, transferred to polyvinylidene fluoride membranes (Millipore Corporation, MA, and U.S.A.) and then blocked for 30 min in Tris-buffered saline with Tween 20 (TBST) and 5% non-fat milk. The blots were incubated at 4°C overnight in a series of antibodies diluted in TBST buffer: BCL11A (Clone: EPR 14943-44, Abcam, London, U.K.) and MDM2 primary antibodies (1:5,000), baculoviral IAP repeat containing 3 (BIRC3) antibody (Clone: E 40, 1:1000 dilution, Abcam), β-2-microglobulin (B2M) antibody (Clone: EP2978Y, 1:5000 dilution, Abcam), STMN1 antibody (Clone: EP1573, 1:50000 dilution, Abcam), SNAI2 antibody (ab75629, 1:50000 dilution, Abcam), haem oxygenase 1 (HMOX1) antibody (Clone: HO-1-1, 1:1000 dilution, Abcam), and protein phosphatase 1 regulatory inhibitor subunit 15A (PPP1R15A) antibody (ab 9869, 1:1000 dilution, Abcam). After washing with TBST, the membranes were incubated in secondary antibodies (1:4,000; KPL, MD, USA) and then analyzed by a chemiluminescence detection kit (Thermo Scientific, Inc., NJ, USA).

Xenograft Studies

The tumor growth of the AMC-HN-8-NC and AMC-HN-8-BCL11A cell lines (1×10^6 cells per cell line) was determined following a subcutaneous injection of cells into the left flank of 6-week-old male nude mice (Department of Laboratory Animal Science, Fudan University), with five animals in each group. The tumor size was analyzed (mm^3) by means of the formula: $0.5 \times (L \times W^2)$. The tumor specimens were fixed using 4% paraformaldehyde for paraffin embedding. Paraffin sections were stained with H&E according to established guidelines. All animal studies were approved by the Animal Center, Eye Ear Nose and Throat Hospital, Fudan University.

Statistical Analysis

The associations between BCL11A and MDM2 status and the recorded clinicopathological characteristics were assessed using a two-sample *t*-test, with $\chi 2$ tests used for categorical variables. A two-tailed *P*-value of 0.05 or less was considered statistically noteworthy. All the data were investigated by SPSS version 19.0 (IBM, Portsmouth, U.K.).

RESULTS

BCL11A Was Highly Expressed in LSCC Patients

Of 69 patients enrolled in this study, immunohistological examination revealed that 52 (75.4%) tumors were classified as high BCL11A expression, while 15 (37.5%) paracancer tissues expressed high BCL11A ($p < 0.01$) (**Figures 1A,B**) (**Table 1**). Although age, smoking and alcohol did not differ significantly between groups, most of the BCL11A high-expression patients were diagnosed in the advanced clinical N1/N2 lymph node metastasis stage ($p = 0.023$) (**Table 2**).

In accordance with previous studies, high expression of BCL11A was associated with significantly higher loco-regional recurrence or mortality (hazard ratio: 12; 95% CI, 1.43–100.8, $P = 0.009$) (**Table 2**).

High BCL11A Levels Promoted LSCC Development

BCL11A, a transcription factor and component of the BRAF complex, has been shown to be involved in regulating cell proliferation, apoptosis and transformation (10). We next investigated the cellular and molecular mechanisms of high levels of BCL11A in LSCC. We started by testing whether BCL11A overexpression affects LSCC cells *in vitro*. We examined the LSCC cell line AMC-HN-8 and found that it expressed low levels of BCL11A (**Figure 1C**). The AMC-HN-8 cell line has been extensively used to study LSCC (11), and we chose to test BCL11A overexpression in AMC-HN-8 cells. The effects of BCL11A overexpression (**Figures 1D,E**) were confirmed at the RNA and protein levels.

BCL11A Promoted LSCC Cell Proliferation *in vitro*

BCL11A overexpression promoted proliferation in AMC-HN-8 cells (**Figure 2A**). Furthermore, the BCL11A-overexpressing

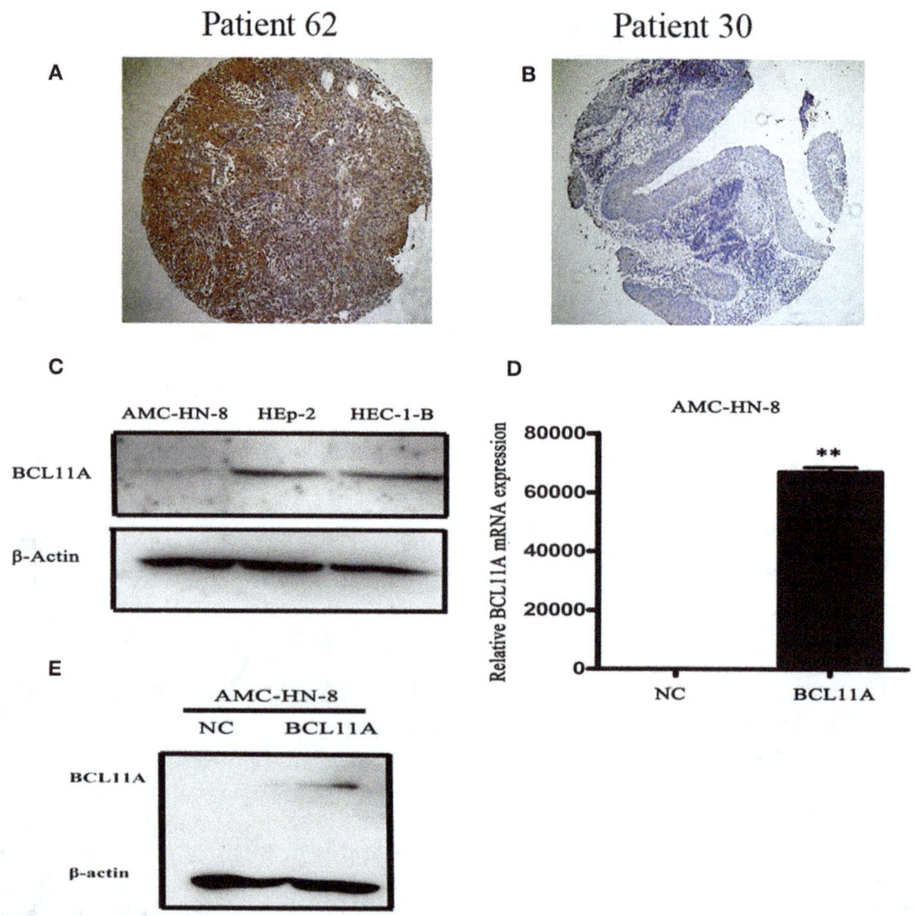

FIGURE 1 | Representative images of BCL11A-positive staining in LSCC cells **(A)** and BCL11A– negative staining in LSCC sections **(B)**. **(C)** A Western blot revealed low expression in the AMC-HN-8 cells. HEC-1-B was used as the positive control for BCL11A expression. **(D,E)** BCL11A overexpression in the AMC-HN-8 cells confirmed by qRT-PCR and Western blot analyses. $^{**}P < 0.01$.

TABLE 1 | Relationship between BCL11A expression and tissue types.

Tissue type	No.	Low	High (%)	OR (95% CI)	*P*-value
Paracancer tissue	40	25	15 (37.5%)		
Carcinoma	69	17	52 (75.4%)	5.1 (2.20–11.84)	<0.01

AMC-HN-8 cells formed more colonies than did the parental cells (**Figures 2B,C**). These results revealed that one important function of BCL11A is to promote LSCC cell proliferation.

Effects of BCL11A Expression on LSCC Cell Migration and Invasion

We next investigated the effect of BCL11A on cell migration and invasion in LSCC cell lines. Transwell assays showed that overexpression of BCL11A significantly increased the migration and invasion capacity of AMC-HN-8 cells (**Figures 3A–D**). The results indicated that overexpression of BCL11A seemed to increase the migration and invasion of these cells.

Change in the Chemosensitivity of Cisplatin After BCL11A Overexpression

We next addressed whether changes in BCL11A in AMC-HN-8 cells could have an impact on chemosensitivity to cisplatin. Overexpression of BCL11A in AMC-HN-8 cells significantly increased their survival or inhibited chemosensitivity to cisplatin (**Figure 4A**). The results show that BCL11A-high tumors could be more resistant to chemotherapies such as cisplatin.

Impact of BCL11A on the Cell Cycle

Overexpression of BCL11A had no significant effect on cell cycle kinetics (**Figure 4B**).

BCL11A Promoted LSCC Growth *in vivo*

The substantial effects of BCL11A expression changes on cell proliferation, cell invasion and chemo-sensitivity prompted us to investigate the consequences of BCL11A expression changes *in vivo*. LSCC cells overexpressing BCL11A were injected into immunocompromised recipient mice to induce tumor development. The tumors in the mice injected with the BCL11A-overexpressing AMC-HN-8 cells were larger and

TABLE 2 | Relationship between BCL11A expression and clinicopathological characteristics.

Parameter	No.	Low (%)	High (%)	OR (95% CI)	*P*-value
AGE					
<60	19	5 (26.3%)	14 (73.7%)	1.13 (0.34–3.79)	0.842
≥60	50	12 (24%)	38 (76%)		
SMOKING					
Never	20	3 (15%)	17 (85%)	0.44 (0.11–1.75)	0.235
Former or current	49	14 (28.6%)	35 (71.4%)		
ALCOHOL					
Never	34	5 (14.7%)	29 (85.3%)	0.33 (0.10–1.07)	0.093
Former or current	35	12 (34.3%)	23 (65.7%)		
LYMPHATIC METASTASIS					
N0	31	12 (38.7%)	19 (61.3%)	4.2 (1.27–12.65)	0.023
N1–2	38	5 (13.2%)	33 (86.8%)		
PATHOLOGICAL STAGE					
Initial (I + II)	14	6 (42.9%)	8 (57.1%)	3 (0.86–10.45)	0.076
Advanced (III+IV)	55	11 (20%)	44 (80%)		
SURVIVAL STATUS (17 PATIENTS WERE LOST TO FOLLOW)					
Survivors	36	16 (44.4%)	20 (55.6%)	12 (1.43–100.8)	0.009
Deceased or recurrence	16	1(6.3%)	15 (93.7%)		

heavier ($P < 0.05$ for both; **Figures 5A–D**). These *in vivo* results demonstrate that BCL11A has important functions for LSCC *in vivo* tumor development.

Correlation of BCL11A and MDM2 in LSCC

It has been shown in breast cancer cells that BCL11A positively regulates MDM2 expression (12). To evaluate the potential association of BCL11A and MDM2 in LSCC, we evaluated BCL11A and MDM2 co-expression by immunochemistry in the same tissue microarrays (TMA) from 69 LSCC patients (**Figures 6A–D**). Each tumor was assigned a BCL11A and MDM2 expression score based on the staining intensity and staining extent. A significant direct correlation was identified between the expression of BCL11A and MDM2 in the samples ($r = 0.442$; $P = 0.001$; **Figure 6E**). Experimentally, overexpression of BCL11A in AMC-HN-8 cells increased the MDM2 protein level (**Figure 6F**). Clinically, the LSCC cases that simultaneously expressed high BCL11A and MDM2 levels exhibited high rates of mortality or recurrence compared to the other patient subgroups (11/23 vs. 5/29). These data suggest that one function of BCL11A in LSCC is the regulation of MDM2.

Regulation of Tumorigenesis Molecules After BCL11A Overexpression

To identify other molecules or pathways that were regulated by BCL11A in LSCC, the Human Cancer PathwayFinder PCR Array analysis of nine different biological pathways (cell cycle, angiogenesis, cell senescence, DNA damage and repair, apoptosis, epithelial-to-mesenchymal transition, metabolism, hypoxia, telomeres and telomerase) (12) was performed (**Figures 6G–I**). The results revealed significant expression changes in several genes, including B2M, HMOX1, SNAI2, STMN1, BIRC3, and PPP1R15A in the AMC-HN-8 cells overexpressing BCL11A (**Figure 6J**). The Western blot analysis verified the expression changes of these proteins, except for STMN1 (**Figure 6K**). The altered gene expression of these molecules could represent additional mechanisms underlying the activity of BCL11A in LSCC.

DISCUSSION

The BCL11A gene, which spans over 102 kb on chromosome 2p16, is associated with various cancers (6, 13). It was initially observed in B-cell chronic lymphocytic leukemia, and it is considered a proto-oncogene of malignant hematological diseases (3, 14). Khaled et al. demonstrated that BCL11A was a new breast tumor gene and an important factor in normal mammary epithelial development (7). Other research indicated that the expression of BCL11A was reduced in bone marrow and brain, lymphoid and fetal liver tissue (15, 16).

BCL11A was also reported to be amplified in lung squamous cell cancer (SCC), with amplification more common among SCC samples of NSCLC without metastases (17). Jiang et al. reported the possible role of BCL11A in identifying and predicting the prognosis of NSCLC patients, particularly those with early-stage SCC. In their study, BCL11A was specifically overexpressed in tumor tissues rather than paracancer tissues. In the present study, BCL11A was also specifically overexpressed at the protein level in LSCC tissues rather than paracancer tissues. These findings are also consistent with the results of Zhang et al. (18), who observed that BCL11A-XL was markedly overexpressed in large cell lung cancer and squamous cell lung cancer.

Khaled et al. reported that knockdown of BCL11A expression in TNBC cells in a mouse model markedly decreased cancer

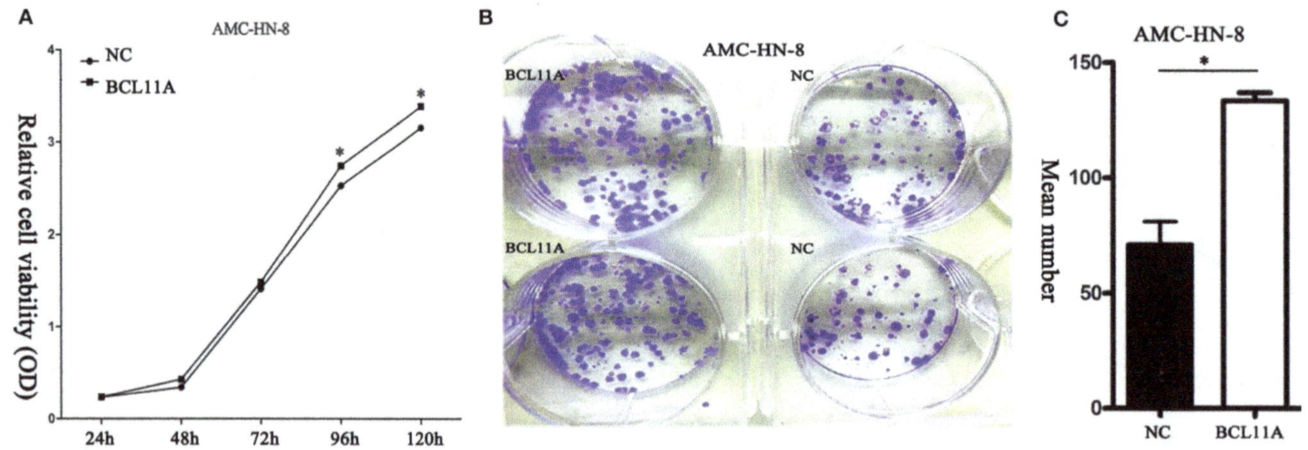

FIGURE 2 | (A) BCL11A overexpression increased AMC-HN-8 cell proliferation. **(B)** Overexpression of BCL11A in the AMC-HN-8 cells significantly increased their colony-forming abilities. **(C)** Quantitative comparison of the colonies formed from the parental AMC-HN-8 cells (NC) and the BCL11A overexpression (BCL11A) ones. $^{*}P < 0.05$.

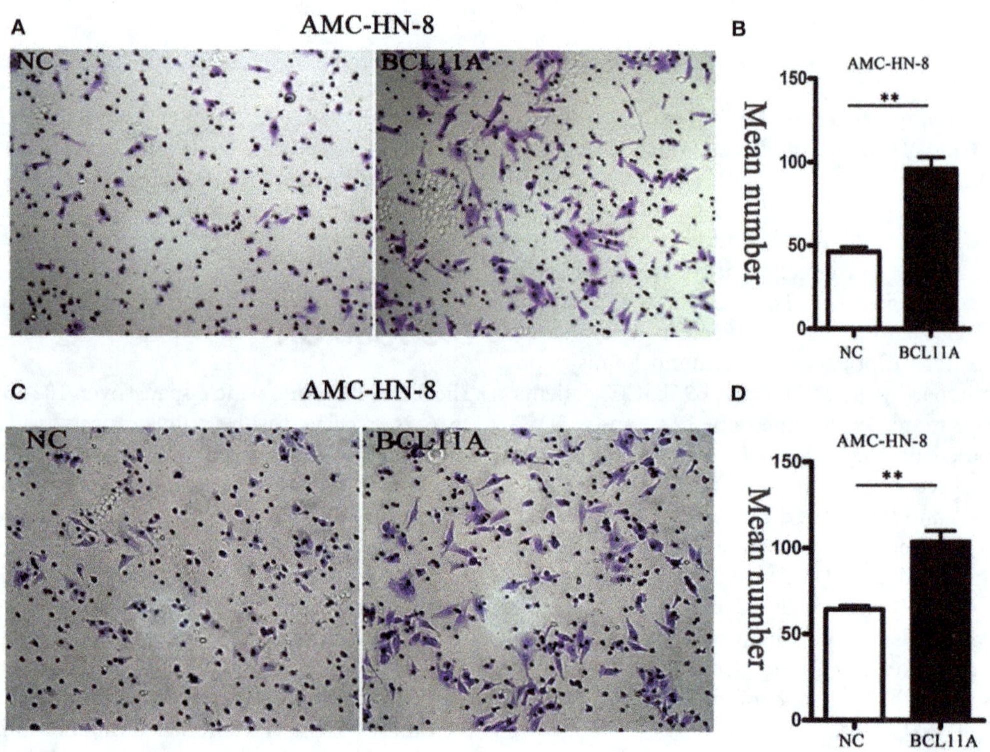

FIGURE 3 | The migration/ invasion ability of LSCC cells with overexpression in the transwell assay. **(A)** Increased migration capability of BCL11A-overexpression AMC-HN-8 cells detected by the transwell assay. Images showing the migrated AMC-HN-8 cells on the lower surface of the transwell membranes. Magnification ×200. **(B)** The numbers of migrated AMC-HN-8 cells in five random fields under the microscope (mean ± SD, $n = 5$). **(C)** Increased invasion capability of BCL11A-overexpression AMC-HN-8 cells. Images showing the invaded BCL11A-overexpresing AMC-HN-8 cells on lower surface of the transwell membranes in different groups. Magnification ×200. **(D)** The number of invaded BCL11A-overexpressing AMC-HN-8 in five random fields under the microscope (mean ± SD, $n = 5$). $^{**}P < 0.01$.

development (7). In this study, BCL11A overexpression in the AMC-HN-8 LSCC cell line increased LSCC proliferation and invasion *in vitro* and promoted the growth of LSCC xenografts *in vivo*. Overexpression of BCL11A had no noteworthy effects on cell cycle kinetics (**Figure 4B**), which is similar to the results presented by Khaled et al. (7). They also reported that the

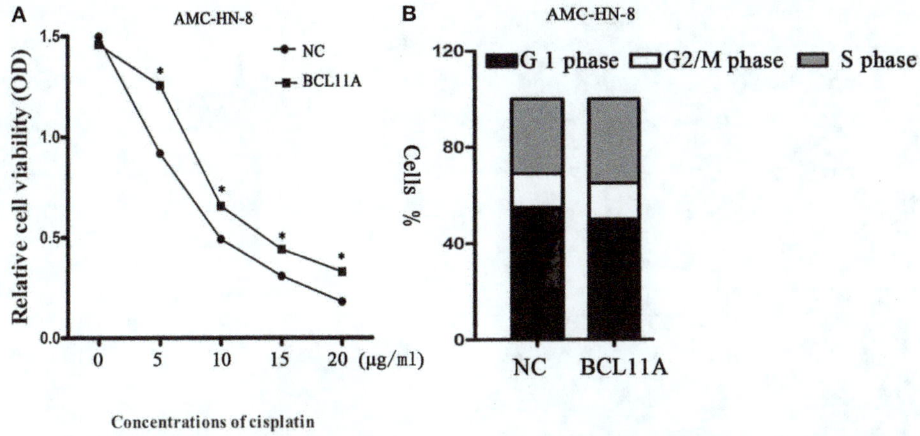

FIGURE 4 | (A) Influence of different concentrations of cisplatin on the cytotoxicity of negative controls (NC) AMC-HN-8 and overexpression BCL11A AMC-HN-8 cell strains. **(B)** Cell cycle investigation, showing that overexpression did not affect cell cycle kinetics in the two cell lines. The data are the mean ± s.d. ($n = 3$).*$P < 0.05$.

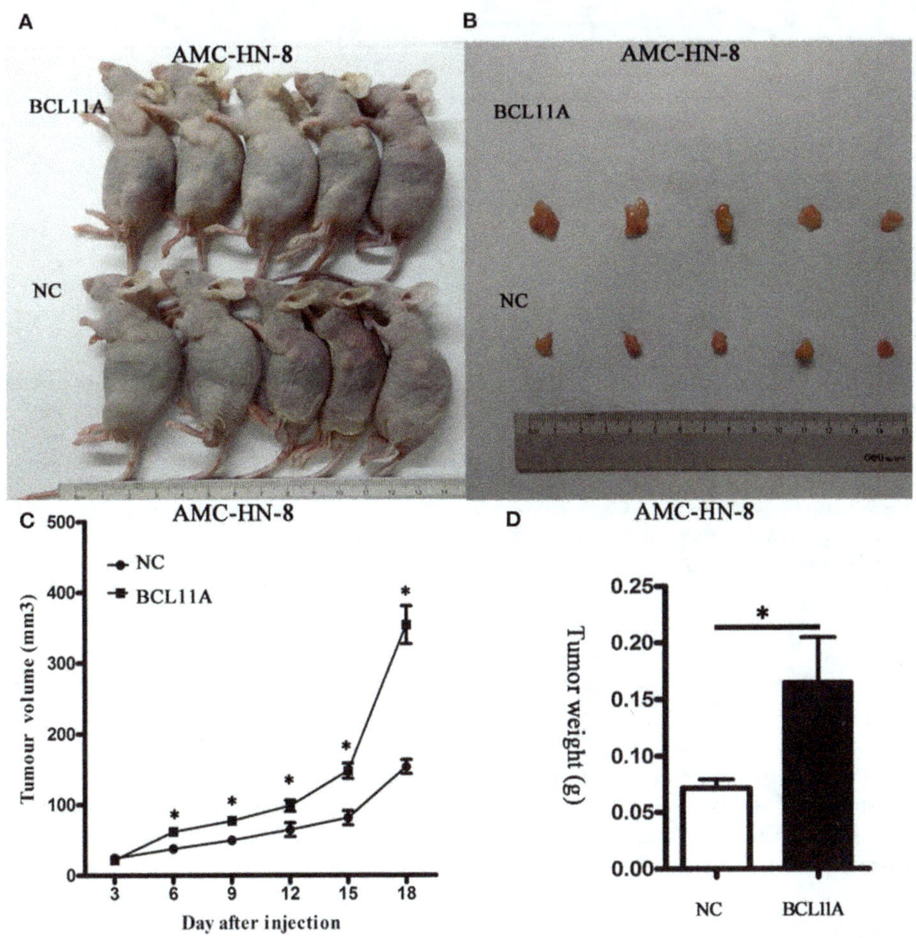

FIGURE 5 | BCL11A regulated AMC-HN-8 cell growth *in vivo*. **(A)** Images of mice with xenograft tumors of BCL11A-overexpression AMC-HN-8 cells and the control cells (NC); **(B)** Image of tumors isolated from nude mice. **(C)** Growth curves of the xenografts in the BCL11A-overexpression AMC-HN-8 cell group and control cells (NC) ($n = 5$, mean ± SEM). **(D)** Comparison of the weight of the xenografts in the BCL11A-overexpression AMC-HN-8 cells and control cells (NC) harvested 18 d after injection of the cells ($n = 5$, mean ± SEM). *$P < 0.05$.

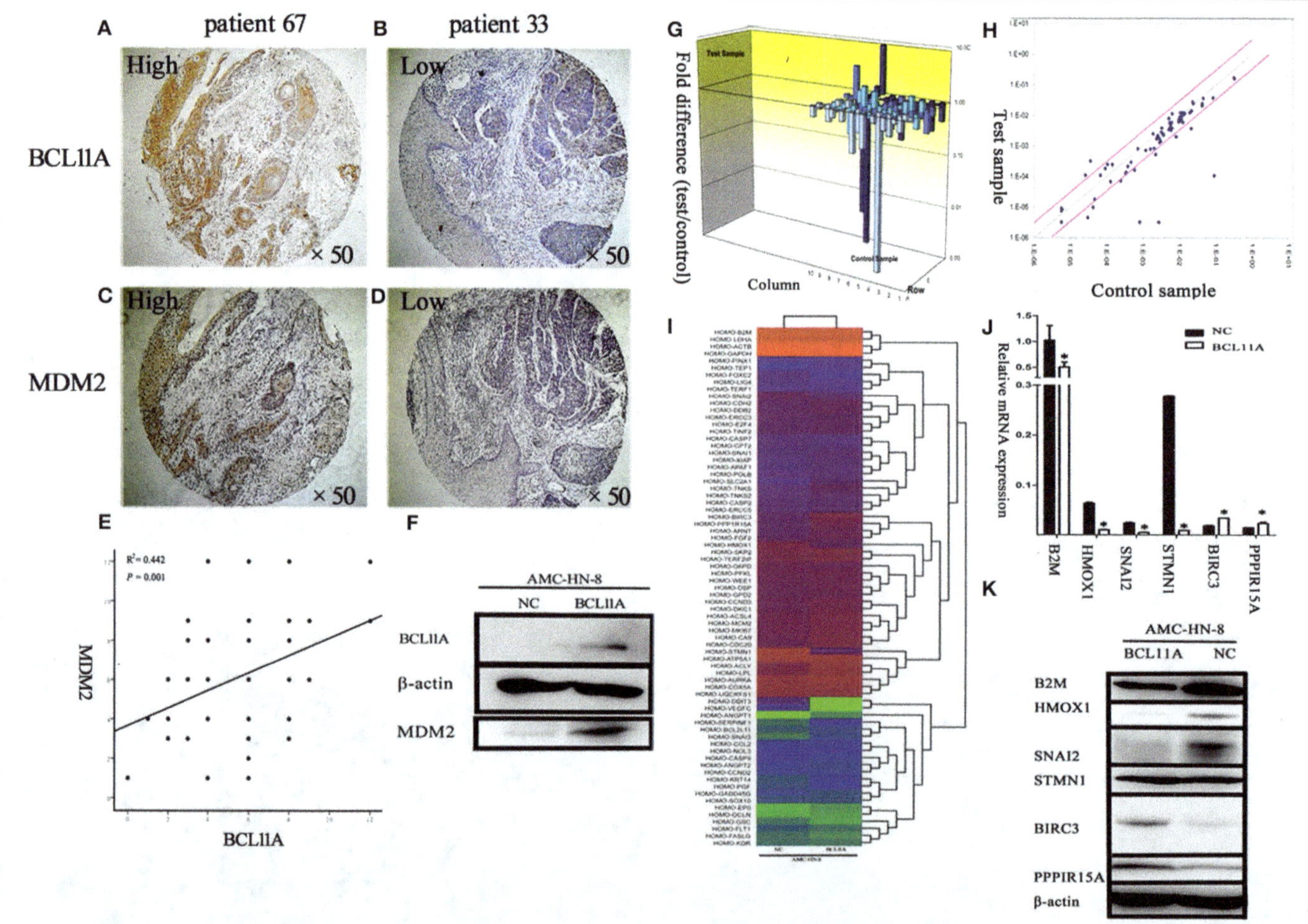

FIGURE 6 | (A–D) Co-expression of BCL11A and MDM2 in some LSCCs, as shown by immunohistochemistry. **(E)** Linear regression analysis of BCL11A vs. MDM2 expression levels (immunohistochemistry scores in the same TMA). **(F)** The Western blot showed that MDM2 was up-regulated in the BCL11A overexpression AMC-HN-8 cell line at the protein level. **(G)** PCR microarray investigation of human cancer pathway genes in the BCL11A-overexpression AMC-HN-8 cells. 3D profile graph displays the fold change in the expression of each gene in the BCL11A-overexpression AMC-HN-8 cells vs. that of the control cells. Columns pointing up (with z-axis values > 1) indicate up-regulation of gene expression, and the columns pointing down (with z-axis values < 1) denote down-regulation of gene expression. **(H)** The corresponding scatter plots display the validity of the test and expression level of every gene in the BCL11A-overexpression AMC-HN-8 cells vs. that of the control cells ($n = 3$). **(I)** Heat map of the 84 probe sets in BCL11A-overexpression AMC-HN-8 cells vs. that of the control cells. **(J)** Six selected genes in the BCL11A-overexpression AMC-HN-8 cells showed a significant change at the mRNA level vs. that of the control cells. **(K)** Western blot verification of the gene expression changes. $^{*}P < 0.05$.

survival rates of triple-negative breast cancer patients with either copy number gains or high expression of BCL11A were poorer than those of the remainder of the group. In addition to lower survival rates, the patients with copy number gains of BCL11A had a higher rate of metastasis and relapse. In our study, LSCC patients with high expression of BCL11A were significantly more likely to suffer loco-regional recurrence or to become moribund than those with low expression of BCL11A (hazard ratio: 12, $P = 0.009$) (**Table 2**). Furthermore, the vast majority of patients with high expression of BCL11A were diagnosed with advanced clinical N1/N2 lymphatic metastasis ($P = 0.023$) (**Table 2**). Previous studies of four other tumor patient data sets reported a similar tendency (19–22). On the other hand, some studies have shown that BCL11A is an independent prognostic factor for both disease-free survival and overall survival (8, 18). The role of BCL11A expression as a biomarker in the clinic requires additional exploration.

It was reported that BCL11A can also upregulate MDM2 expression, which hinders p53 activities (23). These molecular changes happen frequently in solid cancers. Yu et al. reported that Mdm2 was downregulated in Bcl11a-deficient B cells. ChIP tests showed that Bcl11a was bound to Mdm2. Furthermore, overexpressing Mdm2 rescued both apoptosis and proliferation defects caused by Bcl11a knockdown in B cells. In addition, Bcl11a deletion resulted in p53 accumulation in lymphocytes, likely due to reduced Mdm2/Mdm4 (24). In the current study, as shown by the BCL11A and MDM2 immunochemistry scores in the LSCC TMA, there was a significant correlation between BCL11A and MDM2 expression ($r = 0.442$; $P = 0.001$; **Figure 6E**). In the LSCC cell line, overexpression of BCL11A caused high expression of MDM2 (**Figure 6F**). However, the relevance of MDM2 expression highly depends on p53 status, and further research will be focused on the relationship between P53 status and MDM2.

We applied the Cancer PathwayFinder PCR array to identify additional genes regulated by BCL11A in LSCC. Among the upregulated genes in the AMC-HN-8-BCL11A cells, some genes are classified as involving apoptosis, DNA damage, and DNA repair; BIRC3 promotes resistance of cancer cells to apoptosis (25, 26). Another gene, PPP1R15A, was previously shown to be involved in apoptosis or cell growth (27). Among the downregulated genes in the AMC-HN-8-BCL11A cells, some genes were associated with the epithelial-to-mesenchymal transition and hypoxia, including B2M, which is a Class I MHC protein that regulates the proliferation of normal cells and carcinoma cells (28). HMOX1, the inducible isoform of the rate-limiting enzyme in haem degradation, neutralizes inflammatory and oxidative injury. HMOX-1 deficiency results in high levels of endothelial damage and prolonged inflammation (29, 30). In addition, SNAI2, which represses E-cadherin (CDH1), was also downregulated. In renal cell tumors, SNAI2-positive renal cell tumors were reported to be associated with lower-stage tumors and a better prognosis than SNAI2-negative tumors (31).

CONCLUSIONS

This study investigated the proto-oncogene BCL11A in LSCC. The results revealed that BCL11A was upregulated in some clinical LSCC tissue samples at the protein level. The statistical analyses showed that BCL11A expression was strongly associated with lymph node status and the survival of LSCC patients. We demonstrated experimentally that BCL11A regulated cell proliferation, cell invasion/migration and chemosensitivity in LSCC cells *in vitro* and in LSCC xenografts *in vivo*. BCL11A also upregulated the expression of MDM2, which is frequently co-expressed in LSCC.

ETHICS STATEMENT

The studies involving human participants were reviewed and approved by the Ethics Committee of Fudan University. The patients/participants provided their written informed consent to participate in this study. The animal study was reviewed and approved by the Ethics Committee of Fudan University.

AUTHOR'S NOTE

We demonstrated that BCL11A expression was strongly associated with lymph node status and the survival of LSCC patients and BCL11A regulated cell proliferation, cell invasion/migration and chemosensitivity in LSCC cells *in vitro* and LSCC xenografts *in vivo*. BCL11A also up-regulated the expression of MDM2, which is frequently co-expressed in LSCC. Our results uncovered important functions of BCL11A in LSCC and identify BCL11A as a prognostic biomarker and potential therapeutic target in LSCC.

AUTHOR CONTRIBUTIONS

LT and L-ML designed and conceived the experiments. JZ, LiaZ, DZ, W-JT, DT, X-LS, and YueY collected samples. JZ, LinZ, FL, and YonY completed the experiment. JZ, LiaZ, and PL analyzed the experimental data. JZ and DZ finished the paper.

ACKNOWLEDGMENTS

We thank the staff of Shanghai Institute of Immunology, Wellcome Trust Sanger Institute, for their technical support and expertise.

REFERENCES

1. Jemal A, Bray F, Center MM, Ferlay J, Ward E, Forman D. Global cancer statistics. *CA Cancer J Clin.* (2011) 61:69–90. doi: 10.3322/caac.20107
2. Alhamarneh O, Agada F, Madden L, Stafford N, Greenman J. Serum IL10 and circulating CD4(+) CD25(high) regulatory T cell numbers as predictors of clinical outcome and survival in patients with head and neck squamous cell carcinoma. *Head Neck.* (2011) 33:415–23. doi: 10.1002/hed.21464
3. Nakamura T, Yamazaki Y, Saiki Y, Moriyama M, Largaespada DA, Jenkins NA, et al. Evi9 encodes a novel zinc finger protein that physically interacts with BCL6, a known human B-cell proto-oncogene product. *Mol Cell Biol.* (2000) 20:3178–86. doi: 10.1128/MCB.20.9.3178-3186.2000
4. Ng SY, Yoshida T, Zhang J, Georgopoulos K. Genome-wide lineage-specific transcriptional networks underscore Ikaros-dependent lymphoid priming in hematopoietic stem cells. *Immunity.* (2009) 30:493–507. doi: 10.1016/j.immuni.2009.01.014
5. Fell HP, Smith RG, Tucker PW. Molecular analysis of the t(2;14) translocation of childhood chronic lymphocytic leukemia. *Science.* (1986) 232:491–4. doi: 10.1126/science.3961491
6. Satterwhite E, Sonoki T, Willis TG, Harder L, Nowak R, Arriola EL, et al. The BCL11 gene family: involvement of BCL11A in lymphoid malignancies. *Blood.* (2001) 98:3413–20. doi: 10.1182/blood.V98.12.3413
7. Khaled WT, Choon Lee S, Stingl J, Chen X, Raza Ali H, Rueda OM, et al. BCL11A is a triple-negative breast cancer gene with critical functions in stem and progenitor cells. *Nat Commun.* (2015) 6:5987. doi: 10.1038/ncomms6987
8. Jiang BY, Zhang XC, Su J, Meng W, Yang XN, Yang JJ, et al. BCL11A overexpression predicts survival and relapse in non-small cell lung cancer and is modulated by microRNA-30a and gene amplification. *Mol Cancer.* (2013) 12:61. doi: 10.1186/1476-4598-12-61
9. Koo CL, Kok LF, Lee MY, Wu TS, Cheng YW, Hsu JD, et al. Scoring mechanisms of p16INK4a immunohistochemistry based on either independent nucleic stain or mixed cytoplasmic with nucleic expression can significantly signal to distinguish between endocervical and endometrial adenocarcinomas in a tissue microarray study. *J Transl Med.* (2009) 7:25. doi: 10.1186/1479-5876-7-25
10. Kasaian K, Wiseman SM, Walker BA, Schein JE, Zhao Y, Hirst M, et al. The genomic and transcriptomic landscape of anaplastic thyroid cancer: implications for therapy. *BMC Cancer.* (2015) 15:984. doi: 10.1186/s12885-015-1955-9
11. Wan G, Zhou L, Xie M, Chen H, Tian J. Characterization of side population cells from laryngeal cancer cell lines. *Head Neck.* (2010) 32:1302–9. doi: 10.1002/hed.21325

12. Winter SC, Buffa FM, Silva P, Miller C, Valentine HR, Turley H, et al. Relation of a hypoxia metagene derived from head and neck cancer to prognosis of multiple cancers. *Cancer Res.* (2007) 67:3441–9. doi: 10.1158/0008-5472.CAN-06-3322
13. Chen Z, Luo HY, Steinberg MH, Chui DH. BCL11A represses HBG transcription in K562 cells. *Blood Cells Mol Dis.* (2009) 42:144–9. doi: 10.1016/j.bcmd.2008.12.003
14. Weniger MA, Pulford K, Gesk S, Ehrlich S, Banham AH, Lyne L, et al. Gains of the proto-oncogene BCL11A and nuclear accumulation of BCL11A(XL) protein are frequent in primary mediastinal B-cell lymphoma. *Leukemia.* (2006) 20:1880–2. doi: 10.1038/sj.leu.2404324
15. Kuo TY, Hsueh YP. Expression of zinc finger transcription factor Bcl11A/Evi9/CTIP1 in rat brain. *J Neurosci Res.* (2007) 85:1628–36. doi: 10.1002/jnr.21300
16. Sankaran VG, Menne TF, Xu J, Akie TE, Lettre G, Van Handel B, et al. Human fetal hemoglobin expression is regulated by the developmental stage-specific repressor BCL11A. *Science.* (2008) 322:1839–842. doi: 10.1126/science.1165409
17. Boelens MC, Kok K, van der Vlies P, van der Vries G, Sietsma H, Timens W, et al. Genomic aberrations in squamous cell lung carcinoma related to lymph node or distant metastasis. *Lung Cancer.* (2009) 66:372–8. doi: 10.1016/j.lungcan.2009.02.017
18. Zhang N, Jiang BY, Zhang XC, Xie Z, Su J, Zhang Q, et al. The BCL11A-XL expression predicts relapse in squamous cell carcinoma and large cell carcinoma. *J Thorac Dis.* (2015) 7:1630–6. doi: 10.3978/j.issn.2072-1439.2015.09.39
19. Desmedt C, Piette F, Loi S, Wang Y, Lallemand F, Haibe-Kains B, et al. Strong time dependence of the 76-gene prognostic signature for node-negative breast cancer patients in the TRANSBIG multicenter independent validation series. *Clin Cancer Res.* (2007) 13:3207–14. doi: 10.1158/1078-0432.CCR-06-2765
20. Hatzis C, Pusztai L, Valero V, Booser DJ, Esserman L, Lluch A, et al. A genomic predictor of response and survival following taxane-anthracycline chemotherapy for invasive breast cancer. *JAMA.* (2011). 305:1873–81. doi: 10.1001/jama.2011.593
21. Ma XJ, Wang Z, Ryan PD, Isakoff SJ, Barmettler A, Fuller A, et al. A two-gene expression ratio predicts clinical outcome in breast cancer patients treated with tamoxifen. *Cancer Cell.* (2004) 5:607–16. doi: 10.1016/j.ccr.2004.05.015
22. Schmidt M, Bohm D, von Torne C, Steiner E, Puhl A, Pilch H, et al. The humoral immune system has a key prognostic impact in node-negative breast cancer. *Cancer Res.* (2008) 68:5405–13. doi: 10.1158/0008-5472.CAN-07-5206
23. Pulford K, Banham AH, Lyne L, Jones M, Ippolito GC, Liu H, et al. The BCL11AXL transcription factor: its distribution in normal and malignant tissues and use as a marker for plasmacytoid dendritic cells. *Leukemia.* (2006) 20:1439–41. doi: 10.1038/sj.leu.2404260
24. Yu Y, Wang J, Khaled W, Burke S, Li P, Chen X, et al. Bcl11a is essential for lymphoid development and negatively regulates p53. *J Exp Med.* (2012) 209:2467–83. doi: 10.1084/jem.20121846
25. Petersen SL, Wang L, Yalcin-Chin A, Li L, Peyton M, Minna J, et al. Autocrine TNFalpha signaling renders human cancer cells susceptible to Smac-mimetic-induced apoptosis. *Cancer Cell.* (2007) 12:445–56. doi: 10.1016/j.ccr.2007.08.029
26. Petersen SL, Peyton M, Minna JD, Wang X. Overcoming cancer cell resistance to Smac mimetic induced apoptosis by modulating cIAP-2 expression. *Proc Natl Acad Sci USA.* (2010) 107:11936–41. doi: 10.1073/pnas.1005667107
27. Tan J, Yang X, Zhuang L, Jiang X, Chen W, Lee PL, et al. Pharmacologic disruption of Polycomb-repressive complex 2-mediated gene repression selectively induces apoptosis in cancer cells. *Genes Dev.* (2007) 21:1050–63. doi: 10.1101/gad.1524107
28. D'Urso CM, Wang ZG, Cao Y, Tatake R, Zeff RA, Ferrone S. Lack of HLA class I antigen expression by cultured melanoma cells FO-1 due to a defect in B2m gene expression. *J Clin Invest.* (1991) 87:284–92. doi: 10.1172/JCI114984
29. Kawashima A, Oda Y, Yachie A, Koizumi S, Nakanishi I. Heme oxygenase-1 deficiency: the first autopsy case. *Hum Pathol.* (2002) 33:125–130. doi: 10.1053/hupa.2002.30217
30. Yachie A, Toma T, Mizuno K, Okamoto H, Shimura S, Ohta K, et al. Heme oxygenase-1 production by peripheral blood monocytes during acute inflammatory illnesses of children. *Exp Biol Med.* (2003) 228:550–6. doi: 10.1177/15353702-0322805-26
31. Mikami S, Katsube K, Oya M, Ishida M, Kosaka T, Mizuno R, et al. Expression of Snail and Slug in renal cell carcinoma: E-cadherin repressor Snail is associated with cancer invasion and prognosis. *Lab Invest.* (2011) 91:1443–58. doi: 10.1038/labinvest.2011.111

15

Rehabilitation Needs of Head and Neck Cancer Patients and Stakeholders

Maria Karampela[1], Talya Porat[2], Vasiliki Mylonopoulou[3] and Minna Isomursu[1]*

[1] *Faculty of Information Technology and Electrical Engineering, University of Oulu, Oulu, Finland,* [2] *Faculty of Engineering, Dyson School of Design Engineering, Imperial College London, London, United Kingdom,* [3] *Department Of Applied Information Technology, Division of Human Computer Interaction, University of Gothenburg, Gothenburg, Sweden*

Correspondence:
Maria Karampela
marwkarab@gmail.com

Background: The incidents of Head and Neck Cancer (HNC) are rising worldwide, suggesting that this type of cancer is becoming more common. The foreseen growth of incidents signifies that future rehabilitation services will have to meet the needs of a wider population.

Objective: The aim of this paper is to explore the needs of patients, caregivers and healthcare professionals during HNC rehabilitation.

Methods: This paper reports the empirical findings from a case study that was conducted in a cancer rehabilitation center in Copenhagen to elicit the needs of HNC cancer patients, informal caregivers and healthcare professionals.

Results: Four areas of needs during the rehabilitation process were identified: service delivery, emotional, social and physical needs. Service delivery needs and emotional needs have been identified as the most prevalent.

Conclusions: Stakeholders' needs during the rehabilitation process were found to be interrelated. All stakeholders faced service delivery challenges in the form of provision and distribution of information, including responsibilities allocation between municipalities, hospitals and rehabilitation services. Emotional and social needs have been reported by HNC patients and informal caregivers, underlining the importance of inclusion of all actors in the design of future healthcare interventions. Connected Health (CH) solutions could be valuable in provision and distribution of information.

Keywords: connected health (CH), head and neck cancer, stakeholders, informal caregivers, rehabilitation

INTRODUCTION

In 2016, a milestone has been reached and for the first time Head and Neck Cancer (HNC) was acknowledged to resemble a chronic illness (1). HNC has been recognized as one of the few cancer types that requires anticipatory treatment and prolonged rehabilitation (2). This can be related to HNC survivorship experience, which is accompanied with high morbidity and reduction in patients' quality of life. Therefore, the main aim of rehabilitation of HNC is to improve quality of life, which

---

Abbreviations: HNC, Head and Neck Cancer; CKSK, Center for Kræft og Sundhed København; GPs, General Practitioners.

is defined by the WHO "as complete physical, mental and social welfare state and not only the absence of the disease" (3). HNC cancer invades both physical and emotional aspects of life causing often facial disfigurements, disrupting the pleasure of eating (taste, smell), compromising respiratory control, sneezing and laughing mechanisms (1).

Dysphagia is the most common long-term side-effect of chemoradiotherapy (4), and is related to the difficulty of swallowing and movement of food through the 'throat' or pharynx (5). Dysphagia is associated among others with prolonged tube feeding and fundamental changes to eating patterns, social activities and consequently poorer quality of life (6, 7). Apart from the physical side-effects patients often experience psychological disorders. Newly diagnosed HNC patients may experience adjustment disorders and major depression (8). Emotional numbing has been reported as a factor that can increase further patients' distress, as sharing feelings with their beloved ones was found to be a challenge on its own (9).

HNC incidence has also implications on the patient's family and friends. Patients' relatives and friends, known as informal caregivers, provide support to patients in the treatment and post-treatment periods (10). Caregiving is a demanding and challenging assignment. Informal caregivers of HNC patients may experience even higher levels of anxiety than patients within the six month interval following diagnosis, a state which is often related to the fear of cancer recurrence (10). Caregivers' psychological health depends on various factors, such as patients' disease severity, but also on their personality and resources (11). The essential role of informal caregivers and the importance of their wellbeing, has led to suggestions for specialized psychosocial interventions. These interventions have been seen as an effective approach to alleviate informal caregivers' psychosocial burden, while also having a positive impact on the quality of patients' lives (12).

Despite the fact that HNC patients have multiple and severe unmet needs compared to other cancer types (13) and that rehabilitation has a significant role in addressing those needs (14–16), rehabilitation is not always part of the clinical practice in HNC care (17).

The Danish healthcare system can be characterized by decentralized administration, distributed to 5 districts and 98 municipalities. As seen in **Figure 1** below, it operates in three levels; the National (Ministry of Health), the Regional (5 regions), the Local level (98 Municipalities). The Danish healthcare may be unique in its care delivery as it allocates the rehabilitation responsibilities between Hospitals and Municipalities. However, in aspects such as healthcare quality and patient safety it is similar to other European systems (18). In addition to emergency treatments, the hospitals also provide rehabilitation services to patients with cancer, while municipalities play a key role in the prevention of the disease (19, 20). Rehabilitation of cancer patients includes a variety of interventions, such as physical therapy, psychosocial support and physical training (21–23). Cancer rehabilitation programs in Danish municipalities have been available since 2007. Municipalities are only responsible for the generalized rehabilitation interventions (24, 25), while the hospitals hold the main responsibility for specialized rehabilitation services for patients with cancer (26).

Previous studies have focused on addressing the rehabilitation needs of HNC patients and stakeholders. Healthcare professionals have reported cases in which lack of expertise to perform medical procedures and gaps in service provision led to poor services related to psychosocial needs of patients and caregivers (27, 28). The unmet information needs have been also discussed from the perspectives of patients and caregivers. Caregivers reported lack of information associated with diagnosis and treatment phases. Studies concluded that patients and caregivers also require more information about self-care, pain and distress management, while the preferable mode of information provision was from healthcare professionals and digital interventions (29). Self-management interventions have been proposed as solutions to facilitate care for patients and caregivers (30). The study of Bard et al. points out that some of the patients and caregivers' needs were interrelated, while peer to peer social support was found to be important (30). Ringash et al. investigated the physical, emotional and cognitive needs of HNC patients and caregivers, concluding that 60% to 70% of the stakeholders reported unmet needs (31). A literature review confirmed that further investigation related to the informational and support needs of stakeholders is necessary, addressing a communication gap between patients, caregivers and healthcare professionals (32). The study of McEwen et al. utilized focus groups to address the needs of patients, caregivers and healthcare professionals, to provide insights pertinent to facilitators and barriers to recuperate functional health (17). While they found a significant amount of interrelated needs between the three stakeholders, healthcare professionals have been acknowledged to have many specific needs compared to the other two groups.

The findings above demonstrate that patients and stakeholders face a number of unmet needs in the course of HNC rehabilitation. A relation between unmet patients' needs and caregiving burdens suggests that interventions should focus their efforts on both stakeholders (33). However, the "equation" of rehabilitation provision also includes the healthcare professionals. The present study reflects upon the studies of (17, 32, 33) by exploring the needs of patients, caregivers and healthcare professionals during HNC rehabilitation. We address the following research question: *What are the needs of the different stakeholders during Head and Neck cancer rehabilitation in the Danish context?* We explored this research question by analyzing a case study that was conducted at the Center for Kræft og Sundhed København (CKSK), during a service design course for a Master's degree. CKSK is the largest and newest rehabilitation center in Denmark that offers rehabilitation services to approximately 1,500 cancer survivors every year. Our case study explores the phenomenon of interrelated needs and the possibility to develop Connected Health (CH) rehabilitation solutions through collaboration of HNC patients, family members and healthcare professionals.

Connected Health (CH) is a conceptual model for health management (usually *via* mobile, wireless, telehealth interventions) (34) where devices and services are designed around patient's needs, and health data is shared, in such a way

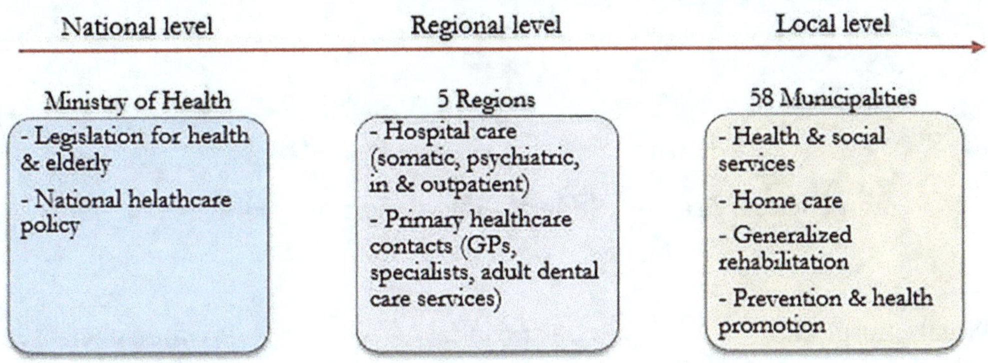

FIGURE 1 | The Danish healthcare system, an overview of responsibilities between the 3 levels (National, Regional and Local) (18).

that patients are able to receive proactive and efficient care (34). CH interventions can enhance the quality of life of patients during cancer care, focusing not only on personalized solutions, but also on multidisciplinary and inclusive approaches for rehabilitation (35).

METHODS

Case Study in CKSK Rehabilitation Center

We conducted a single-case study in the second half of 2017, where the unit of analysis was the CKSK head and neck cancer rehabilitation center. According to Yin, case study is an empirical inquiry that explores a contemporary phenomenon within its real-life context utilizing multiple sources of evidence in order to understand and explore the phenomenon under investigation (36). While most of the data collection was done in the context of Center for Kræft og Sundhed København (CKSK), supplementing data was also collected through an organization called Sundhed.dk. Sundhed.dk is a national and publicly funded health data and information portal in Denmark, complementing the service delivery needs from the viewpoint of a provider of digital solutions for rehabilitation service.

The selection of the case partners for this study reflected upon a need. Only a few municipalities in the Danish district offer rehabilitation programs for HNC patients, therefore CKSK center has to share professional expertise and knowledge with other municipalities that lack rehabilitation expertise. This problem has inspired CKSK and Sundhed.dk to collaborate in order to create a digitally assisted solution that can overcome this problem and share rehabilitation expertise and knowledge to other parts of Denmark. Before initiating the project, the case partners wanted to explore and fully comprehend the needs of the stakeholders to develop a CH solution which would serve its purpose. **Figure 2** presents a simplified version of a cancer patient's pathway in Denmark.

Data Collection

Data collection was performed by five groups of service design students (24 individuals), who were instructed and supervised by three service design researchers from design, engineering and information systems disciplines (one of the supervisors is a co-author of this paper). The 24 students who participated in the course were divided into five groups. Each group selected one of its members to conduct the interviews. As the goal of the case study was to collect rich, detailed information about the needs, the data collection was qualitative in nature.

The stakeholder participants were selected, as a convenience sample, by the center. The selection was based upon the following three criteria: (1) patients in their first year of rehabilitation; (2) diversity of roles of healthcare professionals; (3) willingness and availability of stakeholders to participate in relatively lengthy interviews in an active way. Data collection and understanding of the HNC domain included two phases: presentations from healthcare professionals and written material, and semi-structured interviews.

Phase 1: Presentations From Healthcare Professionals and Written Material

Written material about HNC rehabilitation was made available to the students to understand the basic concepts, and the rehabilitation center management and nurses introduced their subjective views on problems and needs. In addition, a management representative and design professional from Sundhed.dk presented their views on possibilities and challenges of digital service delivery for cancer rehabilitation. Following this, a session with rehabilitation professionals was arranged to collect data about the needs of different areas of rehabilitation. Healthcare professionals, namely an occupational therapist, a physiotherapist, a social worker, a dietician and a nurse, gave short presentations to the groups describing their work practices and relationships to patients, as well as their specific needs in regards to their occupation. By identifying the different stakeholders and the interplay between them, the student groups were able to characterize their roles and values pertinent to the rehabilitation process (37).

Phase 2: Semi-Structured Interviews

Four HNC patients, five healthcare professionals and four informal caregivers were interviewed face-to- face by all the groups of students at the premises of the center. Participants were advised to express and elaborate on their personal

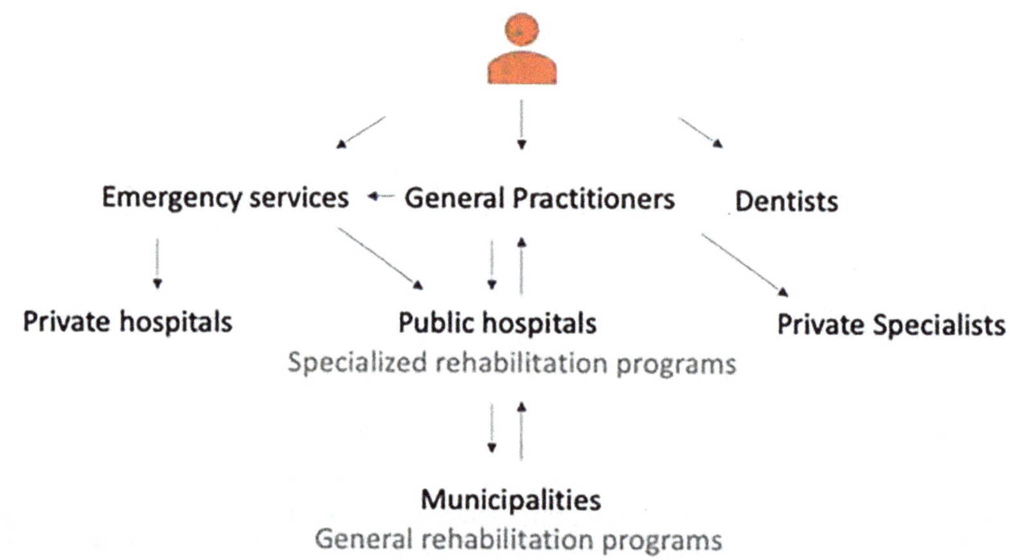

FIGURE 2 | A simplified version of a cancer patient's journey in the Danish healthcare system. The care process starts with GP's who are the gatekeepers of the secondary care, then moves to Hospitals for provision of medical treatment and specialized rehabilitation and finally to Municipalities for generalized rehabilitation services. Dentists are self-referred specialists.

experiences during their rehabilitation and encouraged to comment about the content of questions, if they felt they were too personal or made them feel uncomfortable. Semi-structured interviews were organized around themes such as rehabilitation, communication, network, and close relations, with the aim to gain knowledge about the stakeholders needs and requirements. Students performed the semi-structured interviews with the different stakeholders. The interview questions were developed together with their supervisors to gain knowledge about their needs and elicit requirements for proposing future CH rehabilitation interventions. Students audio recorded the interviews and transcribed them verbatim, applying thematic analysis methods (38). Semi-structured interviews with the different stakeholders lasted between 30 minutes to 1 hour, depending on the preference of the stakeholder. All patients were interviewed in Danish (see example questions in Multimedia Appendix 1). To explore the rehabilitation services provided in municipal districts other than Copenhagen, one of the student groups conducted phone interviews with cancer coordinators from four municipalities of different sizes across Denmark. Desk research, also known as secondary research, was also used by all the groups to collect information about the relevant stakeholders and to acquire general technical and medical knowledge concerning patients with HNC (39). The students were in their final year of their master degree and were sufficiently trained to utilize the aforementioned methods as they have received specialized courses to attain this knowledge. Data collection methods were developed and implemented under the supervision of their teachers and teaching assistants. **Figure 3** presents an overview of the data analysis process from the viewpoints of the students and authors.

Participants' Characteristics

Four HNC patients during their rehabilitation were recruited from CKSK. Three males and one female patient, age ranged from 34 to 74, in their first year of rehabilitation provided consent to participate in this study. Patients during their first year of rehabilitation were chosen to be included, as that is the phase they have frequent interactions with the rehabilitation service. Patients with severe challenges in communication were excluded from the study. Inclusion/exclusion criteria was made by the healthcare professionals of the rehabilitation center. **Table 1** presents the patients characteristics.

Four informal caregivers and five healthcare professionals were also recruited. The informal caregivers were three females (spouses of the patients) and one male (father of the patient). The Healthcare professionals who participated in the study were an occupational therapist, a physiotherapist, a social worker, a dietician and a nurse, who was acting as a contact person for the patients. To explore the rehabilitation services provided in municipal districts other than Copenhagen, one of the groups also conducted phone interviews with cancer coordinators from four municipalities of different sizes across Denmark.

Data Analysis

For the purpose of this paper, a meta-synthesis of the qualitative data was conducted by the authors to abstract and generalize through the process of translation and synthesis (40, 41) - to thin out (42) - from the thick descriptions generated by the 5 groups of students (n=24). This was not a process of secondary data analysis of the primary data collected by the groups (e.g. recordings of group discussions, or transcripts of interviews), but an analysis of thick descriptions generated by the groups during the data collection

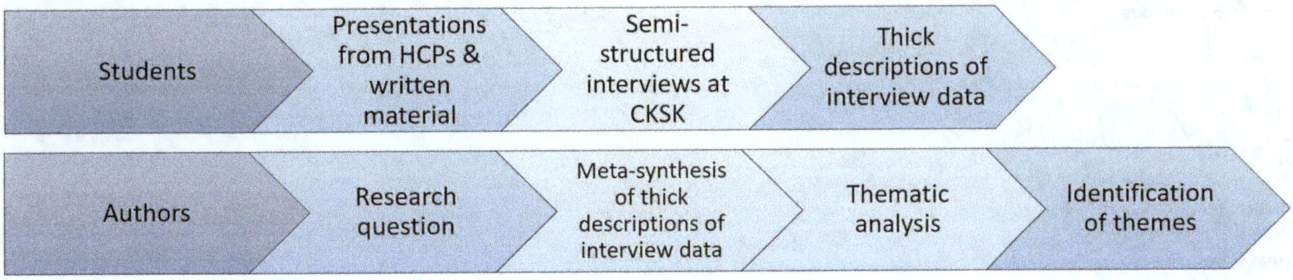

FIGURE 3 | Overview of the data analysis process from the perspectives of the students and authors.

TABLE 1 | HNC patients' characteristics.

ID	Participant #1	Participant #2	Participant #3	Participant #4
Gender	Male	Male	Male	Female
Age	74	67	34	56
Education[a]	BA[b]	MA[c]	MA	HD[d]
Employment[e]	No	Yes	Yes	No
Living condition	Single	With family	With family	Single
Rehab. time	9 months	12 months	3 months	10 months
HNC type	N/D[f]	N/D	Salivary glands	HPV[g]
Treatment	Surgery 33 x radiation	Surgery 35 x radiation 3 x chemotherapy	Surgery 35 x radiation	35 x radiation 2 x chemotherapy

[a]*Education completed,* [b]*Bachelor's Degree,* [c]*Master's Degree,* [d]*Higher Degree,* [e]*Employment status,* [f]*Not Defined,* [g]*Human papillomavirus.*

process. The meta-synthesis was done through a thematic analysis, where the thick descriptions created by the data collection groups were analyzed to identify themes and sub-themes (43) that would be descriptive for identifying and understanding the needs of stakeholders. "Thick description refers to the researcher's task of both describing and interpreting observed social action (or behavior) within its particular context" (39). Coding was used as an interpretive instrument for dealing with the content (44). We used the resulting thick description as an articulation of how we jointly see and understand the phenomenon we were studying, intertwining it with the analysis process for not merely including detail, but also interpreting and translating the detailed description of observations in the social, physical, organizational, technical and physiological context (45). All the four authors read and reviewed the thick descriptions created by the data collection groups. The authors adopted a collaborative process to analyze the thick descriptions, which was performed in two phases. Initially, the first two authors had two sessions in which the findings were discussed and themes and sub-themes were defined. In the second phase, the third and fourth authors were involved in the data analysis process to validate and discuss the justifications and choices done. After a briefing by the first author, all the authors had an additional session, in which a discussion on the themes took place and the data were grouped into the final themes and sub-themes.

Ethical Considerations

The ethics committee of the IT-University of Copenhagen follows the principles of the Danish Code of Conduct for Research Integrity (46). An email approval for the use of data collected by the students and the analysis and interpretation work they did was asked before meta-analysis. The ethics approval process of the Center for Kræft og Sundhed København was followed in approaching and working with patients and care professionals. The participants were presented an informed consent form which they signed prior to the study, they were provided contact information of a contact person, and they were informed regarding their right to withdraw from the study at any time.

RESULTS

The findings below are presented as follows: (1) HNC patients' needs, (2) Informal caregivers' needs and (3) Healthcare professionals' needs. The following four sub-themes have been identified: service delivery needs, emotional needs, physical needs and social needs. **Table 2** provides a summary of the results.

HNC Patients' Needs

Patients' rehabilitation needs are unique, as the physical and emotional symptoms are comprehensive and diverse. Four areas of needs have been identified: service delivery, emotional, social and physical.

Service Delivery Needs

Lack of information and organizational challenges were reported by the patients. More specifically, they addressed lack of

TABLE 2 | Summary of needs - HNC patients, informal caregivers and healthcare professionals.

Service Delivery needs	Emotional needs	Social needs	Physical needs
HNC Patients			
Lack of information and organizational challenges Dissatisfaction caused by paper format Information management Tight rehabilitation schedule	Need for emotional support Support fuels HNC Patients motivation Need for a disease free space	Need for socializing with people they identify with Socialization fuels their motivation	Need for practical suggestions relating to nutrition and eating difficulties
Informal Caregivers			
Lack of information Information management	Need for support in dealing with their anxiety, stress	Need for support in dealing with their anxiety and feelings of guilt and shame	N/A
Healthcare Professionals			
Lack of contextual knowledge, experience and reliable information Organizational and structural challenges Need for technological support to share knowledge between municipalities	N/A	N/A	N/A[a]

[a]*Not applicable.*

information at hospitals concerning the rehabilitation services provided by the municipalities.

A considerable 'pain point' for patients was related to unanswered questions. They felt that they do not have the opportunity to receive answers to questions that may suddenly arise.

The findings highlighted issues arising from the service provision. Patients were dissatisfied receiving information regarding the rehabilitation process mostly on paper:

"Yes, they could come up with something better. Something people can see on a screen, you know? That would help me, definitely."

Another point of contention was related to information management. It was hard for patients to keep track of all the information and translate it to relevant knowledge and actions, especially during the cancer diagnosis phase:

"[…] it is insanely hard before the treatment period to understand what is going to happen. So really really hard. Hmm, and there was very much information overload."

The experience of another patient concerning the management of medical information during the diagnosis period was the following:

"I could not tell them [the parents] anything because I did not have the information. I was totally far away when I was given the information."

These findings indicate how important it is for patients to receive information in a comprehensive way in order to have an overview of their cancer treatment and rehabilitation process. The majority of them found it demanding and difficult to manage and keep control of their tight treatment schedule.

Emotional Needs

Alongside with the physical support, patients highlighted the paramount importance of communication and psychological support from relatives, friends and healthcare professionals throughout the treatment and post-treatment periods:

"[…] find that person, who can coach you. It does not need to be a coach […]. But find that person, who can help you to take care of your mind."

Some of the patients underwent the rehabilitation process without having direct support from relatives or friends. They praised the experience of rehabilitation at CSCK and explained how crucial was the emotional support they received from healthcare professionals and other cancer patients.

The emotional support could trigger motivation. The need for motivation and sense of duty to participate actively in the rehabilitation process has been addressed by the HNC patients. A concrete example is pertinent to physical activities, as patients mentioned that they have to perform exercises regularly, which required a lot of discipline especially after the end of the rehabilitation program and when they were outside the center:

"My sister has completed the exercises alongside me every day when I stayed with her. It became a habit."

They argued that the provision of emotional support is also essential as the nature of the detrimental side-effects of HNC require long-term efforts to appreciate their progress. Struggling to monitor their own progress was reported to be a demotivating factor, especially if they do not have insight into their own progress.

Finally, HNC patients expressed a demand for a disease-free space. They addressed the need to hold conversations about everyday life out of the cancer context, as they felt that they were constantly being reminded of their medical condition:

"I would rather talk about anything else [than my disease] […] I had a hard time talking to my regular friends about this. Because I didn't want to be "the sick one". I didn't want to talk about my cancer."

This could pinpoint that when patients are engaging in their pre-cancer environment they desire to be again their disease-free selves.

HNC patients valued the support from relatives and family as an essential factor that had a positive impact on their life. They argued that informal caregivers supported them in coping with the burden that the disease posed and to manage their stress levels:

"My mother and wife were completely destroyed. My father also for that matter - and my brother. The whole family. It was a huge shock."

A contact person in the rehabilitation center was considered to be a key individual. The contact person utilizes informal conversations, specialist knowledge and emotional support to customize the rehabilitation program to the patient's specific needs:

"I've always been able to call her [my contact person] at any point in time - if I've had a bad episode - and talk to her. She has been there 100% of the time. […] And if I couldn't get a hold of her, she has always called me back […]."

HNC patients asserted that the contact person was highly appreciated and acted as a motivation trigger for the patients.

Social Needs

Apart from emotional needs, patients addressed a need for social interaction with other HNC patients. Socializing with patients that faced similar life-threatening disease considered to be essential for patients with HNC:

"[…] we talked during breaks at the training session, while waiting on the [workout] machines […] and we talked about "what have you been operated for?" and "what have you experienced". It was pretty comforting to get to know each other, and it encouraged me to go exercising."

Socializing with other HNC patients enabled them to communicate their concerns pertinent to treatment and their rehabilitation challenges, including common side- effects of radiation therapy, such as sore mouth and swallowing problems. Patients argued that social support is an important part of their rehabilitation and act as a motivator to perform swallowing exercises on a regular basis:

"It has been helpful to have someone there to get me to do them [exercises]. If I had only received papers for the exercises I wouldn't have done them."

The demand for social support found to be higher in areas outside the capital where there is lower concentration of HNC cancer patients and lack of specialized rehabilitation centers.

Nevertheless, a few patients reported as a barrier to social support the lack of identification with other cancer patients due to issues such as age gap. A patient expressed the need to identify himself with other patients in a similar age group. Since he could not find any groups/events he felt comfortable in, he searched for videos on YouTube to learn from and identify with patients more resembling his own life situation and/or age group.

Physical Needs

The majority of patients reported eating challenges after treatments as a side-effect of radiation therapy. Effects such as dental problems, swallowing difficulties and taste changes, along with pain and fear associated with food consumption:

"It's not that smart, you cannot eat in public. Sometimes you swallow it down the wrong pipe. Then grab a napkin and stand and cough it up at a speed of hell. It's not that smart to eat in public."

Eating challenges faced by patients are typically long-term. They start from the beginning of the medical treatment, lasting long after the end of the rehabilitation period:

"[…] I wish it was recommended to me from the beginning, as I later learnt, that many people appreciate blueberries before and after treatment."

Informal Caregivers' Needs

The needs of informal caregivers of HNC patients were pertinent to the patients' mental health and to the practical aspects of everyday life.

Service Delivery Needs

In terms of practical information, informal caregivers argued that there were times they felt that they missed the knowledge of how to accommodate the patients' needs in order to establish a supportive relationship during the rehabilitation process. In addition, they experienced distress due to lack of information about the available rehabilitation options at hospital, as well as during the rehabilitation process. For example, one of the common side-effects of the radiation therapy is tooth decay, nevertheless, they argued that they were not aware that dental treatment is not part of the rehabilitation process. Another challenge that was identified related to food preparation and oral exercises. Food preparation for HNC is particularly challenging due to their new nutritional needs after the radiation therapy. Side-effects such as swallowing disorders and pain posed challenges to food preparation and required the adoption of a specific diet.

Emotional Needs

The majority of informal caregivers often experienced stress and anxiety, which negatively affected their mental health in daily life. They experienced difficulties in expressing their feelings in the context of cancer. More specifically, relatives revealed that feelings of guilt and shame often remained unspoken, while taboo subjects such as sexual intercourse were neglected.

Social Needs

Social needs were related to the emotional support of HNC patients. The informal caregivers expressed the desire to speak and connect with someone that understands their point of view without criticizing them:

"You're left with forbidden feelings. Things you do not like to say out loud."

Healthcare Professionals' Needs

Healthcare professionals' needs were also acknowledged, as their input was considered valuable in having a holistic overview of the service ecology. The findings represent different healthcare professional specialties views relevant to HNC rehabilitation and were focused on service delivery needs.

Service Delivery Needs

Healthcare professionals who were located outside the capital area stated that they lack contextual knowledge, experience and information pertinent to HNC:

"In other municipalities they need concrete knowledge about what to do with this type of patients […] because they don't have the same opportunities."

The majority of them did not have previous experience and knowledge in treating HNC patients, indicating that these cases require specialized interventions. A desire for reliable information among healthcare professionals highlighted the potential value of interventions which are reliable, trustworthy and accurate. In some cases, healthcare professionals from municipalities in Jutland had to arrange phone consultations with CKSK to find answers to their questions:

"How do we train the musculature?", "What kind of exercises should the physiotherapist use?"

Healthcare professionals agreed that digital solutions for knowledge sharing could have a positive impact on their performance. When healthcare professionals sought knowledge the main source of information was their colleagues. If their colleagues were not available, then they would seek knowledge through Sundhed.dk, Promedicin.dk or other sources of information. In the same vein, the value of knowledge and experience sharing between patients highlighted by healthcare professionals as a means that would facilitate their work. However, healthcare professionals mentioned that it is challenging to convince patients to gather and share their experiences in a formal setting.

While knowledge sharing is a common practice in the secondary sector, healthcare professionals highlighted that knowledge sharing practices are not common in the primary sector:

"In the secondary sector we shared a lot of data, insights and discussed a lot across different departments. In the primary care there is no such thing as knowledge sharing or discussion."

Another finding indicates that vital treatments such as dental treatment, and rehabilitation responsibilities are allocated at various authorities on different governmental levels. A healthcare professional from a municipality in Jutland said:

"This [the dentists] we have nothing to do with. So, I believe that it is the responsibility of the hospital. We have nothing to do with that."

This impedes the already decentralized municipal rehabilitation offer even further due to the uncertainty of distribution of responsibilities.

DISCUSSION

The aim of this study was to elicit the needs of stakeholders during HNC rehabilitation in a Danish context. Our findings suggest that HNC patients and stakeholders have interrelated needs. Service delivery needs have been addressed by the patients and the stakeholders as the area that posed multiple challenges. A need for emotional support has been addressed by both the patients and informal caregivers, while social needs have been reported from the perspective of patients. The main physical challenge that has been found in this study concerns dysphagia.

Service Delivery Needs

Joint service delivery challenges have been addressed by HNC patients and stakeholders. These challenges concern unmet needs related to lack and organization of information. We found a relationship between the lack and organization of information provided for the patients in different phases of rehabilitation, and the paper format and volume of information. The provision of information in paper copies, has been seen as a factor that can lower the usability and the perceived value of information (47). Digital interactive interventions and tailor-made communication have been proposed as effective approaches for information provision to patients and informal caregivers (48–51). Digital information delivery could provide means to tackle information overload, for example, through personalization and contextualization of content. A recent multi-institutional study concluded that HNC patients prefer multiple modes of information delivery (72%), with one-to-one consultation being the most preferred method for cancer education followed by internet-based interventions (52).

Cancer patients have specific information requirements, requesting oftentimes to receive as much information as possible related to their cancer and its treatment (29, 53, 54). Information about diagnostic tests and treatment options have been reported as those areas in which patients and caregivers request to receive more information than they currently get. However, there is a lack of specialized learning resources and services to cover these ongoing needs (17, 33, 55). In line with this, our participants expressed a need for reception of supplementary or more comprehensive information in regards to swallowing exercises and dental treatments, confirming findings of other researchers (56). The provision of explanatory context and support from healthcare professionals, as well as information consistency have been valued as factors that could increase patients' satisfaction (57). The design of information systems for HNC patients is a highly complex process underpinned not only by the complexity of the disease itself, but also from the unique requirements and needs of each patient (31, 58–61).

Another endorsed problem concerns information management from the perspective of patients and informal caregivers. They argued that managing and having an overview of information has been challenging. Information management issues, such as the difficulty to keep track of all the treatments and interventions needed during rehabilitation can be attributed to the non-digital format of information and the lack of an efficient information management service. Journeys that cancer patients undergo are often fragmented and highly individual (62). Personalization of services and patients' involvement in the design process of interventions has been suggested as a way to identify changing needs within rehabilitation processes and to point out the specific moments that patients experience challenges (59, 63, 64). Effective communication between healthcare professionals and patients have been seen to have positive effects on patients' health, highlighting therefore that inclusion of patients in the design of services could be beneficial in different aspects (65).

Stakeholders participation in the design of rehabilitation services could also contribute towards more efficient re-allocation of organizational and structural responsibilities. In Denmark the responsibilities are allocated at various authorities on different governmental levels, with municipalities holding the responsibility for the generalized rehabilitation interventions, while the hospitals for the specialized rehabilitation services for patients with cancer (24, 25). This organizational structure had been seen as a factor that can cause dissatisfaction, confusion and decreased the trust of patients, as it is not always transparent who holds each responsibility. The municipalities do not possess specialized proficiency needed to elaborate rehabilitation of HNC patients, due to discrepancies in the number of cancer incidences across the country (66). Knowledge and professional skills are divided across great distances, which often hinders closer collaboration across professional groups. Seamless collaboration between hospitals and municipalities could improve patients' experience and contribute towards establishing a trustful relationship between the two parties (66).

Besides organizational and structural problems, healthcare professionals who are working in municipalities located outside the Danish capital, point out an unmet need for knowledge sharing between healthcare professionals. They proposed that peer-to-peer knowledge sharing could elicit essential and updated treatment information. Knowledge generation practices through reflection on clinical experiences, or working relationships are sources of information that healthcare professionals can benefit from, nevertheless under-utilization of sharing professional experiences and communication gaps between healthcare professionals are common practices in healthcare (17, 67). Treatment decisions in HNC are critical and require the establishment of a multidisciplinary team of healthcare professionals (68). The challenges of providing consistent speech pathology care to regional/rural patients, as well as supporting clinicians with less experience in services or with less exposure to HNC utilizing telehealth is an approach used in other countries such as Australia (69). In addition, healthcare professionals argued that knowledge input from HNC patients about their rehabilitation experience and needs, could lead towards service improvements. Based on these findings Sundhed.dk and CKSK are planning to create an information portal for patients with HNC, which will facilitate patients, informal caregivers and healthcare professionals during HNC rehabilitation.

Emotional Needs

Emotional needs from the perspective of patients and informal caregivers include a desire for mutual psychological support. Emotional support is positively related to quality of life among cancer patients (70). Patients with deterioration in quality of life perceived a larger decrease in emotional support than patients with a positive course. HNC patients argued that emotional support enables them to continue practicing the swallowing and physical exercises. Therefore, motivation for rehabilitation and emotional support were found to have a positive relation. Similar to McEwen et al.'s findings, our HNC patients asserted also that a contact person motivated them to keep up with rehabilitation and supported them to coordinate all the interventions (17). Nevertheless, the emotional distress of newly diagnosed patients is related also to other factors such as the marital status and patients' lifestyle (8). Half of our participants stated that they were living alone, a fact that can have a negative impact on their emotional needs. As for informal caregivers, they felt that the burden of supporting their beloved ones had an impact on their wellbeing. Literature supports that caregivers often neglect their own health as they have the notion that the patient should be the center of attention (71), therefore an increasing attention should be given to comprehend the effects this has on the mental and psychological aspects of HNC caregiving. Due to the severity of side-effects such as the ability to speak (72), HNC caregiving poses a high risk of post-traumatic stress disorders and anxiety (17, 73–75). According to Howren et al. (76), interventions for HNC caregivers is still in its infancy, therefore future healthcare interventions should be focusing on accommodating their needs.

Social Needs

In line with previous studies, a need for social support has been also expressed by the informal caregivers and patients that participated in our study (32, 33). Informal caregivers can support and encourage patients that undergo post-treatment changes such as speech disorders, nutrition difficulties or facial features changes. Besides that, social inclusion of patients can contribute towards better functionality and better quality of life after treatment (77). As for patient-to-patient support, according to our findings, patients reported that the social support from peers had a positive impact on motivating them to continue performing physical exercises (78). HNC patients prefer to socialize with patients perceived as similar to them (30). The similarity of characteristics is based on individuals and on variables that patients perceive as relevant to their condition e.g. age, treatment, common experiences etc. (79). For example, breast cancer patients might identify themselves with everyday women, who cope with cancer rather than with the super-copers presented on television programs. These super-copers are usually famous women with cancer, who present that nothing has changed after cancer treatment (79). Moreover, the need to socialize with other patients similar to them is connected to minimization of feelings of deviance (80, 81). This also relates directly to the disease-free space the patients wish to have. Healthy people may ask more questions about a patient's condition or even start treating them differently than before the diagnosis. This behavior change is related to various reasons such as feelings that the other person is sick and therefore in need of help, difficulties to understand the condition or fear of feeling uncomfortable. The reaction of the social environment to the person with the diagnosed condition can be a reminder of the condition to the patients.

The social aspect during rehabilitation of HNC patients has been found to be influential also for informal caregivers, as they reported negative feelings such as guilt and shame. These feelings may be common to people close to a victimized person (i.e. a person who presided as a victim by a particular situation in this case cancer). Husbands of female breast cancer patients seem to deal with their negative feelings by perceiving themselves to be better than the norm, even if that was untrue (75, 78). According to Taylor et al. (82), only 4% of female breast cancer patients were abandoned by their husbands (82). However, the husband who is leaving his sick wife was believed to be the norm by the informal caregivers (i.e. husbands). In general, comparing with people worse than one-self can lead to self-enhancement and better coping with the difficult situation (83). Psychosocial interventions have been concentrating on providing support to patients only for a limited time after the end of treatment. Nevertheless, in the cases of patients with HNC the development of long-term interventions is crucial (33, 84).

The need for social connections is in line with the Self-Determination Theory (85) arguing that 'relatedness' - the feeling of being understood, trusted and cared for by others, is one of the most important basic psychological needs for fostering wellbeing and enhancing motivation and sustainable behavior change.

Physical Needs

The main physical challenge that emerged in this study concerns eating difficulties, as a side-effect of medical treatment. This should be related to the fact that all four participants of our study received radiation therapy. Interventions that may improve the problems associated with nutrition after HNC treatments are essential and have direct effects on quality of patients' life (86). Current practice for managing dysphagia in HNC can include structured swallowing exercises usually given by a speech and language therapist prior and following cancer treatment (5, 21). In addition, mobile interventions, asynchronous telepractice applications for swallowing therapy like "SwallowIT" or screening tools for detection of swallowing, nutrition and distress status have been proposed as possible solutions to facilitate HNC patients' needs (87–89). Strength-based exercises and range of movement exercises (maneuvers) aimed at the swallowing musculature may prevent muscle atrophy and improve prognosis for oral intake (90–92). However, patient adherence to swallowing exercises is often poor (93–95). Devices supporting the exercises have proven efficient e.g. IQoro (96), however, improved adherence may be achieved by facilitating a change in patient behavior (5) and focusing on the psychological and/or social aspects of eating and drinking and not only on the functional aspect (92, 93). A recent systematic review to identify behavioral strategies in swallowing interventions, has found that behavior change techniques that occurred more frequently in effective interventions were; practical social support, behavioral practice, self-monitoring of behavior and credible source, such as a skilled clinician delivering the intervention (5).

Implications for Design and Future Work

The findings of this study highlight the different stakeholders' needs in the rehabilitation process, and pave the way for different and specific CH interventions that could address some of the HNC needs. For example, based on the findings, students identified several design opportunities in the form of questions: How do we ensure that patients have the opportunity to receive answers for spontaneous questions? How might we 'educate' relatives to behave more naturally and not pity or feel sorry for the patient? How might we support patients to overcome the social challenges related to eating in public? How can we better prepare patients for their individual treatment and the challenges that come with it? How might we help caregivers to feel less guilty and more supported? How can we create a service that encourages patients to perform their exercises outside the center? Students also proposed initial design ideas and concepts such as developing a "digital colleague" that provides professional knowledge for healthcare professionals about HNC and creating an online community for both healthcare professionals and patients, to share their experience on HNC rehabilitation. CH interventions have the potential to support the creation of holistic, personalized and inclusive solutions to tackle the diverse and complex needs of HNC patients (35).

Based on our findings, future research should explore possibilities of CH solutions to support the psychological wellbeing of both the informal caregivers (a safe place that enables them to share their thoughts, frustrations and guilt feelings) and for patients to gain strength from people in a similar situation. In addition, digital solutions to smoothen the care pathways would be a promising area of research. Especially, the transition from cancer care to rehabilitation could be eased with digital solutions that would guide the patient through the transition. The first steps of the rehabilitation process which are characterized by overload of information could benefit from solutions that would gradually personalize the rehabilitation information and actions by integrating them into the everyday lives of the patients. The current Covid-19 outbreak poses new challenges, such as the minimization of patient-staff contact time to reduce the risk of virus transmission (97). The pandemic outbreak is an opportunity to reconsider HNC cancer management, focusing on delivering CH solutions that will support the provision of rehabilitation support from a multidisciplinary team of healthcare professionals (98, 99). For example, CH solutions for swallowing-therapy exercises utilizing video communication and sensors during HNC rehabilitation is a successful intervention used in the postCovid-19 period (35). The value of such CH rehabilitation solutions for HNC is recognized during the pandemic, paving the way to novel care delivery methods (98).

We plan to continue our collaboration with the stakeholders and take forward some of the proposed concepts and ideas. In addition, we are considering a follow-up study with HNC in the UK to evaluate if some of the proposed solutions could be relevant or adjusted to the UK population.

Limitations

Our study has a number of limitations. The limited number of participants and the specific types of HNC and medical treatments might have introduced a bias in the findings. In addition, omitting information with regards to the patients' surgery and treatment type (e.g., type of surgery, site of tumor or radiation dose) may have resulted in exclusion of specific patients' rehabilitation needs. For example, a patient who underwent total laryngectomy could have different needs compared to a patient who underwent partial glossectomy. Similarly, including only patients who were capable of conducting lengthy and rigorous interviews may have excluded participants with severe communication difficulties, who may have additional needs that were not captured. However, rehabilitation needs are unique in nature and depend on a variety of factors (e.g., age, severity, treatment type, family support, socio-economic state, individual characteristics, etc). Our aim was to elicit and identify the more holistic needs that might be common across different HNC patients. The qualitative nature of this research increases the credibility of the results, as it provides in-depth content focusing on the needs of a group. One can argue that our findings represent the primary needs of stakeholders during the rehabilitation of HNC patients. In addition, the secondary synthesis of data, the multiple different data collection processes and people engaged to collect the data might have introduced bias. Further research could observe later stages of the service design process, for example observing experiences of stakeholders after the implementation of a digital intervention supporting the rehabilitation process. Despite these limitations, the study is a baseline for future endeavors, as research addressing the interrelated needs of stakeholders during rehabilitation of HNC patients is still in its early stages.

CONCLUSIONS

While preliminary, this study offers insights related to the needs of patients and stakeholders during the HNC rehabilitation. Our findings point out that stakeholders' needs are interrelated. All the stakeholders faced service delivery challenges contextual to lack and organization of information, as well as to information sharing and management. The distribution of responsibilities between municipalities, hospitals and rehabilitation services raised additional challenges, suggesting that reallocation of responsibilities could alleviate this issue. Interrelated emotional and social needs have been found for HNC patients and informal caregivers, underlining the importance of inclusion of all actors in the design of future healthcare interventions.

ETHICS STATEMENT

Ethical review and approval was not required for the study on human participants in accordance with the local legislation and institutional requirements. Written informed consent for participation was not required for this study in accordance with the national legislation and the institutional requirements.

AUTHOR CONTRIBUTIONS

All the authors have been involved in analysis and interpretation of data. MK has been responsible for drafting the first version of the manuscript and coordinating writing. TP, VM, and MI have been involved in revising the manuscript critically for important intellectual content. Portions of this manuscript were presented at the 13th EAI International Conference on Pervasive Computing Technologies for Healthcare (100). All authors contributed to the article and approved the submitted version.

ACKNOWLEDGMENTS

We would like to thank Center for Kræft og Sundhed København and Sundhed.dk for the collaboration with IT-University of Copenhagen. We would also like to thank the students of IT-University of Copenhagen who took part in data collection activities.

REFERENCES

1. Jacobson MC. The Experience of Head and Neck Cancer Survivorship (Including Laryngectomy): An Integrated Biopsychosocial Model. *Curr Opin Supportive Palliative Care* (2018) 12(1):65–73. doi: 10.1097/SPC.0000000000000322
2. Meyers E. Rehabilitation and Treatment of Head and Neck Cancer. *Cancer* (1986).
3. World Health Organisation. *Rehabilitation* (Accessed: September 2018).
4. Patterson JM, McColl E, Wilson J, Carding P, Rapley T. Head and Neck Cancer Patients' Perceptions of Swallowing Following Chemoradiotherapy. *Supportive Care Cancer* (2015) 23(12):3531–8. doi: 10.1007/s00520-015-2715-8
5. Govender R, Smith CH, Gardner B, Barratt H, Taylor SA. Improving Swallowing Outcomes in Patients With Head and Neck Cancer Using a Theory-Based Pretreatment Swallowing Intervention Package: Protocol for a Randomised Feasibility Study. *BMJ Open* (2017) 7(3):014167. doi: 10.1136/bmjopen-2016-014167
6. McQuestion M, Fitch M, Howell D. The Changed Meaning of Food: Physical, Social and Emotional Loss for Patients Having Received Radiation Treatment for Head and Neck Cancer. *Eur J Oncol Nurs* (2011) 15(2):145–51. doi: 10.1016/j.ejon.2010.07.006
7. Semenov YR, Starmer HM, Gourin CG. The Effect of Pneumonia on Short-Term Outcomes and Cost of Care After Head and Neck Cancer Surgery. *Laryngoscope* (2012) 122(9):1994–2004. doi: 10.1002/lary.23446
8. Kugaya A, Akechi T, Okuyama T, Nakano T, Mikami I, Okamura H, et al. Prevalence, Predictive Factors, and Screening for Psychologic Distress in Patients With Newly Diagnosed Head and Neck Cancer. *Cancer* (2000) 88(12):2817–23. doi: 10.1002/1097-0142(20000615)88:12<2817::AID-CNCR22>3.0.CO;2-N
9. Verdonckde Leeuw IM, Eerenstein SE, van der Linden MH, Kuik DJ, de Bree R, Leemans CR. Distress in Spouses and Patients After Treatment for Head and Neck Cancer. *Laryngoscope* (2007) 117(2):238–41. doi: 10.1097/01.mlg.0000250169.10241.58
10. Longacre ML, Ridge JA, Burtness BA, Galloway TJ, Fang CY. Psychological Functioning of Caregivers for Head and Neck Cancer Patients. *Oral Oncol* (2012) 48(1):18–25. doi: 10.1016/j.oraloncology.2011.11.012
11. Sherwood PR, Given BA, Donovan H, Baum A, Given CW, Bender CM, et al. Guiding Research in Family Care: A New Approach to Oncology Caregiving. *Psycho-Oncol: J Psychol Soc Behav Dimensions Cancer* (2008) 17(10):986–96. doi: 10.1002/pon.1314
12. Applebaum AJ, Farran CJ, Marziliano AM, Pasternak AR, Breitbart W. Preliminary Study of Themes of Meaning and Psychosocial Service Use Among Informal Cancer Caregivers. *Palliative Supportive Care* (2014) 12 (2):139–48. doi: 10.1017/S1478951513000084
13. Holm LV, Hansen DG, Johansen C, Vedsted P, Larsen PV, Kragstrup J, et al. Participation in Cancer Rehabilitation and Unmet Needs: A Population-Based Cohort Study. *Supportive Care Cancer* (2012) 20(11):2913–24. doi: 10.1007/s00520-012-1420-0
14. Retèl VP, van der Molen L, Hilgers FJ, Rasch CR, l'Ortye AA, Steuten LM, et al. A Cost-Effectiveness Analysis of a Preventive Exercise Program for Patients With Advanced Head and Neck Cancer Treated With Concomitant Chemo-Radiotherapy. *BMC Cancer* (2011) 11(1):475 doi: 10.1186/1471-2407-11-475

15. Kotz T, Federman AD, Kao J, Milman L, Packer S, Lopez-Prieto C, et al. Prophylactic Swallowing Exercises in Patients With Head and Neck Cancer Undergoing Chemoradiation: A Randomized Trial. *Arch Otolaryngol–Head Neck Surg* (2012) 138(4):376–82. doi: 10.1001/archoto.2012.187
16. Eades M, Murphy J, Carney S, Amdouni S, Lemoignan J, Jelowicki M, et al. Effect of an Interdisciplinary Rehabilitation Program on Quality of Life in Patients With Head and Neck Cancer: Review of Clinical Experience. *Head Neck* (2013) 35(3):343–9. doi: 10.1002/hed.22972
17. McEwen S, Rodriguez AM, Martino R, Poon I, Dunphy C, Rios JN, et al. I Didn't Actually Know There Was Such a Thing as Rehabilitation?: Survivor, Family, and Clinician Perceptions of Rehabilitation Following Treatment for Head and Neck Cancer. *Supportive Care Cancer* (2016) 24(4):1449–53. doi: 10.1007/s00520-015-3021-1
18. Ministry of Health. *Healthcare in Denmark: An Overview.* (2016) (Accessed: July 2020).
19. Pedersen KM, Christiansen T, Bech M. The Danish Health Care System: Evolution-Not Revolution-In a Decentralized System. *Health economics* (2005) 14(S1):41–57. doi: 10.1002/hec.1028
20. *Patients Cancer Plan, [In Danish]* (Accessed: September 2018).
21. McEwen SE, Davis AM, Jones JM, Martino R, Poon I, Rodriguez AM, et al. Development and Preliminary Evaluation of a Rehabilitation Consult for Survivors of Head and Neck Cancer: An Intervention Mapping Protocol. *Implementation Sci* (2015) 10(1):6. doi: 10.1186/s13012-014-0191-z
22. Egan MY, McEwen S, Sikora L, Chasen M, Fitch M, Eldred S. Rehabilitation Following Cancer Treatment. *Disability Rehabil* (2013) 35(26):2245–58. doi: 10.3109/09638288.2013.774441
23. *Program for Rehabilitation and Palliation in Connection With Cancer [In Danish]* (Accessed: September 2018).
24. Christiansen T. Ten Years of Structural Reforms in Danish Healthcare. *Health Policy* (2012) 106(2):114–9. doi: 10.1016/j.healthpol.2012.03.019
25. Strandberg-Larsen M, Nielsen MB, Krasnik A, Vrangbæk K. Is Denmark Prepared to Meet Future Health Care Demands? *Eurohealth* (2006) 12(4):7–10.
26. The Danish Health Authority. *Cancer Pathways* (Accessed: September 2018).
27. Wells M, Semple C, Lane C. A National Survey of Healthcare Professionals' Views on Models of Follow-Up, Holistic Needs Assessment and Survivorship Care for Patients With Head and Neck Cancer. *Eur J Cancer Care* (2015) 24 (6):873–83. doi: 10.1111/ecc.12285
28. Breen LJ, O'Connor M, Calder S, Tai V, Cartwright J, Beilby JM. The Health Professionals' Perspectives of Support Needs of Adult Head and Neck Cancer Survivors and Their Families: A Delphi Study. *Supportive Care Cancer* (2017) 25(8):2413–20. doi: 10.1007/s00520-017-3647-2
29. Longacre ML, Galloway TJ, Parvanta CF, Fang CY. Medical Communication-Related Informational Need and Resource Preferences Among Family Caregivers for Head and Neck Cancer Patients. *J Cancer Educ* (2015) 30 (4):786–91. doi: 10.1007/s13187-015-0814-3
30. Badr H, Lipnick D, Diefenbach MA, Posner M, Kotz T, Miles B, et al. Development and Usability Testing of a Web-Based Self-Management Intervention for Oral Cancer Survivors and Their Family Caregivers. *Eur J Cancer Care* (2016) 25(5):806–21. doi: 10.1111/ecc.12396
31. Ringash J, Bernstein LJ, Devins G, Dunphy C, Giuliani M, Martino R, et al. Head and Neck Cancer Survivorship: Learning the Needs, Meeting the Needs. *Semin Radiat Oncol* (2018) 28(1):64–74. doi: 10.1016/j.semradonc.2017.08.008
32. Fang CY, Heckman CJ. Informational and Support Needs of Patients With Head and Neck Cancer: Current Status and Emerging Issues. *Cancers Head Neck* (2016) 1(1):15. doi: 10.1186/s41199-016-0017-6
33. Chen S-C, Tsai M-C, Liu C-L, Yu W-P, Liao C-T, Chang JT-C. Support Needs of Patients With Oral Cancer and Burden to Their Family Caregivers. *Cancer Nurs* (2009) 32(6):473–81. doi: 10.1097/NCC.0b013e3181b14e94
34. Karampela M, Isomursu M, Porat T, Maramis C, Mountford N, Giunti G, et al. The Extent and Coverage of Current Knowledge of Connected Health: Systematic Mapping Study. *J Med Internet Res* (2019) 21(9):e14394. doi: 10.2196/14394
35. Signorelli GR, Lehocki F, Fernández MM, O'Neill G, O'Connor D, Brennan L, et al. A Research Roadmap: Connected Health as an Enabler of Cancer Patient Support. *J Med Internet Res* (2019) 21(10):e14360. doi: 10.2196/14360
36. Yin RK. *Case Study Research and Applications: Design and Methods.* (2017). 22–6.
37. Kouprie M, Visser FS. A Framework for Empathy in Design: Stepping Into and Out of the User's Life. *J Eng Design* (2009) 20(5):437–48. doi: 10.1080/09544820902875033
38. Virginia B, Clarke V. What Can "Thematic Analysis" Offer Health and Wellbeing Researchers? *Int J Qual Stud Health Well-Being* (2014) 9:26152. doi: 10.3402/qhw.v9.26152
39. Ponterotto JG. Brief Note on the Origins, Evolution, and Meaning of the Qualitative Research Concept Thick Description. *Qual Rep* (2006) 11(3):538–49. doi: 10.46743/2160-3715/2006.1666
40. Walsh D, Downe S. Meta-Synthesis Method for Qualitative Research: A Literature Review. *J Adv Nurs* (2005) 50(2):204–11. doi: 10.1111/j.1365-2648.2005.03380.x
41. Zimmer L. Qualitative Meta-Synthesis: A Question of Dialoguing With Texts. *J Adv Nurs* (2006) 53(3):311–8. doi: 10.1111/j.1365-2648.2006.03721.x
42. Sandelowski M, Docherty S, Emden C. Qualitative Metasynthesis: Issues and Techniques. *Res Nurs Health* (1997) 20(4):365–71. doi: 10.1002/(SICI)1098-240X(199708)20:4<365::AID-NUR9>3.0.CO;2-E
43. Braun V, Clarke V. Using Thematic Analysis in Psychology. *Qual Res Psychol* (2006) 3(2):77–101. doi: 10.1191/1478088706qp063oa
44. Evers JC. Elaborating on Thick Analysis: About Thoroughness and Creativity in Qualitative Analysis. *Forum Qual Sozialforsch* (2015) 17(1). doi: 10.17169/fqs-17.1.2369
45. Freeman M. The Hermeneutical Aesthetics of Thick Description. *Qual Inq* (2014) 20(6):827–33. doi: 10.1177/1077800414530267
46. Ministry of Higher Education and Science. *Danish Code of Conduct for Research Integrity.* (2014). Available at: https://ufm.dk/en/publications/2014/the-danish-code-of-conduct-for-research-integrity [Accessed September 04, 2021].
47. Harjumaa M, Saraniemi S, Pekkarinen S, Lappi M, Similä H, Isomursu M. Feasibility of Digital Footprint Data for Health Analytics and Services: An Explorative Pilot Study. *BMC Med Inf Decision Making* (2016) 16(1):139. doi: 10.1186/s12911-016-0378-0
48. Dsouza V, Serrao M, Watson E, Blouin E, Zeitouni A, Allison PJ. Information Service in Head and Neck Cancer Care - A Qualitative Study. *Supportive Care Cancer* (2018) 26(1):91–8. doi: 10.1007/s00520-017-3818-1
49. Dsouza V, Blouin E, Zeitouni A, Muller K, Allison P. Multimedia Information Intervention and Iits Benefits in Partners of the Head and Neck Cancer Patients. *Eur J Cancer Care* (2017) 26(4):12440. doi: 10.1111/ecc.12440
50. van Dulmen S. The Value of Tailored Communication for Person-Centred Outcomes. *J Eval Clin Pract* (2011) 17(2):381–3. doi: 10.1111/j.1365-2753.2010.01586.x
51. Brennan DM, Mawson S, Brownsell S. Telerehabilitation: Enabling the Remote Delivery of Healthcare, Rehabilitation, and Self Management. *Stud Health Technol Inform* (2009) 145:231–48. doi: 10.3233/978-1-60750-018-6-231
52. Jabbour J, Milross C, Sundaresan P, Ebrahimi A, Shepherd HL, Dhillon HM, et al. Education and Support Needs in Patients With Head and Neck Cancer: A Multi-Institutional Survey. *Cancer* (2017) 123(11):1949–57. doi: 10.1002/cncr.30535
53. Cox A, Jenkins V, Catt S, Langridge C, Fallowfield L. Information Needs and Experiences: An Audit of UK Cancer Patients. *Eur J Oncol Nurs* (2006) 10 (4):263–72. doi: 10.1016/j.ejon.2005.10.007
54. Morrison V, Henderson B, Zinovieff F, Davies G, Cartmell R, Hall A, et al. Common, Important, and Unmet Needs of Cancer Outpatients. *Eur J Oncol Nurs* (2012) 16(2):115–23. doi: 10.1016/j.ejon.2011.04.004
55. Herrmann T, Peters PM, Van Laar ES. Online Education Needs and Preferences of Patients With Cancer and Their Caregivers. *Am Soc Clin Oncol* (2017) 35:15. doi: 10.1200/JCO.2017.35.15_suppl.e21669
56. Fang CY, Longacre ML, Manne SL, Ridge JA, Lango MN, Burtness BA. Informational Needs of Head and Neck Cancer Patients. *Health Technol* (2012) 2(1):57–62. doi: 10.1007/s12553-012-0020-9
57. Mills ME, Sullivan K. The Importance of Information Giving for Patients Newly Diagnosed With Cancer: A Review of the Literature. *J Clin Nurs* (1999) 8(6):631–42. doi: 10.1046/j.1365-2702.1999.00296.x
58. Semple CJ, McGOWAN B. Need for Appropriate Written Information for Patients, With Particular Reference to Head and Neck Cancer. *J Clin Nurs* (2002) 11(5):585–93. doi: 10.1046/j.1365-2702.2002.00641.x

59. Llewellyn C, McGurk M, Weinman J. How Satisfied Are Head and Neck Cancer (HNC) Patients With the Information They Receive Pre-Treatment? Results From the Satisfaction With Cancer Information Profile (SCIP). *Oral Oncol* (2006) 42(7):726–34. doi: 10.1016/j.oraloncology.2005.11.013
60. Pollock K, Cox K, Howard P, Wilson E, Moghaddam N. Service User Experiences of Information Delivery After a Diagnosis of Cancer: A Qualitative Study. *Supportive Care Cancer* (2008) 16(8):963–73. doi: 10.1007/s00520-007-0363-3
61. Brockbank S, Miller N, Owen S, Patterson JM. Pretreatment Information On? Dysphagia: Exploring the Views of Head and Neck Cancer Patients. *J Pain Symptom Manage* (2015) 49(1):89–97. doi: 10.1016/j.jpainsymman.2014.04.014
62. Hägglund M, Bolin P, Koch S. Living With Lung Cancer-Patients' Experiences as Input to Ehealth Service Design. *In: MedInfo* (2015) 47(5):391–5. doi: 10.3233/978-1-61499-564-7-391
63. Barnhart MK, Ward EC, Cartmill B, Nund R, Robinson RA, Chandler SJ, et al. Content Analysis of Rehabilitation Goals for Patients Following non-Surgical Head and Neck Cancer Treatment. *Supportive Care Cancer* (2019) 27(2):639–47. doi: 10.1007/s00520-018-4364-1
64. Halldórsdóttir S, Hamrin E. Caring and Uncaring Encounters Within Nursing and Health Care From the Cancer Patient's Perspective. *Cancer Nurs* (1997) 20(2):120–8. doi: 10.1097/00002820-199704000-00007
65. Street RL Jr, Makoul G, Arora NK, Epstein RM. How Does Communication Heal? Pathways Linking Clinician–Patient Communication to Health Outcomes. *Patient Educ Couns* (2009) 74(3):295–301. doi: 10.1016/j.pec.2008.11.015
66. Kristiansen M, Adamsen L, Piil K, Halvorsen I, Nyholm N, Hendriksen C. A Three-Year National Follow-Up Study on the Development of Community-Level Cancer Rehabilitation in Denmark. *Scandinavian J Public Health* (2017) 47(5):511–8. doi: 10.1177/1403494817746535
67. Kinsella EA. Professional Knowledge and the Epistemology of Reflective Practice. *Nurs Philosophy* (2010) 11(1):3–14. doi: 10.1111/j.1466-769X.2009.00428.x
68. Cognetti DM, Weber RS, Lai SY. Head and Neck Cancer. *Cancer* (2008) 113 (S7):1911–32. doi: 10.1002/cncr.23654
69. Burns CL, Kularatna S, Ward EC, Hill AJ, Byrnes J, Kenny LM. Cost Analysis of a Speech Pathology Synchronous Telepractice Service for Patients With Head and Neck Cancer. *Head Neck* (2017) 39(12):2470–80. doi: 10.1002/hed.24916
70. Courtens A, Stevens F, Crebolder H, Philipsen H. Longitudinal Study on Quality of Life and Social Support in Cancer Patients. *Cancer Nurs* (1996) 19 (3):162–9. doi: 10.1097/00002820-199606000-00002
71. Bevans M, Sternberg EM. Caregiving Burden, Stress, and Health Effects Among Family Caregivers of Adult Cancer Patients. *Jama* (2012) 307 (4):398–403. doi: 10.1001/jama.2012.29
72. Nund RL, Rumbach AF, Debattista BC, Goodrow MN, Johnson KA, Tupling LN, et al. Communication Changes Following non-Glottic Head and Neck Cancer Management: The Perspectives of Survivors and Carers. *Int J Speech-Language Pathol* (2015) 17(3):263–72. doi: 10.3109/17549507.2015.1010581
73. Richardson AE, Morton R, Broadbent E. Caregivers' Illness Perceptions Contribute to Quality of Life in Head and Neck Cancer Patients at Diagnosis. *J Psychosocial Oncol* (2015) 33(4):414–32. doi: 10.1080/07347332.2015.1046011
74. Posluszny DM, Dougall AL, Johnson JT, Argiris A, Ferris RL, Baum A, et al. Posttraumatic Stress Disorder Symptoms in Newly Diagnosed Patients With Head and Neck Cancer and Their Partners. *Head Neck* (2015) 37(9):1282–9. doi: 10.1002/hed.23760
75. Balfe M, O'brien K, Timmons A, Butow P, O'sullivan E, Gooberman-Hill R, et al. Informal Caregiving in Head and Neck Cancer: Caregiving Activities and Psychological Well-Being. *Eur J Cancer Care* (2018) 27(2):12520. doi: 10.1111/ecc.12520
76. Howren MB, Christensen AJ, Karnell LH, Funk GF. Psychological Factors Associated With Head and Neck Cancer Treatment and Survivorship: Evidence and Opportunities for Behavioral Medicine. *J Consulting Clin Psychol* (2013) 81(2):299. doi: 10.1037/a0029940
77. Karnell LH, Christensen AJ, Rosenthal EL, Magnuson JS, Funk GF. Influence of Social Support on Health-Related Quality of Life Outcomes in Head and Neck Cancer. *Head Neck: J Sci Specialties Head Neck* (2007) 29(2):143–6. doi: 10.1002/hed.20501
78. Govender R, Wood CE, Taylor SA, Smith CH, Barratt H, Gardner B. Patient Experiences of Swallowing Exercises After Head and Neck Cancer: A Qualitative Study Examining Barriers and Facilitators Using Behaviour Change Theory. *Dysphagia* (2017) 32(4):559–69. doi: 10.1007/s00455-017-9799-x
79. Wood JV, Taylor SE, Lichtman RR. Social Comparison in Adjustment to Breast Cancer. *J Pers Soc Psychol* (1985) 49(5):1169. doi: 10.1037/0022-3514.49.5.1169
80. Coates D, Winston T. Counteracting the Deviance of Depression: Peer Support Groups for Victims. *J Soc Issues* (1983) 39(2):169–94. doi: 10.1111/j.1540-4560.1983.tb00147.x
81. Boinon D, Sultan S, Charles C, Stulz A, Guillemeau C, Delaloge S, et al. Changes in Psychological Adjustment Over the Course of Treatment for Breast Cancer: The Predictive Role of Social Sharing and Social Support. *Psycho-Oncology* (2014) 23(3):291–8. doi: 10.1002/pon.3420
82. Taylor SE, Wood JV, Lichtman RR. It Could Be Worse: Selective Evaluation as a Response to Victimization. *J Soc Issues* (1983) 39(2):19–40. doi: 10.1111/j.1540-4560.1983.tb00139.x
83. Wills TA. Downward Comparison Principles in Social Psychology. *psychol Bull* (1981) 90(2):245. doi: 10.1037/0033-2909.90.2.245
84. Stanton AL. Psychosocial Concerns and Interventions for Cancer Survivors. *J Clin Oncol* (2006) 24(32):5132–7. doi: 10.1200/JCO.2006.06.8775
85. Deci EL, Ryan RM. The "What" and "Why" of Goal Pursuits: Human Needs and the Self-Determination of Behavior. *Psychol Inq* (2000) 11(4):227–68. doi: 10.1207/S15327965PLI1104_01
86. Daugaard R, Kjaer T, Johansen C, Christiansen J, Andersen E, Nielsen AL, et al. Association Between Late Effects Assessed by Physicians and Quality of Life Reported by Head-And-Neck Cancer Survivors. *Acta Oncol* (2017) 56 (2):342–7. doi: 10.1080/0284186X.2016.1267873
87. Cowie J, Boa S, King E, Wells M, Cairns D. Electronic Swallowing Intervention Package to Support Swallowing Function in Patients With Head and Neck Cancer: Development and Feasibility Study. *JMIR Form Res* (2018) 2(2):e15. doi: 10.2196/formative.9703
88. Wall LR, Ward EC, Cartmill B, Hill AJ, Porceddu SV. Examining User Perceptions of SwallowIT: A Pilot Study of a New Telepractice Application for Delivering Intensive Swallowing Therapy to Head and Neck Cancer Patients. *J Telemed Telecare* (2017) 23(1):53–9. doi: 10.1177/1357633X15617887
89. Wall L, Ward E, Cartmill B, Hill A, Isenring E, Byrnes J, et al. Computerised Screening of Swallowing, Nutrition and Distress in Head and Neck Cancer Patients and Their Carers. *Dysphagia* (2015) 30(5):667–7. doi: 10.1007/s00455-015-9633-2
90. Duarte VM, Chhetri DK, Liu YF, Erman AA, Wang MB. Swallow Preservation Exercises During Chemoradiation Therapy Maintains Swallow Function. *Otolaryngol–Head Neck Surg* (2013) 149(6):878–84. doi: 10.1177/0194599813502310
91. Hutcheson KA, Bhayani MK, Beadle BM, Gold KA, Shinn EH, Lai SY, et al. Eat and Exercise During Radiotherapy or Chemoradiotherapy for Pharyngeal Cancers: Use It or Lose It. *JAMA Otolaryngol–Head Neck Surg* (2013) 139 (11):1127–34. doi: 10.1001/jamaoto.2013.4715
92. King SN, Dunlap NE, Tennant PA, Pitts T. Pathophysiology of Radiation-Induced Dysphagia in Head and Neck Cancer. *Dysphagia* (2016) 31(3):339–51. doi: 10.1007/s00455-016-9710-1
93. Mortensen H, Jensen K, Aksglæde K, Lambertsen K, Eriksen E, Grau C. Prophylactic Swallowing Exercises in Head and Neck Cancer Radiotherapy. *Dysphagia* (2015) 30(3):304–14. doi: 10.1007/s00455-015-9600-y
94. Lazarus C, Husaini H, Falciglia D, DeLacure M, Branski R, Kraus D, et al. Effects of Exercise on Swallowing and Tongue Strength in Patients With Oral and Oropharyngeal Cancer Treated With Primary Radiotherapy With or Without Chemotherapy. *Int J Oral Maxillofacial Surg* (2014) 43(5):523–30. doi: 10.1016/j.ijom.2013.10.023
95. Shinn EH, Basen-Engquist K, Baum G, Steen S, Bauman RF, Morrison W, et al. Adherence to Preventive Exercises and Self-Reported Swallowing Outcomes in Post-Radiation Head and Neck Cancer Patients. *Head Neck* (2013) 35(12):1707–12. doi: 10.1002/hed.23255

96. *IQoro, Breath, Eat, Smille, Talk* (Accessed: September 2018).
97. Vukkadala N, Qian ZJ, Holsinger FC, Patel ZM, Rosenthal E. COVID-19 and the Otolaryngologist: Preliminary Evidence-Based Review. *Laryngoscope* (2020) 130(11):2537–43. doi: 10.1002/lary.28672
98. Han AY, Miller JE, Long JL, St John MA. Time for a Paradigm Shift in Head and Neck Cancer Management During the COVID-19 Pandemic. *Otolaryngol–Head Neck Surg* (2020) 163(3):447–54. doi: 10.1177/0194599820931789
99. Song K, Fary K. Cancer Rehabilitation During the COVID-19 Pandemic: An Overview of Special Considerations. *J Int Soc Phys Rehabil Med* (2020) 3.2:38. doi: 10.4103/jisprm.jisprm_10_20
100. Karampela M, Porat T, Mylonopoulou V. May. Needs of Head and Neck Cancer Patients and Stakeholders During Rehabilitation. In: *In Proceedings of the 13th EAI International Conference on Pervasive Computing Technologies for Healthcare*. New York, NY, USA: Association for Computing Machinery (2019). p. 415–21. doi: 10.1145/3329189.3329236

16

Combinatorial Low Dose Arsenic Trioxide and Cisplatin Exacerbates Autophagy via AMPK/STAT3 Signaling on Targeting Head and Neck Cancer Initiating Cells

Wei-Chun Hu[1†], *Wan-Huai Teo*[1†], *Tung-Fu Huang*[2,3,4], *Te-Chang Lee*[5] *and Jeng-Fan Lo*[1,6,7,8*]

[1] Institute of Oral Biology, National Yang-Ming University, Taipei, Taiwan, [2] School of Medicine, National Yang-Ming University, Taipei, Taiwan, [3] Department of Orthopedics and Traumatology, Taipei Veterans General Hospital, Taipei, Taiwan, [4] Department of Exercise and Health Science, National Taipei University of Nursing and Health Sciences, Taipei, Taiwan, [5] Institute of Biomedical Sciences, Academia Sinica, Taipei, Taiwan, [6] Department of Dentistry, School of Dentistry, National Yang-Ming University, Taipei, Taiwan, [7] Cancer Progression Research Center, National Yang-Ming University, Taipei, Taiwan, [8] Department of Dentistry, Taipei Veterans General Hospital, Taipei, Taiwan

Correspondence:
Jeng-Fan Lo
jflo@ym.edu.tw

†These authors have contributed equally to this work

Head and neck squamous cell carcinoma (HNSCC) is a highly lethal disease with high-level of epidemic both in the world and Taiwan. Previous studies support that head and neck cancer-initiating cells (HN-CICs), a subpopulation of cancer cells with enhanced stemness properties, contribute to therapy resistance and tumor recurrence. Arsenic trioxide (As_2O_3; ATO) has shown to be an effective anti-cancer drug targeting acute promyelocytic leukemia (APL). Combinatorial treatment with high dose of ATO and cisplatin (CDDP) exert synergistic apoptotic effects in cancer cell lines of various solid tumors, however, it may cause of significant side effect to the patients. Nevertheless, none has reported the anti-cancerous effect of ATO/CDDP targeting HN-CICs. In this study, we aim to evaluate the low dose combination of ATO with conventional chemo-drugs CDDP treatment on targeting HN-CICs. We first analyzed the inhibitory tumorigenicity of co-treatment with ATO and chemo-drugs on HN-CICs which are enriched from HNSCC cells. We observed that ATO/CDDP therapeutic regimen successfully synergized the cell death on HN-CICs with a Combination Index (CI) <1 by Chou-Talalay's analysis *in vitro*. Interestingly, the ATO/CDDP regimen also induced exaggerated autophagy on HN-CICs. Additionally, this drug combination strategy also empowered both preventive and therapeutic effect by *in vivo* xenograft assays. Finally, we provide the underlying molecular mechanisms of ATO-based therapeutic regimen on HN-CICs. Together, low dose of combinatorial ATO/CDDP regimen induced cell death as well as exacerbated autophagy via AMPK-STAT3 mediated pathway in HN-CICs.

Keywords: head and neck cancer-initiating cells, arsenic trioxide, combination index, autophagy, synergistic effects

BACKGROUND

Head and neck cancer (HNC), a disease with a major worldwide burden. About 95% of HNC is squamous cell carcinoma (HNSCC) which make up the sixth most common cause of cancer death. It is responsible for 300,000 deaths annually (1). HNSCC is considered one of the most common cancers leading to significant mortality and morbidity in Taiwan. Treatment for HNSCC usually involves therapies with surgery, radiation, or chemotherapy alone or concurrent chemotherapy/radiation. However, the overwhelming majority of HNSCC patients' survival outcomes still remain poor. The 5-year overall survival rate of HNSCC's patients is about 40–50% (2), thus, illustrating the urgent need to develop novel therapeutic options to prolong the patients survival.

In the past decade, the hierarchical model of cancer stem cells (CSCs) or cancer initiating cells (CICs) has raised an intense topic in cancer biology or treatment. The CICs are a subpopulation of cancer cells with differentiation ability to maintain the bulk cells population of the tumor with heterogeneous phenotypes and to trigger tumor-initiating activity. Besides, the self-renewal ability of CICs also attributes to the cancer relapse, drug resistance and radio-resistance (3). Most of the therapeutic agents are capable of eliminating the more rapidly proliferating bulk cells, however, the CICs may lay dormant after the therapies (4). After the interruption of treatment, CICs may remerge as they are intrinsically resistant to the therapy agents or they have required mutations that confer resistance to the therapy agents (5). Previously, we have successfully enriched HN-CICs by spheroid cultivation (6), and have identified a subset of HN-CICs with low intracellular reactive oxygen species levels (ROS^{Low}) which sustain the stemness properties and tumorigenicity (7). The HN-CICs have demonstrated chemo-resistant phenotype. Interestingly, this subpopulation cells also can be enriched in cisplatin-resistance cell line (7). Thus, development of novel therapeutic agents to target HN-CICs is required, and it would benefit for future HNSCC therapy.

Arsenic Trioxide As_2O_3 (ATO) has been used in traditional Chinese medicine as pharmaceutical agents for over 2400 years (8). It has shown promising results in the treatment of hematopoietic malignancies (9, 10). In year 2000, Food and Drug Administration (11) have approved arsenic trioxide (Trisenox^{TM}) for treatment of acute promyelocytic leukemia (APL) (12). Studies have shown that ATO was an effective therapeutic agent in APL with 63.8 to 93% high remission rate and could prolong patients' survival rate (13). A number of studies also have revealed a pro-apoptotic activity of ATO in solid tumors, including breast cancer, gastric cancer, hepatocellular carcinomas and sarcoma (14–17). Although ATO is able to improve the disease outcome, of note, ATO also introduces to common side effects such as gastrointestinal disorders, cough, fatigue, skin rash, myelosuppression and the most burden are the liver function failure and cardiac toxicity (18). Previous studies have revealed that ATO has been correlated to many anticancer mechanisms, such as promoting tumor cell differentiation, inhibition of tumor cell growth and induce cells apoptosis. ATO also shows to reduce chemo-resistance in tumor cells via inducing the apoptosis mechanism (19). ATO has been reported to induce partial differentiation and apoptosis in APL cells (20, 21). Although ATO anti-cancer activity has utterly studied in various solid tumors such as hepatocellular carcinoma (HCC), colorectal cancer (CRC), breast cancer and gliomas, it's only effective in APL treatment and less successful in other malignancies. Clinically, high dose of ATO is required to accomplish the anti-cancer activity in solid tumors in comparison with hematological malignancies (22). Instead of attempting on ATO single treatment, researchers are looking toward the combinatorial therapeutic regimen. It has been reported that ATO enhances the therapeutic efficacy of cisplatin treatment on both oral and ovarian cancers (23, 24). ATO treatment has been carried out in HNSCC (25, 26), however the results indicating that high doses of single ATO is required to eliminate the cancer cells. Impractical high doses usage of ATO will cause strong side effects in heart and vascular toxicity. Concerning these side effects, the combination regimens of ATO treatments are applied to various cancers (27).

ATO can induce autophagy cell death in various solid tumors (28). Autophagy is referred to an intracellular degradation system in cytoplasmic components and act as cytoprotective to overcome various stress condition. The interplay of autophagy and cancer is complicate and remain controversy. There are evidences implicating that autophagy may play a role as a tumor suppressor (29), while some suggest that it may promote tumorigenesis (30). Interestingly, our previous finding shows that YMGK-1 from *Antrodia cinnamomea* successfully eliminates HN-CICs via autophagy mediated cell death (31).

In this study, we performed a combinatorial low dose ATO/cisplatin (CDDP) treatment targeting the HN-CICs as well as HNSCC cisplatin-resistant cells (HNSCC-CisPt^R). We examined the cytotoxicity effects of low dose ATO/CDDP treatment both *in vitro* and *in vivo* assays. The experimental results revealed that the combinatorial of low dose ATO/CDDP treatment has a great potential to promote cell death in HN-CICs. In addition, we further investigated the cellular mechanism underlying ATO-base therapeutic regimen induced cell death. We found that ATO/CDDP not only induced cell differentiation but also exaggerated autophagy mediated cell death. The combinatorial low dose of ATO/CDDP treatment provided a potential therapeutic application, which can efficiently eradicate the HN-CICs.

MATERIALS AND METHODS

Cell Lines Cultivation and Enrichment of HN-CICs From HNSCCs

The oral cavity HNSCC cell lines, SAS obtained from Japanese Collection Research Bioresources (Tokyo, Japan), OECM1 provided by Prof. Ching-Liang Meng of National Defense Medical College, (Taipei, Taiwan) and SAS-CisPt^R cells were used in this study. SAS, SAS-CisPt^R and OECM1 cells were cultured in DMEM and RPMI supplemented with 10% FBS (GIBCO, Mexico), respectively (6, 7). The enrichment of HN-CICs were performed by cultivating both cell lines in tumor sphere condition medium consisting of serum-free DMEM/F12 medium (GIBCO, UK), N2 supplement (GIBCO, USA), 10 ng/mL human recombinant basic fibroblast growth factor (bFGF), and 10 ng/mL Epidermal Growth Factor (EGF) (PEPROTECH, USA). The cells were plated at a density of 7.5×10^4 live cells per 100 mm dishes as per experimental requirement. The cells were monitored and the medium was changed every other day until the tumor sphere cells were formed in about 4 weeks. All cells were cultured under the condition of 37°C with 5% CO_2 (6).

Western Blot

Protein extracts were prepared from cells by using RIPA buffer, and the protein concentration was measured by protein assay kit (Bio-Rad, USA). Protein extracts were denatured in sample buffer and subjected to SDS-PAGE gel electrophoresis. The electrophoretic proteins were then transferred to the nitrocellulose (NC) membrane. Nitrocellulose membranes were blocked in 5% skimmed milk and probed with primary antibodies. NC membrane were then washed and incubated with HRP-conjugated secondary anti-rabbit IgG or anti-mouse IgG at room temperature in TBST containing 5% milk for 1 h. After extensive washes in TBST, the signals were visualized by the enhanced chemiluminescence system as described by the manufacturer (Millipore, Germany) in conjunction with in LAS-4000 image analyzer (GE Healthcare, Japan). The immunoblotting signals from anti-Beta-actin (BA3R, Thermo Fisher Scientific, USA) or anti-GAPDH (GA1R, Thermo Fisher Scientific, USA) antibodies were used as a loading control.

Annexin V Apoptotic Assay

Apoptotic cells were detected with an Annexin V-FITC kit (Calbiochem, Darmstadt, Germany). 1×10^6 cells were stained with Annexin V–FITC and analyzed by FACS Calibur apparatus (Becton Dickinson, USA).

Anchorage Independent Growth Assay

Each well (35 mm) of a six-well culture dish was coated with 2 ml bottom agar (Sigma-Aldrich, USA) mixture [DMEM, 10% (v/v) FCS, 0.6% (w/v) agar]. After the bottom layer was solidified, 1 ml top agar-medium mixture [DMEM, 10% (v/v) FCS, 0.3% (w/v) agar] containing 1×10^4 cells with ATO or CDDP single treatment and ATO/CDDP combined treatment was added, and the dishes were incubated at 37°C for 15 days. The colonies were counted over five fields per well for 15 fields in triplicate experiments.

Subcutaneous Xenografts in Nude Mice

All the animal practices in this study were approved and treated in accordance with the Institutional Animal Care and Use Committee (IACUC No. 1020504) of National Yang-Ming University, Taipei, Taiwan. HN-CICs cells were subcutaneously injected into BALB/c nude mice (6–8 weeks). Tumor volume (TV) was calculated using the following formula: TV (cm^3) = (Length × Width ^{2})/2.

Inmmunohistochemistry

After deparaffinization and rehydration, the tissue sections were processed with antigen retrieval by boiling the slides in sodium citrate buffer (10 mM, pH 6.0). The slides were immersed in 3% H_2O_2 for 10 min and washed thrice with PBST. The tissue sections were then blocked with serum (Vestastain Elite ABC kit, Vector Laboratories, USA) for 30 min, followed by incubating with the primary antibody, in PBS solution at room temperature for 2 h in a container. Tissue slides were washed with PBS and incubated with biotin-labeled secondary antibody for 30 min, followed by 30 min streptavidin-horse radish peroxidase conjugates incubation. The slides were washed thrice with PBS. Subsequently, the tissue sections were immersed with AEC substrate kit as described by the manufacturer (Dako Corporation, USA) for 10 min. Hematoxylin was applied for counter-staining. Finally, the tumor sections were mounted with Gurr® (BDH Laboratory Supplies, U.K.) and examined under a microscope.

RESULTS

Combinatorial Low Dose ATO/CDDP Treatment Synergistically Promotes Cell Death in HN-CICs and Diminishes the Stemness Properties

In order to evaluate the anti-cancerous efficacy of low dose combinatorial treatment with ATO/CDDP, we performed the co-treatment on HN-CICs by combining different doses of ATO with different doses of conventional chemo-drug, CDDP. Annexin V/PI double staining was used to examine the apoptotic effects by ATO/CDDP co-treatment. The flow cytometry analyses indicated that the cell number of Annexin V/PI positive staining under the co-treatment of ATO/CDDP was substantially higher than that of HN-CICs with single treatment (**Figure 1A**). Cells treated with low dose of ATO (3 μM) in combination with 8 μM CDDP revealed strong cell death. These results indicate that low dose of combinatorial ATO/CDDP can promote cell death of HN-CICs. However, we found that co-treatment of ATO/CDDP did not cause cell death in normal human keratinocyte cells (NHOK) (**Supplementary 1**). In additional, either SAS-CICs or OECM1-CICs showed more resistant to ATO single treatment when compared with parental cell lines (data not shown). To determine the synergistic effects of the combinatorial ATO/CDDP treatment, we performed the Chou-Talalay's method analyses, and the combination index value (CI value) was calculated by using CompuSyn software. As shown in **Figure 1B** and **Table S1**, most of combinational regimens were reside on synergism sections (CI < 1). For the following experiments conducted we used the combinatorial ATO/CDDP dosages with synergism. Additionally, the protein level of stemness markers such as Nanog and Oct4 was downregulated in ATO/CDDP co-treated SAS derived HN-CICs (SAS-CICs) in comparison to that of the untreated cells or cisplatin/ATO single treated cells (**Figure 1C**). The above mentioned findings indicate that the stemness properties of SAS-CICs were abrogated after the ATO/CDDP combinatorial treatment.

ATO/CDDP Treatment Re-sensitizes the Cisplatin-Resistance Cell Line

As we have demonstrated that HN-CICs are more chemoresistant (7). Here, we would like to investigate whether combinatorial

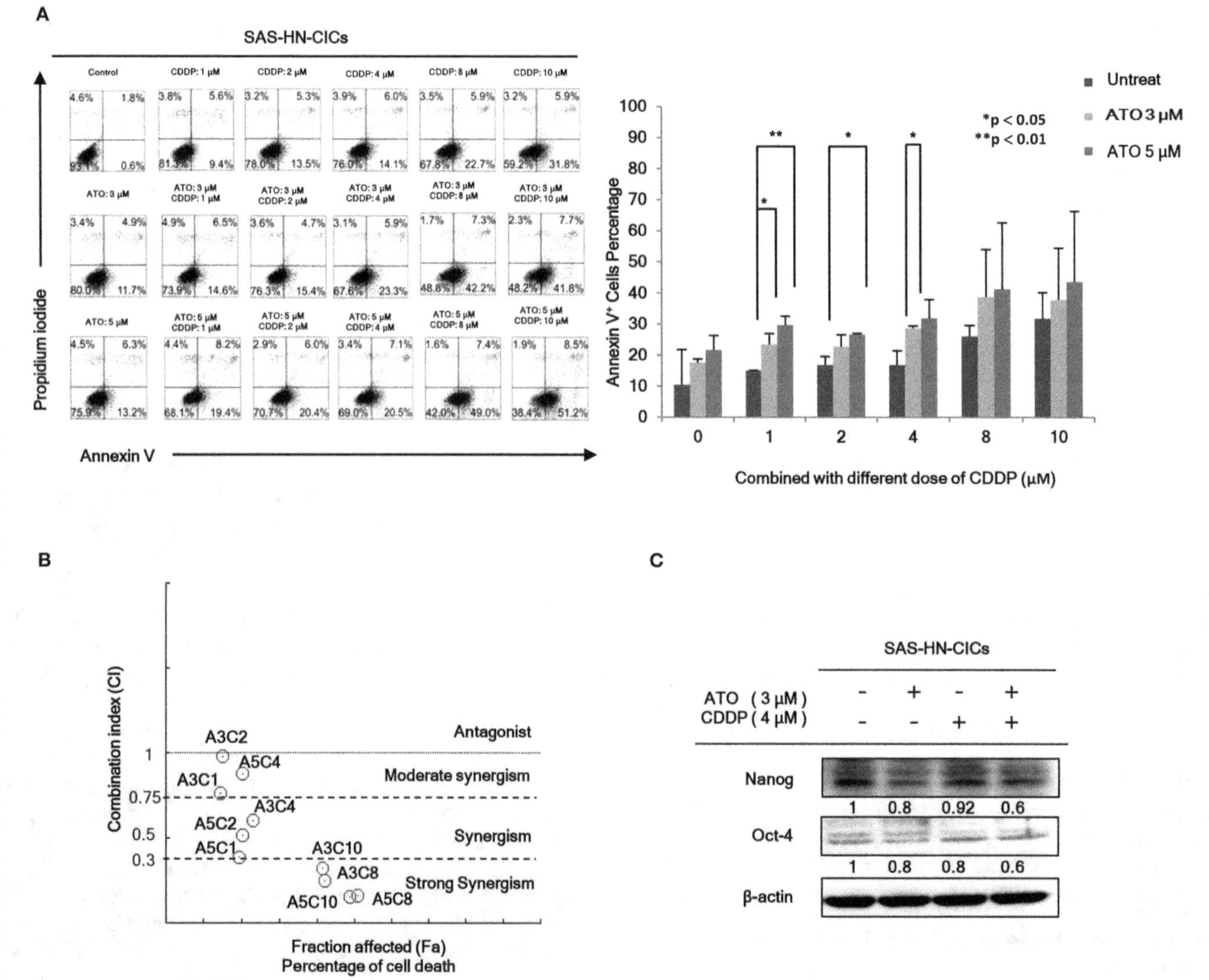

FIGURE 1 | Synergistic effect of combinatorial low dose ATO/CDDP treatment on promoting cell death and diminishing the stemness properties of HN-CICs. **(A)** HN-CICs treated with ATO/CDDP, ATO, and CDDP alone for 24 h, respectively. The cell death was examined by Annexin V/PI staining. Statistical analysis was performed by student's *t*-tests. $^*p < 0.05$ and $^{**}p < 0.01$. **(B)** Synergistic effect of combination ATO/CDDP on HN-CICs was calculated by using Chou–Talalay analysis. Different doses of combination ATO/CDDP treatment induced cell death of HN-CICs (percentage) and combination index (CI value), Y axis. Each point represents different doses of combination ATO/CDDP CI value. CI values were generated by using Compusyn Software, X axis indicates the effects (Fa, fractioned effected, % inhibition), and symbols represent CI values derived from actual data points (CI = 1, activity; CI > 1, antagonism; CI < 1, synergy). **(C)** Immunoblot assay to examine the expression of the stemness markers, Nanog and Oct-4, of HN-CICs after single or combined treatment of ATO (3 μM) or CDDP (4 μM) on HN-CICs for 48 h, respectively. β-actin signal was used as loading control.

low dose ATO/CDDP treatment can re-sensitize the chemo-resistant cells by co-treating the Cisplatin resistant SAS-CisPt^R cells (7) which possessing the HN-CICs characters with ATO/CDDP regimen. The combinatorial low dose ATO/CDDP treatment not only re-sensitized to CDDP but also induced cell death on the treated SAS-CisPt^R cells (**Figure 2A**). Consistent to SAS-CICs results, the stemness properties of SAS-CisPt^R cells were also diminished after the combined treatment with ATO/CDDP (**Figure 2B**).

ATO/CDDP Treatment Induces Autophagic Cell Death and Promotes Cell Differentiation in HN-CICs

According to our previous research, autophagy mediated cell death can be a major molecular mechanism to induce cell death in HN-CICs (31). In fact, the role of ATO in promoting cellular autophagy are reported in other cancer cell line (27). Initially, we found that the cell death numbers were increased when HN-CICs were treated with low dose ATO/CDDP through

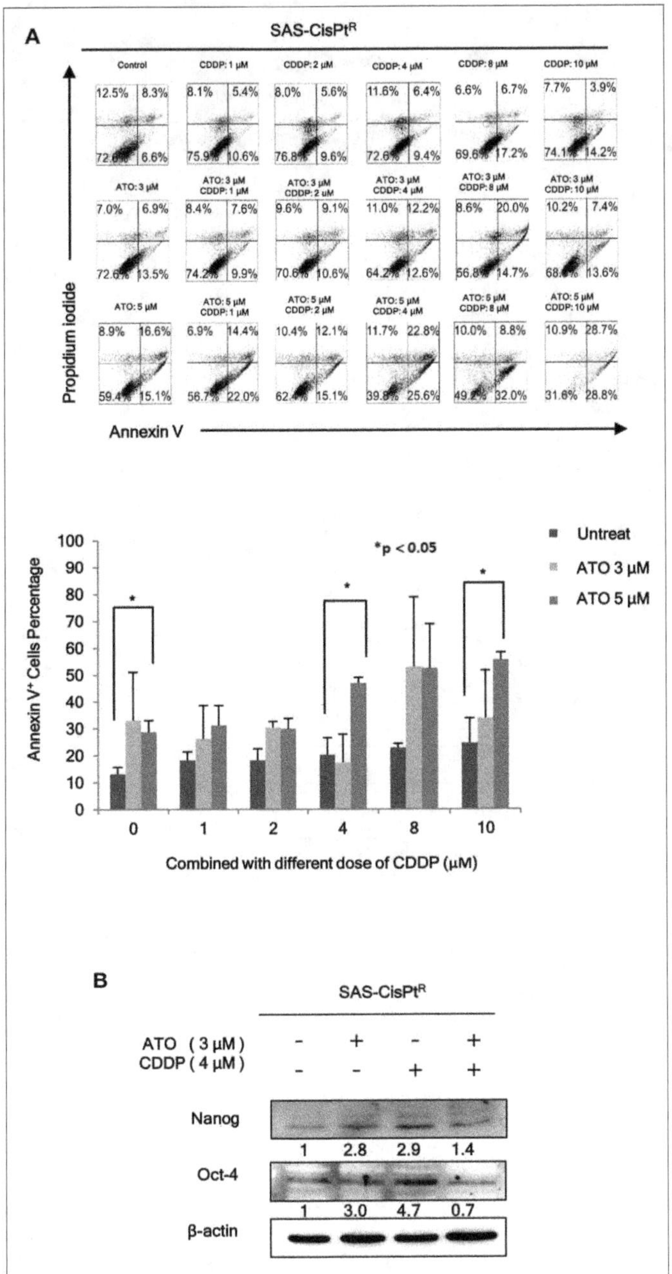

FIGURE 2 | Low dose ATO/CDDP co-treatment re-sensitizing the SAS-CisPt^R cells. **(A)** Cell death of the SAS-CisPt^R cells treated with single or combined ATO and CDDP for 24 h was examined by Annexin V/PI staining. Statistical analyses were performed by student's *t*-tests. $^*p < 0.05$. **(B)** Immunoblot analyses were used to detected the expression profile of stemness markers, Nanog and Oct-4, of SAS-CisPt^R cells after single or combined treatment of ATO (3 μM) or CDDP (4 μM), respectively. β-actin signal was used as loading control.

Annexin V/PI double staining analyses. However, this induced cell death caused by ATO/CDDP co-treatment was reversed when the autophagic cell death inhibitor, 3-Methyladenine (3-MA), was simultaneously co-treated (**Figure 3A**). Further, we determined the protein LC-3B I/II ratio, a autophagic marker, by immunoblotting assay (**Figure 3B**). ATO single treatment induced expression of autophagy marker, LC-3B-II. The expression of LC-3B-II was further elevated in cells under ATO/CDDP treatment, interestingly, addition of 3-MA also reversed the expression of LC-3B-II. Moreover, the expression of both apoptotic markers [poly (ADP ribose) polymerase (PARP1) and cleaved-caspase3] was also significantly increased, and this induction of apoptotic markers can be reversed by 3-MA co-treatment. We also observed the elevated protein level of the differentiation markers (cytokeratin 18 and involucrin) in ATO/CDDP combinatorial treated cells compared to the protein level of single treated or untreated cells (**Figure 3C**). Taken together, these results suggest that low dose of combinatorial ATO/CDDP promotes cell death by exaggerating autophagy to promote both cell apoptosis and differentiation.

Combinatorial Low Dose ATO/CDDP Suppresses the Malignancy of HN-CICs *in vitro* and *in vivo*

To further characterize the anti-cancerous effects of ATO/CDDP combined treatment in HN-CICs, we first performed anchorage independent growth assay. The colony number of the untreated cells was similar to that of the ATO or CDDP singly treated HN-CICs (**Figure 4A**). However, combined treatment with 2 or 4 μM ATO and CDDP significantly reduced the colony number (**Figure 4A**). These results indicate that low dose of ATO combined treatment with CDDP impairs malignancy and self-renewal ability of HN-CICs. To further elucidate the anti-cancerous growth effects of the combined treatment of ATO/CDDP *in vivo*, we used xenograft mouse models to analyze the attenuated tumorigeneity of HN-CICs by ATO/CDDP regimen treatment. Here, we carried out two animal models, the first one was administrated as the cancer preventive model (**Figure 4B**). To do so, the 8-week old nude mice were first subcutaneously injected with HN-CICs which were pre-treated with single or combined regimen of ATO/CDDP. The size of tumor generated from the pre-treated HN-CICs was measured continuously after cell inoculation (**Figure 4C**). We observed that HN-CICs under single treatment with ATO or CDDP did not significantly affect their tumor growth ability but delay the tumor initiating timing of HN-CICs during tumor formation. However, HN-CICs pretreated with ATO/CDDP regimen showed dramatic loss of tumor initiating ability. Secondly, we performed the cancer therapeutic model (**Figure 4D**). Nude mice were first injected with enriched HN-CICs. When mice bearing HN-CICs derived tumor, with primary tumor growing to around 0.1 cm^3, they were administrated with single ATO, CDDP or combinatorial regimen. In the therapeutic model, we found that the effect of cisplatin single treatment was similar to the placebo group on day 36 (**Figure 4E**). Additionally, ATO single treatment compared to CDDP single and placebo treatment showed an anti-cancerous effect but without the statistical significance. Unsurprisingly, we observed that the combined ATO/CDDP treatment had significant effect on inhibiting tumor growth. The above mentioned results implicate that combinatorial of low dose ATO/CDDP has a therapeutic potential on targeting

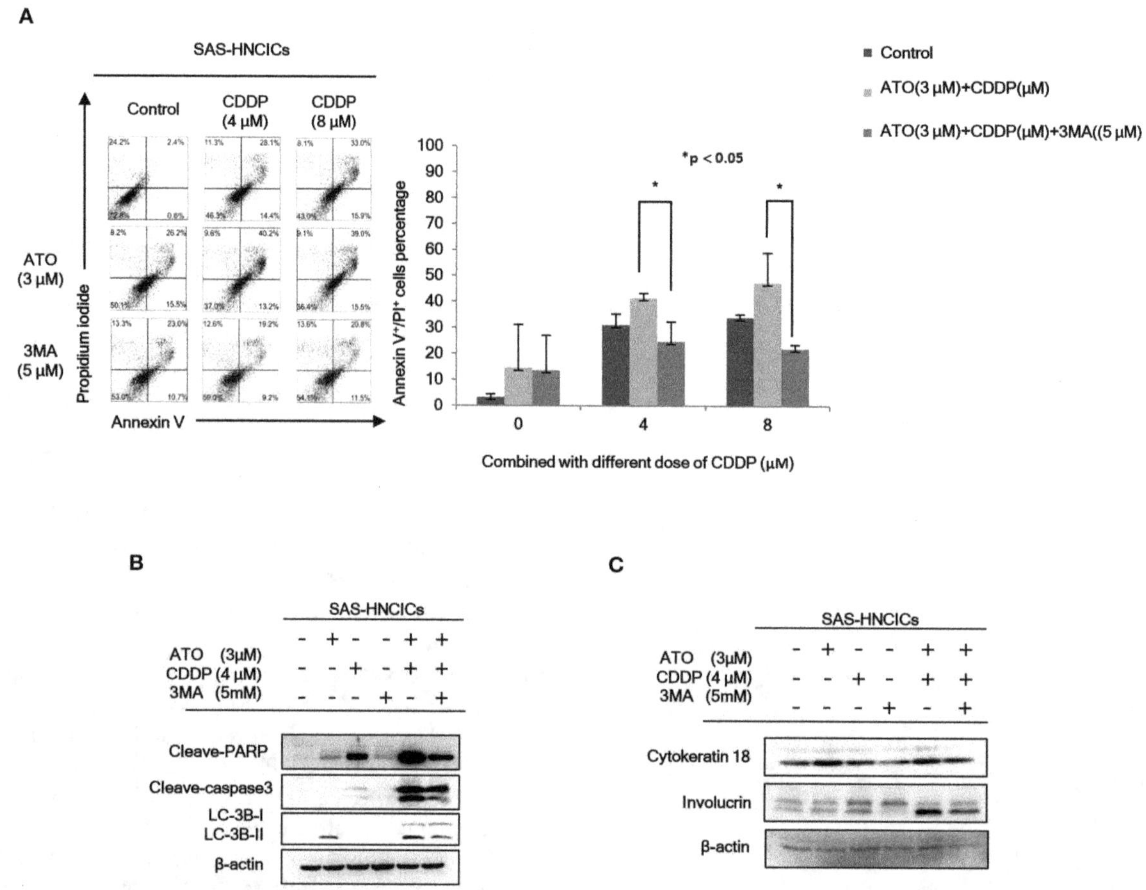

FIGURE 3 | Low dose ATO/CDDP co-treatment inducing autophagy and differentiation in HN-CICs. **(A)** SAS-CICs cells were treated with different doses of ATO, CDDP and/or 3-Methylamphetamine (3-MA) for 24 h and analyzed by annexin V/PI staining. The bar chart revealed the amount of Annexin V^+/PI^+ cells. **(B)** Immunoblot analyses indicated expression of autophagy related markers such as PARP, cleaved caspase3 and LC3B. **(C)** SAS-CICs cells were treated with single or combined treatment of ATO (3 μM), CDDP (4 μM), and/or 3-MA (5 mM) for 48 h. Immunoblot analyses were used to detected the expression profile of epithelial differentiation marker such as Cytokeratin 18 and Involucrin. β-actin signal was used as loading control. Statistical analyses were performed by student's *t*-tests. $^*p < 0.05$.

HN-CICs. To further verify the cell death response to drug treatment, we performed TUNEL assay to detect the dying cells of tumor mass with drug treatment (**Figure 4F**). The TUNEL signal was highly displayed in the combined ATO/CDDP administrated tumor sections. We also observed a strong cytokeratin 18 staining, and a mild decrease of NANOG signal on IHC staining of ATO/ CDDP combined treated tumor sections (**Figure 4G**). Taken together, the results suggest that low dose of ATO/CDDP therapy is able to suppress tumor growth by inducing cell death and abolishing cancer stemness in xenografted mouse model.

The Molecular Mechanisms of ATO-Based Therapeutic Regimen Promote Cell Death in HN-CICs

According to our previous studies, dysregulation of autophagy could be the main molecular mechanism to induce the cell death in HN-CICs (31, 32). Further, we showed that ATO/CDDP treatment induced autophagic cell death and promotes cell differentiation in HN-CICs. Hence, we first examined the autophagy signaling pathway to uncover this molecular mechanism whether it is dysregulated in inducing cell death by ATO/CDDP regimen treatment. When the combination treatment applied, we observed a decrease of phospho-PI3K and phospho-mTOR in both SAS-HNCICs (**Figure 5A**) and SAS-CisPt^R (**Figure 5C**) but not in OECM1-CICs by immunoblot analyses (**Figure 5B**). Additionally, the ATO/CDDP combined treatment suppressed the expression of phospho-STAT3 in SAS-CICs, OECM1-CICs, and SAS-CisPt^R. Interestingly, a significant elevation of p-AMPK was observed in these SAS-CICs, OECM1-CICs and SAS-CisPt^R cells under ATO/CDDP treatment. Together, the dysregulation of autophagy of HN-CICs are regulated through AMPK, STAT3 signaling pathways under ATO/CDDP treatment.

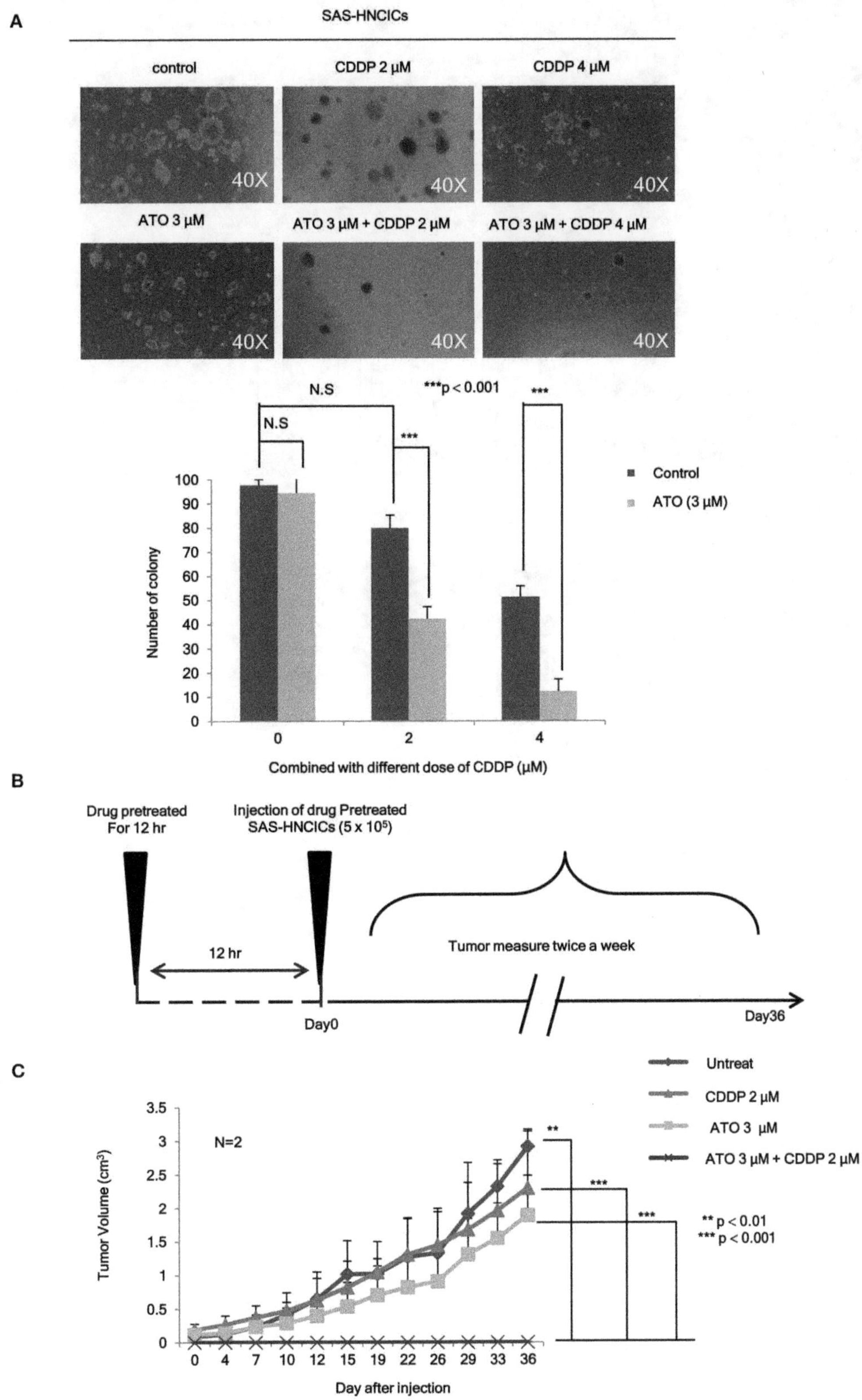

FIGURE 4 | Continued

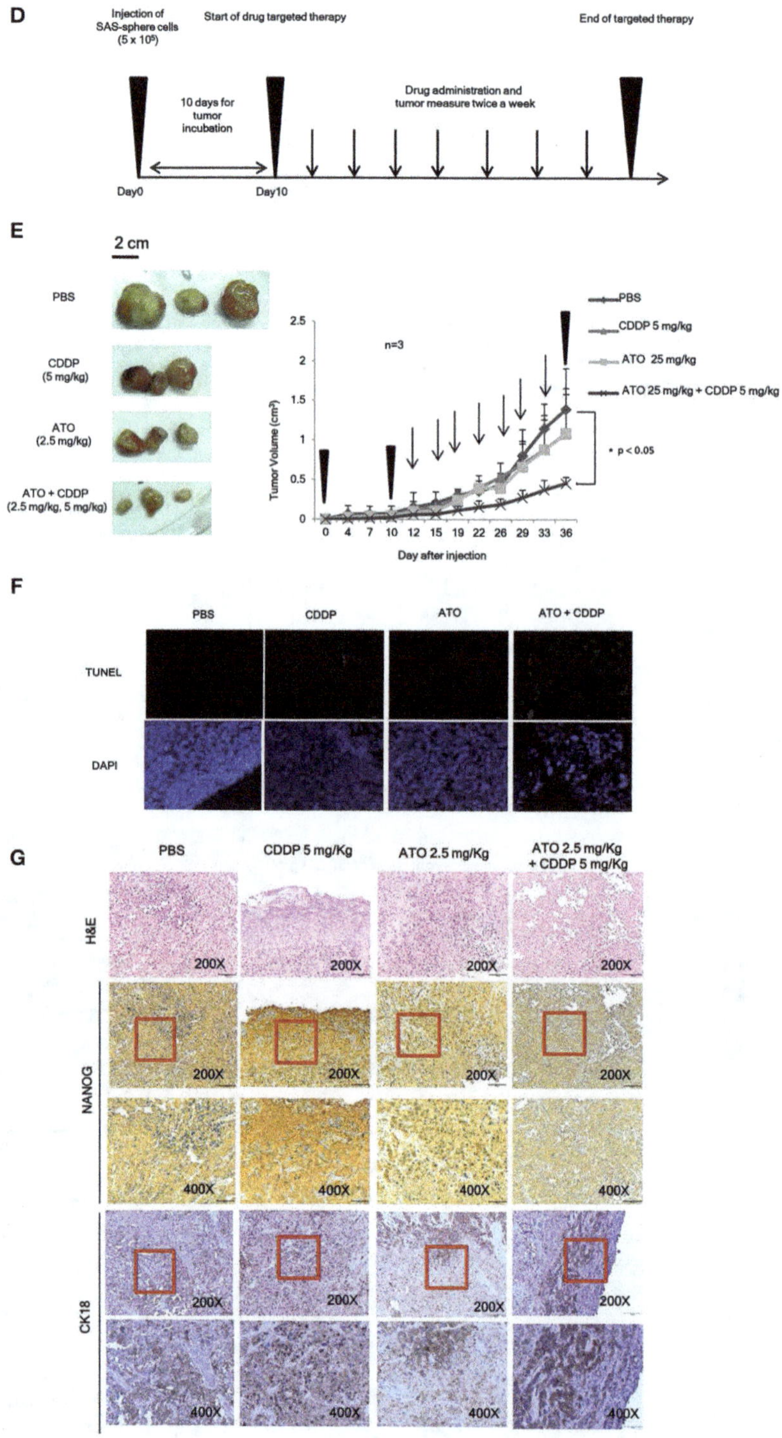

FIGURE 4 | Low dose ATO/CDDP treatment suppressing the malignancy of HN-CICs both *in vitro* and *in vivo*. **(A)** SAS-CICs cells were treated with single or combined treatment of ATO and CDDP for 12 h. The treated cells were then plated on soft agar for 15 days. The colony formation ability of the SAS-CICs cell under distinct condition was collected as shown in the representative images. The bar graphs showed the amounts of colonies with a diameter ≥ 100 μm over 5 fields per assay. The data are the mean ± SD from three independent experiments and analyzed by Student's *t*-test ($^*p < 0.05$). **(B)** The schematic of preventive model;

(Continued)

FIGURE 4 | SAS-CICs cells were singly or combinatorically pretreated with ATO (3 μM) and of CDDP (2 μM) for 12 h. These cells were subcutaneously injected into the back of nude mice. **(C)** The tumor growth generated from the treated SAS-CICs cells was recorded and analyzed. **(D)** The schematic of therapeutic model was used to demonstrate the anti-tumorous ability of low doses ATO/CDDP regimen. SAS-CICs cells were first subcutaneously inoculated onto the back of nude mice. When the tumor size reached around 0.1 cm^3, ATO (2.5 mg/kg) and CDDP (5 mg/kg) were either singly or combinatorically intraperitoneal injected into the nude mice. PBS was used as placebo. **(E)** The mice were sacrificed on day 36, and the images of the generated tumors were collected. Tumor growth curves were also recorded and analyzed. **(F)** TUNEL assay was performed to analyze the cell death among the collected xenograft tumors. DAPI dye was used as counter staining. **(G)** Xenograft tumors generated from SAS-CICs cells treated with ATO/CDDP regimen were collected. Subsequently, immunohistochemistry staining was performed to detect the expression of stemness marker (Nanog) and differentiation marker (CK18). H&E; hematoxylin and eosin stain.

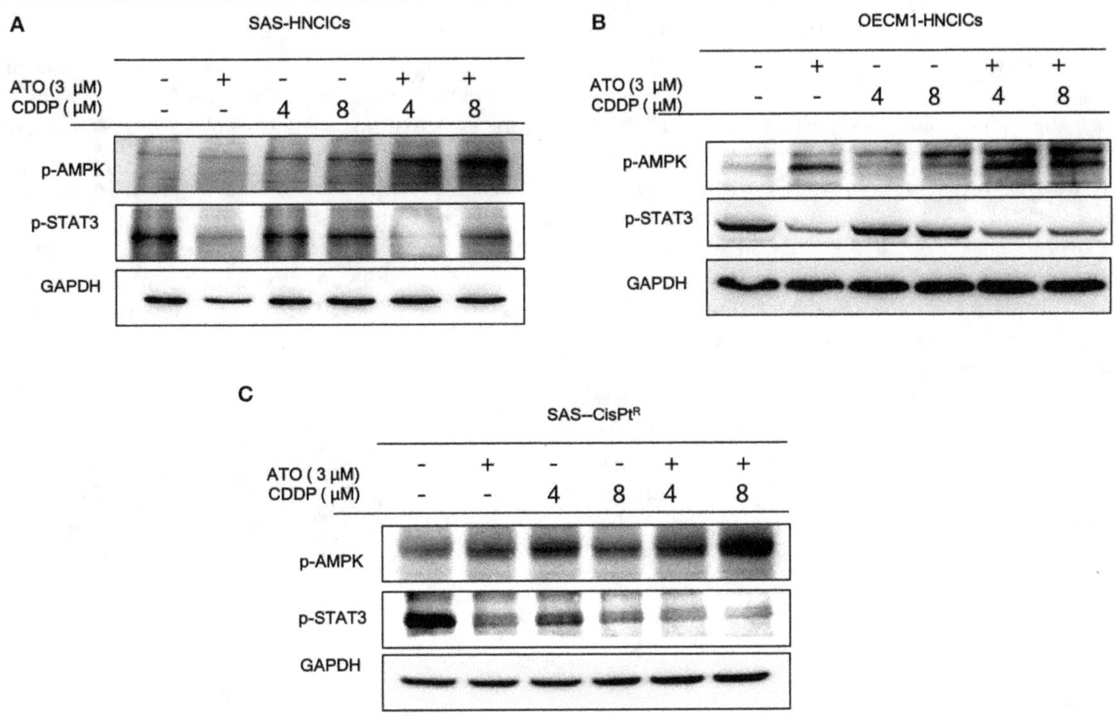

FIGURE 5 | The molecular targets of ATO/CDDP regimen. **(A)** SAS-CICs, **(B)** OECM1-CICs, and **(C)** SAS-CisPtR administrated with single or combined treatment of ATO and CDDP treated were harvested and analyzed by immunoblot assay by targeting the cancerous related molecules, p-AMPK and p-STAT3. GAPDH was used as loading control.

DISCUSSION

Arsenic trioxide is well-known of its anti-cancer activity to treat acute promyelocytic leukemia (APL) patients (33). In previous studies, 0.16 mg/kg/day ATO is administered to APL patient; the treatment course takes about 6 weeks and the dosage of ATO is nearly 6–8 μM in the plasma (34). In the conventional ATO therapy, it requires a high dose to induce the apoptotic effect. In this study, we have successfully demonstrated a low dose of combinatorial ATO/CDDP treatment synergistically induced the exaggerated autophagy mediated cell death in HN-CICs. The CI analysis indicates that the combinatorial effect of ATO/CDDP exhibits a wide range of synergism (CI < 1) in HN-CICs, ranging from 0.15 to 0.98. Further, we found that the low dose ATO (3 μM) combined with 4 μM cisplatin effectively induced apoptotic cell death in HN-CICs (**Figure 1A**). This combinational regimen also inhibited the HN-CICs self-renewal ability. Importantly, we observed the inhibitory tumorigenicity of HN-CICs in the therapeutic nude mice model *in vivo* which was administrated with low dose ATO/CDDP. Moreover, the combinatorial low doses of both ATO and CDDP in our study were effective even in the cisplatin-resistant cells.

HNSCC patients are still facing the relapse after therapy (35). This may due to the conventional treatments cannot efficiently eliminate CICs, which are involved in the tumor progression, metastasis, and chemo/radio resistance (36). Recent clinical studies showed that conventional chemotherapeutics generally affect proliferative cells, potentially eliminate proliferating cancer cells but not targeting the slow dividing cells CICs (37). CICs have exhibited quiescent slow-cycling phenotype and have been shown to be involved in tumor progression, cancer recurrence and metastasis because of their therapeutic resistance (31, 38). Thus, in this study we focused on ATO/CDDP combinatorial therapy targeting the HN-CICs. This ATO-based therapeutic regimen seems to promote the HN-CICs differentiation (**Figures 3C, 4G**) as we observed the enhanced expression of differentiation markers Cytokeratin 18 and Involucrin. It has been reported, ATO can diminish stemness properties in leukemia or hepatocellular carcinoma derived cancer initiating cells (39, 40). In addition, Tomuleasa et al. have reported that low concentration of ATO lead to differentiation in glioblastoma multiforme (GBM) stem-like cells (41). Cisplatin is a standard therapeutic agent of HNSCC through specifically targeting highly proliferation cells (2, 11, 42). Indeed, cumulative evidence suggested CDDP could not suppress the high stemness properties of cancer cells. Together, the combinatorial low dose ATO/CDDP regimen seems to facilitate HN-CICs differentiation into highly proliferated cells and subsequently underwent cell apoptosis.

We observed the induced autophagy when the ATO/CDDP was applied to HN-CICs. The expression of LC3 II (**Figure 3B**), a well-known marker for autophagy, was enhanced in this combinatorial treated HN-CICs. Similar results are seen in our early discovery that exaggerated induction of autophagy abolishes the stemness properties of HN-CICs, in the mean times, loss of stemness properties of HN-CICs can promote the cell differentiation ability (31). During the cancer progression and metastasis stage, autophagy emerges as a pro-tumoral role in order to eliminate the ROS-induced metabolic stress (43, 44). Intriguingly, we observed a consistency of up-regulation of p-AMPK in combinatorial treated cells. AMPK is a conserve energy-sensing kinase. AMPK is activated in response to metabolic stress and shortage of energy. Once activated, AMPK globally promotes catabolic processes. In accordance, AMPK has be linked to the regulation of autophagy (45, 46). Here, we showed that the activation of AMPK seems to increase the autophagic flux in ATO/CDDP treated cells (**Figure 5**). In this case, the excessive autophagy in these treated cells reverse the protective role of pro-tumoral but promoting the CICs to undergo autophagic cell death.

Another crucial issue of current HNSCC therapeutic is an emerging of drug resistance. This is most likely due to the existence of CICs which are resistant to chemo-drugs. Our previous publications (7, 32) have demonstrated that CDDP-resistance cells (SAS-CisPt^{R}) consist of highly stemness properties. The combination of ATO/CDDP regimen synergistically induced cell death in SAS-CisPt^{R} cells (**Figure 2A**). Although the dose used to diminish the SAS-CisPt^{R} cell lines was higher than the dose used in HN-CICs, the dosage is relatively lower than clinical administrated dosage. The anti-tumorous effect of the combined ATO/CDDP treatment to ovarian cancer (24) or oral squamous cell carcinoma (OSCC) (23) has been studied by others. However, the used dose of ATO/CDDP is higher than that in our current study. Furthermore, we had successfully eradicated both the HN-CICs and SAS-CisPtR cells by using low dose of ATO/CDDP regimen.

Cisplatin induced drug resistance effects are connected with mTOR signaling up-regulated (47). Our results also revealed that the treatment of ATO/CDDP in HN-CICs could reverse the cisplatin induced mTOR upregulation in SAS-CICs and OECM1-CICs (**Figure 5**). Phosphatidylinositol 3-kinase (PI3K)/mammalian target of rapamycin (mTOR) pathway is a well-known signaling for controlling cell survival through autophagy regelation. This crucial survival pathway can affect cells proliferation, angiogenesis, metabolism, and differentiation. Interesting, our result revealed that the phosphorylated PI3K expression only suppressed in SAS derived HN-CICs and SAS-CisP^{R} but not in OECM1-CICs under ATO/CDDP regimen treatment. This may refer to the conversed sensitivity of PI3K between SAS-CICs and OECM1-CICs. In other autophagy inhibitor study also perform different PI3K effects during their drug treatment (48). Together, the upstream of mTOR signal may not derive from PI3K in OECM1 cells. Finally, SAS-CisPt^{R} cells did not decrease mTOR under ATO/CDDP treatment. However, PI3K signaling is becoming more sensitive in CDDP single and ATO/CDDP combined treatment in this resistance line. This phenotype may refer to drug-resistance of SAS-CisPt^{R} cells. To overcome cisplatin cytotoxicity, this cell line obtained other mTOR upstream signaling to maintain cell survive but not derived fromPI3K. However, we still can successfully promote cell death in these cells via ATO/CDDP treatment (**Figure 2**). The PI3K/mTOR

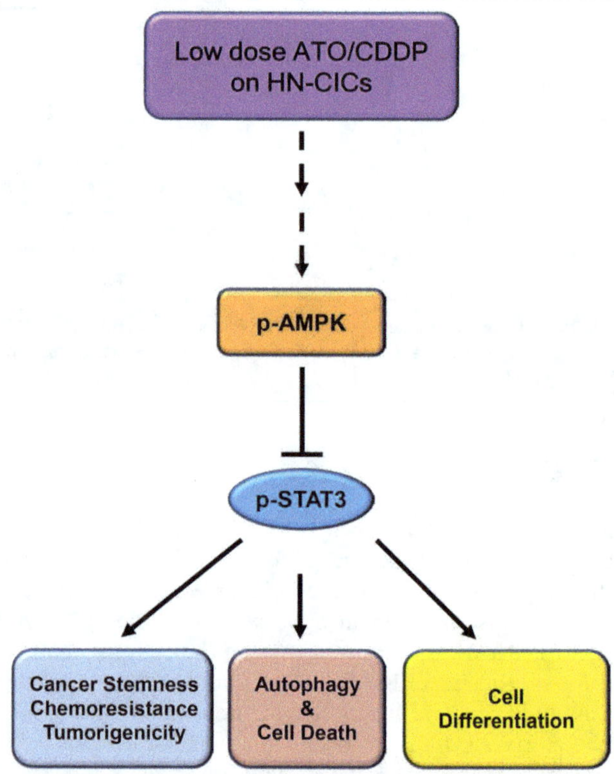

FIGURE 6 | Schematic of molecular signaling targeted by low dose ATO/CDDP regimen. Overall, the low dose ATO/CDDP regimen diminishes the stemness properties, and promotes cell differentiation in HN-CICs. Exaggerated autophagy mediated cell death is induced by the low dose ATO/CDDP regimen to inhibit the tumorigenicity of HN-CICs. Tumor suppressor AMPK expression increased may participate in this molecular mechanism regulation. However, this therapeutic regimen direct or indirect targets are still unknown; (----) refers to unknown relationship or factors.

is shown in dysregulation pathway in various cancer cells (49). Recently in glioblastoma stem-like cells research, mTOR pathway is link to the self-renewal ability and tumorigenicity of CICs. In addition, cellular key energy sensor kinase AMP activated protein (AMPK) was reported that it could promote autophagy by mTOR inactivation. In our data also suggested ATO-based therapeutic regimen can induced AMPK activity.

High concentrations of ATO can activate Jun N-terminal kinase (JNK) (50). In addition, in adipocyte study that JNK/STAT3 signaling can be suppressed by AMPK (51). In breast CICs study, STAT3 has been suggested as a specific marker, which can mediate the Nanog regulation. In our previous publication, YMGKI-2 showed to restore the chemosensitivity and promoting differentiation in CICs through targeting the Src/STAT3/c-Myc pathway (31, 32). Taken together, these evidences support that STAT3 play a critical role in HN-CICs. STAT3 signaling is constitutively activated in various cancer types (32, 52, 53). Its diverse pro-tumoral role has been widely reported. Thus, STAT3 signaling has been chosen as cancer therapeutic target. STAT3 has been proposed as CDDP sensitivity converse key factor (54). There are reports showing some potential molecules could affect the JAK-STAT3 cancerous pathway (55) to promote cell apoptosis effects. Fascinatingly, our data revealed the ATO single treatment, or ATO combined with CDDP could significantly block STAT3 activity in HN-CICs.

CONCLUSION

Overall, the low dose combinatorial treatment of ATO/CDDP provokes a synergistic cell death effect in both HN-CICs and SAS-CisPt^R cells. Although the proposed dosage is lower than the clinical dosage, it could effectively diminish the HN-CICs. Strikingly, with this low dose combinatorial ATO/CDDP, we showed either both *in vitro* and *in vivo* study, the tumorigenesis was inhibited. Finally, the ATO/CDDP treated HN-CICs and/or SAS-CisPt^R cells underwent cell differentiation, autophagy, and cell death might through the activation of p-AMPK and inhibition of STAT3 signaling pathway (**Figure 6**).

ETHICS STATEMENT

The animal study was reviewed and approved by All the experimental procedures regarding animal handling were approved by the Institutional Animal Care and Use Committee (IACUC) of the National Yang-Ming University (IACUC No. 1020504).

AUTHOR CONTRIBUTIONS

W-CH, W-HT, and J-FL: study design and manuscript drafting. W-CH and W-HT: experimental work. T-FH, T-CL, and J-FL: reviewed the manuscript and discussed results.

REFERENCES

1. Jemal A, Bray F, Center MM, Ferlay J, Ward E, Forman D. Global cancer statistics. *CA Cancer J Clin.* (2011) 61:69–90. doi: 10.3322/caac.20107
2. Leemans CR, Braakhuis BJ, Brakenhoff RH. The molecular biology of head and neck cancer. *Nat Rev Cancer.* (2011) 11:9–22. doi: 10.1038/nrc2982
3. De Angelis ML, Francescangeli F, La Torre F, Zeuner A. Stem cell plasticity and dormancy in the development of cancer therapy resistance. *Front Oncol.* (2019) 9:626. doi: 10.3389/fonc.2019.00626
4. Baillie R, Tan ST, Itinteang T. Cancer stem cells in oral cavity squamous cell carcinoma: a review. *Front Oncol.* (2017) 7:112. doi: 10.3389/fonc.2017.00112
5. McCubrey JA, Chappell WH, Abrams SL, Franklin RA, Long JM, Sattler JA, et al. Targeting the cancer initiating cell: the Achilles' heel of cancer. *Adv Enzyme Regul.* (2011) 51:152–62. doi: 10.1016/j.advenzreg.2010.09.002
6. Chiou SH, Yu CC, Huang CY, Lin SC, Liu CJ, Tsai TH, et al. Positive correlations of Oct-4 and Nanog in oral cancer stem-like cells and high-grade oral squamous cell carcinoma. *Clin Cancer Res.* (2008) 14:4085–95. doi: 10.1158/1078-0432.CCR-07-4404
7. Chang CW, Chen YS, Chou SH, Han CL, Chen YJ, Yang CC, et al. Distinct subpopulations of head and neck cancer cells with different levels of intracellular reactive oxygen species exhibit diverse stemness, proliferation, and chemosensitivity. *Cancer Res.* (2014) 74:6291–305. doi: 10.1158/0008-5472.CAN-14-0626
8. Rao Y, Li R, Zhang D. A drug from poison: how the therapeutic effect of arsenic trioxide on acute promyelocytic leukemia was discovered. *Sci China Life Sci.* (2013) 56:495–502. doi: 10.1007/s11427-013-4487-z
9. Au WY, Li CK, Lee V, Yuen HL, Yau J, Chan GC, et al. Oral arsenic trioxide for relapsed acute promyelocytic leukemia in pediatric patients. *Pediatr Blood Cancer.* (2012) 58:630–2. doi: 10.1002/pbc.23306
10. Carney DA. Arsenic trioxide mechanisms of action–looking beyond acute promyelocytic leukemia. *Leuk Lymph.* (2008) 49:1846–51. doi: 10.1080/10428190802464745
11. Safdari Y, Khalili M, Farajnia S, Asgharzadeh M, Yazdani Y, Sadeghi M. Recent advances in head and neck squamous cell carcinoma–a review. *Clin Biochem.* (2014) 47:1195–202. doi: 10.1016/j.clinbiochem.2014.05.066
12. Lengfelder E, Hofmann WK, Nowak D. Impact of arsenic trioxide in the treatment of acute promyelocytic leukemia. *Leukemia.* (2012) 26:433–42. doi: 10.1038/leu.2011.245
13. Kitamura K, Kiyoi H, Yoshida H, Tobita T, Takeshita A, Ohno R, et al. New retinoids and arsenic compounds for the treatment of refractory acute

promyelocytic leukemia: clinical and basic studies for the next generation. *Cancer Chemother Pharmacol.* (1997) 40:S36–41.
14. Zhang YC, Zhou YQ, Yan B, Shi J, Xiu LJ, Sun YW, et al. Secondary acute promyelocytic leukemia following chemotherapy for gastric cancer: a case report. *World J Gastroenterol.* (2015) 21:4402–7. doi: 10.3748/wjg.v21.i14.4402
15. Wang Y, Wang L, Yin C, An B, Hao Y, Wei T, et al. Arsenic trioxide inhibits breast cancer cell growth via microRNA-328/hERG pathway in MCF-7 cells. *Mol Med Rep.* (2015) 12:1233–8. doi: 10.3892/mmr.2015.3558
16. Luo Q, Li Y, Lai Y, Zhang Z. The role of NF-kappaB in PARP-inhibitor-mediated sensitization and detoxification of arsenic trioxide in hepatocellular carcinoma cells. *J Toxicol Sci.* (2015) 40:349–63. doi: 10.2131/jts.40.349
17. Chiu HW, Tseng YC, Hsu YH, Lin YF, Foo NP, Guo HR, et al. Arsenic trioxide induces programmed cell death through stimulation of ER stress and inhibition of the ubiquitin-proteasome system in human sarcoma cells. *Cancer Lett.* (2015) 356(Pt. B):762–72. doi: 10.1016/j.canlet.2014.10.025
18. Soignet SL, Frankel SR, Douer D, Tallman MS, Kantarjian H, Calleja E, et al. United States multicenter study of arsenic trioxide in relapsed acute promyelocytic leukemia. *J Clin Oncol.* (2001) 19:3852–60. doi: 10.1200/JCO.2001.19.18.3852
19. Zhai B, Jiang X, He C, Zhao D, Ma L, Xu L, et al. Arsenic trioxide potentiates the anti-cancer activities of sorafenib against hepatocellular carcinoma by inhibiting Akt activation. *Tumour Biol.* (2015) 36:2323–34. doi: 10.1007/s13277-014-2839-3
20. Soignet SL, Maslak P, Wang ZG, Jhanwar S, Calleja E, Dardashti LJ, et al. Complete remission after treatment of acute promyelocytic leukemia with arsenic trioxide. *N Engl J Med.* (1998) 339:1341–8. doi: 10.1056/NEJM199811053391901
21. Gianni M, Koken MH, Chelbi-Alix MK, Benoit G, Lanotte M, Chen Z, et al. Combined arsenic and retinoic acid treatment enhances differentiation and apoptosis in arsenic-resistant NB4 cells. *Blood.* (1998) 91:4300–10.
22. Subbarayan PR, Ardalan B. In the war against solid tumors arsenic trioxide needs partners. *J Gastrointest Cancer.* (2014) 45:363–71. doi: 10.1007/s12029-014-9617-8
23. Nakaoka T, Ota A, Ono T, Karnan S, Konishi H, Furuhashi A, et al. Combined arsenic trioxide-cisplatin treatment enhances apoptosis in oral squamous cell carcinoma cells. *Cell Oncol.* (2014) 37:119–29. doi: 10.1007/s13402-014-0167-7
24. Zhang N, Wu ZM, McGowan E, Shi J, Hong ZB, Ding CW, et al. Arsenic trioxide and cisplatin synergism increase cytotoxicity in human ovarian cancer cells: therapeutic potential for ovarian cancer. *Cancer Sci.* (2009) 100:2459–64. doi: 10.1111/j.1349-7006.2009.01340.x
25. Seol JG, Park WH, Kim ES, Jung CW, Hyun JM, Kim BK, et al. Effect of arsenic trioxide on cell cycle arrest in head and neck cancer cell line PCI-1. *Biochem Biophys Res Commun.* (1999) 265:400–4. doi: 10.1006/bbrc.1999.1697
26. Kotowski U, Heiduschka G, Brunner M, Erovic BM, Martinek H, Thurnher D. Arsenic trioxide enhances the cytotoxic effect of cisplatin in head and neck squamous cell carcinoma cell lines. *Oncol Lett.* (2012) 3:1326–30. doi: 10.3892/ol.2012.643
27. Pastorek M, Gronesova P, Cholujova D, Hunakova L, Bujnakova Z, Balaz P, et al. Realgar. (As4S4) nanoparticles and arsenic trioxide. (As2O3) induced autophagy and apoptosis in human melanoma cells *in vitro*. *Neoplasma.* (2014) 61:700–9. doi: 10.4149/neo_2014_085
28. Toepfer N, Childress C, Parikh A, Rukstalis D, Yang W. Atorvastatin induces autophagy in prostate cancer PC3 cells through activation of LC3 transcription. *Cancer Biology Ther.* (2011) 12:691–9. doi: 10.4161/cbt.12.8.15978
29. Zeng X, Kinsella TJ. Impact of autophagy on chemotherapy and radiotherapy mediated tumor cytotoxicity: "To Live or not to Live". *Front Oncol.* (2011) 1:30. doi: 10.3389/fonc.2011.00030
30. Perera RM, Stoykova S, Nicolay BN, Ross KN, Fitamant J, Boukhali M, et al. Transcriptional control of autophagy-lysosome function drives pancreatic cancer metabolism. *Nature.* (2015) 524:361–5. doi: 10.1038/nature 14587
31. Chang C-W, Chen C-C, Wu M-J, Chen Y-S, Chen C-C, Sheu S-J, et al. Active component of *Antrodia cinnamomea* mycelia targeting head and neck cancer initiating cells through exaggerated autophagic cell death. *Evid Based Complement Altern Med.* (2013) 2013:946451. doi: 10.1155/2013/946451
32. Chang CW, Chen YS, Chen CC, Chan IO, Chen CC, Sheu SJ, et al. Targeting cancer initiating cells by promoting cell differentiation and restoring chemosensitivity via dual inactivation of STAT3 and src activity using an active component of antrodia cinnamomea mycelia. *Oncotarget.* (2016) 7:73016–31. doi: 10.18632/oncotarget.12194
33. Mi JQ, Chen SJ, Zhou GB, Yan XJ, Chen Z. Synergistic targeted therapy for acute promyelocytic leukaemia: a model of translational research in human cancer. *J Intern Med.* (2015) 278:627–42. doi: 10.1111/joim. 12376
34. Shen ZX, Chen GQ, Ni JH, Li XS, Xiong SM, Qiu QY, et al. Use of arsenic trioxide. (As2O3) in the treatment of acute promyelocytic leukemia (APL): II. Clinical efficacy and pharmacokinetics in relapsed patients. *Blood.* (1997) 89:3354–60.
35. Siegel RL, Miller KD, Jemal A. Cancer statistics, 2015. *CA Cancer J Clin.* (2015) 65:5–29. doi: 10.3322/caac.21254
36. Frank NY, Schatton T, Frank MH. The therapeutic promise of the cancer stem cell concept. *J Clin Invest.* (2010) 120:41–50. doi: 10.1172/JCI41004
37. Moore N, Lyle S. Quiescent, slow-cycling stem cell populations in cancer: a review of the evidence and discussion of significance. *J Oncol.* (2011) 2011:396076. doi: 10.1155/2011/3 96076
38. Koukourakis MI, Giatromanolaki A, Tsakmaki V, Danielidis V, Sivridis E. Cancer stem cell phenotype relates to radio-chemotherapy outcome in locally advanced squamous cell head-neck cancer. *Br J Cancer.* (2012) 106:846–53. doi: 10.1038/bjc.2012.33
39. Ito K, Bernardi R, Morotti A, Matsuoka S, Saglio G, Ikeda Y, et al. PML targeting eradicates quiescent leukaemia-initiating cells. *Nature.* (2008) 453:1072–8. doi: 10.1038/nature 07016
40. Li L, Liu Y, Guo Y, Liu B, Zhao Y, Li P, et al. Regulatory MiR-148a-ACVR1/BMP circuit defines a cancer stem cell-like aggressive subtype of hepatocellular carcinoma. *Hepatology.* (2015) 61:574–84. doi: 10.1002/hep.27543
41. Tomuleasa C, Soritau O, Kacso G, Fischer-Fodor E, Cocis A, Ioani H, et al. Arsenic trioxide sensitizes cancer stem cells to chemoradiotherapy. A new approach in the treatment of inoperable glioblastoma multiforme. *J BUON.* (2010) 15:758–62.
42. Li H, Zhu X, Zhang Y, Xiang J, Chen H. Arsenic trioxide exerts synergistic effects with cisplatin on non-small cell lung cancer cells via apoptosis induction. *J Exp Clin Cancer Res.* (2009) 28:110. doi: 10.1186/1756-9966-28-110
43. Guo JY, Chen H-Y, Mathew R, Fan J, Strohecker AM, Karsli-Uzunbas G, et al. Activated Ras requires autophagy to maintain oxidative metabolism and tumorigenesis. *Genes Dev.* (2011) 25:460–70. doi: 10.1101/gad.2016311
44. Guo JY, Karsli-Uzunbas G, Mathew R, Aisner SC, Kamphorst JJ, Strohecker AM, et al. Autophagy suppresses progression of K-ras-induced lung tumors to oncocytomas and maintains lipid homeostasis. *Genes Dev.* (2013) 27:1447–61. doi: 10.1101/gad.219642.113
45. Luo Z, Zang M, Guo W. AMPK as a metabolic tumor suppressor: control of metabolism and cell growth. *Fut Oncol.* (2010) 6:457–70. doi: 10.2217/fon.09.174
46. Sanli T, Steinberg GR, Singh G, Tsakiridis T. AMP-activated protein kinase (AMPK) beyond metabolism: a novel genomic stress sensor participating in the DNA damage response pathway. *Cancer Biol Ther.* (2014) 15:156–69. doi: 10.4161/cbt.26726
47. Yang H, Gao Y, Fan X, Liu X, Peng L, Ci X. Oridonin sensitizes cisplatin-induced apoptosis via AMPK/Akt/mTOR-dependent autophagosome accumulation in A549 cells. *Front Oncol.* (2019) 9:769. doi: 10.3389/fonc.2019.00769
48. Cheng MF, Lin SR, Tseng FJ, Huang YC, Tsai MJ, Fu YS, et al. The autophagic inhibition oral squamous cell carcinoma cancer growth of 16-hydroxy-cleroda-3,14-dine-15,16-olide. *Oncotarget.* (2017) 8:78379–96. doi: 10.18632/oncotarget. 18987
49. Zhou J, Wulfkuhle J, Zhang H, Gu P, Yang Y, Deng J, et al. Activation of the PTEN/mTOR/STAT3 pathway in breast cancer stem-like cells is required for viability and maintenance. *Proc Natl Acad Sci USA.* (2007) 104:16 158–63. doi: 10.1073/pnas.0702596104

50. Wen J, Cheng HY, Feng Y, Rice L, Liu S, Mo A, et al. P38 MAPK inhibition enhancing ATO-induced cytotoxicity against multiple myeloma cells. *Br J Haematol.* (2008) 140:169–80. doi: 10.1111/j.1365-2141.2007.06895.x
51. Mancini SJ, White AD, Bijland S, Rutherford C, Graham D, Richter EA, et al. Activation of AMP-activated protein kinase rapidly suppresses multiple pro-inflammatory pathways in adipocytes including IL-1 receptor-associated kinase-4 phosphorylation. *Mol Cell Endocrinol.* (2017) 440:44–56. doi: 10.1016/j.mce.2016.11.010
52. Chang L, Gong F, Cai H, Li Z, Cui Y. Combined RNAi targeting human Stat3 and ADAM9 as gene therapy for non-small cell lung cancer. *Oncol Lett.* (2016) 11:1242–50. doi: 10.3892/ol.2015.4018
53. Zheng M, Cao MX, Yu XH, Li L, Wang K, Wang SS, et al. STAT3 Promotes invasion and aerobic glycolysis of human oral squamous cell carcinoma via inhibiting FoxO1. *Front Oncol.* (2019) 9:1175. doi: 10.3389/fonc.2019.01175
54. Fang L, Gao L, Xie L, Xiao G. GC7 enhances cisplatin sensitivity via STAT3 signaling pathway inhibition and eIF5A2 inactivation in mesenchymal phenotype oral cancer cells. *Oncol Rep.* (2018) 39:1283–91. doi: 10.3892/or.2017.6161
55. Luo F, Xu Y, Ling M, Zhao Y, Xu W, Liang X, et al. Arsenite evokes IL-6 secretion, autocrine regulation of STAT3 signaling, and miR-21 expression, processes involved in the EMT and malignant transformation of human bronchial epithelial cells. *Toxicol Appl Pharmacol.* (2013) 273:27–34. doi: 10.1016/j.taap.2013.08.025

17

MMP25 Regulates Immune Infiltration Level and Survival Outcome in Head and Neck Cancer Patients

Yujie Liang [1,2*†], *Chenyu Guan* [1,2†], *Kan Li* [1,2], *Guangsen Zheng* [1,2], *Tao Wang* [1,2], *Sien Zhang* [1,2] *and Guiqing Liao* [1,2*]

[1] *Department of Oral and Maxillofacial Surgery, Guanghua School of Stomatology, Hospital of Stomatology, Sun Yat-sen University, Guangzhou, China,* [2] *Guangdong Province Key Laboratory of Stomatology, Sun Yat-sen University, Guangzhou, China*

***Correspondence:**
Yujie Liang
yujie0350@126.com
Guiqing Liao
drliaoguiqing@hotmail.com

† *These authors have contributed equally to this work*

Background: MMP25 is a critical gene of matrix metalloproteinases (MMPs). However, the molecular mechanism of MMP25 in head and neck cancer pathogenesis remains unclear.

Methods: MMP25 expression was analyzed using The Cancer Genome Atlas (TCGA) database, and its influence on clinical prognosis was performed using Kaplan–Meier and Cox regression analyses. The correlation between MMP25 and immune infiltration was investigated by CIBERSORT, TIMER, and ESTIMATE. In addition, the relationship between MMP25 expression and molecular mechanisms was analyzed by gene set enrichment analysis (GSEA), gene ontology (GO), and weighted gene co-expression network analysis (WGCNA).

Results: MMP25 expression level correlated with prognosis and immune infiltrating levels, especially activated $CD4^+$ memory T cells, in head and neck cancer. Moreover, MMP25 expression potentially mediated genes, such as IRF8, IKZF1, and DOCK2, and tumor-associated pathways, including p53 signaling, PI3K/AKT/mTOR signaling, and JAK/STAT signaling pathway.

Conclusions: These findings suggested that MMP25 plays a critical role in the prognosis and immune infiltration level of head and neck cancer. In addition, MMP25 expression significantly correlated with the regulation of various oncogenes and tumor-related pathways.

Keywords: MMP25, head and neck cancer, immune infiltration level, TCGA, bioinformatics

INTRODUCTION

Head and neck cancer was the seventh most common cancer worldwide (1), originating from multiple anatomical structures:the oral cavity, sinonasal cavity, pharynx, and larynx (2). Advanced disease carries a high risk of local recurrence and metastasis, with poor prognosis (3, 4). Immune checkpoint inhibitors have been considered as a promising strategy for the treatment of head and neck cancer (5). Clinical trials have shown a clear prognostic advantage in head and neck cancer patients treated with immunotherapy (6). However, an increasing number of studies found that some types of head and neck cancer were insensitive to current immunotherapies (7). Moreover, a recent study has found that tumor-infiltrating immune cells, such as tumor-associated macrophages (TAMs) and regulatory T cells (Tregs) (8), impaired the prognosis and efficacy of immunotherapy in head and neck cancer.

MMPs are calcium-dependent zinc-containing endopeptidases which can degrade the extracellular matrix of tumor tissues and regulate tumor immune environment, and promote cancer invasion and metastasis (9, 10). MMP25 is a member of the matrix metalloproteinase family that is able to degrade collagens, gelatin, and fibrin (11). However, the underlying functions of MMP25 in the head and neck cancer still require further investigation. In this study, we comprehensively analyzed the mechanism by which MMP25 expression influences the prognosis of head and neck cancer patients. Our results showed that MMP25 high expression was related to head and neck cancer patients' better outcome, and that was regulated by oncogenes and cancer-associated pathways. In addition, we found that MMP25 had a significant effect on immune infiltration level in head and neck cancer. The findings shed light on the role of MMP25 in head and neck cancer by providing a potential correlation and a precise mechanism between MMP25 and tumor immune microenvironment.

MATERIALS AND METHODS

Data Source

Expression data and corresponding clinical information of head and neck cancer patients were downloaded from The Cancer Genome Atlas (TCGA) (Tumor samples: $n = 502$, Normal samples: $n = 44$).

Transcriptional Expression of Matrix Metalloproteinases

MMP1, MMP2, MMP3, MMP7, MMP8, MMP9, MMP10, MMP11, MMP12, MMP13, MMP14, MMP15, MMP16, MMP17, MMP19, MMP20, MMP21, MMP23B, MMP24, MMP24OS, MMP25, MMP26, MMP27, and MMP28 were formed with the FPKM of each mRNA expression of samples. Then, comparisons between tumor tissues and normal tissues were analyzed.

Prognostic Analysis of Head and Neck Patients

The clinical outcome of head and neck patients was determined using the Kaplan–Meier method, the log-rank test, and univariate Cox proportional hazards regression. The samples were stratified as high or low expression around the quartile of each MMPs' expression.

Identification of Differentially Expressed Genes

Differentially expressed genes (DEGs) were identified in head and neck cancer tissues by comparison with MMP25 high and low expression groups and using the "edgeR" package in R (R version 3.5.2). $|\text{Fold Change}| > 2$ and adjusted $p < 0.05$ were set as the statistical threshold value of DEGs. The heatmap, volcano plot with clustering for the significantly differentially expressed mRNAs in head and neck cancer between MMP25 high and low expression groups, was generated with the "ggplot2" package in R. GO analysis was constructed by "enrichplot" in R.

Gene Set Enrichment Analysis (GSEA)

The molecular mechanisms underlying the association between MMP25 expression were explored with GSEA. The number of permutations was set at 1,000, and the $p < 0.05$ and a false discovery rate (FDR) <0.25 were considered statistically significant. Multiple GSEA plots were produced by "plyr," "ggplot2," and "grid" packages in R.

The Clinical Features Correlated With MMP25 Expression Level

Clinical information from head and neck cancer patients, including age, gender, tumor grade, and clinical stage, was downloaded from TCGA. Samples were divided into two groups and according to the quartile of MMP25 expression level. Multivariate Cox regression and nomogram were used to analyze the role of MMP25 in the head and neck cancer patients' clinical features.

Immune Landscape Related to MMP25 Expression Level

The samples were analyzed by CIBERSORT to define 22 immune cell subtypes (12). Immune scores were calculated by ESTIMATE algorithm of immune cells (13). The correlations between MMP25 expression levels and immune infiltration level was estimated by TIMER, which is a comprehensive resource for analysis of immune infiltrates of gene expression profiles (14).

Weighted Gene Co-expression Network Analysis

The weighted gene co-expression network analysis (WGCNA) (15, 16) package was used to identify key modules associated with prognosis and clinical stage based on MMP25 expression levels. The module is a cluster of closely interconnected genes, based on the dendrogram height. The module eigengenes of clinical features were hierarchically clustered into different color modules.

Statistical Analysis

The analyses were carried out using "R" software (version 3.5.3), GraphPad Prism 8, and IBM SPSS Statistics 19; $p < 0.05$ was considered statistically significant. $^{***}p < 0.001$, $^{**}p < 0.01$ $^{*}p < 0.05$.

RESULTS

Expression of Matrix Metalloproteinases Family in Head and Neck Cancer

The expression levels of matrix metalloproteinases family genes are shown in **Figure 1**. Except for MMP24OS, the transcription level of other MMP family genes, including MMP1, MMP2, MMP3, MMP7, MMP8, MMP9, MMP10, MMP11, MMP12, MMP13, MMP14, MMP15, MMP16, MMP17, MMP19, MMP20, MMP21, MMP23B, MMP24, MMP25, MMP26, MMP27, and MMP28, in the tumor tissues was significantly higher than those in normal tissues.

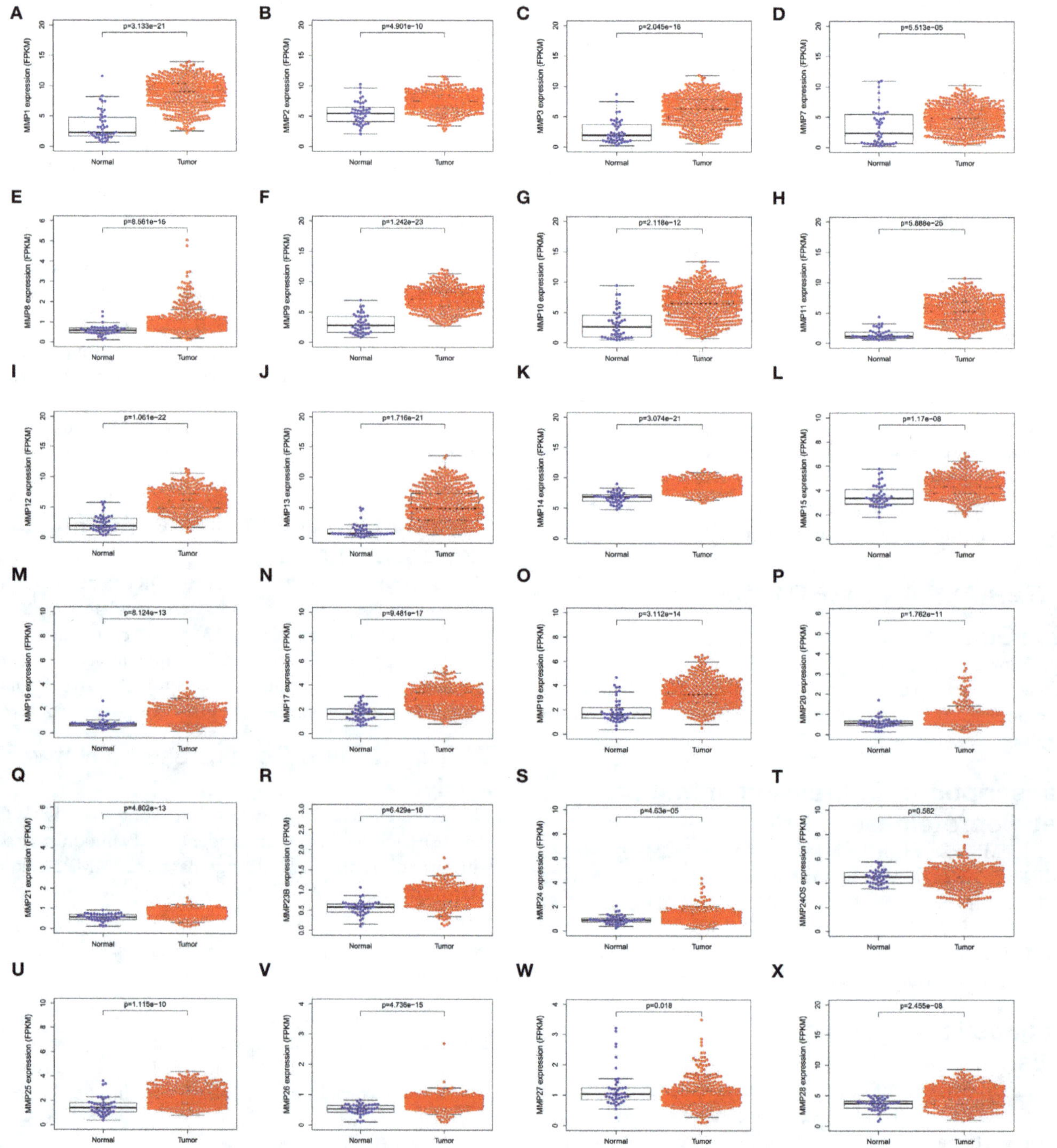

FIGURE 1 | Scatter plots showing the expression levels of matrix metalloproteinases family genes of normal tissues (blue) and tumor tissues (red) in head and neck cancer. **(A)** MMP1; **(B)** MMP2; **(C)** MMP3; **(D)**MMP7; **(E)** MMP8; **(F)** MMP9; **(G)**MMP10; **(H)** MMP11; **(I)** MMP12; **(J)** MMP13; **(K)**MMP14; **(L)**MMP15; **(M)**MMP16; **(N)** MMP17; **(O)** MMP19; **(P)** MMP20; **(Q)** MMP21; **(R)**MMP23B; **(S)** MMP24; **(T)** MMP24OS; **(U)** MMP25; **(V)** MMP26; **(W)** MMP27; **(X)** MMP28.

Analysis of the Prognosis Associated With MMPs Expression Levels in TCGA Cohort of Head and Neck Cancer

Expression levels of MMP10, MMP19, MMP24, and MMP25, which were associated with prognosis in head and neck cancer, were identified using Kaplan–Meier method and log-rank test (**Figure 2**, **Table 1**). Univariate Cox regression analysis showed that there was no significant dereference between expression levels of MMP10 ($p = 0.16$), MMP19 ($p = 0.06$), and MMP24 ($p = 0.30$). Eventually, MMP25 was identified.

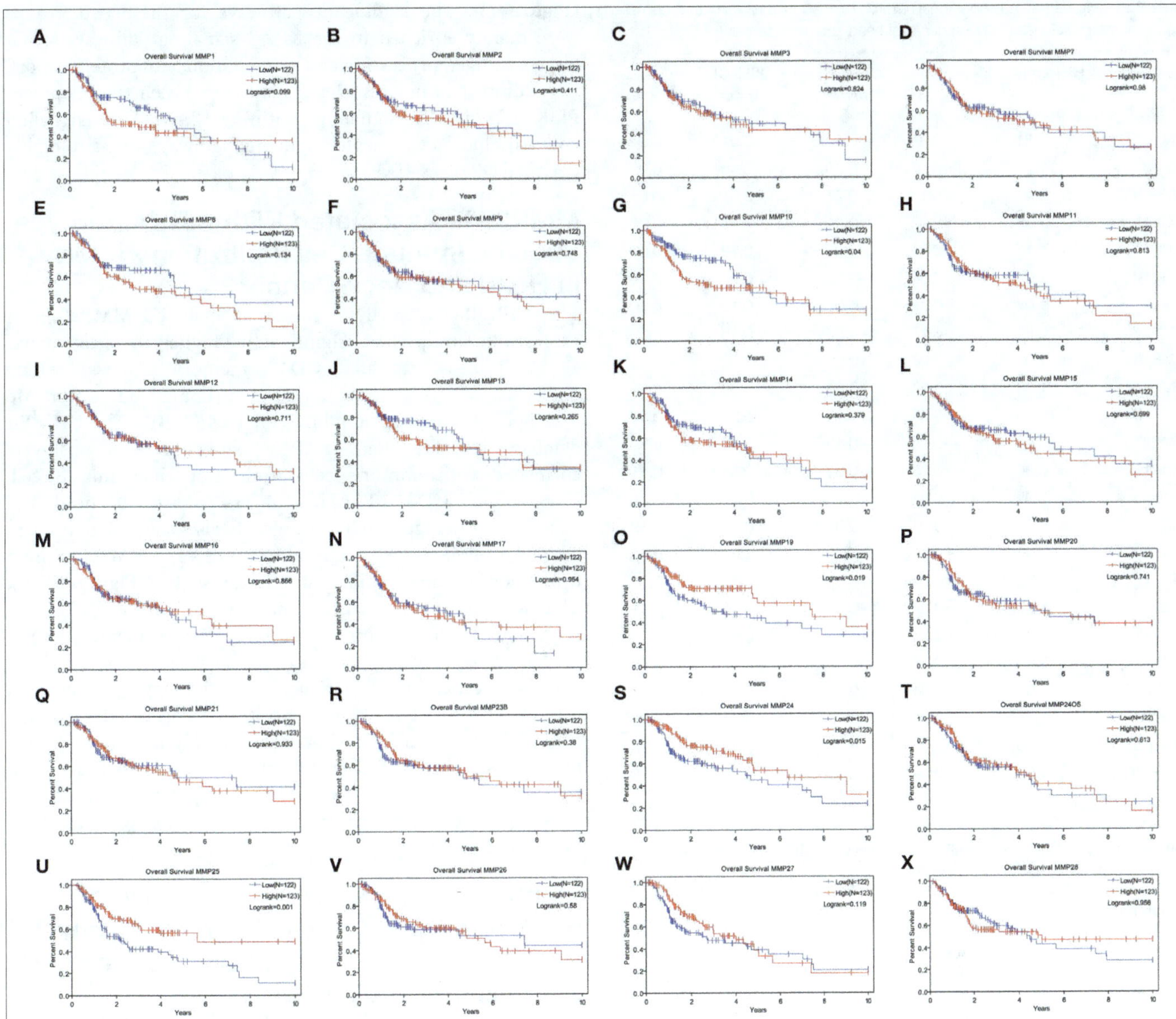

FIGURE 2 | Analysis of the role of MMPs genes in the overall survival in head and neck cancer patients by Kaplan–Meier method and the log-rank test. **(A)** MMP1; **(B)** MMP2; **(C)** MMP3; **(D)** MMP7; **(E)** MMP8; **(F)** MMP9; **(G)**MMP10; **(H)** MMP11; **(I)** MMP12; **(J)** MMP13; **(K)** MMP14; **(L)** MMP15; **(M)** MMP16; **(N)** MMP17; **(O)** MMP19; **(P)** MMP20; **(Q)** MMP21; **(R)** MMP23B; **(S)** MMP24; **(T)** MMP24OS; **(U)** MMP25; **(V)** MMP26; **(W)** MMP27; **(X)** MMP28.

Analysis of the Clinical Features Associated With MMP25 Expression Levels in TCGA Cohort of Head and Neck Cancer

In TCGA cohort, multivariate Cox regression model indicated that MMP25 expression was correlated with clinical stage with prognosis of head and neck cancer patients in terms of overall survival in the TCGA cohort (**Table 2**). In view of the prognostic value of MMP25 in head and neck cancer, we tried to construct the nomogram for predicting 1-, 3-, and 5-year survival. The result illustrated that clinical stages shared the largest contribution to overall survival, followed by MMP25 expression group (**Figure 3**).

Analysis of the Differential Expressed Genes With MMP25 High and Low Expression Group of Head and Neck Cancer

A total of 433 differential expressed genes, including 239 upregulated and 194 downregulated DEGs, was screened with MMP25 high and low expression group ($|\log FC| > 2$ and adjusted $p < 0.05$) (**Figure 4B**). The top 20 differential expressed genes were TIFAB, CLEC6A, PPP1R16B, IRF8, ITGAL, IKZF1, DOCK2, PTPRC, FGL2, MPEG1, IL10RA, ITK, CD226, TLR8, MMP25, LILRB2, PRKCB, SIGLEC10, RHOH, and CXCR6 (**Figure 4A**). The expression levels of

TABLE 1 | Univariate Cox proportional hazards regression analysis of the role of matrix metalloproteinases (MMPs) genes of head and neck cancer (HNSC).

Gene	HR[exp(coef)]	coef	95% CI lower	95% CI upper	*p*-value
MMP25	0.81	−0.21	−0.41	−0.01	0.04
MMP8	1.26	0.23	0.00	0.46	0.05
MMP19	0.88	−0.13	−0.27	0.01	0.06
MMP1	1.06	0.06	−0.01	0.12	0.08
MMP14	1.15	0.14	−0.02	0.29	0.09
MMP10	1.04	0.04	−0.02	0.10	0.16
MMP3	1.04	0.04	−0.02	0.10	0.20
MMP24	0.84	−0.17	−0.50	0.15	0.30
MMP13	1.03	0.03	−0.03	0.08	0.33
MMP7	1.02	0.02	−0.05	0.09	0.52
MMP15	1.05	0.05	−0.12	0.22	0.56
MMP27	0.91	−0.10	−0.45	0.25	0.58
MMP17	0.96	−0.05	−0.22	0.13	0.61
MMP16	0.95	−0.05	−0.27	0.18	0.68
MMP9	1.02	0.02	−0.07	0.10	0.69
MMP20	0.93	−0.07	−0.43	0.29	0.71
MMP12	1.02	0.02	−0.07	0.10	0.71
MMP2	1.02	0.02	−0.08	0.11	0.71
MMP21	1.14	0.13	−0.60	0.85	0.73
MMP11	0.99	−0.01	−0.08	0.07	0.88
MMP23B	1.04	0.04	−0.60	0.69	0.89
MMP26	1.04	0.04	−0.71	0.78	0.92
MMP28	1.00	0.00	−0.09	0.09	0.98
MMP24OS	1.00	0.00	−0.18	0.18	0.98

TABLE 2 | Multivariate Cox regression of clinical characteristics of HNSC patients in The Cancer Genome Atlas (TCGA) cohort.

Variables	MMP25		
	High ($n = 100$)	Low ($n = 101$)	*p*-value
Age			0.91
≤60	46	46	
>60	54	55	
Gender			0.59
Male	64	74	
Female	36	27	
Grade			0.95
Grade (1+2)	70	82	
Grade (3+4)	30	19	
Stage			0.019
Stage (I+II)	32	13	
Stage (III+IV)	68	88	

these genes were positively correlated with the expression level of MMP25. The GO analysis showed that the differentially expressed genes were highly associated with T cell activation, external side of plasma membrane, and receptor ligand activity (**Figure 4C**). The significant pathways for these two groups were mainly enriched in the KRAS signaling pathway, MYC-targets, antigen processing and presentation, and protein export. In addition, tumor-associated pathways, such as apoptosis, PI3K/AKT/mTOR signaling pathway, JAK/STAT signaling pathway, and T cell receptor signaling pathway, were also highly enriched (**Figures 4D,E**).

MMP25 Is Associated With mRNA Subtype Specific Immune Cell Infiltration Patterns in Head and Neck Cancer

The CIBERSORT analysis indicated that the MMP25 high expression group had significantly higher B cells naïve, $CD8^+$ T cells, activated $CD4^+$ memory T cells, resting NK cells, M1 macrophage, and neutrophils, but lower M0 macrophage and eosinophil (**Figures 5A,B**). The TIMER database revealed that MMP25 expression was positively correlated with immune cells infiltration, including B cell, $CD8^+$T cell, $CD4^+$ T cell, and macrophage in head and neck cancers (**Figure 5C**). The graph also showed that there has been an increase of immune scores in the MMP25 high expression group of different clinical stages (**Figures 5D,E**). The Kaplan–Meier method analysis of CIBERSORT data suggested that the infiltration level of activated memory $CD4^+$ T cells was significantly related to the survival outcome of head and neck cancer patients. The infiltration level of activated memory $CD4^+$ T cells was positively correlated with the MMP25 expression level (**Supplemental Figures 1A,B**). These findings showed that a high infiltration level of activated memory $CD4^+$ T cells played an important role in the better prognosis of cancer patients in the MMP25 high expression group.

Identify Key Modules Associated With Head and Neck Cancer Patients' Survival Ratio and Clinical Stage Based on the Expression Levels of MMP25

Gene modules were analyzed using the WGCNA in the MMP25 high and low expression groups, respectively. In the high expression group, soft power 4 and the minimum module size cut-off 30 were chosen as the threshold to identify co-expressed gene modules (**Figure 6A**). Gene color modules that were related to the clinical stage were identified (**Supplemental Figure 2**). These significant gene color modules were further used for GO analysis to display the gene pathway enrichment, gene symbols, and their character in KEGG, as shown in **Supplemental Tables 1, 2**. The genes were related to many pathways in cancer, such as PI3K-Akt signaling pathway, p53 signaling pathway, Ras signaling pathway, MAPK signaling pathway, and TNF signaling pathway. In addition, genes were also enriched in cell cycle, DNA replication, and mismatch in cancer. Hub genes ADCY6, APP, TNC, MFGE8, MFI2, ANO8, APLP2, LTBP1, SERPINA1, and PROC were highly related to the survival outcome of patients. IFIT3, OAS2, OAS1, HLA-C, HLA-E, IRF1, GBP2, IRF2, OAS3, and IFIT1 were closely associated with the patients' clinical stages. However, in the

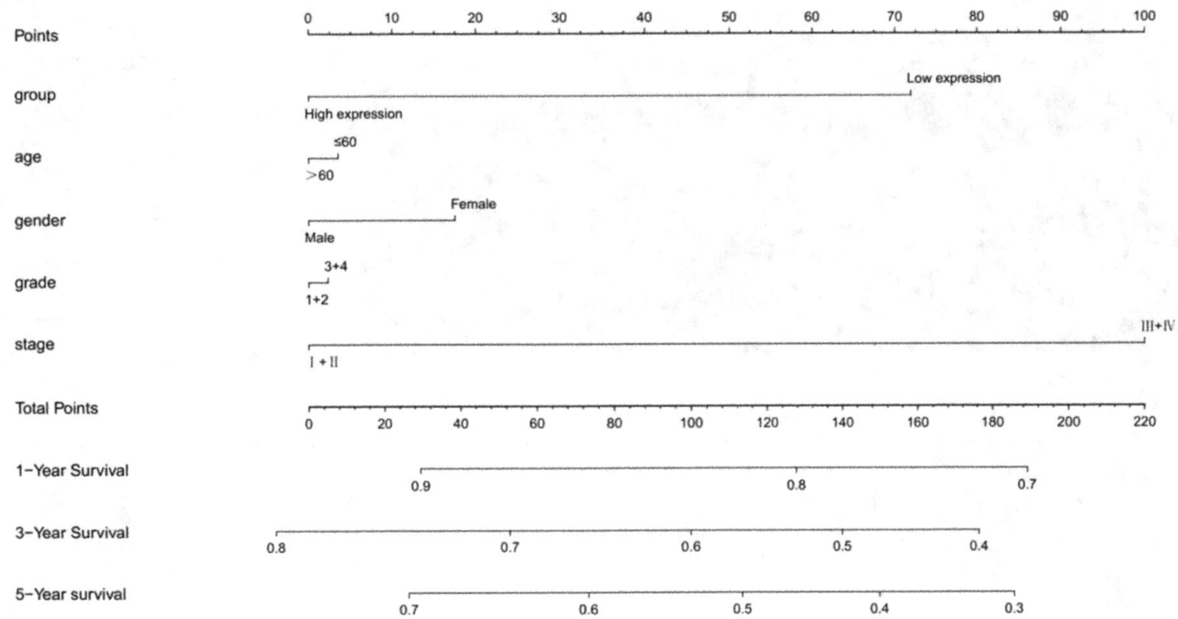

FIGURE 3 | Nomogramfor predicting 1-, 3-, or 5-year survival in head and neck cancer patients. The top row shows the point value for each variable. Rows indicate the variables included in the nomogram. Each variable corresponds to a point value based on head and neck cancer characteristics. The sum of these values is located on the Total Points, and the line drawn downward to the survival axes is used to determine the likelihood of 1-, 3-, or 5-year survival.

low expression group, hub genes CDC34, UBE2D3, GAN, FZR1, CUL3, KLHL2, FBXL8, CDC16, FBXW11, and LMO7 were highly related to the survival outcome. CDSN, LCE1D, LCE3B, LCE1E, LCE3C, LCE1B, LCE2A, LCE1A, LCE2B, and LCE2C were associated with the patients' clinical stages (**Figures 6E–H**).

DISCUSSION

MMP25 is a member of the matrix metalloproteinase family which is frequently connected to embryonic development, reproduction, and tissue remodeling, as well as tumorigenesis. Although MMP25 has not been extensively investigated, research showed that MMP25 could regulate the chemotaxis of neutrophil and monocyte and generate "eat-me" signals to increase the phagocytic removal of neutrophils (17). MMP25 is highly expressed in human cancer cells, such as colon cancer cells and gastric cancer cells (18, 19). In addition, MMP25 was highly expressed and promoted tumor growth in colon cancer (18). Here, we report that the expression level of MMP25 correlated to the activated $CD4^+$ memory T cells and prognosis in head and neck cancer. High expression levels of MMP25 were associated with a better survival outcome. Increased MMP25 expression level could impact the clinical stages of head and neck cancer patients, indicating that MMP25 expression could be used as a potential predictor of clinical stage and prognosis. Moreover, our analysis suggested that immune infiltration levels and diverse tumor-associated pathways were correlated with levels of MMP25 expression. Therefore, our study provides an insight into understanding the role of MMP25 in tumor immune environment and molecular mechanism in head and neck cancer.

In this research, we first analyzed the expression levels of MMPs and prognostic landscape in head and neck cancer. The differential expression between cancer and normal tissues was observed in many matrix metalloproteinase family genes. Expression levels of MMP10, MMP19, MMP24, and MMP25 were associated with prognosis in TCGA cohort of head and neck cancer by Kaplan-Meier analysis. Chongshan Wu demonstrated that the high expression of MMP19 was determined to be a poor prognostic factor in colorectal cancer (20). Trever G Bivona also suggested that MMP24 was a biomarker of tumor progression and worse outcomes in lung and/or gastric cancer patients (21). Univariate Cox proportional hazards regression demonstrated a significant correlation between MMP25 (HR=0.81, $p = 0.04$) and MMP8 (HR=1.26, $p = 0.05$) and prognosis of head and neck cancer patients. Notably, we observed that MMP25 was the only one gene that not only significantly expressed compared to the normal tissues but also played a significant role in the survival outcome of head and neck cancer patients by analysis of Kaplan–Meier method and univariate Cox proportional hazards regression. Likewise, recent evidence also revealed that high MMP25 expression levels were correlated with a better overall survival in ovarian cancer (22). Clinicopathological features from TCGA cohort of head and neck cancer showed that high levels of MMP25 expression were correlated with patients' clinical stages in our study. This important role of MMP25 has not been reported yet so far. Together, these findings suggest that high MMP25 expression levels may be used as a potential prognostic indicator in head and neck cancer.

Differential expressed genes analysis showed that the expression level of MMP25 was related to genes, such as IRF8, IKZF1, and DOCK2. Jason B. Muhitch et al. showed that high

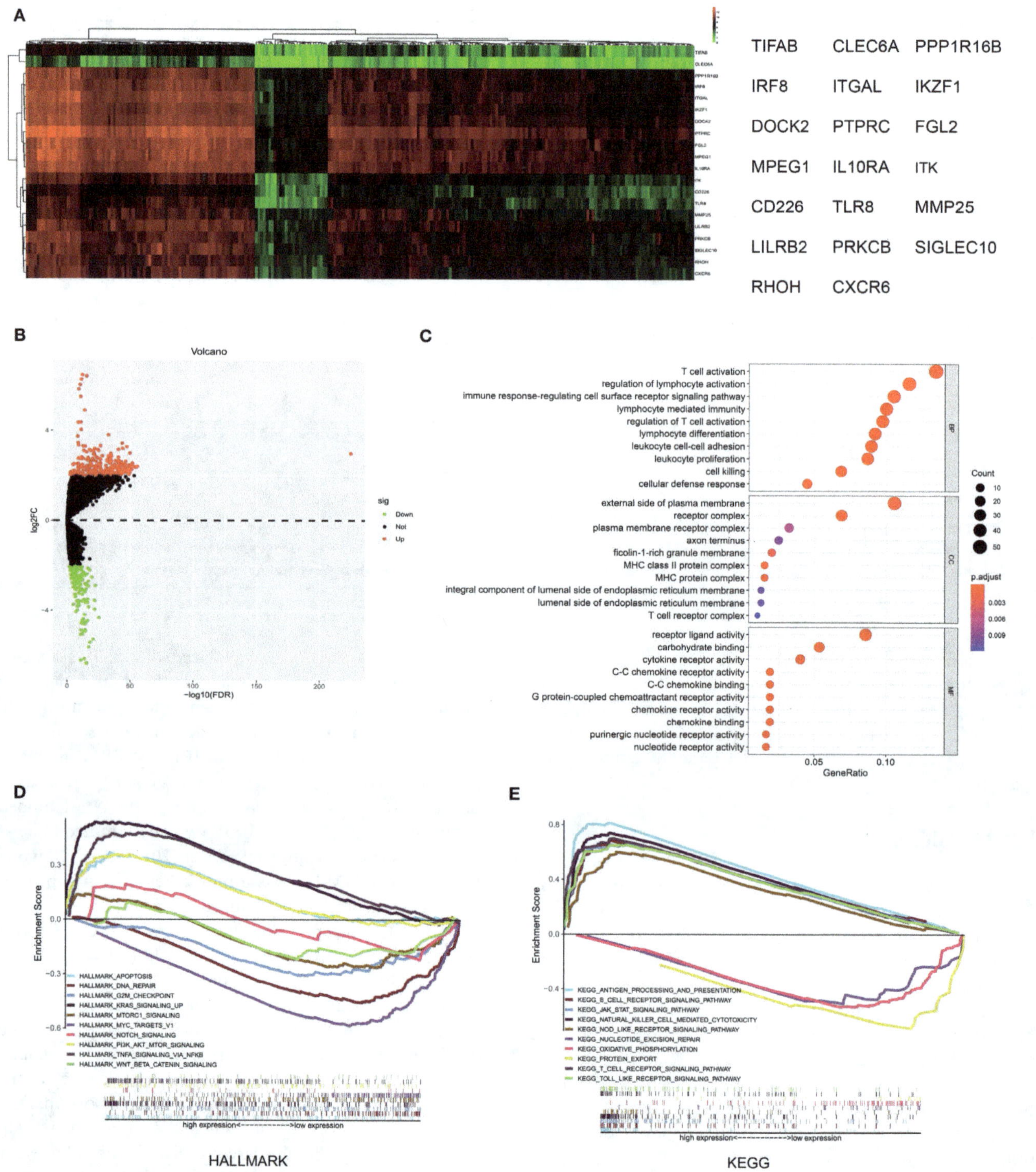

FIGURE 4 | Differential expressed genes and gene set enrichment analysis (GSEA) with MMP25 high and low expression group. **(A)** Heatmap of differential expressed genes analysis by "edgeR" package in R. **(B)** Volcano plot of differential expressed genes with MMP25 high and low expression group. **(C)** GO analysis of differential expressed genes. **(D)** Hallmark enrichment analysis by GSEA. **(E)** KEGG enrichment analysis by GSEA.

expression levels of IRF8 within metastatic sites prolonged overall survival of renal cell carcinoma compared to low levels of IRF8 expression (23). Overexpression of IKZF1 in melanomas enhanced the recruitment of immune infiltration and sensitivity to PD1 and CTLA4 inhibitors (24). Another study also showed that DOCK2 was significantly associated with survival outcome

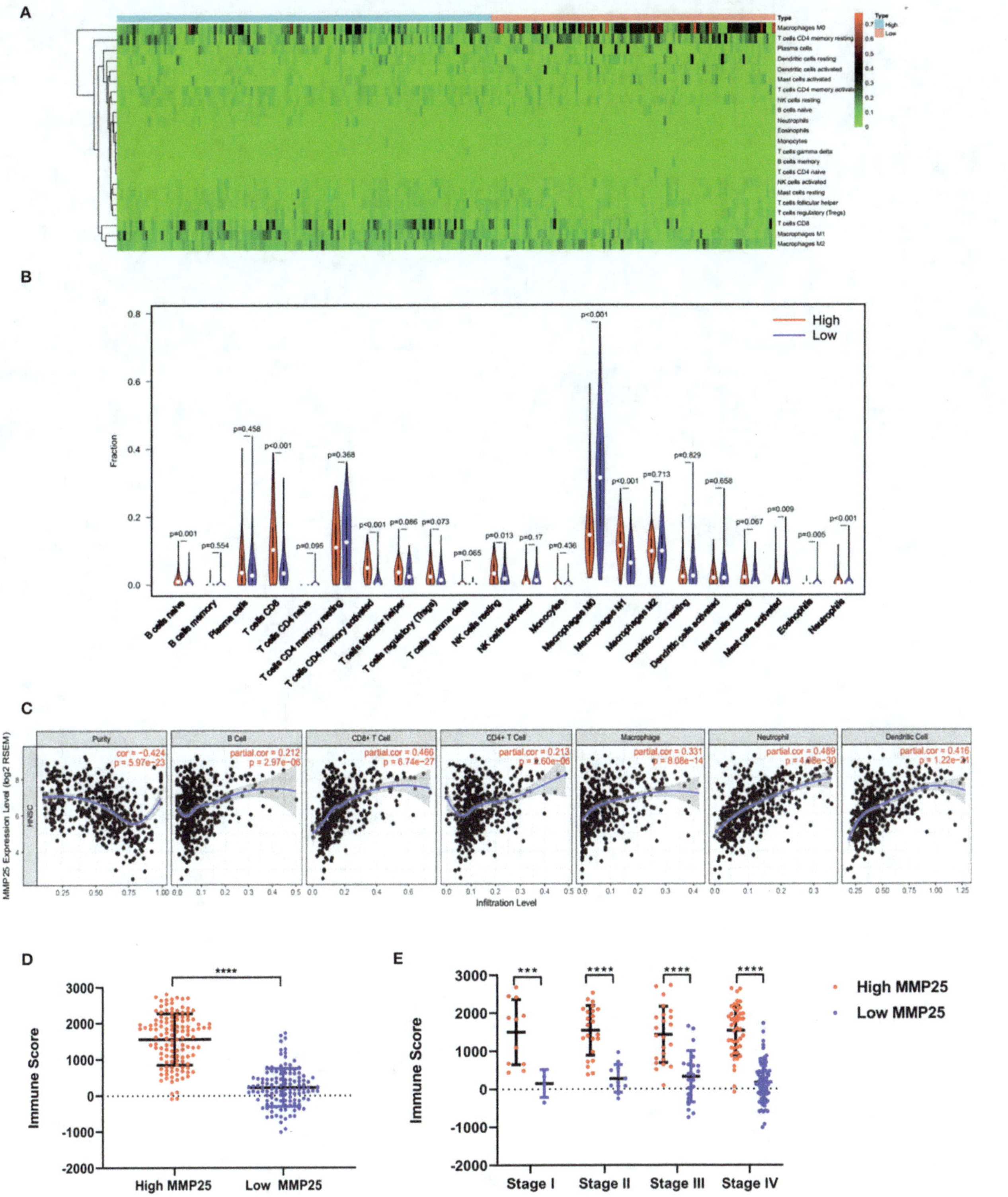

FIGURE 5 | Immune cell infiltration patterns and scores between MMP25 high and low expression group. **(A)** Heatmap of immune infiltration level. **(B)** Violin plot of immune infiltration level between MMP25 high (red) and low (blue) expression group. **(C)** The correlation between the MMP25 expression level and immune infiltration level by TIMER database. **(D)** Difference of immune scores between two groups. **(E)** Difference of immune scores among clinical stages.

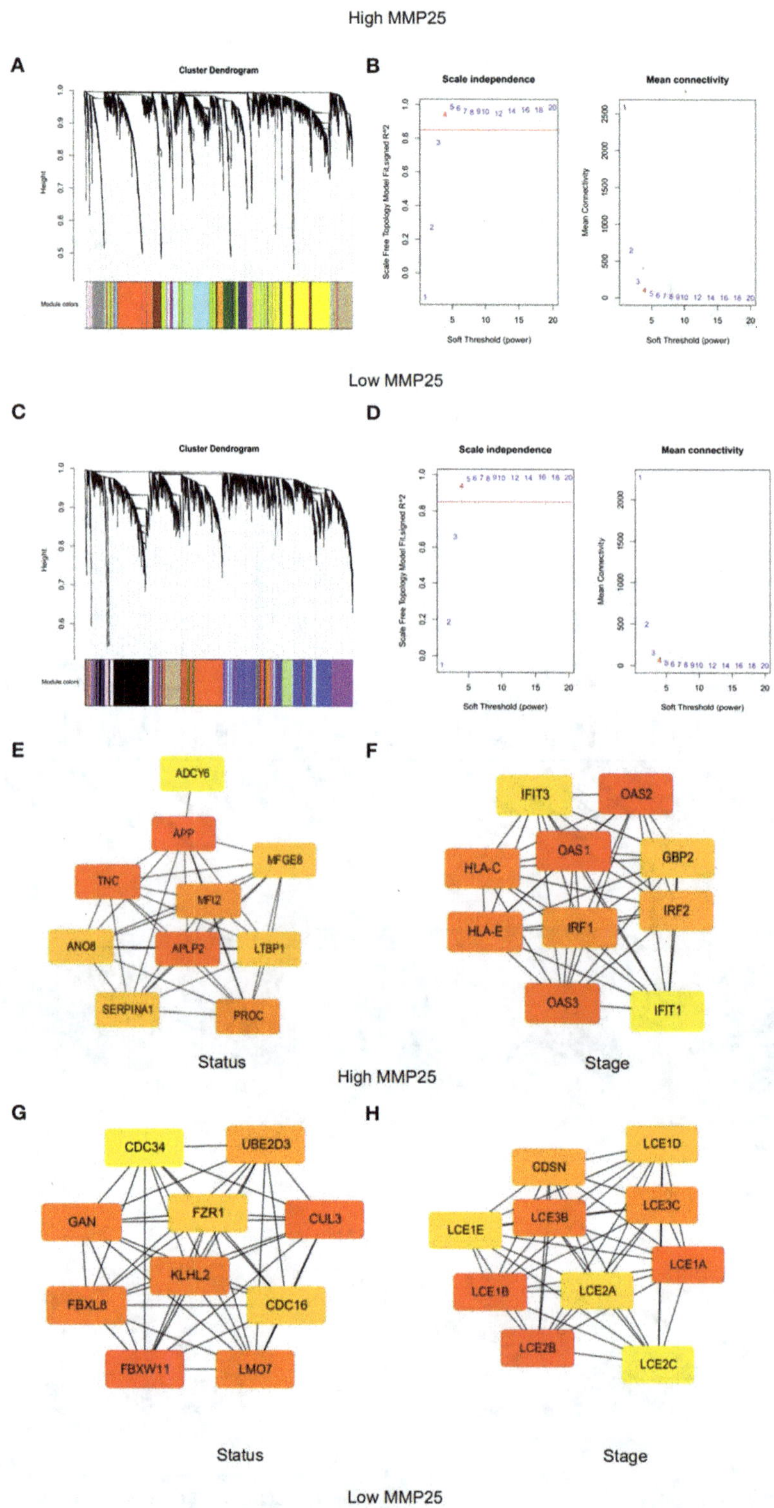

FIGURE 6 | Weighted gene co-expression network analysis of module eigengenes of grade correlated with **(A)** Clustering dendrograms of genes in the MMP25 high expression group. **(B)** The scale-free topology model fit for various soft-thresholding powers (β) in MMP25 high expression group. **(C)** Clustering dendrograms of genes in the MMP25 low expression group. **(D)** The scale-free topology model fit for various soft-thresholding powers (β) in MMP25 low expression group. **(E)** Hub genes protein interaction network of the significant modules for patients' status in MMP25 high expression group. **(F)** Hub genes protein interaction network of the significant modules for patients' stages in MMP25 high expression group. **(G)** Hub genes protein interaction network of the significant modules for patients' status in MMP25 low expression group. **(H)** Hub genes protein interaction network of the significant modules for patients' stages in MMP25 low expression group.

in colorectal cancer (25). In our study, the GO analysis of these differential expressed genes revealed that they were enriched in critical immune biological processes, including T cell activation, regulation of lymphocyte activation, immune response-regulating cell surface receptor signaling pathway, and so on. This partly explained the role of MMP25 in the activation of the $CD4^+$ T memory cell by CIBERSORT analysis. Juric et al. revealed that MMP9 inhibition was able to promote T cell response by disruption of biochemical and physical barriers (26). The MMP23 expression of primary melanoma also demonstrated a trend toward an increased proportion of immunosuppressive Foxp3+ regulatory T cells. These results provided further support for the hypothesis that MMP25 could regulate the immune infiltration level due to the activation of downstream immunological molecules.

Furthermore, high expression levels of MMP25 were associated with many pathways in cancer, for instance, KRAS signaling pathway, apoptosis, PI3K/AKT/mTOR signaling pathway, and JAK/STAT signaling pathway. It has been revealed that JAK/STAT and mTOR pathways were significantly associated with poor overall survival (27, 28). Immune regulatory processes are largely driven by JAK-STAT signaling by a wide range of downstream cellular effectors, including oncogenes, miRNAs, DNA methylation, and other co-regulatory factors (29). Kozaki et al. found that PIK3CA mutations were relatively high in the late stage of oral cancer (30). Recent studies describe that the activation of KRAS signaling on cancer cells extends to the cancer microenvironment (31). Apoptosis is a mechanism that may contribute to cancer. Defects can occur at any point along apoptosis-associated pathways, leading to malignant transformation of the affected cells, tumor metastasis, and resistance (32). In addition, we identified key modules associated with head and neck cancer (HNSCC) patient's survival ratio and clinical stage based on the weighted gene co-expression network analysis (WGCNA). Hub genes have been identified, for example, APLP2, IFIT1, IFIT3, and CDC34. APLP2 expression was significantly related to disease-specific survival in renal cell carcinoma (33). It could be hypothesized that MMP25 was able to interact with multiple key genes to affect the progression of head and neck cancer. Taken together, it is possible that the regulation of cancer-associate genes and signaling pathways may be involved in the regulatory role of MMP25 in the clinical stages and prognosis in HNSCC.

Another important result of this study is that MMP25 expression correlated with diverse immune infiltration levels in head and neck cancer. Our results indicated that there was a correlation between MMP25 expression level and infiltration level of macrophages and B cells naïve, $CD8^+$ T cells, activated $CD4^+$ memory T cells, resting NK cells, M1 macrophage, and neutrophils, but lower M0 macrophage and eosinophil. Univariate Cox proportional hazards regression of these types of immune cells showed that activated $CD4^+$ memory T cells correlated with lower hazard ratio (HR) for better overall survival (OS). Oberg showed that in patients with colon cancer, higher percentages of $CD4^+$ memory T cells may be indicative of a better prognosis (34). Meanwhile, $CD4^+$ memory T cells are associated with tumor cell metastasis to lymph nodes and tumor progression (35). Immune score was an algorithm providing scores of the immune infiltration level by ESTIMATE (13). In the present study, the high expression level of MMP25 showed a strong relationship with the immune scores between tumor tissues and normal tissues, as well as in different clinical stages. It is known that the immune scores could predict patients' clinical outcomes (36).

In summary, increased MMP25 expression correlates with better prognosis and increased immune infiltration levels in head and neck cancer, especially activated CD4+ memory T cells. Moreover, the expression of MMP25 potentially contributes to the regulation of tumor-associated pathway and oncogenes. Therefore, we propose that MMP25 probably plays an integral correlative role in immune cell infiltration and can be a potential prognosis biomarker in head and neck cancer. Further exploration of MMP25 function in clinical cohort study or *in vivo* and *in vitro* model will probably contribute to confirm these results.

AUTHOR CONTRIBUTIONS

YL and CG contributed to conception and design of the study and data analysis. KL, GZ, TW, and SZ contributed to data acquisition. GL and YL critically revised the manuscript. All authors contributed to the article and approved the submitted version.

REFERENCES

1. Bray F, Ferlay J, Soerjomataram I, Siegel RL, Torre LA, Jemal A. Global cancer statistics 2018: GLOBOCAN estimates of incidence and mortality worldwide for 36 cancers in 185 countries. *CA Cancer J Clin.* (2018) 68:394–424. doi: 10.3322/caac.21492
2. Chow LQM. Head and neck cancer. *N Engl J Med.* (2020) 382:60–72. doi: 10.1056/NEJMra1715715
3. Ahmad P, Sana J, Slavik M, Slampa P, Smilek P, Slaby O. MicroRNAs involvement in radioresistance of head and neck cancer. *Dis Markers.* (2017) 2017:8245345. doi: 10.1155/2017/8245345
4. Luo X, Qiu Y, Jiang Y, Chen F, Jiang L, Zhou Y, et al. Long non-coding RNA implicated in the invasion and metastasis of head and neck cancer: possible function and mechanisms. *Mol Cancer.* (2018) 17:14. doi: 10.1186/s12943-018-0763-7
5. Xu B, Jungbluth AA, Frosina D, Alzumaili B, Aleynick N, Slodkowska E, et al. Immune microenvironment and expression of PD-L1, PD-1, cancer testis antigen PRAME and MHC I in salivary duct carcinoma. *Histopathology.* (2019) 75:672–82. doi: 10.1111/his.13944
6. Mandal R, Senbabaoglu Y, Desrichard A, Havel JJ, Dalin MG, Riaz N, et al. The head and neck cancer immune landscape and its immunotherapeutic implications. *JCI Insight.* (2016) 1:e89829. doi: 10.1172/jci.insight.89829
7. Mehra R, Seiwert TY, Gupta S, Weiss J, Gluck I, Eder JP, et al. Efficacy and safety of pembrolizumab in recurrent/metastatic head and neck squamous cell

carcinoma: pooled analyses after long-term follow-up in KEYNOTE-012. *Br J Cancer.* (2018) 119:153–9. doi: 10.1038/s41416-018-0131-9

8. Jie HB, Schuler PJ, Lee SC, Srivastava RM, Argiris A, Ferrone S, et al. CTLA-4^+ Regulatory T cells increased in cetuximab-treated head and neck cancer patients suppress NK cell cytotoxicity and correlate with poor prognosis. *Cancer Res.* (2015) 75:2200–10. doi: 10.1158/0008-5472.CAN-14-2788
9. Liotta LA, Stetler-Stevenson WG. Metalloproteinases and cancer invasion. *Semin Cancer Biol.* (1990) 1:99–106.
10. Vayrynen O, Astrom P, Nyberg P, Alahuhta I, Pirila E, Vilen ST, et al. Matrix metalloproteinase 9 inhibits the motility of highly aggressive HSC-3 oral squamous cell carcinoma cells. *Exp Cell Res.* (2019) 376:18–26. doi: 10.1016/j.yexcr.2019.01.018
11. English WR, Velasco G, Stracke JO, Knauper V, Murphy G. Catalytic activities of membrane-type 6 matrix metalloproteinase (MMP25). *FEBS Lett.* (2001) 491:137–42. doi: 10.1016/S0014-5793(01)02150-0
12. Newman AM, Liu CL, Green MR, Gentles AJ, Feng W, Xu Y, et al. Robust enumeration of cell subsets from tissue expression profiles. *Nat Methods.* (2015) 12:453–7. doi: 10.1038/nmeth.3337
13. Yoshihara K, Shahmoradgoli M, Martinez E, Vegesna R, Kim H, Torres-Garcia W, et al. Inferring tumour purity and stromal and immune cell admixture from expression data. *Nat Commun.* (2013) 4:2612. doi: 10.1038/ncomms3612
14. Li T, Fan J, Wang B, Traugh N, Chen Q, Liu JS, et al. TIMER: a web server for comprehensive analysis of tumor-infiltrating immune cells. *Cancer Res.* (2017) 77:e108–e110. doi: 10.1158/0008-5472.CAN-17-0307
15. Zhang B, Horvath S. A general framework for weighted gene co-expression network analysis. *Stat Appl Genet Mol Biol.* (2005) 4:Article17. doi: 10.2202/1544-6115.1128
16. Langfelder P, Horvath S. WGCNA: an R package for weighted correlation network analysis. *BMC Bioinformatics.* (2008) 9:559. doi: 10.1186/1471-2105-9-559
17. Starr AE, Bellac CL, Dufour A, Goebeler V, Overall CM. Biochemical characterization and N-terminomics analysis of leukolysin, the membrane-type 6 matrix metalloprotease (MMP25): chemokine and vimentin cleavages enhance cell migration and macrophage phagocytic activities. *J Biol Chem.* (2012) 287:13382–95. doi: 10.1074/jbc.M111.314179
18. Sun Q, Weber CR, Sohail A, Bernardo MM, Toth M, Zhao H, et al. MMP25 (MT6-MMP) is highly expressed in human colon cancer, promotes tumor growth, and exhibits unique biochemical properties. *J Biol Chem.* (2007) 282:21998–2010. doi: 10.1074/jbc.M701737200
19. Wang Y, Yu SJ, Li YX, Luo HS. Expression and clinical significance of matrix metalloproteinase-17 and−25 in gastric cancer. *Oncol Lett.* (2015) 9:671–6. doi: 10.3892/ol.2014.2747
20. Chen Z, Wu G, Ye F, Chen G, Fan Q, Dong H, et al. High expression of MMP19 is associated with poor prognosis in patients with colorectal cancer. *BMC Cancer.* (2019) 19:448. doi: 10.1186/s12885-019-5673-6
21. Okimoto RA, Breitenbuecher F, Olivas VR, Wu W, Gini B, Hofree M, et al. Inactivation of capicua drives cancer metastasis. *Nat Genet.* (2017) 49:87–96. doi: 10.1038/ng.3728
22. Zeng L, Qian J, Zhu F, Wu F, Zhao H, Zhu H. The prognostic values of matrix metalloproteinases in ovarian cancer. *J Int Med Res.* 2019:300060519825983. doi: 10.1177/0300060519825983
23. Muhitch JB, Hoffend NC, Azabdaftari G, Miller A, Bshara W, Morrison CD, et al. Tumor-associated macrophage expression of interferon regulatory factor-8 (IRF8) is a predictor of progression and patient survival in renal cell carcinoma. *J Immunother Cancer.* (2019) 7:155. doi: 10.1186/s40425-019-0630-0
24. Chen JC, Perez-Lorenzo R, Saenger YM, Drake CG, Christiano AM. IKZF1 Enhances immune infiltrate recruitment in solid tumors and susceptibility to immunotherapy. *Cell Syst.* (2018) 7:92–103.e104. doi: 10.1016/j.cels.2018.05.020
25. Yu J, Wu WK, Li X, He J, Li XX, Ng SS, et al. Novel recurrently mutated genes and a prognostic mutation signature in colorectal cancer. *Gut.* (2015) 64:636–45. doi: 10.1136/gutjnl-2013-306620
26. Juric V, O'Sullivan C, Stefanutti E, Kovalenko M, Greenstein A, Barry-Hamilton V, et al. MMP-9 inhibition promotes anti-tumor immunity through disruption of biochemical and physical barriers to T-cell trafficking to tumors. *PLoS ONE.* (2018) 13:e0207255. doi: 10.1371/journal.pone.0207255
27. Marques AE, Elias ST, Porporatti AL, Castilho RM, Squarize CH, De Luca Canto G, et al. mTOR pathway protein immunoexpression as a prognostic factor for survival in head and neck cancer patients: a systematic review and meta-analysis. *J Oral Pathol Med.* (2016) 45:319–28. doi: 10.1111/jop.12390
28. Khanna P, Chua PJ, Bay BH, Baeg GH. The JAK/STAT signaling cascade in gastric carcinoma (review). *Int J Oncol.* (2015) 47:1617–26. doi: 10.3892/ijo.2015.3160
29. Owen KL, Brockwell NK, Parker BS. JAK-STAT signaling: a double-edged sword of immune regulation and cancer progression. *Cancers.* (2019) 11:2002. doi: 10.3390/cancers11122002
30. Kozaki K, Imoto I, Pimkhaokham A, Hasegawa S, Tsuda H, Omura K, et al. PIK3CA mutation is an oncogenic aberration at advanced stages of oral squamous cell carcinoma. *Cancer Sci.* (2006) 97:1351–8. doi: 10.1111/j.1349-7006.2006.00343.x
31. Dias Carvalho P, Guimaraes CF, Cardoso AP, Mendonca S, Costa AM, Oliveira MJ, et al. KRAS oncogenic signaling extends beyond cancer cells to orchestrate the microenvironment. *Cancer Res.* (2018) 78:7–14. doi: 10.1158/0008-5472.CAN-17-2084
32. Wong RS. Apoptosis in cancer: from pathogenesis to treatment. *J Exp Clin Cancer Res.* (2011) 30:87. doi: 10.1186/1756-9966-30-87
33. Gao L, Zhao H, Zhang D, Zhou C, Wang H, Ren C, et al. Role of APLP2 in the prognosis and clinicopathology of renal cell carcinoma. *Oncol Lett.* (2019) 17:508–13. doi: 10.3892/ol.2018.9577
34. Oberg A, Samii S, Stenling R, Lindmark G. Different occurrence of CD8+, CD45R0+, and CD68+ immune cells in regional lymph node metastases from colorectal cancer as potential prognostic predictors. *Int J Colorectal Dis.* (2002) 17:25–29. doi: 10.1007/s003840100337
35. Vahidi Y, Faghih Z, Talei AR, Doroudchi M, Ghaderi A. Memory $CD4^+$ T cell subsets in tumor draining lymph nodes of breast cancer patients: a focus on T stem cell memory cells. *Cell Oncol.* (2018) 41:1–11. doi: 10.1007/s13402-017-0352-6
36. Liu W, Ye H, Liu YF, Xu CQ, Zhong YX, Tian T, et al. Transcriptome-derived stromal and immune scores infer clinical outcomes of patients with cancer. *Oncol Lett.* (2018) 15:4351–7. doi: 10.3892/ol.2018.7855

18

The Role of Akt in Acquired Cetuximab Resistant Head and Neck Squamous Cell Carcinoma: An *In Vitro* Study on a Novel Combination Strategy

Hannah Zaryouh[1†], Ines De Pauw[1†], Hasan Baysal[1], Patrick Pauwels[1,2], Marc Peeters[1,3], Jan Baptist Vermorken[1,3], Filip Lardon[1‡] and An Wouters[1‡]*

[1] Center for Oncological Research (CORE), Integrated Personalized & Precision Oncology Network (IPPON), University of Antwerp, Antwerp, Belgium, [2] Department of Pathology, Antwerp University Hospital, Antwerp, Belgium, [3] Department of Medical Oncology, Antwerp University Hospital, Antwerp, Belgium

***Correspondence:**
Hannah Zaryouh
Hannah.Zaryouh@uantwerpen.be

†These authors share first authorship

‡These authors share senior authorship

The epidermal growth factor receptor (EGFR) is a therapeutic target in head and neck squamous cell carcinoma (HNSCC). Resistance to EGFR-targeted therapies, such as cetuximab, poses a challenging problem. This study aims to characterize acquired cetuximab resistance mechanisms in HNSCC cell lines by protein phosphorylation profiling. Through this, promising combination treatments can be identified to possibly overcome acquired cetuximab resistance in HNSCC. Protein phosphorylation profiling showed increased phosphorylation of Akt1/2/3 after cetuximab treatment in acquired cetuximab resistant cells compared to cetuximab sensitive cells, which was confirmed by western blotting. Based on this protein phosphorylation profile, a novel combination treatment with cetuximab and the Akt1/2/3 inhibitor MK2206 was designed. Synergy between cetuximab and MK2206 was observed in two cetuximab sensitive HNSCC cell lines and one acquired cetuximab resistant variant in simultaneous treatment schedules. In conclusion, this study demonstrates that increased Akt1/2/3 phosphorylation seems to be characteristic for acquired cetuximab resistance in HNSCC cell lines. Our results also show an additive to synergistic interaction between cetuximab and MK2206 in simultaneous treatment schedules. These data support the hypothesis that the combination of cetuximab with PI3K/Akt pathway inhibition might be a promising novel therapeutic strategy to overcome acquired cetuximab resistance in HNSCC patients.

Keywords: PI3K/Akt pathway, cetuximab, EGFR, HNSCC, Akt inhibitor, resistance

INTRODUCTION

Head and neck squamous cell carcinoma (HNSCC) is the sixth most common cancer type worldwide and remains one of the most challenging malignancies to treat (1, 2). Through our increasing knowledge regarding the molecular biology of HNSCC, several therapeutic strategies have been developed. The introduction of targeted therapies that inhibit oncogenic signaling pathways, as well as the development of immunotherapies that activate a patient's immune system are now at the forefront of personalized medicine in cancer treatment.

Over the past decades, research has revealed that the epidermal growth factor receptor (EGFR, HER1) plays an integral role in the tumorigenesis of HNSCC. Increased or sustained activation of the EGFR signaling pathway can induce malignant transformation through sustained signaling for cell proliferation, anti-apoptotic signaling, angiogenesis and metastasis (3). Furthermore, EGFR is highly expressed in a wide range of malignancies, including HNSCC. As a result, EGFR is considered as a compelling drug target (3, 4).

In 2006, the anti-EGFR monoclonal antibody (mAb) cetuximab, was approved by the Food and Drug Administration (FDA) in combination with radiotherapy for locoregionally advanced HNSCC (median overall survival (OS) of 4.1 years versus 2.4 years with radiotherapy alone) and in combination with platinum-based therapy and infusional 5-fluorouracil (EXTREME regimen) for the first-line treatment of patients with recurrent/metastatic (R/M) HNSCC (median OS 10.1 months versus 7.4 months with chemotherapy alone) (5–7). To date, the therapeutic landscape of HNSCC is changing as the anti-programmed death-1 (PD-1) immune checkpoint inhibitor pembrolizumab has been FDA-approved in June 2019 as a first-line treatment of R/M HNSCC. The Keynote-048 study demonstrated that pembrolizumab with platinum and 5-fluorouracil significantly improved median OS versus the EXTREME regimen with cetuximab in the total population of HNSCC patients (13.0 months versus 10.7 months) (8). In particular, patients expressing programmed death ligand-1 (PD-L1) (85% of HNSCC patients has combined positive score ≥ 1) show an increased benefit from treatment with pembrolizumab plus platinum and 5-fluorouracil (median OS 13.6 months versus 10.4 months). However, response rates to this treatment regimen are 36% and thus still limited and comparable to the EXTREME regimen with cetuximab (8, 9). Hence, to date, management of R/M HNSCC relies on combination treatment involving platinum, 5-fluorouracil and the addition of pembrolizumab or cetuximab. However, as mentioned, only a fraction of HNSCC patients respond to these treatment regimens.

The reason for resistance to pembrolizumab treatment in HNSCC remains largely unknown. In this regard, several biomarkers, such as PD-L1 expression, immune infiltration, tumor mutational burden and immune-gene expression profiling, have been explored for their predictive potential. However, none of them could be validated in HNSCC so far (10). Concerning cetuximab, this resistance is partly attributable to lack and/or loss of sensitivity of tumor cells to EGFR inhibition, which develops during treatment and compromises the therapeutic outcome. If resistance to cetuximab therapy is present at baseline, this is defined as intrinsic (primary) resistance and can be explained by resistance-conferring factors pre-existing in the bulk of tumor cells. Moreover, nearly all patients whose tumors initially respond inevitably become acquired (secondary) resistant. Acquired resistance refers to disease progression during ongoing treatment that was initially effective (11). In these scenarios, targeting EGFR alone may not be efficacious and requires the addition of a supplementary targeting agent to maximize the therapeutic response.

Therefore, the present study aims to investigate a novel combination strategy to overcome acquired cetuximab resistance. We hypothesized that acquired cetuximab resistance in HNSCC may arise from the activation of compensatory signaling pathways following cetuximab treatment, which are able to reverse the inhibitory effects of cetuximab through phosphorylation of key proteins, thereby promoting cell survival. Pharmacological inhibition of these phosphorylated proteins might be essential to overcome acquired cetuximab resistance in HNSCC. Therefore, we first characterized the protein phosphorylation profile of two cetuximab sensitive (Cet_{Sens}) HNSCC cell lines and their acquired cetuximab resistant (Acq_{Res}) variants. Based on this protein phosphorylation profile, a novel combination treatment was designed to overcome acquired therapy resistance.

MATERIAL AND METHODS

Cell Culture

HPV-negative human HNSCC cell lines SC263 and SCC22b were kindly provided by Prof. Dr. Sandra Nuyts (University Hospital Leuven, Leuven, Belgium) and Prof. Dr. Olivier De Wever (Laboratory of Experimental Cancer Research, Ghent University Hospital, Ghent, Belgium). These HNSCC cell lines were previously identified as Cet_{Sens} following cetuximab treatment for 168h using the colorimetric sulforhodamine B (SRB) assay. Isogenic Acq_{Res} HNSCC cell lines (SC263-R and SCC22b-R) were previously generated by chronically exposing these initially Cet_{Sens} cell lines (parental) to cetuximab, starting with the IC_{50} concentration of cetuximab (12–14). In parallel, control cell lines (SC263-S and SCC22b-S) were established by exposure to the vehicle control (PBS). After 10 dose doublings, dose-response studies demonstrated that cetuximab-exposed cells developed resistance towards cetuximab (12–14). All cell lines were cultured in DMEM, supplemented with 10% fetal bovine serum, 1% penicillin/streptomycin and 1% L-glutamine (Life Technologies, Merelbeke, Belgium). Resistant cell lines were exposed to the highest doubling dose of cetuximab every four weeks. Cells were grown as monolayers and maintained in exponential growth in 5% CO_2/95% air in a humidified incubator at 37°C. All cell lines were confirmed free of mycoplasma infection through regular testing (MycoAlert Mycoplasma Detection Kit, Lonza, Verviers, Belgium). The identity of each cell line was validated through short tandem repeat profiling (Centre of Medical Genetics, University of Antwerp, Antwerp, Belgium).

Human Protein Phosphorylation Antibody Array

Human phospho-kinase antibody array kit (ARY003B, Proteome Profiler, R&D Systems, Minneapolis, MN, USA) was used to determine the relative levels of protein phosphorylation in the Cet_{Sens} and Acq_{Res} cell lines after cetuximab treatment. The human phospho-kinase antibody array was performed according to the manufacturer's protocol. In short, cells were lysed on 6-well plates after treatment with cetuximab (0 and 100 nM, 2 hours, diluted in sterile PBS, Merck, Darmstadt, Germany). Twenty minutes before lysis, epidermal growth factor (EGF, 50 ng/ml, Sigma-Aldrich, Diegem, Belgium) was added to the medium. Protein concentrations were determined using the Pierce BCA protein kit (Thermo Scientific, Erembodegem, Belgium). Next, samples were prepared and 450 µg of proteins were incubated overnight with nitrocellulose membranes which are spotted with 46 capture antibodies in duplicate. The specific target proteins (**Supplementary Table 1**), if present in the sample, bind to these capture antibodies, leading to protein-antibody interactions. These protein-antibody interactions are then visualized using chemiluminescent detection reagents on the Lumi-Imager (Roche Diagnostics, Vilvoorde, Belgium). The antibodies of this kit bind to all isoforms of the target proteins and are therefore not isoform-specific. The signal is proportional to the amount phosphorylation in the bound analyte. Quantification of phosphorylation levels was executed following the manufacturer's protocol. In short, the integrated optical density of each spot was measured and corrected for background signal using Image J software (15). Only proteins that gave rise to an integrated optical density at least 1.5-fold above background were further used for data processing. Mean integrated optical densities were obtained by averaging the integrated optical density of the duplicates on the array. The fold changes were calculated by dividing the mean integrated optical densities of the treatment and control groups.

Western Blot

In order to validate findings of the human phospho-kinase antibody array with western blot, cell lysates were three times independently prepared as described above. Twenty micrograms of proteins were separated by SDS-page (10% polyacrylamide gel, 100V, 2h) and western blot was performed (100V, 1h). Blocking of non-specific binding sites was done by incubation of the membrane with Odyssey blocking buffer TBS (Li-Cor, Leusden, The Netherlands) for 1h at room temperature while shaking. Next, primary and secondary antibody incubation and washing was performed using the SNAP id 2.0 protein detection system (Merck Millipore) according to the manufacturer's instructions. Membranes were incubated with the following antibodies: phospho-Akt (S473) rabbit mAb (1:1000, no. 193H12, Cell Signaling Technology, Leiden, The Netherlands) and total Akt (pan) rabbit mAb (1:1000, no. 11E7, Cell Signaling Technology). Anti-β-actin was used as an internal standard (1:5000, no. A5441, Sigma Aldrich). Goat-anti-rabbit (1:10000, no. 926-32211, Li-Cor) or goat-anti-mouse (1:10000, no. 926-68070, Li-Cor) fluorescently labeled secondary antibodies were used and fluorescent detection was performed using the Odyssey imaging system (Li-Cor). Protein levels were quantified using Image Studio™ Lite, a software program available on the Odyssey imaging system. Phospho-Akt and Akt expression levels were corrected for loading differences based on beta-actin expression. Fold changes were calculated by dividing the mean fluorescent signal of the treatment and control groups.

In Silico Analysis of Akt1, Akt2 and Akt3 Expression

The baseline mRNA expression of Akt1/2/3 in HNSCC patients was examined using the RNA sequencing data from The Cancer Genome Atlas (TCGA) dataset (Provisional, 522 sequenced HNSCC patients). RNASeqV2 from TCGA was processed and normalized using the software package RNA-Seq by Expectation Maximization (RSEM) in order to generate transcripts per million. This dataset was downloaded from cBioportal.

Sulforhodamine B Assay

Cell survival was assessed using the colorimetric SRB assay, as previously described (16, 17). This assay is used for cell density determination, based on the measurement of cellular protein content, whereby it is not possible to make a distinction between inhibition of proliferation (cytostatic effect) and cell death (cytotoxic effect). Optimal seeding densities for each cell line were determined in order to ensure exponential growth during the whole duration of the assay. Cells were counted with a TC20 Automated Cell Counter (Biorad, Temse, Belgium). After overnight incubation, cells were treated with MK2206 (72h, 0-5 µM, pan-Akt inhibitor, Selleck Chemicals, Houston, USA) in combination with cetuximab (0-50 nM). Hereby, two simultaneous combination schedules were tested:

1. Cetuximab plus MK2206 with total treatment duration of 72h
2. Cetuximab for 168h with MK2206 added during the last 72h of treatment

MK2206 was diluted in DMSO (Merck Millipore SA/NV, Overijse, Belgium) and further dilutions were made in cell culture medium. IC_{50} values (i.e. drug concentration causing 50% growth inhibition) were calculated using Graphpad Prism 9 software. Possible synergism between cetuximab and MK2206 was determined by calculation of the combination index (CI) using the Additive Model as described by others (18–20). $CI < 0.800$, $CI = 1.000 \pm 0.200$ and $CI > 1.200$ indicated synergism, additivity and antagonism, respectively.

Statistical Analysis

We performed all experiments at least three times independently, unless otherwise stated. In cytotoxicity experiments, each condition was tested in triplicate in each of the three experiments. Differences in total and phosphorylated Akt1/2/3, determined with western blot, were statistically analyzed using the non-parametric Kruskal-Wallis test. Significant values were adjusted by the Bonferroni correction for multiple testing. One-way ANOVA with Tukey-Kramer HSD posthoc analysis was used to assess significant differences in Akt1/2/3 mRNA expression of HNSCC patients (RNASeqV2 TCGA data). The influence of cetuximab treatment on the effect of MK2206 alone was evaluated for each cell line using linear mixed models in case of non-independent observations. More specifically, combination treatment was set as fixed effect. A random intercept for experimental replicates was added in order to account for the dependence of observations between experiments. The influence of cetuximab resistance status on the effect of MK2206 alone was also evaluated using linear mixed models. Resistance status was set as fixed effect and a random intercept for cell line and experimental replicates was added to account for the dependence of observations between cell lines and experiments. GraphPad Prism 9 was used for data comparison and artwork. All statistical analyses were performed in JMP Pro 15 and SPSS v25. P-values below 0.050 were considered significant.

RESULTS

Acquired Cetuximab Resistant HNSCC Cell Lines Show Increased Phosphorylation of Akt After Cetuximab Treatment

In order to characterize acquired cetuximab resistance, a protein phosphorylation profile was established using the human phospho-kinase antibody array. Hereby, the effect of cetuximab treatment on the phosphorylation of various proteins (**Supplementary Table 1**) was determined in two Cet_{Sens} HNSCC cell lines and their isogenic Acq_{Res} variants. Data analysis of the protein phosphorylation profile revealed a differential response of Cet_{Sens} HNSCC cell lines and Acq_{Res} variants to cetuximab treatment. As this change was most pronounced in substrates involved in the Akt signaling pathway, we focused further on the interpretation of these results in the next paragraph.

The effects of cetuximab treatment on the phosphorylation of EGFR, Akt and other substrates involved in the Akt pathway were quantified in Cet_{Sens} HNSCC cell lines and Acq_{Res} variants (**Figure 1**). Following cetuximab treatment, activating phosphorylation of EGFR was decreased in all HNSCC cell lines, suggesting inhibition of EGFR signaling. Both Cet_{Sens} HNSCC cell lines (i.e. SC263-S and SCC22b-S) demonstrated decreased phosphorylation of Akt1/2/3 at T308 after cetuximab treatment. T308 is phosphorylated by phosphoinositide-dependent kinase-1 (PDK1) in the phosphoinositide 3-kinase (PI3K)/Akt pathway, leading to Akt activation (21). As a result, the PI3K/Akt pathway is inhibited by cetuximab in Cet_{Sens} HNSCC cell lines. In contrast, a considerable increase in Akt1/2/3 phosphorylation at T308 was observed after cetuximab treatment in both Acq_{Res} variants. Furthermore, phosphorylation of Akt1/2/3 at S473, by mammalian target of rapamycin complex 2 (mTORC2) (21), was also enhanced in both Acq_{Res} variants, particularly in SCC22b-R. In addition, cetuximab treatment induced an increased phosphorylation of several downstream substrates of the Akt pathway [e.g. mTOR, p70 S6 kinase, glycogen synthase kinase-3 α/ß (GSK-3α/ß), proline-rich Akt substrate 40kDa (PRAS40) and WNK lysine deficient protein kinase-1 (WNK1)] in Acq_{Res} variants, especially in SCC22b-R. This means that the Akt pathway is still activated in Acq_{Res} cells following cetuximab treatment, leading to anti-apoptotic and pro-proliferative effects.

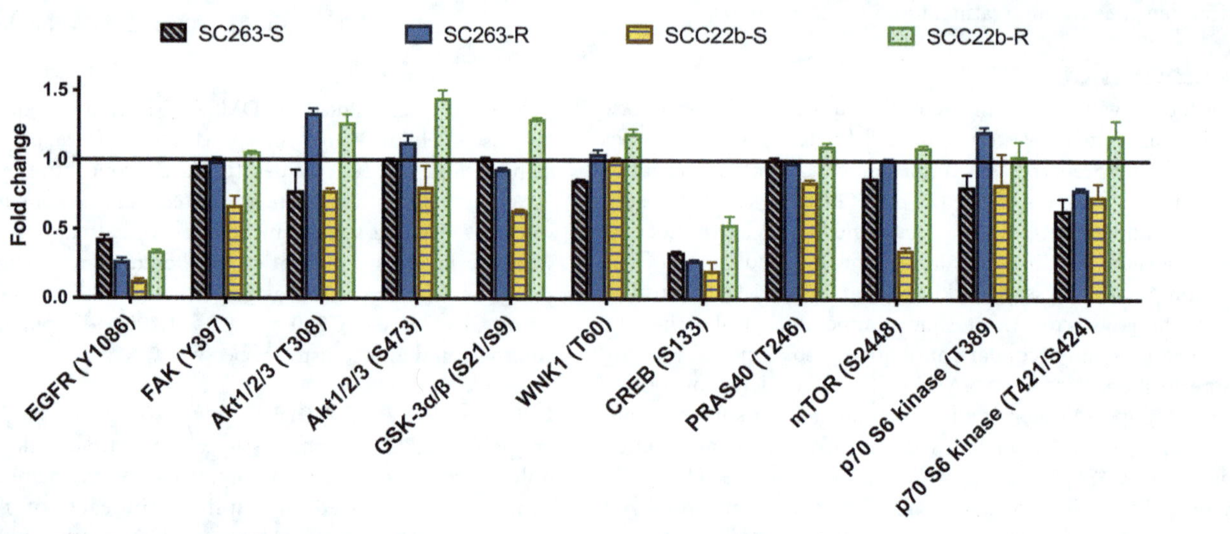

FIGURE 1 | Quantification of the human phospho-kinase array blots of cetuximab sensitive (SC263-S and SCC22b-S) HNSCC cell lines and corresponding acquired cetuximab resistant (SC263-R and SCC22b-R) variants. Graph represents the fold change of selected substrates, i.e. phosphorylated EGFR, Akt1/2/3 and other substrates involved in the Akt pathway, after cetuximab treatment. Protein phosphorylation profiling was conducted with one cell lysate. The fold changes were calculated by the ratio of the mean integrated optical density (duplicates) in treatment versus control groups. Error bars were calculated based on differences between duplicates. Suffix -S: cetuximab sensitive cell line and suffix -R: acquired cetuximab resistant cell line.

Western Blot Analysis Confirms Increased Akt1/2/3 Phosphorylation Following Cetuximab Treatment in Acquired Cetuximab Resistant HNSCC Cell Lines

Results from the protein phosphorylation profiling were first validated using western blot. Protein levels of total Akt1/2/3 and phosphorylated Akt1/2/3 at S473 were determined after cetuximab treatment in Cet_{Sens} HNSCC cell lines and Acq_{Res} variants (**Figures 2A, B**). Regarding the expression of total Akt 1/2/3, no change was observed following cetuximab treatment in the SC263-S and the Acq_{Res} SC263-R variant. Cetuximab treatment resulted in a small decrease in total Akt1/2/3 in SCC22b-S, while it resulted in a considerable increase in the Acq_{Res} variant (i.e. SCC22b-R). There was no statistical difference in the change of expression of total Akt1/2/3 following cetuximab treatment across cell lines ($p = 0.130$, **Figure 2B**). Cetuximab treatment did not induce any change in the phosphorylation of Akt1/2/3 at S473 in SC263-S, while a clear decrease in phosphorylated Akt1/2/3 was observed in SCC22b-S after cetuximab treatment. Cetuximab treatment induced a very small increase in the phosphorylation of Akt1/2/3 in SC263-R, while a considerable increase was observed in SCC22b-R. These results suggest a compensatory activation of the PI3K/Akt pathway in reaction to cetuximab treatment in Acq_{res} variants. Statistical analysis showed a significant difference in the change of Akt1/2/3 phosphorylation at S473 after cetuximab treatment between SCC22b-S and SCC22b-R ($p = 0.023$), but not between SC263-S and SC263-R ($p = 1.000$, **Figure 2B**). Comparison of the results of the protein phosphorylation profiling and western blot showed good similarity between both assays. Hence, the increase in Akt1/2/3 phosphorylation after cetuximab treatment in the Acq_{Res} HNSCC cell lines, detected with protein phosphorylation profiling, was confirmed with western blot (**Figure 2C**).

In conclusion, protein phosphorylation profiling demonstrated increased phosphorylation of Akt1/2/3 after cetuximab treatment in the Acq_{Res} HNSCC cell lines. This increase in phosphorylation was confirmed with western blot and was found significantly different between SCC22b-S and SCC22b-R. These results suggest that the combination of cetuximab with an Akt1/2/3 inhibitor might be a potential novel therapeutic combination strategy to overcome acquired cetuximab resistance in HNSCC cell lines.

HNSCC Patients Demonstrate Akt Expression

Before investigating the cytotoxic effect of the combination treatment with the EGFR inhibitor cetuximab and the

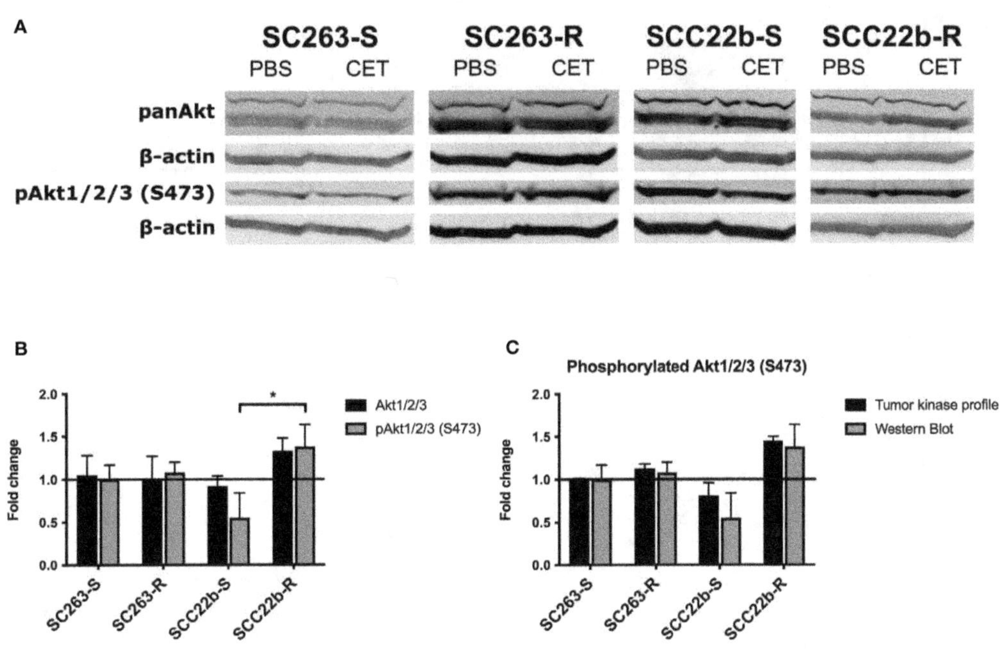

FIGURE 2 | Protein levels of total and phosphorylated Akt1/2/3 in cetuximab sensitive (SC263-S and SCC22b-S) HNSCC cell lines and corresponding acquired cetuximab resistant (SC263-R and SCC22b-R) variants. **(A)** Western blot was used to determine the levels of total and phosphorylated Akt1/2/3 (S473) after cetuximab treatment in cetuximab sensitive and acquired cetuximab resistant HNSCC cell lines. β-actin detection served as loading control. **(B)** Quantification of western blot results for total and phosphorylated Akt1/2/3. Signals were corrected for β-actin and the effect of cetuximab treatment is presented as fold change. Fold changes were calculated by dividing the mean fluorescent signal of the treatment and control groups. The graph represents the average fold change of three independent experiments. **(C)** Fold change of phosphorylated Akt1/2/3 at S473 following cetuximab treatment observed with protein phosphorylation profiling and western blot. CET, cetuximab; pAkt1/2/3, phosphorylated Akt1/2/3; *p-value ≤ 0.050. Suffix -S: cetuximab sensitive cell line and suffix -R: acquired cetuximab resistant cell line.

Akt1/2/3 inhibitor MK2206, we determined the expression of Akt isoforms in HNSCC patients using RNA sequencing data from the TCGA dataset (Provisional, RNASeqV2 RSEM, 522 sequenced HNSCC patients). This data demonstrated that there is a significant difference in mRNA expression between Akt1, Akt2 and Akt3 ($p < 0.0001$, **Supplementary Table 2**) in HNSCC patients (**Supplementary Figure 1**). As substantial Akt1, Akt2 and Akt3 mRNA levels were detected in the majority of tumor samples of HNSCC patients, we can conclude that the target of MK2206 is present in HNSCC patients. Therefore, this drug can play a potential role in the treatment of HNSCC patients.

Combining Cetuximab With MK2206 Shows Additive to Synergistic Effects in HNSCC Cell Lines

Possible synergistic effects of treatment with cetuximab and MK2206 were investigated in two Cet_{Sens} HNSCC cell lines and their isogenic Acq_{Res} variants. Two simultaneous combination schedules were evaluated. First, cells were treated simultaneously for 72h with 0-5 μM MK2206 and fixed doses of cetuximab. Fixed doses of cetuximab were based on the outcome of previous monotherapy experiments with total treatment duration of 72h (data not shown). As mentioned above, we previously identified Cet_{Sens} cell lines based on the outcomes of experiments with a total treatment time of 168h (14). After 72h of cetuximab treatment, there was only a limited effect on cell survival. Therefore, we chose two high concentrations of cetuximab (i.e. 25 nM and 50 nM) to use in these simultaneous combination experiments with MK2206. Based on results reported in clinical trials, these concentrations are considered clinically relevant in *in vitro* studies (22). Regarding MK2206, based on early phase clinical trials, clinically relevant concentrations with manageable side effects were estimated at ≤1 μM for *in vitro* studies (23).

The dose-response curves of the Cet_{Sens} HNSCC cell lines and their Acq_{Res} variants are shown in **Figures 3A–D**. A clear concentration-dependent effect of MK2206 after 72 hours of treatment was observed in all HNSCC cell lines. The IC_{50} values for MK2206 monotherapy ranged from 1.752 ± 0.084 μM to 4.764 ± 0.436 μM (**Supplementary Figure 2A** and **Table 1**).

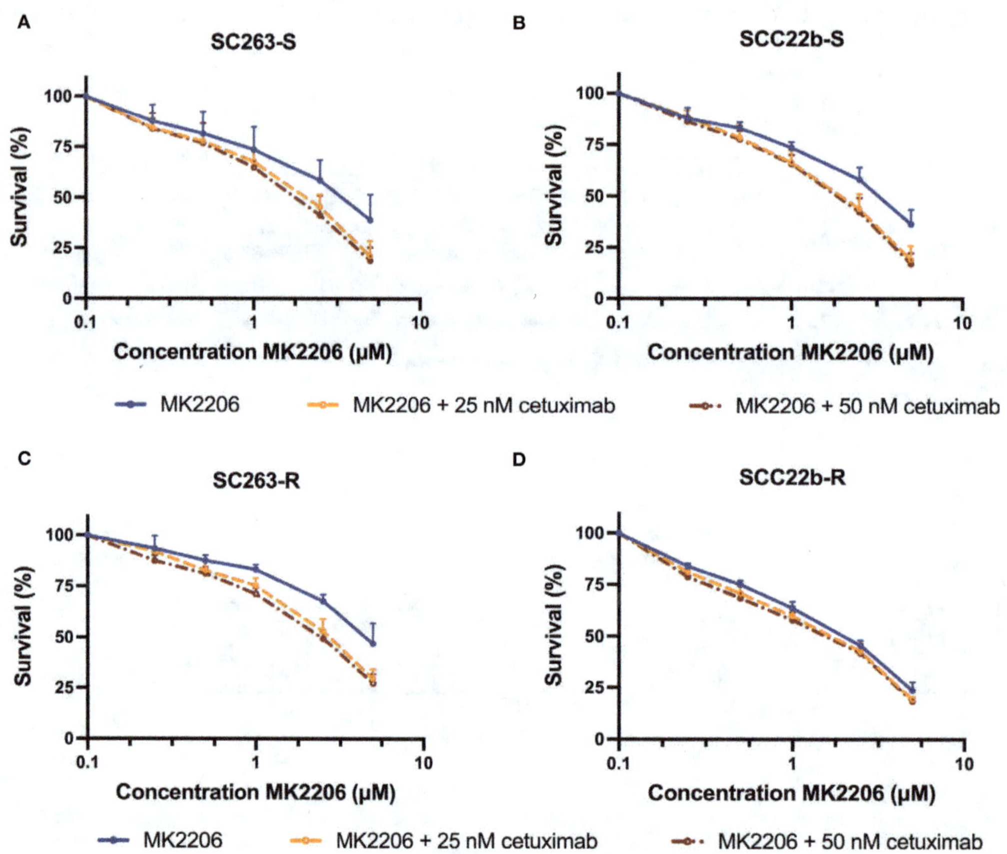

FIGURE 3 | The cytotoxic effect of cetuximab plus MK2206 with a total treatment duration of 72h. Dose-response curves for the cetuximab sensitive HNSCC cell lines SC263-S **(A)** and SCC22b-S **(B)** show a synergistic effect. Regarding the acquired cetuximab resistant variants, dose-response curves indicate a synergistic and additive effect in SC263-R **(C)** and SCC22b-R **(D)**, respectively. Survival curves were corrected for the cytotoxic effect of cetuximab alone. Cells were treated with fixed concentrations of cetuximab, which were chosen based on the outcome of previous monotherapy experiments. Suffix -S: cetuximab sensitive cell line and suffix -R: acquired cetuximab resistant cell line.

Acquired cetuximab resistance had no significant influence on the inhibitory potential of MK2206 ($p = 0.954$). Compared to MK2206 treatment alone, simultaneous treatment with cetuximab caused a significant decrease in IC_{50} value ($p \leq 0.048$) in Cet_{Sens} HNSCC cell lines and the Acq_{Res} variants (**Supplementary Figure 2A** and **Table 1**). Furthermore, the CI ranged from 0.707 to 0.917 (**Table 2**). Synergy between cetuximab and 2.5 μM MK2206 was observed in two Cet_{Sens} HNSCC cell lines and one Acq_{Res} variant (i.e. in SC263-S, SC263-R and SCC22b-S with CI ≤ 0.783, **Supplementary Figure 2B** and **Table 2**) after 72h of simultaneous treatment. Combining MK2206 with higher cetuximab concentrations resulted in an increased synergistic or additive effect.

Next, the cytotoxic effect of the second treatment schedule was investigated. Hereby, the cells were treated with fixed doses of cetuximab for 168h and MK2206 (0-2.5 μM) was added during the last 72h of treatment. The goal of this prolonged treatment schedule was to decrease the used drug concentrations. In contrast to the first treatment schedule, Cet_{Sens} HNSCC cell lines were treated with lower concentrations of cetuximab (i.e. 0.5 nM, 1 nM and 5 nM) due to prolonged treatment duration. These fixed concentrations were based on the outcome of previous monotherapy experiments with a total treatment duration of 168h (14).

Figures 4A–D shows the dose-response curves of the Cet_{Sens} HNSCC cell lines and their Acq_{Res} variants. The addition of MK2206 during the last 72h of treatment still resulted in a concentration-dependent cytotoxic effect of this compound. The IC_{50} values for MK2206 ranged from 1.073 ± 0.038 μM to 4.372 ± 1.182 μM (**Supplementary Figures 3A, B** and **Table 3**). Compared to MK2206 treatment alone, simultaneous treatment with cetuximab resulted in a decrease in IC_{50} value ($0.033 \leq p \leq 0.127$). Furthermore, in this treatment regimen, the CI ranged from 0.578 to 0.867 (**Table 4**). Synergy between cetuximab and 1 μM MK2206 was observed in two Cet_{Sens} HNSCC cell lines and one Acq_{Res} variant (i.e. in SC263-S, SC263-R and SCC22b-S with CI ≤ 0.796, **Supplementary Figures 3C, D** and **Table 4**). Combining MK2206 with higher cetuximab concentrations increased the synergistic interaction in Cet_{Sens} cell lines. As this synergistic effect was reached using lower concentrations of both MK2206 and cetuximab, we consider this treatment schedule as the most interesting for further investigation.

DISCUSSION

Targeted therapies are key for the personalized treatment of cancer patients (3). Although treatment with the EGFR-inhibitor cetuximab improves OS in HNSCC patients, therapeutic resistance poses a challenging problem and limits the success of effective anti-EGFR cancer therapies in the clinic (24). Therefore, it is of utmost importance to rationally develop novel combination strategies to overcome this therapy resistance.

Increased or sustained stimulation of EGFR mediates the activation of various signal transduction pathways. Proteins involved in these signaling pathways are potential contributors to the development of acquired resistance to drugs inhibiting EGFR signaling (25). In order to identify the signaling pathways characteristic for acquired cetuximab resistance, protein phosphorylation profiling was performed in HNSCC cell lines. This technique has already been successfully applied in other

TABLE 2 | CI for HNSCC cell lines after treatment with cetuximab plus 2.5 μM MK2206 for 72h.

Cell line	Condition	CI
SC263-S	2.5 μM MK2206 + 25 nM cetuximab	**0.775**
	2.5 μM MK2206 + 50 nM cetuximab	**0.707**
SCC22b-S	2.5 μM MK2206 + 25 nM cetuximab	**0.757**
	2.5 μM MK2206 + 50 nM cetuximab	**0.730**
SC263-R	2.5 μM MK2206 + 25 nM cetuximab	**0.783**
	2.5 μM MK2206 + 50 nM cetuximab	**0.728**
SCC22b-R	2.5 μM MK2206 + 25 nM cetuximab	0.937
	2.5 μM MK2206 + 50 nM cetuximab	0.917

CI < 0.800, CI = 1.000 ± 0.200, and CI > 1.200 indicate synergism, additivity or antagonism, respectively. CI < 0.800 are indicated in bold. Suffix -S: cetuximab sensitive cell line and suffix -R: acquired cetuximab resistant cell line.

TABLE 1 | IC_{50} and standard errors for HNSCC cell lines after treatment with MK2206 plus cetuximab for 72h.

Cell line	Condition	IC_{50} MK2206 (μM)	P-value
SC263-S	MK2206	3.311 ± 0.537	–
	MK2206 + 25 nM cetuximab	1.816 ± 0.134	0.068
	MK2206 + 50 nM cetuximab	1.609 ± 0.154	**0.048**
SCC22b-S	MK2206	3.086 ± 0.239	–
	MK2206 + 25 nM cetuximab	1.749 ± 0.120	**0.006**
	MK2206 + 50 nM cetuximab	1.646 ± 0.101	**0.004**
SC263-R	MK2206	4.764 ± 0.436	–
	MK2206 + 25 nM cetuximab	2.545 ± 0.135	**0.015**
	MK2206 + 50 nM cetuximab	2.212 ± 0.109	**0.010**
SCC22b-R	MK2206	1.752 ± 0.084	–
	MK2206 + 25 nM cetuximab	1.446 ± 0.085	**0.020**
	MK2206 + 50 nM cetuximab	1.327 ± 0.082	**0.006**

P < 0.050, significant difference in IC_{50} compared to MK2206 monotherapy. P < 0.050 are indicated in bold. -, cannot be calculated. Suffix -S: cetuximab sensitive cell line and suffix -R: acquired cetuximab resistant cell line.

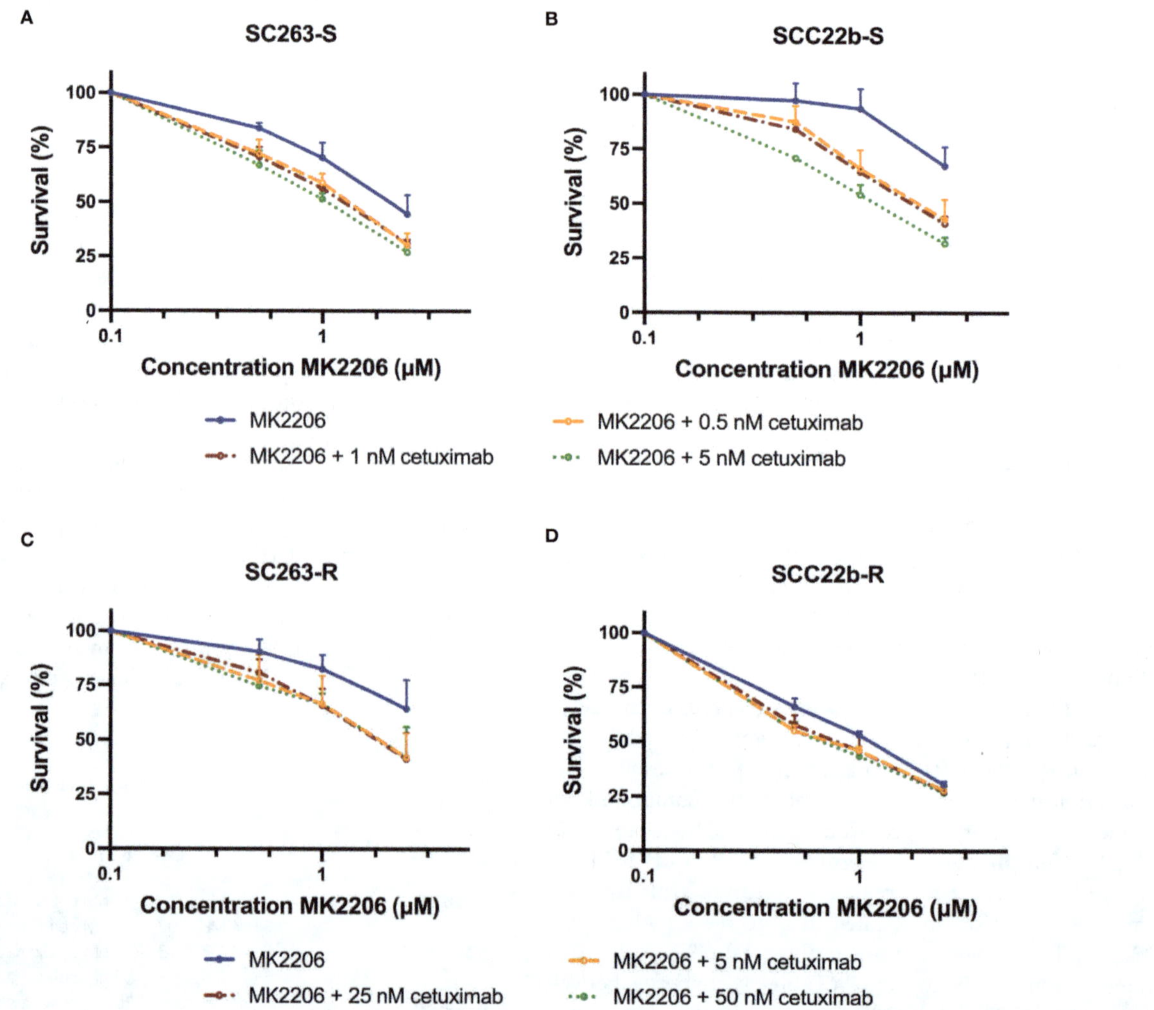

FIGURE 4 | The cytotoxic effect of cetuximab for 168h with MK2206 added during the last 72h of treatment. Dose-response curves for the cetuximab sensitive HNSCC cell lines SC263-S **(A)** and SCC22b-S **(B)** show a synergistic interaction. Regarding the acquired cetuximab resistant variants, dose-response curves indicate a synergistic and additive effect in SC263-R **(C)** and SCC22b-R **(D)**, respectively. Survival curves were corrected for the cytotoxic effect of cetuximab alone. Cells were treated with fixed concentrations of cetuximab, which were based on the outcome of previous monotherapy experiments. Suffix -S: cetuximab sensitive cell line and suffix -R: acquired cetuximab resistant cell line.

studies to identify drug resistance mechanisms (26–28). In the present study, the effect of cetuximab treatment on the phosphorylation of several proteins was determined in two Cet_{Sens} HNSCC cell lines and their isogenic Acq_{Res} variants. Based on this protein phosphorylation profiling, novel rationally designed combination strategies were investigated to overcome drug resistance.

Protein phosphorylation profiling showed a differential response of Cet_{Sens} HNSCC cell lines and their Acq_{Res} variants to EGFR inhibition by cetuximab. This profile strongly suggested that increased phosphorylation of Akt1/2/3 following cetuximab treatment is characteristic for Acq_{Res} HNSCC cell lines. In general, Cet_{Sens} HNSCC cell lines demonstrated decreased phosphorylation of EGFR (Y1086), Akt1/2/3 (T308 and S473) and downstream substrates after cetuximab treatment. Although EGFR phosphorylation was decreased, Akt1/2/3 was still phosphorylated and activated following cetuximab treatment in Acq_{Res} HNSCC cell lines. This was supported by the observed increase in phosphorylation of several downstream substrates of Akt, such as mTOR, p70S6 kinase, GSK-3α/β, PRAS40 and WNK1. Thus, in Acq_{Res} HNSCC cell lines, the Akt pathway was still able to exerts its anti-apoptotic and pro-proliferative effects under cetuximab treatment, possibly leading to therapy resistance. Importantly, it is worth mentioning that the number of cell lines used in this study is a limiting factor. Therefore, our data needs to be validated in additional isogenic HNSCC cell lines (and ideally in HNSCC patient samples) in order to strengthen the results. Although further confirmation in

TABLE 3 | IC_{50} and standard errors for HNSCC cell lines after treatment with cetuximab for 168h with MK2206 added during the last 72h of treatment.

Cell line	Condition	IC_{50} MK2206 (μM)	P-value
SC263-S	MK2206	2.067 ± 0.177	-
	MK2206 + 0.5 nM cetuximab	1.253 ± 0.078	0.127
	MK2206 + 1 nM cetuximab	1.200 ± 0.043	0.102
	MK2206 + 5 nM cetuximab	1.002 ± 0.049	0.051
SCC22b-S	MK2206	3.541 ± 0.540	-
	MK2206 + 0.5 nM cetuximab	1.919 ± 0.197	0.112
	MK2206 + 1 nM cetuximab	1.787 ± 0.071	0.082
	MK2206 + 5 nM cetuximab	1.187 ± 0.043	**0.027**
SC263-R	MK2206	4.372 ± 1.182	-
	MK2206 + 5 nM cetuximab	1.851 ± 0.315	**0.045**
	MK2206 + 25 nM cetuximab	1.815 ± 0.201	0.054
	MK2206 + 50 nM cetuximab	1.51 ± 0.264	0.090
SCC22b-R	MK2206	1.073 ± 0.038	-
	MK2206 + 5 nM cetuximab	0.710 ± 0.034	0.052
	MK2206 + 25 nM cetuximab	0.769 ± 0.061	0.102
	MK2206 + 50 nM cetuximab	0.670 ± 0.033	**0.033**

$P < 0.050$, significant difference in IC_{50} compared to MK2206 monotherapy. $P < 0.050$ are indicated in bold. -, cannot be calculated. Suffix -S: cetuximab sensitive cell line and suffix -R: acquired cetuximab resistant cell line.

TABLE 4 | CI for HNSCC cell lines after treatment with cetuximab for 168h with 1 μM MK2206 added during the last 72h of treatment.

Cell line	Condition	CI
SC263-S	1 μM MK2206 + 0.5 nM cetuximab	0.838
	1 μM MK2206 + 1 nM cetuximab	0.801
	1 μM MK2206 + 5 nM cetuximab	**0.732**
SCC22b-S	1 μM MK2206 + 0.5 nM cetuximab	**0.705**
	1 μM MK2206 + 1 nM cetuximab	**0.688**
	1 μM MK2206 + 5 nM cetuximab	**0.578**
SC263-R	1 μM MK2206 + 5 nM cetuximab	0.805
	1 μM MK2206 + 25 nM cetuximab	**0.796**
	1 μM MK2206 + 50 nM cetuximab	0.806
SCC22b-R	1 μM MK2206 + 5 nM cetuximab	0.867
	1 μM MK2206 + 25 nM cetuximab	0.865
	1 μM MK2206 + 50 nM cetuximab	0.818

CI < 0.800, CI = 1.000 ± 0.200, and CI > 1.200 indicate synergism, additivity or antagonism, respectively. CI < 0.800 are indicated in bold. Suffix -S: cetuximab sensitive cell line and suffix -R: acquired cetuximab resistant cell line.

HNSCC cell lines and patient samples is still needed, based on our results, Akt represents a potential target to improve outcome of cetuximab-based treatment in HNSCC patients.

The PI3K/Akt pathway has been shown to regulate various normal biological processes, such as cellular survival, migration, proliferation, differentiation, angiogenesis, protein synthesis and glucose metabolism. Activation of Akt can be initiated by several events, mainly through a receptor-ligand interaction on the cell membrane. This receptor activation results in activation of PI3K, which phosphorylates phosphatidylinositol 3,4-biphosphate (PIP_2) to generate phosphatidylinositol 3,4,5-triphosphate (PIP_3). The binding of PIP_3 to Akt locates Akt to the plasma membrane and allows its phosphorylation and activation by PDK1. Akt can also be phosphorylated by other substrates and in response to cellular stress, such as ischemia, hypoxia and oxidative stress. The tumor suppressor phosphatase and tensin homolog (PTEN) catalyzes the dephosphorylation of PIP_3 and is the major negative regulator of Akt signaling. Activated Akt exerts its effects by phosphorylating various downstream substrates, all resulting in anti-apoptotic or pro-proliferative effects (29–32). However, the pathway is also associated with a number of oncogenic processes. Indeed, the PI3K/Akt pathway is one of the most frequently dysregulated signaling pathways in cancer, including HNSCC (33, 34).

The present study demonstrates that increased Akt activation (not isoform-specific) is characteristic for acquired cetuximab resistance in HNSCC cell lines. Importantly, this observation needs to be validated in a cohort of HNSCC patient samples in order to elucidate its clinical value. Nevertheless, previous research has already suggested that enhanced Akt activation can play a role in resistance to cetuximab, not only in HNSCC but also in colorectal cancer and non-small cell lung cancer (35–39). Increased activation of the Akt signaling pathway has been associated with genetic alterations in the *PIK3CA* gene (40). For instance, Rebucci et al. have demonstrated that treatment of cetuximab resistant HNSCC cells with cetuximab did not result in the decreased levels of phosphorylated Akt that were seen in cetuximab sensitive HNSCC cells. A mutation in exon 20 of the *PIK3CA* gene, that encodes for the catalytic p110 α subunit of PI3K, was responsible for this persistent Akt activation (36). According to the TCGA dataset, respectively 18.4% and 20.8% of HNSCC patients demonstrate *PIK3CA* mutations or amplification (41, 42). In addition, loss of the tumor suppressor *PTEN* can also lead to persistent activation of the PI3K/Akt pathway (43, 44). According to TCGA, deep and shallow deletions in the *PTEN* gene occur in 3.4% and 24.0% of HNSCC patients, respectively (41, 42). Based on these findings, the genetic background of the HNSCC cell lines used in this study was determined using whole-exome sequencing (data not shown). Both Cet_{Sens} HNSCC cell lines and their Acq_{Res} variants display no mutations, deletions and/or insertions in the *PI3KCA* and *PTEN* genes. As such, the persistent Akt activation in Acq_{Res} HNSCC cell lines following cetuximab treatment cannot be explained by the genetic background of the cell lines. However, genetic alterations in *PIK3CA* and *PTEN*, possibly leading to persistent Akt activation, are present in a significant number of HNSCC patients in the TCGA cohort. Interestingly, both Cet_{Sens} HNSCC cell lines and their Acq_{Res} variants have *TP53* gene mutations that are predicted to have a deleterious effect on protein function. Functional p53 inhibits the PI3K/Akt pathway by regulating the transcription of four genes, which all have an inhibitory effect on Akt and mTOR (45, 46). As a result, mutant p53 can cause sustained activation of the PI3K/Akt pathway. However, as not only Acq_{Res} cell lines, but also Cet_{Sens} cell lines display mutations in *TP53*, the underlying mechanism behind the observed increased phosphorylation of Akt after cetuximab treatment in Acq_{Res} HNSCC cell lines remains unclear. To define the exact role of genetic alterations in the PI3K/Akt pathway, regarding response to cetuximab, more in-depth studies are needed with HNSCC patient samples.

As we found that increased Akt1/2/3 phosphorylation is characteristic for Acq_{Res} HNSCC cell lines and Akt1, Akt2 and

Akt3 are expressed in HNSCC patients, we hypothesized that the combination of cetuximab with an Akt inhibitor might be a potential novel therapeutic strategy to overcome acquired cetuximab resistance. To date, Akt inhibitors are not yet included in clinical practice (32). A phase II study with the pan-Akt inhibitor MK2206 in R/M HNSCC patients showed promising results (i.e. partial responses), but was not moved to phase III so far (NCT01349933). This might be due to the fact that pan-Akt inhibitors targeting all isoforms of Akt have shown to enhance the invasiveness of cancer cells in some cases. In this regard, Brolih et al. demonstrated that Akt1 inhibition leads to a more invasive phenotype in HNSCC tumors that primarily express Akt1 (47). Consistently, the latter was also observed in several studies for breast cancer (48–51). This suggests that the expression of specific Akt isoforms can influence the outcome of pharmacological Akt inhibition. Therefore, Akt isoform analysis may be necessary in order to predict the outcome of pan-Akt inhibitors (47). Alternatively, the use of isoform-selective Akt inhibitors, which have recently been developed (52), may also offer a solution to overcome the potential limitations of the pan-Akt inhibitor MK2206. On the other hand, it has been suggested that future studies should explore mechanism-based combination strategies with chemotherapy or other molecular targeted agents (53).

In the present study, our results provide a rationale to combine cetuximab with MK2206 to overcome acquired cetuximab resistance in HNSCC. To test our hypothesis, we examined the effects of treatment with cetuximab and the Akt inhibitor MK2206 in Cet_{Sens} HNSCC cell lines and Acq_{Res} variants. Hereby, two simultaneous combination schedules were tested. Synergy between cetuximab and MK2206 was observed in two Cet_{Sens} HNSCC cell lines and one Acq_{Res} variant in both simultaneous treatment schedules. An additive effect was observed in the Acq_{Res} SCC22b-R HNSCC cell line. Interestingly, MK2206 monotherapy demonstrated already a large cytotoxic effect in the SCC22b-R cell line compared to the other three cell lines used in this study. A possible explanation is that the SCC22b-R cell line demonstrated the largest increase in phosphorylation of Akt1/2/3 in the protein phosphorylation profiling analysis. As a result, the increased cytotoxic effect of MK2206 treatment alone might explain the observed additive interaction with cetuximab. Additional research is required to further elucidate the molecular mechanisms underlying the additive to synergistic effect between cetuximab and MK2206. Overall, this study demonstrated the potential of Akt inhibition in combination treatments to overcome acquired cetuximab resistance in HNSCC.

Besides the rational design of novel combination strategies, characterization of cetuximab resistance mechanisms can also lead to the identification of predictive biomarkers. To date, no definitive biomarkers have been identified to predict the efficacy of EGFR-targeting agents in patients with HNSCC (25, 54). We found in literature that phosphorylation of Akt at S473 serves as an independent prognostic marker for radiosensitivity in advanced HNSCC and that inhibition of Akt phosphorylation with pharmacological compounds might circumvent resistance to radiotherapy (55). Moreover, it has already been reported that phosphorylated Akt might be a potential predictive biomarker for EGFR-targeted therapies. For instance, lower phosphorylated Akt was observed in cetuximab sensitive HNSCC tumors in cell line xenograft models (56). Furthermore, Lyuo et al. analyzed a cohort with 50 oral squamous cell carcinoma patients who received cetuximab-based induction chemotherapy and found that lower expression of phosphorylated Akt was associated with better disease-free survival (57). In addition, the ECOG2303 phase II trial showed that biomarker signatures consistent with activation of the PI3K/Akt pathway are associated with inferior outcomes to cetuximab-containing chemoradiotherapy regimen (37). These results encourage additional research to precisely define the role of the PI3K/Akt pathway as predictive biomarker for EGFR-targeting agents in HNSCC.

CONCLUSION

In conclusion, protein phosphorylation analysis demonstrated that increased Akt1/2/3 phosphorylation is characteristic for acquired cetuximab resistance in HNSCC cell lines. Furthermore, we observed an additive to synergistic interaction between the EGFR inhibitor cetuximab and the pan-Akt inhibitor MK2206 in cetuximab sensitive and acquired cetuximab resistant HNSCC cell lines. Overall, these data support the hypothesis that downstream effectors of the PI3K/Akt pathway serve as promising drug targets in the search for novel therapeutic combination strategies that are able to overcome resistance to anti-EGFR treatment in HNSCC patients.

ETHICS STATEMENT

Ethical review and approval was not required for the study on human participants in accordance with the local legislation and institutional requirements. Written informed consent for participation was not required for this study in accordance with the national legislation and the institutional requirements.

AUTHOR CONTRIBUTIONS

Conceptualization, HZ, IDP, JBV, and AW. Data curation, IDP and HZ. Formal analysis, IDP and HZ. Funding acquisition, MP, FL, and AW. Investigation, IDP, HZ, and HB. Methodology, IDP and AW. Project administration, IDP, HZ, and AW. Resources, PP, FL, and AW. Supervision, IDP and AW. Visualization, IDP, HZ, and AW. Writing—original draft, IDP, and HZ. Writing—review & editing, HZ, IDP, HB, MP, JBV, FL, and AW. All authors contributed to the article and approved the submitted version.

ACKNOWLEDGMENTS

This work was performed with the support of 'Kom op tegen Kanker' (Stand up to Cancer), the Flemish Cancer Society.

SUPPLEMENTARY MATERIAL

Supplementary Figure 1 | mRNA expression level of Akt1/2/3 in HNSCC patients, available from TCGA. The graph shows the log transformed mRNA expression (mean and standard deviation) of Akt1/2/3 from 522 HNSCC patients (individual dots). This dataset (TCGA Provisional, RNASeqV2) was downloaded from cBioportal. *, p-value ≤ 0.050.

Supplementary Figure 2 | The cytotoxic effect of cetuximab plus MK2206 with a total treatment duration of 72h. **(A)** IC_{50} of MK2206 for HNSCC cell lines after treatment with MK2206 alone and in combination with cetuximab. **(B)** Combination index (CI) versus fraction affected (FA) plot of 2.5 μM MK2206 with fixed doses of cetuximab (25 nM and 50 nM) in SC263-S (red), SCC22b-S (blue), SC263-R (green) and SCC22b-R (orange). *, significant difference in IC_{50} compared to MK2206 monotherapy ($p < 0.050$). CI < 0.800, CI = 1.000 ± 0.200 and CI > 1.200 indicated synergism, additive effect and antagonism, respectively. Suffix -S: cetuximab sensitive cell line and suffix -R: acquired cetuximab resistant cell line.

Supplementary Figure 3 | The cytotoxic effect of cetuximab for 168h with MK2206 added during the last 72h of treatment. **(A)** IC_{50} of MK2206 for cetuximab sensitive HNSCC cell lines after combination treatment. **(B)** IC_{50} of MK2206 for acquired cetuximab sensitive HNSCC cell lines after combination treatment. **(C)** Combination index (CI) versus fraction affected (FA) plot of 1 μM MK2206 with fixed doses of cetuximab (0.5 nM, 1 nM and 5 nM) in SC263-S (red) and SCC22b-S (blue). **(D)** Combination index (CI) versus fraction affected (FA) plot of 1 μM MK2206 with fixed doses of cetuximab (5 nM, 25 nM and 50 nM) in SC263-R (green) and SCC22b-R (orange). *, significant difference in IC_{50} compared to MK2206 monotherapy ($p < 0.050$). CI < 0.800, CI = 1.000 ± 0.200 and CI > 1.200 indicated synergism, additive effect, and antagonism, respectively. Suffix -S: cetuximab sensitive cell line and suffix -R: acquired cetuximab resistant cell line.

REFERENCES

1. Bray F, Ferlay J, Soerjomataram I, Siegel RL, Torre LA, Jemal A. Global Cancer Statistics 2018: GLOBOCAN Estimates of Incidence and Mortality Worldwide for 36 Cancers in 185 Countries. *CA Cancer J Clin* (2018) 68 (6):394–424. doi: 10.3322/caac.21492
2. Ferlay J, Colombet M, Soerjomataram I, Mathers C, Parkin DM, Piñeros M, et al. Estimating the Global Cancer Incidence and Mortality in 2018: GLOBOCAN Sources and Methods. *Int J Cancer* (2019) 144(8):1941–53. doi: 10.1002/ijc.31937
3. Mahipal A, Kothari N, Gupta S. Epidermal Growth Factor Receptor Inhibitors: Coming of Age. *Cancer Control: J Moffitt Cancer Center* (2014) 21(1):74–9. doi: 10.1177/107327481402100111
4. Wieduwilt MJ, Moasser MM. The Epidermal Growth Factor Receptor Family: Biology Driving Targeted Therapeutics. *Cell Mol Life Sci: CMLS* (2008) 65 (10):1566–84. doi: 10.1007/s00018-008-7440-8
5. Bonner JA, Harari PM, Giralt J, Azarnia N, Shin DM, Cohen RB, et al. Radiotherapy Plus Cetuximab for Squamous-Cell Carcinoma of the Head and Neck. *New Engl J Med* (2006) 354(6):567–78. doi: 10.1056/NEJMoa053422
6. Bonner JA, Harari PM, Giralt J, Cohen RB, Jones CU, Sur RK, et al. Radiotherapy Plus Cetuximab for Locoregionally Advanced Head and Neck Cancer: 5-Year Survival Data From a Phase 3 Randomised Trial, and Relation Between Cetuximab-Induced Rash and Survival. *Lancet Oncol* (2010) 11 (1):21–8. doi: 10.1016/S1470-2045(09)70311-0
7. Vermorken JB, Mesia R, Rivera F, Remenar E, Kawecki A, Rottey S, et al. Platinum-Based Chemotherapy Plus Cetuximab in Head and Neck Cancer. *N Engl J Med* (2008) 359(11):1116–27. doi: 10.1056/NEJMoa0802656
8. Burtness B, Harrington KJ, Greil R, Soulieres D, Tahara M, de Castro GJr., et al. Pembrolizumab Alone or With Chemotherapy Versus Cetuximab With Chemotherapy for Recurrent or Metastatic Squamous Cell Carcinoma of the Head and Neck (KEYNOTE-048): A Randomised, Open-Label, Phase 3 Study. *Lancet (London England)* (2019) 394(10212):1915–28. doi: 10.1016/S0140-6736(19)32591-7.31679945
9. Cohen EEW, Bell RB, Bifulco CB, Burtness B, Gillison ML, Harrington KJ, et al. The Society for Immunotherapy of Cancer Consensus Statement on Immunotherapy for the Treatment of Squamous Cell Carcinoma of the Head and Neck (HNSCC). *J Immunother Cancer* (2019) 7(1):184. doi: 10.1186/s40425-019-0662-5
10. Oliva M, Spreafico A, Taberna M, Alemany L, Coburn B, Mesia R, et al. Immune Biomarkers of Response to Immune-Checkpoint Inhibitors in Head and Neck Squamous Cell Carcinoma. *Ann Oncol: Off J Eur Soc Med Oncol* (2019) 30(1):57–67. doi: 10.1093/annonc/mdy507
11. Leto SM, Trusolino L. Primary and Acquired Resistance to EGFR-Targeted Therapies in Colorectal Cancer: Impact on Future Treatment Strategies. *J Mol Med (Berl)* (2014) 92(7):709–22. doi: 10.1007/s00109-014-1161-2
12. Boeckx C, Blockx L, de Beeck KO, Limame R, Camp GV, Peeters M, et al. Establishment and Characterization of Cetuximab Resistant Head and Neck Squamous Cell Carcinoma Cell Lines: Focus on the Contribution of the AP-1 Transcription Factor. *Am J Cancer Res* (2015) 5(6):1921–38.
13. De Pauw I, Wouters A, Van den Bossche J, Deschoolmeester V, Baysal H, Pauwels P, et al. Dual Targeting of Epidermal Growth Factor Receptor and HER3 by MEHD7945A as Monotherapy or in Combination With Cisplatin Partially Overcomes Cetuximab Resistance in Head and Neck Squamous Cell Carcinoma Cell Lines. *Cancer Biother Radiopharm* (2017) 32(7):229–38. doi: 10.1089/cbr.2017.2216
14. De Pauw I, Lardon F, Van den Bossche J, Baysal H, Fransen E, Deschoolmeester V, et al. Simultaneous Targeting of EGFR, HER2, and HER4 by Afatinib Overcomes Intrinsic and Acquired Cetuximab Resistance in Head and Neck Squamous Cell Carcinoma Cell Lines. *Mol Oncol* (2018) 12 (6):830–54. doi: 10.1002/1878-0261.12197
15. Schneider CA, Rasband WS, Eliceiri KW. NIH Image to ImageJ: 25 Years of Image Analysis. *Nat Methods* (2012) 9(7):671–5. doi: 10.1038/nmeth.2089
16. Pauwels B, Korst AE, de Pooter CM, Pattyn GG, Lambrechts HA, Baay MF, et al. Comparison of the Sulforhodamine B Assay and the Clonogenic Assay for *In Vitro* Chemoradiation Studies. *Cancer Chemother Pharmacol* (2003) 51 (3):221–6. doi: 10.1007/s00280-002-0557-9
17. Limame R, Wouters A, Pauwels B, Fransen E, Peeters M, Lardon F, et al. Comparative Analysis of Dynamic Cell Viability, Migration and Invasion Assessments by Novel Real-Time Technology and Classic Endpoint Assays. *PloS One* (2012) 7(10):e46536. doi: 10.1371/journal.pone.0046536
18. Valeriote F, Lin H. Synergistic Interaction of Anticancer Agents: A Cellular Perspective. *Cancer Chemother Rep* (1975) 59(5):895–900.
19. Jonsson E, Fridborg H, Nygren P, Larsson R. Synergistic Interactions of Combinations of Topotecan With Standard Drugs in Primary Cultures of Human Tumor Cells From Patients. *Eur J Clin Pharmacol* (1998) 54(7):509–14. doi: 10.1007/s002280050505

20. Deben C, Lardon F, Wouters A, Op de Beeck K, Van den Bossche J, Jacobs J, et al. APR-246 (PRIMA-1(MET)) Strongly Synergizes With AZD2281 (Olaparib) Induced PARP Inhibition to Induce Apoptosis in non-Small Cell Lung Cancer Cell Lines. *Cancer Lett* (2016) 375(2):313–22. doi: 10.1016/j.canlet.2016.03.017
21. Hornbeck PV, Zhang B, Murray B, Kornhauser JM, Latham V, Skrzypek E. PhosphoSitePlus, 2014: Mutations, PTMs and Recalibrations. *Nucleic Acids Res* (2015) 43(Database issue):D512–20. doi: 10.1093/nar/gku1267
22. Shibata K, Naito T, Okamura J, Hosokawa S, Mineta H, Kawakami J. Simple and Rapid LC-MS/MS Method for the Absolute Determination of Cetuximab in Human Serum Using an Immobilized Trypsin. *J Pharm Biomed Anal* (2017) 146:266–72. doi: 10.1016/j.jpba.2017.08.012
23. Yap TA, Yan L, Patnaik A, Fearen I, Olmos D, Papadopoulos K, et al. First-In-Man Clinical Trial of the Oral Pan-AKT Inhibitor MK-2206 in Patients With Advanced Solid Tumors. *J Clin Oncol: Off J Am Soc Clin Oncol* (2011) 29 (35):4688–95. doi: 10.1200/JCO.2011.35.5263
24. Cohen RB. Current Challenges and Clinical Investigations of Epidermal Growth Factor Receptor (EGFR)- and ErbB Family-Targeted Agents in the Treatment of Head and Neck Squamous Cell Carcinoma (HNSCC). *Cancer Treat Rev* (2014) 40(4):567–77. doi: 10.1016/j.ctrv.2013.10.002
25. Boeckx C, Baay M, Wouters A, Specenier P, Vermorken JB, Peeters M, et al. Anti-Epidermal Growth Factor Receptor Therapy in Head and Neck Squamous Cell Carcinoma: Focus on Potential Molecular Mechanisms of Drug Resistance. *Oncologist* (2013) 18(7):850–64. doi: 10.1634/theoncologist.2013-0013
26. Davies KD, Mahale S, Astling DP, Aisner DL, Le AT, Hinz TK, et al. Resistance to ROS1 Inhibition Mediated by EGFR Pathway Activation in non-Small Cell Lung Cancer. *PloS One* (2013) 8(12):e82236. doi: 10.1371/journal.pone.0082236
27. Baumgartner U, Berger F, Hashemi Gheinani A, Burgener SS, Monastyrskaya K, Vassella E. miR-19b Enhances Proliferation and Apoptosis Resistance *via* the EGFR Signaling Pathway by Targeting PP2A and BIM in non-Small Cell Lung Cancer. *Mol Cancer* (2018) 17(1):44. doi: 10.1186/s12943-018-0781-5
28. Fan PD, Narzisi G, Jayaprakash AD, Venturini E, Robine N, Smibert P, et al. YES1 Amplification is a Mechanism of Acquired Resistance to EGFR Inhibitors Identified by Transposon Mutagenesis and Clinical Genomics. *Proc Natl Acad Sci USA* (2018) 115(26):E6030–e8. doi: 10.1073/pnas.1717782115
29. Rogers SJ, Box C, Harrington KJ, Nutting C, Rhys-Evans P, Eccles SA. The Phosphoinositide 3-Kinase Signalling Pathway as a Therapeutic Target in Squamous Cell Carcinoma of the Head and Neck. *Expert Opin Ther Targets* (2005) 9(4):769–90. doi: 10.1517/14728222.9.4.769
30. Engelman JA, Luo J, Cantley LC. The Evolution of Phosphatidylinositol 3-Kinases as Regulators of Growth and Metabolism. *Nat Rev Genet* (2006) 7 (8):606–19. doi: 10.1038/nrg1879
31. Vander Broek R, Mohan S, Eytan DF, Chen Z, Van Waes C. The PI3K/Akt/mTOR Axis in Head and Neck Cancer: Functions, Aberrations, Cross-Talk, and Therapies. *Oral Dis* (2015) 21(7):815–25. doi: 10.1111/odi.12206
32. Nitulescu GM, Margina D, Juzenas P, Peng Q, Olaru OT, Saloustros E, et al. Akt Inhibitors in Cancer Treatment: The Long Journey From Drug Discovery to Clinical Use (Review). *Int J Oncol* (2016) 48(3):869–85. doi: 10.3892/ijo.2015.3306
33. Liu P, Cheng H, Roberts TM, Zhao JJ. Targeting the Phosphoinositide 3-Kinase Pathway in Cancer. *Nat Rev Drug Discovery* (2009) 8(8):627–44. doi: 10.1038/nrd2926
34. Simpson DR, Mell LK, Cohen EE. Targeting the PI3K/AKT/mTOR Pathway in Squamous Cell Carcinoma of the Head and Neck. *Oral Oncol* (2015) 51 (4):291–8. doi: 10.1016/j.oraloncology.2014.11.012
35. Silva-Oliveira RJ, Melendez M, Martinho O, Zanon MF, de Souza Viana L, Carvalho AL, et al. AKT Can Modulate the *In Vitro* Response of HNSCC Cells to Irreversible EGFR Inhibitors. *Oncotarget* (2017) 8(32):53288–301. doi: 10.1158/1538-7445.AM2017-4091
36. Rebucci M, Peixoto P, Dewitte A, Wattez N, De Nuncques MA, Rezvoy N, et al. Mechanisms Underlying Resistance to Cetuximab in the HNSCC Cell Line: Role of AKT Inhibition in Bypassing This Resistance. *Int J Oncol* (2011) 38(1):189–200.
37. Psyrri A, Lee JW, Pectasides E, Vassilakopoulou M, Kosmidis EK, Burtness BA, et al. Prognostic Biomarkers in Phase II Trial of Cetuximab-Containing Induction and Chemoradiation in Resectable HNSCC: Eastern Cooperative Oncology Group E2303. *Clin Cancer Res* (2014) 20(11):3023–32. doi: 10.1158/1078-0432.CCR-14-0113
38. Yamatodani T, Ekblad L, Kjellen E, Johnsson A, Mineta H, Wennerberg J. Epidermal Growth Factor Receptor Status and Persistent Activation of Akt and P44/42 MAPK Pathways Correlate With the Effect of Cetuximab in Head and Neck and Colon Cancer Cell Lines. *J Cancer Res Clin Oncol* (2009) 135 (3):395–402. doi: 10.1007/s00432-008-0475-2
39. Kim SM, Kim JS, Kim JH, Yun CO, Kim EM, Kim HK, et al. Acquired Resistance to Cetuximab Is Mediated by Increased PTEN Instability and Leads Cross-Resistance to Gefitinib in HCC827 NSCLC Cells. *Cancer Lett* (2010) 296(2):150–9. doi: 10.1016/j.canlet.2010.04.006
40. Pedrero JM, Carracedo DG, Pinto CM, Zapatero AH, Rodrigo JP, Nieto CS, et al. Frequent Genetic and Biochemical Alterations of the PI 3-K/AKT/PTEN Pathway in Head and Neck Squamous Cell Carcinoma. *Int J Cancer J Int du Cancer* (2005) 114(2):242–8. doi: 10.1002/ijc.20711
41. Cerami E, Gao J, Dogrusoz U, Gross BE, Sumer SO, Aksoy BA, et al. The Cbio Cancer Genomics Portal: An Open Platform for Exploring Multidimensional Cancer Genomics Data. *Cancer Discovery* (2012) 2(5):401–4. doi: 10.1158/2159-8290.CD-12-0095
42. Gao J, Aksoy BA, Dogrusoz U, Dresdner G, Gross B, Sumer SO, et al. Integrative Analysis of Complex Cancer Genomics and Clinical Profiles Using the Cbioportal. *Sci Signaling* (2013) 6(269):pl1. doi: 10.1126/scisignal.2004088
43. Kondo N, Tsukuda M, Taguchi T, Nakazaki K, Sakakibara A, Takahashi H, et al. Gene Status of Head and Neck Squamous Cell Carcinoma Cell Lines and Cetuximab-Mediated Biological Activities. *Cancer Sci* (2011) 102(9):1717–23. doi: 10.1111/j.1349-7006.2011.01999.x
44. Mriouah J, Boura C, Pinel S, Chretien AS, Fifre A, Merlin JL, et al. Cellular Response to Cetuximab in PTEN-Silenced Head and Neck Squamous Cell Carcinoma Cell Line. *Int J Oncol* (2010) 37(6):1555–63. doi: 10.3892/ijo_00000809
45. Feng Z, Hu W, de Stanchina E, Teresky AK, Jin S, Lowe S, et al. The Regulation of AMPK β1, TSC2, and PTEN Expression by P53: Stress, Cell and Tissue Specificity, and the Role of These Gene Products in Modulating the IGF-1-AKT-mTOR Pathways. *Cancer Res* (2007) 67(7):3043. doi: 10.1158/0008-5472.CAN-06-4149
46. Feng Z, Zhang H, Levine AJ, Jin S. The Coordinate Regulation of the P53 and mTOR Pathways in Cells. *Proc Natl Acad Sci USA* (2005) 102(23):8204–9. doi: 10.1073/pnas.0502857102
47. Brolih S, Parks SK, Vial V, Durivault J, Mostosi L, Pouysségur J, et al. AKT1 Restricts the Invasive Capacity of Head and Neck Carcinoma Cells Harboring a Constitutively Active PI3 Kinase Activity. *BMC Cancer* (2018) 18(1):249. doi: 10.1186/s12885-018-4169-0
48. Dillon RL, Marcotte R, Hennessy BT, Woodgett JR, Mills GB, Muller WJ. Akt1 and Akt2 Play Distinct Roles in the Initiation and Metastatic Phases of Mammary Tumor Progression. *Cancer Res* (2009) 69(12):5057–64. doi: 10.1158/0008-5472.CAN-08-4287
49. Hutchinson JN, Jin J, Cardiff RD, Woodgett JR, Muller WJ. Activation of Akt-1 (PKB-Alpha) Can Accelerate ErbB-2-Mediated Mammary Tumorigenesis But Suppresses Tumor Invasion. *Cancer Res* (2004) 64(9):3171–8. doi: 10.1158/0008-5472.CAN-03-3465
50. Li CW, Xia W, Lim SO, Hsu JL, Huo L, Wu Y, et al. AKT1 Inhibits Epithelial-To-Mesenchymal Transition in Breast Cancer Through Phosphorylation-Dependent Twist1 Degradation. *Cancer Res* (2016) 76(6):1451–62. doi: 10.1158/0008-5472.CAN-15-1941
51. Riggio M, Perrone MC, Polo ML, Rodriguez MJ, May M, Abba M, et al. AKT1 and AKT2 Isoforms Play Distinct Roles During Breast Cancer Progression Through the Regulation of Specific Downstream Proteins. *Sci Rep* (2017) 7:44244. doi: 10.1038/srep44244
52. Quambusch L, Landel I, Depta L, Weisner J, Uhlenbrock N, Müller MP, et al. Covalent-Allosteric Inhibitors to Achieve Akt Isoform-Selectivity. *Angew Chem Int Ed Engl* (2019) 58(52):18823–9. doi: 10.1002/anie.201909857
53. Oki Y, Fanale M, Romaguera J, Fayad L, Fowler N, Copeland A, et al. Phase II Study of an AKT Inhibitor MK2206 in Patients With Relapsed or Refractory Lymphoma. *Br J Haematol* (2015) 171(4):463–70. doi: 10.1111/bjh.13603
54. Kim BJ, Jeong JH, Kim HS, Kim JH. The Role of Anti-EGFR Agents in Patients With Locoregionally Advanced Head and Neck Cancer: A Meta-

Analysis of Randomized Trials. *Oncotarget* (2017) 8(60):102371–80. doi: 10.18632/oncotarget.21987

55. Freudlsperger C, Horn D, Weissfuss S, Weichert W, Weber KJ, Saure D, et al. Phosphorylation of AKT(Ser473) Serves as an Independent Prognostic Marker for Radiosensitivity in Advanced Head and Neck Squamous Cell Carcinoma. *Int J Cancer J Int du Cancer* (2015) 136(12):2775–85. doi: 10.1002/ijc.29328
56. Stein AP, Swick AD, Smith MA, Blitzer GC, Yang RZ, Saha S, et al. Xenograft Assessment of Predictive Biomarkers for Standard Head and Neck Cancer Therapies. *Cancer Med* (2015) 4(5):699–712. doi: 10.1002/cam4.387
57. Lyu J, Song H, Tian Z, Miao Y, Ren G, Guo W. Predictive Value of pAKT/PTEN Expression in Oral Squamous Cell Carcinoma Treated With Cetuximab-Based Chemotherapy. *Oral Surg Oral Med Oral Pathol Oral Radiol* (2016) 121(1):67–72. doi: 10.1016/j.oooo.2015.09.002

19

When the Loss Costs too Much: A Systematic Review and Meta-Analysis of Sarcopenia in Head and Neck Cancer

Xin Hua [1,2†], Shan Liu [3†], Jun-Fang Liao [4†], Wen Wen [1,2†], Zhi-Qing Long [1,2], Zi-Jian Lu [1,5], Ling Guo [1,5†] and Huan-Xin Lin [1,2*†]*

[1] State Key Laboratory of Oncology in South China, Collaborative Innovation Center for Cancer Medicine, SunYat-sen University Cancer Center, Guangzhou, China, [2] Department of Radiotherapy, Sun Yat-sen University Cancer Center, Guangzhou, China, [3] Department of Radiation Oncology, Sichuan Cancer Hospital & Institute, Sichuan Cancer Center, School of Medicine, University of Electronic Science and Technology of China, Chengdu, China, [4] Department of Radiation Oncology, National Cancer Center/National Clinical Cancer Research Center for Cancer/Cancer Hospital & Shenzhen Hospital, Chinese Academy of Medical Sciences and Peking Union Medical College, Shenzhen, China, [5] Guangdong Key Laboratory of Nasopharyngeal Carcinoma Diagnosis and Therapy, Department of Nasopharyngeal Carcinoma, Sun Yat-sen University Cancer Center, Guangzhou, China

***Correspondence:**
Ling Guo
guoling@sysucc.org.cn
Huan-Xin Lin
linhx@sysucc.org.cn

† These authors have contributed equally to this work

Purpose: Whether or not skeletal muscle mass (SMM) depletion, known as sarcopenia, has significant negative effects on the prognosis of patients with head and neck cancer (HNC) is both new and controversial. In this meta-analysis, we aimed to determine the prognostic significance of sarcopenia in HNC.

Methods: We searched PubMed, the Cochrane Library, Embase, and Web of Science, which contain trial registries and meeting proceedings, to identify related published or unpublished studies. We used the Newcastle–Ottawa Scale (NOS) to appraise the risk of bias of the included retrospective studies. Pooled hazard ratios (HR) and the I^2 statistic were estimated for the impact of sarcopenia on overall survival (OS) and relapse-free survival (RFS).

Results: We analyzed data from 11 studies involving 2,483 patients (39.4% on average of whom had sarcopenia). Based on the univariate analysis data, the sarcopenia group had significantly poorer OS compared to the non-sarcopenia group [HR = 1.97, 95% confidence interval (CI): 1.71–2.26, I^2 = 0%]. In the cutoff value subgroup, group 1, defined as skeletal muscle index (SMI) of 38.5 cm^2/m^2 for women and 52.4 cm^2/m^2 for men (HR = 2.41, 95% CI: 1.72–3.38, I^2 = 0%), had much poorer OS. In the race subgroup, the results were consistent between the Asia (HR = 2.11, 95% CI: 1.59–2.81) and non-Asia group (HR = 1.92, 95% CI: 1.64–2.25). The sarcopenia group also had significantly poorer RFS (HR = 1.74, 95% CI: 1.43–2.12, I^2 = 0%).

Conclusions: Presence of pre-treatment sarcopenia has a significant negative impact on OS and RFS in HNC compared with its absence. Further well-conducted studies with detailed stratification are needed to complement our findings.

Keywords: head and neck cancer, sarcopenia, meta-analysis, prognostic factor, skeletal muscle mass (SMM)

INTRODUCTION

Head and neck cancer (HNC) is a complex heterogeneous disease; numerous covariates affect its survival outcomes. According to National Comprehensive Cancer Network (NCCN) guidelines, radiotherapy (RT) with or without chemotherapy is the main treatment method for locally advanced HNC (1). Due to the local toxic effects of RT and chemoradiotherapy, patients with HNC may experience significant progressive weight loss and muscle mass depletion, which eventually lead to poor prognosis (2–4). Although weight loss is commonly used in clinical settings to screen for the risk of adverse outcomes in HNC, there are no universally recognized clear and reliable conclusions on the association of skeletal muscle mass (SMM) depletion and prognosis in HNC.

The main factors affecting treatment outcome are tumor characteristics and host-related factors (including age, sex, and nutritional status). Patients with HNC have a much higher risk of malnutrition than patients with other malignancies (5). Cancer patients with malnutrition typically lose lean body mass and muscle mass, while fat mass may remain or even increase (6). Muscle mass depletion, known as sarcopenia, can theoretically affect the treatment tolerance and prognosis of patients with HNC.

Sarcopenia is officially defined as generalized and progressive low SMM and function, and is related to physical disability and functional impairment (7). Sarcopenia in HNC can be quantified by the cross-sectional area in square centimeters (cm^2) divided by the squared height in meters (m^2) at the third lumbar (L3) or cervical (C3) vertebra level using computed tomography (CT) imaging (8). Recent studies have shown that sarcopenia is associated with increased risk of complications after tumor therapy and reduced disease-free survival (DFS) and overall survival (OS) (9–12). Sarcopenia and its effect on treatment-related complications and the clinical prognosis of HNC have recently attracted research attention. However, underestimation of the importance of sarcopenia continues to evolve when compared to the large number of studies that have been focused on different patient- and disease-related variables affecting the prognosis of patients with HNC (13–16).

Currently, whether sarcopenia in HNC can act as a prognostic factor is both little well-known and controversial (17, 18). Accordingly, we conducted this meta-analysis to investigate the prevalence of sarcopenia in patients with HNC and to determine its impact on clinical prognosis.

METHODS

Search Strategy

The prospective registration number of this meta-analysis on PROSPERO was CRD42019128406. This study was approved by the Ethics Committee of Sun Yat-sen University Cancer Center. Databases such as PubMed, the Cochrane Library, Embase, and Web of Science, which contain trial registries and meeting proceedings, were searched before August 30, 2019. In each database, we used the same search term: ("sarcopenia" or "fragility" or "sarcopenic" or "muscle index" or "muscle mass" or "muscle depletion" or "muscular atrophy") and ("head and neck cancer" or "head and neck neoplasm" or "HNSCC"). The language restriction was English; there were no other filters.

Study Selection

At the full-text screening step, two reviewers (X.H. and S.L.) assessed the relevant literature independently for inclusion. The κ statistic was used for inter-rater reliability (19). The inclusion criteria were as follows: (1) cohort and case–control study; (2) studied patients with HNC(s); (3) reported SMM or function measurement; and (4) reported prognostic data such as OS, progression-free survival (PFS), or DFS. Studies were excluded if data on the impact of sarcopenia on survival outcomes were unavailable.

Data Extraction

The two reviewers (S.L. and X.H.) extracted data from primary texts and Supplementary Appendixes independently and summarized them in a standardized data abstraction form. The extracted items are partly listed in **Table 1**. The results were reconciled and a third reviewer (J.F.L.) was consulted if there were discrepancies. In the case of missing data, the authors of the study in question were contacted via e-mail. If the authors did not reply, data from the published articles were used.

Risk of Bias Assessment

Two reviewers (W.W. and Z.Q.L.) assessed the bias independently. We used the modified Newcastle–Ottawa Scale (NOS) (35), which involves patient selection, study group comparability, and assessment of outcomes, to appraise the methodological quality of the included retrospective studies. The quality of each cohort study was scored 0–9, and case–control studies were scored 0–10; studies with scores of at least 6 were deemed good quality (19).

Meta-Analysis

We calculated and subsequently pooled in standard meta-analyses and hazard ratios (HRs) with corresponding 95% confidence intervals (95% CIs) for survival outcomes. HR and its 95% CI were directly used if these values were reported; otherwise, the natural logarithm of the HR (lnHR) and standard error of the lnHR [se(lnHR)] were calculated to determine the pooled HRs and 95% CIs according to the method of Parmar et al. (36) and Tierney et al. (37). The χ^2 and I^2 tests were used to appraise statistical heterogeneity between studies, with significance set at $P < 0.10$. The random-effects model was consistently used to maintain a conservative conclusion. Exploratory subgroup analyses were also performed. Potential publication bias was quantitatively assessed by funnel plot and quantified by the Egger test (38) and the trim-and-fill method (39) using Stata 14.0 (Stata Corp, College Station, TX, USA). The meta-analyses were performed using Review Manager 5.3 (Cochrane Collaboration, Oxford, UK).

TABLE 1 | Characteristics of included studies.

Author year	Country	Cancer	Stage	No. of patients	Age	Follow-up (months)	Sarcopenia assessment	Cut point (cm^2/m^2)			Sarcopenia (%)	Treatment	Outcome	Adjusted major confounders	NOS score
								Female	Male	Methods					
Ganju et al. (20)	America	Head and neck excluding p16+ oropharynx cancer	AJCC 7th III–IVB	246	60 (19–88)	35.1 (1–83)	*L3 SMI	41	43 or 53 by BMI	Martin et al. (12)	58	CCRT/IC+ CCRT, Surgery+	OS PFS	Baseline BMI, Age, Sex, Race, Site, Stage, Smoke, Treatment	**7**
Stone et al. (21)	America	Head and neck	AJCC I–IVB	260	61.1 (±11)	ND	L3 SMI	38.5	52.4	Prado et al. (6)	55.4	Surgery ± RT/CRT	OS	Baseline BMI, Stage, Smoke, ALB, HPV, Treatment	**7**
Bril et al. (22)	Netherlands	Larynx and Hypopharynx	AJCC 6/7th 0–IV	235	64.7 (±9.1)	62.4	*L3 SMI	43.2	43.2	Wendrich et al. (23)	46.4	Surgery ± pre Chemo/RT ± adjuvant treatment	OS	Baseline BMI, Sex, Smoke, Site, Treatment	**7**
Jung et al. (24)	Korea	Head and neck	AJCC 7th III–IV	258	64 (56–73)	53.6 (26.3–70.5)	L3 SMI	38.5	52.4	Prado et al. (6), Mourtzakis et al. (25)	6.6	Surgery ± RT/CCRT	OS DFS	Baseline Age, CCI, ALB, Site, HPV-P16, Smoke, Treatment	**7**
†Van Rijn-Dekker et al. (26)	Netherlands	HNSCC	AJCC I–IVB	750	ND	ND	*L3 SMI	30.6	42.4	Lowest gender-specific quartile	25	Chemo/RT	OS DFS	Baseline Age, WHO score, stage, site	**6**
Cho et al. (17)	Korea	Head and neck	AJCC III–IVB	221	59 (18–94)	30 (1–110)	L3 SMI	31	49	Go et al. (27), Kim et al. (28)	48.0	RT/ CCRT/ IC+CCRT	OS, PFS	Univariate analysis	**7**
‡Fattouh et al. (29)	America	HNSCC	AJCC 6/7th M0	113	ND	≥60	L3 SMI	38.5	52.4	Prado et al. (30), Mokdad et al. (31)	64.6	Chemo/RT, Surgery+	OS	Baseline BMI, Age, Sex, Stage, Treatment	**8**
Grossberg et al. (18)	ND	HNSCC	AJCC 7th M0	190	57.7 (±9.4)	68.6	L3 SMI	38.5	52.4	Prado et al. (6), Parsons et al. (32)	35.3	RT/CCRT/IC+ CCRT, Surgery+	OS,	Baseline BMI, Age, Sex, Smoke, Site, Stage, Treatment, HIV, Diabetes, Cardiovascular disease	**8**
Nishikawa et al. (33)	Japan	HNSCC	M0	85	66 (28–89)	29.6 (1–40.7)	L3 SMI	30.3	46.7	Prado et al. (6)	46.0	RT/ CCRT/ BioRT/Surgery, NACT+	OS	Baseline weight loss, ALB, CRP	**6**
Tamaki et al. (34)	Japan	SCC of oropharyngeal	AJCC II–IVC	113	Non-sarcopenia 57.63 (±10.25); sarcopenia 63.5 (±12.91)	0–120	L3 SMI	41	41or 43	Martin et al. (12)	28.3	CCRT/surgery ± adjuvant treatment	OS DFS	Baseline BMI, HPV-P16, Sex, Smoke, Alcohol	**6**
Wendrich et al. (23)	Dutch	HNSCC	AJCC III-IV (locally advanced)	112	54.5 (±9.4)	15–90	*L3 SMI	43.2	43.2	Non-gender-specific optimal stratification	54.5	CCRT	OS	Univariate analysis	**6**

**L3 SMI was calculated by C3 SMI using the method from Swartz et al. (8).*
†Research as a conference meeting paper and the author provided information about sarcopenia (%).
‡Research does not have a univariate analyzed OS data.
AJCC, American Joint Committee on Cancer; BMI, body mass index; HNSCC, head and neck squamous cell carcinoma; CCRT, concurrent chemoradiotherapy; IC, induction chemotherapy; L3, the third lumbar vertebra; No., number; ND, no description; OS, overall survival; DFS, disease-free survival; DSS, disease-specific survival; M, metastasis; NOS, Newcastle–Ottawa Scale; PFS, progression-free survival; RT, radiation therapy; SMI, skeletal muscle index. Bold represents the value of NOS-Score.

RESULTS

Search Strategy

After the initial literature search on August 30, 2019, 11 studies (17, 18, 20–24, 26, 29, 33, 34), including one nested case-control study (29) and a meeting abstract (26), assessing 2,483 patients were pooled in the present meta-analysis. Of the patients involved, an average of 39.4% had sarcopenia (979 patients and 1,504 patients had and did not have sarcopenia, respectively, according to different cutoff values; **Figure 1**). The kappa coefficient was 0.842 (**Figure S1**).

Characteristics of the Studies

Table 1 summarizes the characteristics of the 11 retrospective studies. Four studies (17, 24, 33, 34) were from Asia, i.e., Japan and Korea. All studies included patients with non-metastatic clinical stage, except the cohort of Tamaki et al. (34), which included four patients with stage IVC disease. All studies used the SMI, quantified by the cross-sectional area in cm^2 divided by m^2 at the L3 or the C3, and then calculated the L3 vertebra level mainly using CT imaging. There were different sarcopenia cutoff definitions (6, 12, 25, 27, 28, 30–32); three studies (22, 23, 26) used self-defined definitions to obtain optimum stratification. Sarcopenia prevalence ranged from 6.6 to 64.6%. The HRs from nine studies were adjusted for major confounders such as baseline body mass index (BMI) etc. The quality of all included studies was fair (**Table S1**). All studies had low risk of bias, with NOS scores of 6–8. HR and 95% CI data from two studies (17, 23) were extracted and estimated from survival curves using indirect methods. Lastly, no authors except Van Rijn-Dekker (26) replied to our query e-mails; therefore, we used only the available published data.

Overall Survival

The meta-analysis of the univariate and multivariate data of the influence of the SMI on OS using the random-effects model is depicted in (**Figures 2A,B**). The sarcopenia group had significantly poorer OS compared to the non-sarcopenia group (in **Figure 2A** HR = 1.97, 95% CI: 1.71–2.26, I^2 = 0% and $P = 0.46$; in **Figure 2B** HR = 2.15, 95% CI: 1.66–2.79, $I^2 = 50\%$ and $P = 0.04$). **Table 2** shows the exploratory subgroup analyses. In the primary SMI subgroup, the L3 SMI calculated from the C3 SMI showed results consistent with the L3 primary SMI (HR = 1.90, 95% CI: 1.60–2.25; HR = 2.12, 95% CI: 1.66–2.71, respectively). In the three subgroups according to cutoff values, group 1, defined as SMI of 38.5 cm^2/m^2 for women and 52.4 cm^2/m^2 for men, had much poorer OS (HR = 2.41, 95% CI: 1.72–3.38, $I^2 = 0\%$). Sarcopenia had a similar impact on the Asia and non-Asia subgroups (HR = 2.11, 95% CI: 1.59–2.81; HR = 1.92, 95% CI: 1.64–2.25, respectively). There was no difference between the high-quality group with NOS ≥ 7 and intermediate-quality group with NOS = 6 (HR = 2.13, 95% CI: 1.74–2.60; HR = 1.83, 95% CI: 1.48–2.26, respectively). As the χ^2 test P-value of 0.46 and an I^2 of 0% indicated consistency between the studies (**Figure 2A**), we did not perform sensitivity analysis except for multivariate meta-analysis for OS (**Table S2**).

Relapse-Free Survival

We defined RFS as the interval between diagnosis to the detection of first progression, death from any cause, or last follow-up that

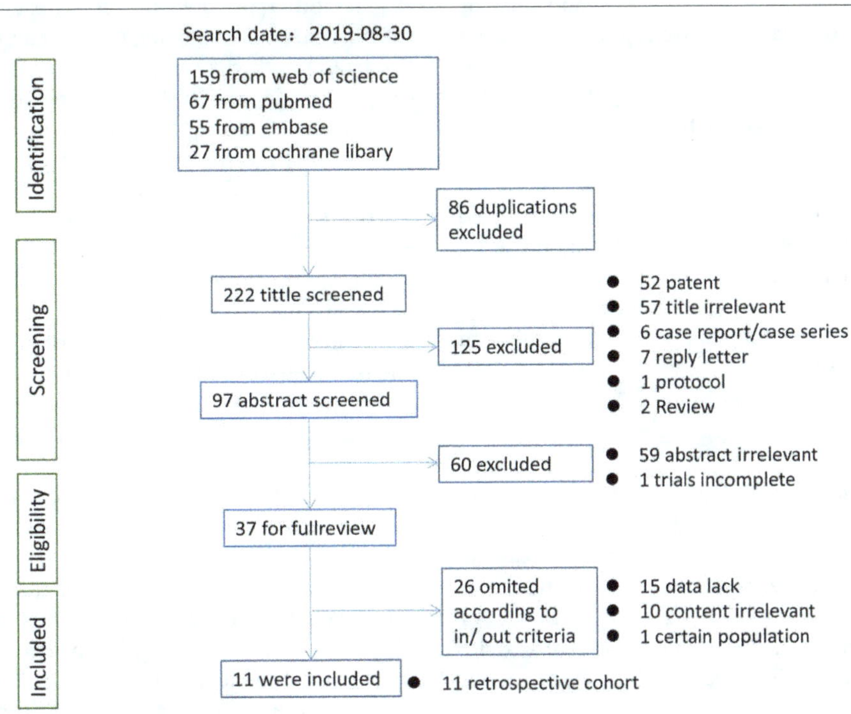

FIGURE 1 | Flow chart of study selection for meta-analysis.

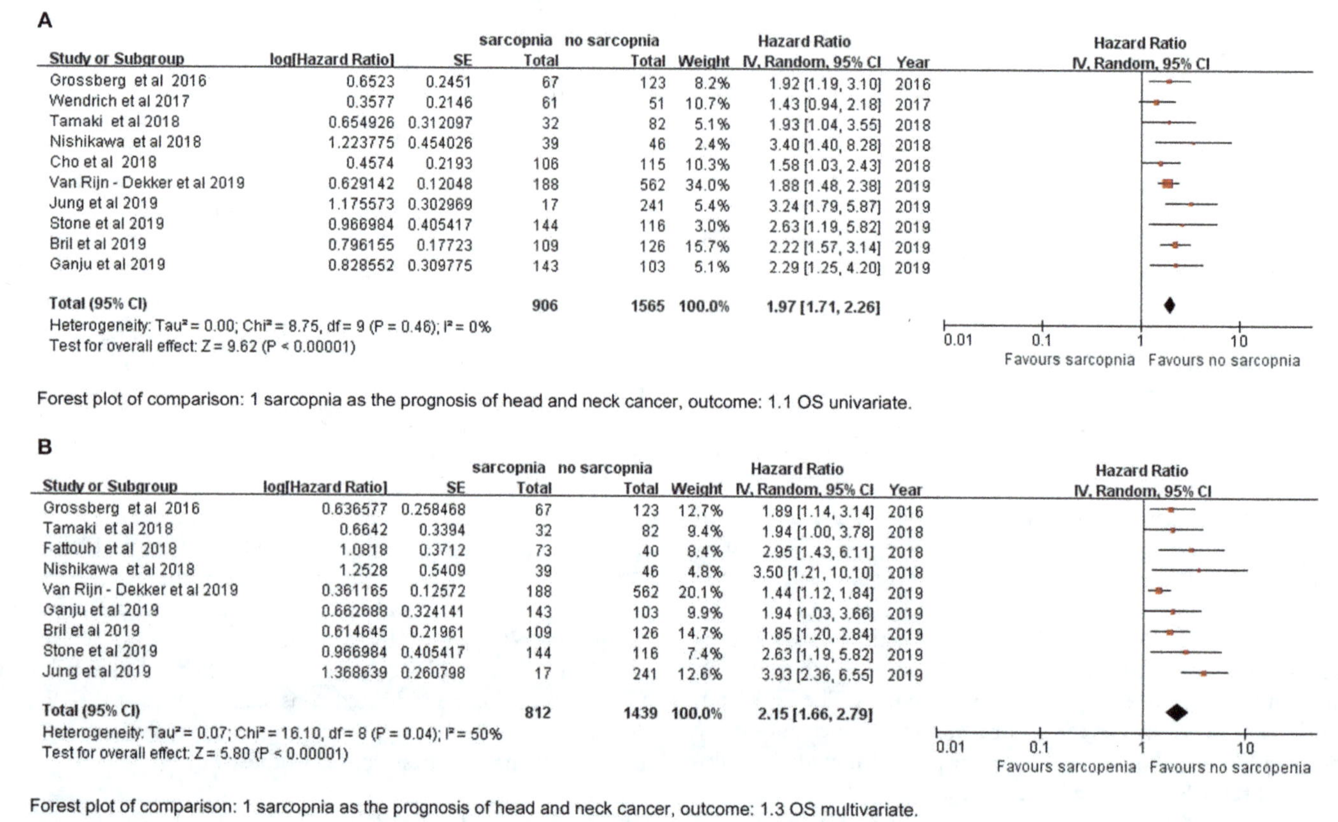

FIGURE 2 | Forest plot of **(A)** univariate data of OS, **(B)** multivariate data of OS.

represented PFS in the study by Cho et al. (17) and DFS by Tamaki et al. (34). The sarcopenia group had significantly poorer RFS based on both univariate and multivariate data (HR = 1.74, 95% CI: 1.43–2.12, $P < 0.00001$, $I^2 = 0\%$; HR = 1.68, 95% CI: 1.27–2.23, $P = 0.003$, $I^2 = 14\%$; **Figures 3A,B**).

Publication Bias

The publication bias test results are not separately reported (**Figures S2, S3**). In accordance with the funnel plot in **Figure S3**, Egger's test indicated a high likelihood of reporting bias ($P =$ 0.035); however, the trim-and-fill method indicated that three hypothetical studies were filled in while the final conclusion remained unchanged (**Figure S2**).

DISCUSSION

Sarcopenia, known as the loss of SMM and function, is common in patients with various solid cancers with incidence ranging from 11 to 74% (40, 41). Following digestive cancer, patients with HNCs have a higher risk of experiencing malnutrition than patients with other cancer types (5, 42), due to the impact of the special tumor location and more serious treatment toxicity on the food intake. Accordingly, several recent studies have further explored the predictive value of sarcopenia in treatment-related complications and the prognosis of survival in HNC. Wendrich et al. (23) found that sarcopenia increased the risk of chemotherapy dose-limiting toxicity (CDLT) in patients with LA-HNSCC receiving chemoradiotherapy (44.3 vs. 13.7%, $P < 0.001$). Achim et al. (43) showed that up to 77% of patients with laryngeal cancer had preoperative sarcopenia and that sarcopenia was an independent predictor for all complications of total laryngectomy. Wendrich et al. (23) did not find a significant OS reduction for low SMM ($P = 0.187$). Grossberg et al. (18) found that, in patients with HNSCC, pre-RT SM depletion was no longer prognostic when BMI was included in the multivariate analysis. Indeed, obese patients without sarcopenia have significantly better prognosis than obese patients with sarcopenia (sarcopenia obesity) (6, 44). Therefore, as a nutrition-related indicator, whether sarcopenia independently affects the prognosis of HNC is appealing.

This is the first meta-analysis to report quantitative assessment of SMI and prognosis in HNC. The pooled HRs show that pre-treatment sarcopenia is significantly associated with poorer OS and RFS. The univariate HRs for survival outcomes were used to derive conclusions because we believed and observed that the multivariate meta-analysis that negative results did not participate in could be a source of publication bias.

We found relatively significant heterogeneity ($I^2 = 50\%$) in the multivariate meta-analysis for OS (**Figure 2B**). It appears that results by Jung et al. (24) and Van Rijn-Dekker et al. (26) are debatable (**Table S2**). The former had a much higher risk than any other research (HR = 3.93, 95% CI; 2.36–6.55). Interestingly,

TABLE 2 | Subgroup analyses of the prognostic effect on OS of the sarcopenia vs. non-sarcopenia group in head and neck cancer.

Variable	Subgroups	Availability		Effect		Heterogeneity	
		Studies (*N*)	Patients (*N*)	HR (95% CI)	*P*-values	I^2 (%)	P^{*}_{inter}
Race	Asian	4	678	2.11 [1.59, 2.81]	<0.00001	39	0.5
	Non-Asian	6	1,793	1.92 [1.64, 2.25]	<0.0001	0	
Stage	Locally advanced	4	837	1.92 [1.35, 2.73]	0.0003	49	0.95
	Non-metastasis	5	1,520	2.04 [1.71, 2.42]	<0.0001	0	
	Contained M1	1	114	1.94 [1.04, 3.55]	0.04	–	
Primary SMI	L3	6	1,128	2.12 [1.66, 2.71]	<0.00001	7	0.47
	C3	4	1,343	1.90 [1.60, 2.25]	<0.00001	0	
†Cutoff	Group1	3	708	2.41 [1.72, 3.38]	<0.0001	0	0.45
	Group2	3	1,056	1.87 [1.47, 2.38]	<0.00001	14	
	Group3	4	707	1.92 [1.53, 2.41]	<0.00001	0	
NOS quality	NOS ≥ 7	6	1,410	2.13 [1.74, 2.60]	<0.0001	0	0.3
	NOS = 6	4	1,061	1.83 [1.48, 2.26]	<0.00001	8	
HR data extract	Directly	8	2,138	2.11 [1.81, 2.47]	<0.00001	0	0.05
	Indirectly	2	333	1.50 [1.11, 2.03]	0.008	0	

P_{inter} represents the significance of heterogeneity between subgroups calculated by Revman software.
†Cutoff value in Group 1: 38.5 cm²/m² for women and 52.4 cm²/m² for men; Group 2: 30.3–31 cm²/m² for women and 42.4–49 cm²/m² for men; Group 3: 41–43.2 cm²/m² for women and 41–43.2 cm²/m² for men.
N, number; HR, hazards ratio; NOS, Newcastle–Ottawa Scale.

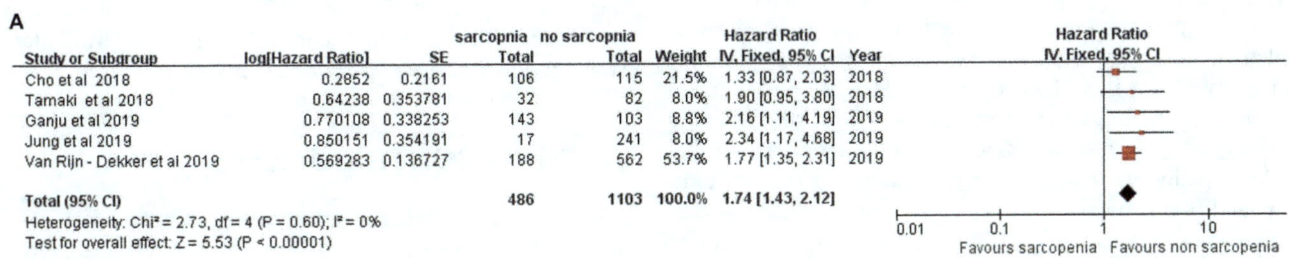

Forest plot of comparison: 1 sarcopnia as the prognosis of head and neck cancer, outcome: 1.2 RFS univariate.

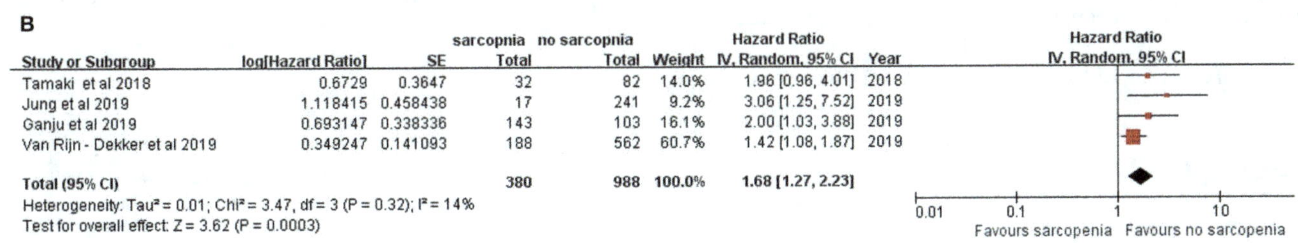

Forest plot of comparison: 1 sarcopnia as the prognosis of head and neck cancer, outcome: 1.4 RFS multivariate.

FIGURE 3 | Forest plot of **(A)** univariate data of RFS, **(B)** multivariate data of RFS.

the cutoff value they used was the same as that from three other included articles (18, 21, 29) (**Table 1**), but the incidence rate of sarcopenia was only 6.6%; the possible reasons for this are as follows: (a) 6.6% is for sarcopenia with visceral obesity in their study, (b) the locally advanced cancer stage is the distinguishing property, or (c) there might be potential bias that affected the incidence. The study by Van Rijn-Dekker et al., which will soon be published in full, was a meeting abstract that investigated a large-scale cohort of 750 patients with HNSCC, the incidence of sarcopenia was also low, i.e., as 25%, and the result was conservative and narrow (HR = 1.44, 95% CI: 1.12–1.84). In their e-mail reply, the cutoff was set by the lowest sex-specific quartile categorized in our Group 2 cutoff subgroup. Group 2 was less good enough to report a prognostic effect of sarcopenia than Group 1, which is based on log-rank statistics to separate patients with sarcopenia (6) (**Table 2**), so we agree that setting a cutoff for sarcopenia by using the log-rank test may be better. It is common to obtain the head and neck CT in HNC, and we also did not observe significant intergroup heterogeneity between the primary site of SMI definition subgroups (C3 or L3) (**Table 2**). We suggest that more studies should explore the effect and cutoff value of neck muscles on HNC prognosis.

In our review, sarcopenia had a similar impact on the Asia and non-Asia subgroups, which suggest that sarcopenia could be widely used. Sarcopenia was not a prognostic factor for p16+ oropharyngeal cancer (34, 45), and maybe different tumor types that caused a wide range of prognosis have specific influence on sarcopenia; thus, it is imperative for further studies on particular and rare types of tumors other than p16+ oropharyngeal cancer to determine the prognostic value of sarcopenia. As for the set of cutoff value, the low intergroup heterogeneity indicates that different cutoffs could all be used (**Table 2**). Therefore, a unitary cutoff is not reasonable, and it can be inferred that using different races, tumor-node-metastasis (TNM) clinical stages, tumor types, age groups, and other features to form the appropriate multi-factor model can identify patients with poor prognosis as accurately as possible.

Our study also aims to turn its attention to the routine evaluation and intervention of sarcopenia for HNC. Many strategies can be attempted to prevent and treat sarcopenia. Among them, lifestyle modification, specific dietary habits, and therapeutic measures have been recommended. Protein supplementation and regular resistance exercise are the mainstream treatments of sarcopenia: to increase muscle mass and help augment muscle strength (46, 47). In addition, drugs that can block the cytokines associated with the muscle atrophy signaling pathways [such as myostatin/activin, interleukin (IL)-6, and tumor necrosis factor (TNF)-α] or medications that induce signals of muscle hypertrophy (such as growth hormone agonists, ghrelin, and anabolic steroids) may be useful for sarcopenia accompanied by visceral obesity (48).

Due to the retrospective nature of the included studies, the present meta-analysis has several limitations. First, only some of those articles included the treatment variable, which is a significant prognostic factor for survival outcomes, into their multivariate analysis, and no matching methods were used, so there might have been interaction effects. Second, there were little data about stratifying the impact of pre-treatment sarcopenia on survival according to clinical stages, which is commonly used for identifying higher-risk groups. For example, Van Rijn-Dekker et al. (26) found that sarcopenia is not a prognostic factor in early-stage HNSCC. Third, because Fattouh et al. (29) only reported the positive HR in their multivariate analysis, the univariate meta-analysis included 10/11 of eligible primary studies; however, according to the principle of Cox regression, there is little chance that the conclusion of the meta-analysis will be affected. Finally, the reasons for the different statistical significance between Egger's test and the trim-and-fill method might derive from the low number of included studies; however, these studies are relatively new, and we did not receive replies from the authors of three conference articles with positive (49, 50) and negative (51) results, which requires further evaluation after their official publication.

CONCLUSION

The presence of pre-treatment sarcopenia has a significant negative impact on OS and RFS in HNC compared with its absence. Further well-conducted studies with detailed stratification are needed to complement our findings.

AUTHOR CONTRIBUTIONS

XH, SL, and J-FL collected, extracted, and analyzed the data and wrote the paper. WW, Z-QL, and Z-JL performed quality assessment and analyzed the data. LG and H-XL conceived and designed this study. All authors reviewed the paper, read, and approved the final manuscript.

REFERENCES

1. Noguchi M, Kakuma T, Uemura H, Nasu Y, Kumon H, Hirao Y, et al. A randomized phase II trial of personalized peptide vaccine plus low dose estramustine phosphate (EMP) versus standard dose EMP in patients with castration resistant prostate cancer. *Cancer Immunol Immun.* (2010) 59:1001–9. doi: 10.1007/s00262-010-0822-4
2. Jager-Wittenaar H, Dijkstra PU, Vissink A, Langendijk JA, van der Laan BF, Pruim J, et al. Changes in nutritional status and dietary intake during and after head and neck cancer treatment. *Head Neck.* (2011) 33:863–70. doi: 10.1002/hed.21546
3. Jackson W, Alexander N, Schipper M, Fig L, Feng F, Jolly S. Characterization of changes in total body composition for patients with head and neck cancer undergoing chemoradiotherapy using dual-energy x-ray absorptiometry. *Head Neck.* (2014) 36:1356–62. doi: 10.1002/hed.23461
4. Langius JA, Bakker S, Rietveld DH, Kruizenga HM, Langendijk JA, Weijs PJ, et al. Critical weight loss is a major prognostic indicator for disease-specific survival in patients with head and neck cancer receiving radiotherapy. *Br J Cancer.* (2013) 109:1093–9. doi: 10.1038/bjc.2013.458
5. Pressoir M, Desne S, Berchery D, Rossignol G, Poiree B, Meslier M, et al. Prevalence, risk factors and clinical implications of malnutrition in French comprehensive cancer centres. *Br J Cancer.* (2010) 102:966–71. doi: 10.1038/sj.bjc.6605578
6. Prado CM, Lieffers JR, McCargar LJ, Reiman T, Sawyer MB, Martin L, et al. Prevalence and clinical implications of sarcopenic obesity in patients with solid tumours of the respiratory and gastrointestinal tracts: a population-based study. *Lancet Oncol.* (2008) 9:629–35. doi: 10.1016/S1470-2045(08)70153-0
7. Cruz-Jentoft AJ, Bahat G, Bauer J, Boirie Y, Bruyere O, Cederholm T, et al. Sarcopenia: revised European consensus on definition and diagnosis. *Age Ageing.* (2019) 48:16–31. doi: 10.1093/ageing/afy169
8. Swartz JE, Pothen AJ, Wegner I, Smid EJ, Swart KM, de Bree R, et al. Feasibility of using head and neck CT imaging to assess skeletal muscle mass in head and neck cancer patients. *Oral Oncol.* (2016) 62:28–33. doi: 10.1016/j.oraloncology.2016.09.006
9. Miyamoto Y, Baba Y, Sakamoto Y, Ohuchi M, Tokunaga R, Kurashige J, et al. Sarcopenia is a negative prognostic factor after curative resection of colorectal cancer. *Ann Surg Oncol.* (2015) 22:2663–8. doi: 10.1245/s10434-014-4281-6

10. Kuroki LM, Mangano M, Allsworth JE, Menias CO, Massad LS, Powell MA, et al. Pre-operative assessment of muscle mass to predict surgical complications and prognosis in patients with endometrial cancer. *Ann Surg Oncol.* (2015) 22:972–9. doi: 10.1245/s10434-014-4040-8
11. Voron T, Tselikas L, Pietrasz D, Pigneur F, Laurent A, Compagnon P, et al. Sarcopenia impacts on short- and long-term results of hepatectomy for hepatocellular carcinoma. *Ann Surg.* (2015) 261:1173–83. doi: 10.1097/SLA.0000000000000743
12. Martin L, Birdsell L, Macdonald N, Reiman T, Clandinin MT, McCargar LJ, et al. Cancer cachexia in the age of obesity: skeletal muscle depletion is a powerful prognostic factor, independent of body mass index. *J Clin Oncol.* (2013) 31:1539–47. doi: 10.1200/JCO.2012.45.2722
13. Du E, Mazul AL, Farquhar D, Brennan P, Anantharaman D, Abedi-Ardekani B, et al. Long-term survival in head and neck cancer: impact of site, stage, smoking, and human papillomavirus status. *Laryngoscope.* (2019) 129:2506–13. doi: 10.1002/lary.27807
14. Giraldi L, Leoncini E, Pastorino R, Wunsch-Filho V, de Carvalho M, Lopez R, et al. Alcohol and cigarette consumption predict mortality in patients with head and neck cancer: a pooled analysis within the International Head and Neck Cancer Epidemiology (INHANCE) consortium. *Ann Oncol.* (2017) 28:2843–51. doi: 10.1093/annonc/mdx486
15. Iyengar NM, Kochhar A, Morris PG, Morris LG, Zhou XK, Ghossein RA, et al. Impact of obesity on the survival of patients with early-stage squamous cell carcinoma of the oral tongue. *Cancer.* (2014) 120:983–91. doi: 10.1002/cncr.28532
16. Rietbergen MM, Brakenhoff RH, Bloemena E, Witte BI, Snijders PJ, Heideman DA, et al. Human papillomavirus detection and comorbidity: critical issues in selection of patients with oropharyngeal cancer for treatment De-escalation trials. *Ann Oncol.* (2013) 24:2740–5. doi: 10.1093/annonc/mdt319
17. Cho Y, Kim JW, Keum KC, Lee CG, Jeung HC, Lee IJ. Prognostic significance of sarcopenia with inflammation in patients with head and neck cancer who underwent definitive chemoradiotherapy. *Front Oncol.* (2018) 8:457. doi: 10.3389/fonc.2018.00457
18. Grossberg AJ, Chamchod S, Fuller CD, Mohamed AS, Heukelom J, Eichelberger H, et al. Association of body composition with survival and locoregional control of radiotherapy-treated head and neck squamous cell carcinoma. *JAMA Oncol.* (2016) 2:782–9. doi: 10.1001/jamaoncol.2015.6339
19. Talwar B, Donnelly R, Skelly R, Donaldson M. Nutritional management in head and neck cancer: United Kingdom National Multidisciplinary Guidelines. *J Laryngol Otol.* (2016) 130:S32–40. doi: 10.1017/S0022215116000402
20. Ganju RG, Morse R, Hoover A, TenNapel M, Lominska CE. The impact of sarcopenia on tolerance of radiation and outcome in patients with head and neck cancer receiving chemoradiation. *Radiother Oncol.* (2019) 137:117–24. doi: 10.1016/j.radonc.2019.04.023
21. Stone L, Olson B, Mowery A, Krasnow S, Jiang A, Li R, et al. Association between sarcopenia and mortality in patients undergoing surgical excision of head and neck cancer. *JAMA Otolaryngol Head Neck Surg.* (2019) 145:647–54. doi: 10.1001/jamaoto.2019.1185
22. Bril SI, Pezier TF, Tijink BM, Janssen LM, Braunius WW, de Bree R. Preoperative low skeletal muscle mass as a risk factor for pharyngocutaneous fistula and decreased overall survival in patients undergoing total laryngectomy. *Head Neck.* (2019) 41:1745–55. doi: 10.1002/hed.25638
23. Wendrich AW, Swartz JE, Bril SI, Wegner I, de Graeff A, Smid EJ, et al. Low skeletal muscle mass is a predictive factor for chemotherapy dose-limiting toxicity in patients with locally advanced head and neck cancer. *Oral oncol.* (2017) 71:26–33.. doi: 10.1016/j.oraloncology.2017.05.012
24. Jung AR, Roh JL, Kim JS, Kim SB, Choi SH, Nam SY, et al. Prognostic value of body composition on recurrence and survival of advanced-stage head and neck cancer. *Eur J Cancer.* (2019) 116:98–106. doi: 10.1016/j.ejca.2019.05.006
25. Mourtzakis M, Prado CM, Lieffers JR, Reiman T, McCargar LJ, Baracos VE. A practical and precise approach to quantification of body composition in cancer patients using computed tomography images acquired during routine care. *Appl Physiol Nutr Metab.* (2008) 33:997–1006. doi: 10.1139/H08-075
26. Van Rijn-Dekker I, Van den Bosch L, Van den Hoek A, Bijl H, Dieters M, Van Aken E, et al. Impact of sarcopenia on survival and late toxicity in head and neck cancer patients treated with RT. *Radiother Oncol.* (2019) 133:S197–8. doi: 10.1016/S0167-8140(19)30813-8
27. Go SI, Park MJ, Song HN, Kang MH, Park HJ, Jeon KN, et al. Sarcopenia and inflammation are independent predictors of survival in male patients newly diagnosed with small cell lung cancer. *Support Care Cancer.* (2016) 24:2075–84. doi: 10.1007/s00520-015-2997-x
28. Kim YS, Lee Y, Chung YS, Lee DJ, Joo NS, Hong D, et al. Prevalence of sarcopenia and sarcopenic obesity in the Korean population based on the Fourth Korean National Health and Nutritional Examination Surveys. *J Gerontol A Biol Sci Med Sci.* (2012) 67:1107–13. doi: 10.1093/gerona/gls071
29. Fattouh M, Chang GY, Ow TJ, Shifteh K, Rosenblatt G, Patel VM, et al. Association between pretreatment obesity, sarcopenia, and survival in patients with head and neck cancer. *Head Neck.* (2018) 41:707–14. doi: 10.1002/hed.25420
30. Prado CM, Baracos VE, McCargar LJ, Reiman T, Mourtzakis M, Tonkin K, et al. Sarcopenia as a determinant of chemotherapy toxicity and time to tumor progression in metastatic breast cancer patients receiving capecitabine treatment. *Clin Cancer Res.* (2009) 15:2920–6. doi: 10.1158/1078-0432.CCR-08-2242
31. Mokdad AH, Ford ES, Bowman BA, Dietz WH, Vinicor F, Bales VS, et al. Prevalence of obesity, diabetes, and obesity-related health risk factors, 2001. *JAMA.* (2003) 289:76–9. doi: 10.1001/jama.289.1.76
32. Parsons HA, Baracos VE, Dhillon N, Hong DS, Kurzrock R. Body composition, symptoms, and survival in advanced cancer patients referred to a phase I service. *PLoS ONE.* (2012) 7:e29330. doi: 10.1371/journal.pone.0029330
33. Nishikawa D, Hanai N, Suzuki H, Koide Y, Beppu S, Hasegawa Y. The impact of skeletal muscle depletion on head and neck squamous cell carcinoma. *ORL.* (2018) 80:1–9. doi: 10.1159/000485515
34. Tamaki A, Manzoor NF, Babajanian E, Ascha M, Rezaee R, Zender CA. Clinical significance of sarcopenia among patients with advanced oropharyngeal cancer. *Otolaryngol Head Neck Surg.* (2018) 160:480–7. doi: 10.1177/0194599818793857
35. Wells G, Shea BJ, O'Connell D, Peterson J, Welch V, Losos M. The Newcastle-Ottawa Scale (NOS) for assessing the quality of nonrandomised studies in meta-analyses. Available online at: http://www.ohri.ca/programs/clinical_epidemiology/oxford.asp
36. Parmar MK, Torri V, Stewart L. Extracting summary statistics to perform meta-analyses of the published literature for survival endpoints. *Stat Med.* (1998) 17:2815–34. doi: 10.1002/(sici)1097-0258(19981230)17:24<2815::aid-sim110>3.0.co;2-8
37. Tierney JF, Stewart LA, Ghersi D, Burdett S, Sydes MR. Practical methods for incorporating summary time-to-event data into meta-analysis. *Trials.* (2007) 8:16. doi: 10.1186/1745-6215-8-16
38. Egger M, Davey Smith G, Schneider M, Minder C. Bias in meta-analysis detected by a simple, graphical test. *BMJ.* (1997) 315:629–34. doi: 10.1136/bmj.315.7109.629
39. Duval S, Tweedie R. Trim and fill: a simple funnel-plot-based method of testing and adjusting for publication bias in meta-analysis. *Biometrics.* (2000) 56:455–63. doi: 10.1111/j.0006-341X.2000.00455.x
40. Shachar SS, Williams GR, Muss HB, Nishijima TF. Prognostic value of sarcopenia in adults with solid tumours: A meta-analysis and systematic review. *Eur J Cancer.* (2016) 57:58–67. doi: 10.1016/j.ejca.2015.12.030
41. Chang KV, Chen JD, Wu WT, Huang KC, Hsu CT, Han DS. Association between loss of skeletal muscle mass and mortality and tumor recurrence in hepatocellular carcinoma: a systematic review and meta-analysis. *Liver Cancer.* (2018) 7:90–103. doi: 10.1159/000484950
42. Gorenc M, Kozjek NR, Strojan P. Malnutrition and cachexia in patients with head and neck cancer treated with (chemo) radiotherapy. *Rep Pract Oncol Radiother.* (2015) 20:249–58. doi: 10.1016/j.rpor.2015.03.001
43. Achim V, Bash J, Mowery A, Guimaraes AR, Li R, Schindler J, et al. prognostic indication of sarcopenia for wound complication after total laryngectomy. *JAMA Otolaryngol Head Neck Surg.* (2017) 143:1159. doi: 10.1001/jamaoto.2017.0547
44. Ozola Zalite I, Zykus R, Francisco Gonzalez M, Saygili F, Pukitis A, Gaujoux S, et al. Influence of cachexia and sarcopenia on survival in pancreatic ductal adenocarcinoma: a systematic review. *Pancreatology.* (2015) 15:19–24. doi: 10.1016/j.pan.2014.11.006
45. Ganju RG, Morse R, Tennapel MJ, Hoover A, Kakarala K, Shnayder L, et al. Skeletal muscle gauge measured at the c3 vertebral body

predicts for outcomes in men with P16-positive oropharynx cancer. *Int J Radiat Oncol Biol Phys.* (2019) 105:E420. doi: 10.1016/j.ijrobp.2019.06.1528

46. Freiberger E, Sieber C, Pfeifer K. Physical activity, exercise, and sarcopenia – future challenges. *Wien Med Wochenschr.* (2011) 161:416–25. doi: 10.1007/s10354-011-0001-z
47. Morley JE, Argiles JM, Evans WJ, Bhasin S, Cella D, Deutz NE, et al. Nutritional recommendations for the management of sarcopenia. *J Am Med Dir Assoc.* (2010) 11:391–6. doi: 10.1016/j.jamda.2010.04.014
48. Cohen S, Nathan JA, Goldberg AL. Muscle wasting in disease: molecular mechanisms and promising therapies. *Nat Rev Drug Discov.* (2015) 14:58–74. doi: 10.1038/nrd4467
49. Chamchod S, Fuller CD, Grossberg AJ, Mohamed AS, Heukelom J, ichelberger H, et al. sarcopenia/cachexia is associated with reduced survival and locoregional control in head and neck cancer patients receiving radiotherapy: results from quantitative imaging analysis of lean body mass. *Oncology.* (2015) 29(4 Suppl 1):205153.
50. Inokuchi H, Okano K, Takehana K, Tsutsui K, Hiraoka M. Prognostic impact of quantitative imaging analysis of lean body mass after chemoradiation therapy for patients with advanced nasopharyngeal cancer. *Int J Radiat Oncol Biol Phys.* (2018) 100:1342. doi: 10.1016/j.ijrobp.2017.12.094
51. Kabarriti R, Ohri N, Bontempo A, Romano M, Modi C, Viswanathan S, et al. The impact of dietary regimen compliance and sarcopenia in head and neck cancer patients treated with definitive radiation therapy. *Int J Radiat Oncol Biol Phys.* (2015) 93:E332–3. doi: 10.1016/j.ijrobp.2015.07.1395

20

MicroRNAs as Therapeutic Targets in Nasopharyngeal Carcinoma

Sumei Wang[1,2,3*], *François-Xavier Claret*[4,5] *and Wanyin Wu*[1,2*]

[1] Guangdong Provincial Key Laboratory of Clinical Research on Traditional Chinese Medicine Syndrome, Guangdong Provincial Hospital of Chinese Medicine, Guangzhou, China, [2] Department of Oncology, The Second Clinical College of Guangzhou University of Chinese Medicine, Guangzhou, China, [3] The Postdoctoral Research Station, Guangzhou University of Chinese Medicine, Guangzhou, China, [4] Department of Systems Biology, The University of Texas MD Anderson Cancer Center, Houston, TX, United States, [5] Experimental Therapeutic Academic Program and Cancer Biology Program, The University of Texas Graduate School of Biomedical Sciences at Houston, Houston, TX, United States

***Correspondence:**
Sumei Wang
wangsumei198708@163.com
Wanyin Wu
wwanyin@126.com

Nasopharyngeal carcinoma (NPC) is a malignancy of epithelial origin that is prone to local invasion and early distant metastasis. Although concurrent chemotherapy and radiotherapy improves the 5-year survival outcomes, persistent or recurrent disease still occurs. Therefore, novel therapeutic targets are needed for NPC patients. MicroRNAs (miRNAs) play important roles in normal cell homeostasis, and dysregulations of miRNA expression have been implicated in human cancers. In NPC, studies have revealed that miRNAs are dysregulated and involved in tumorigenesis, metastasis, invasion, resistance to chemo- and radiotherapy, and other disease- and treatment-related processes. The advantage of miRNA-based treatment approaches is that miRNAs can concurrently target multiple effectors of pathways involved in tumor cell differentiation and proliferation. Thus, miRNA-based cancer treatments, alone or combined with standard chemotherapy and/or radiotherapy, hold promise to improve treatment response and cure rates. In this review, we will summarize the dysregulation of miRNAs in NPC initiation, progression, and treatment as well as NPC-related signaling pathways, and we will discuss the potential applications of miRNAs as biomarkers and therapeutic targets in NPC patients. We conclude that miRNAs might be potential promising therapeutic targets in nasopharyngeal carcinoma.

Keywords: microRNA, Nasopharyngeal Carcinoma (NPC), therapeutic target, biomarker, application

INTRODUCTION

Nasopharyngeal Carcinoma (NPC)

Nasopharyngeal carcinoma is a non-lymphomatous squamous cell carcinoma that arises from the epithelial lining of the nasopharynx. Local invasion and early distant metastasis are common in NPC. Etiologic factors for NPC include Epstein-Barr virus (EBV) infection, genetic predisposition, and environmental factors (1, 2). It is extremely difficult to detect early because of its deep location and lack of obvious clinical signs in its early stages. Concurrent chemotherapy and radiotherapy is a standard treatment for late-stage NPC (3). Nevertheless, despite the effectiveness of concurrent chemotherapy and radiotherapy in treating NPC, local or regional failure in the form of persistent or recurrent disease occurs in some patients. Therefore, novel biomarkers and therapeutic strategies to improve treatment outcomes are urgently required for NPC patients.

MicroRNAs (miRNAs)

MiRNAs are a class of endogenous non-coding RNA molecules that are typically 22–25 nucleotides long (4, 5). They are transcribed from intragenic or intergenic regions by RNA polymerase II into pri-miRNAs (at a length between 1 and 3 kb) (6), and further processed by the RNase III ribonucleases Drosha and DiGeorge syndrome critical region gene 8, *DGCR8*, complex in the nucleus into a hairpin intermediate pre-miRNA (consisting in a stem-loop structure of about 70 nucleotides) (7). The pre-miRNA is then transported from the nucleus to the cytoplasm by exportin 5 (8). After strand separation, the mature double-stranded miRNA, also known as the guide strand, is incorporated into an RNA-induced silencing complex (RISC), whole the passenger strand (miRNA*) is typically degraded. The RISC is the effector complex of the miRNA pathway and comprises miRNA, Argonaute proteins (Argonaute 1 to Argonaute 4) and other proteins. The mature strand is important for target recognition and for the incorporation of specific target mRNAs into RISC (8, 9). Each miRNA can potentially target many genes (about 500 on average), and about 60% of mRNAs have at least 1 evolutionarily conserved sequence that is believed to be targeted by miRNAs (10, 11).

Usually, miRNAs target the 3 prime untranslated region (3′UTR) of their target genes, most often causing mRNA deadenylation and degradation and subsequent translational repression (5, 12). However, other miRNA-mediated mechanisms of modulating mRNA expression have also been reported. Some miRNAs bind to the open reading frame or the 5′UTR of their target genes; in some cases, miRNAs have been shown to activate gene expression rather than suppress it (13). For example, Jopling et al. reported that miR-122 can bind to 5′UTR, inhibiting translation of its target genes (14). In 2008, another miRNA, miR-10a, was reported to enhance translation by binding to ribosomal protein mRNA at the 5′UTR (which is known to regulate translation) downstream of the conserved 5′TOP motif (13). In 2016, we demonstrated that miR-24 could bind to both 3′UTR and 5′UTR of *COPS5* (also named *JAB1* and COP9 signalosome subunit 5), leading to *COPS5* mRNA degradation and translational suppression (15). Besides, miRNAs can also regulate gene expression at the transcriptional level by binding directly to the DNA (16, 17). Moreover, proteins can also be targeted by miRNAs (18) (**Figure 1**).

Exosomal miRNAs

Exosomes are microvesicles that are 40–100 nm long. They originate in intracellular endosomal compartment and are secreted by cells into their microenvironment. Exosomes transport DNA fragments, proteins, mRNAs, and miRNAs from donor cells to recipient cells and are therefore crucial to intercellular communication. Exosomal miRNAs miR-21 and miR-29a are secreted by tumor cells and can bind to toll-like receptors on nearby immune cells, thus initiating an inflammatory response that promotes metastasis (19). Furthermore, miR-21 was observed at a higher level in exosomes from the serum of patients with esophageal squamous cell carcinoma than in serum from patients with benign diseases without systemic inflammation, and an association was found between exosomal miR-21 and the presence of metastasis with inflammation (20). In addition, exosomal miR-223 was reported to be elevated in breast cancer cells and promote breast cancer invasion (21). In NPC, exosomal miR-9 was found to inhibit angiogenesis through regulating PDK/AKT pathway (22). And exosomal miR-24-3p serves as a potential biomarker for NPC prognosis (23). Therefore, exosomal miRNAs are involved in the initiation and progression of cancers including NPC, and could be biomarkers for NPC patients.

EBV-Encoded miRNAs

EBV, a herpesvirus that infects the majority of the population worldwide asymptomatically (24), was the first human virus reported to encode miRNAs (25). More than 44 viral miRNAs are encoded from EBV. In NPC, EBV expresses EBNA1, LMP1, and LMP2A, EBERs, and BARTs (26). miR-BARTs, which are EBV-encoded miRNAs derived from BamH1-A rightward transcripts, are highly expressed in NPC and promote its development. A recent study showed that EBV-encoded miR-BARTS, including BART5-5p, BART7-3p, BART9-3p, and BART14-3p, downregulated the expression of a key DNA double-strand break repair gene, ataxia telangiectasia mutated (*ATM*), by targeting several sites on its 3′-UTR (27). Thus, those 4 EBV-encoded miRNAs work cooperatively to suppress *ATM* activity in response to DNA damage, contributing to NPC tumorigenesis. Those findings indicate that EBV-encoded miRNAs can be used as a novel therapeutic strategy for NPC.

THE MECHANISM OF miRNA REGULATION IN CANCERS

Genes encoding miRNAs are often located at or near fragile sites and in minimal regions of loss of heterozygosity, in minimal regions of amplification, and in common cancer-related breakpoints (28). Upregulated expression of miRNAs can be caused by genomic alterations such as translocations o amplification, and loss of function can be caused by alterations such as deletions, insertions, or mutations (29). For example, the mir-17-92 cluster, which is made up of mir-17, mir-18a, mir-19b,

Abbreviations: A20/TNFAIP3, tumor necrosis factor alpha-induced protein 3; ABCB1, ATP binding cassette subfamily B member 1; ATM, ataxia telangiectasia mutated; BRD7, bromodomain containing 7; CAPN4/CAPNS1, calpain small subunit 1; circRNA, circular RNA; COPS5, COP9 signalosome subunit 5; CXCL12, C-X-C motif chemokine ligand 12; CXCR4, C-X-C motif chemokine receptor 4; DGCR8, Drosha and DiGeorge syndrome critical region gene 8; E2F3, E2F transcription factor 3; EBV, Epstein-Barr virus; EMT, epithelial-mesenchymal transition; EZH2, enhancer of zeste homolog 2; *FGF5*, fibroblast growth factor 5; IL-17, interleukin-17; ITGA3, integrin subunit alpha 3; KLF12, Kruppel-like factor 12; LASP1, LIM and SH3 protein 1; lncRNA, long non-coding RNA; MALAT1, metastasis-associated lung adenocarcinoma transcript-1; AP3K5/ASK1, apoptosis signal-regulating kinasel; miRNA, microRNA; MIF, macrophage migration inhibitory factor; mTOR, mechanistic target of rapamycin kinase; NF-κB, nuclear factor κB; NPC, nasopharyngeal carcinoma; PDRG1, p53 and DNA damage regulated 1; PTEN, phosphatase and tensin homolog; RISC, RNA-induced silencing complex; RP, ribosomal protein; SP1, specificity protein 1; TIAM1, T cell lymphoma invasion and metastasis 1; TRIAP1, TP53-regulated inhibitor of apoptosis 1; TSGA10, testis-specific gene antigen 10; UTR, untranslated region; WNT2B, Wnt family member 2B; XIST, X inactivate-specific transcript.

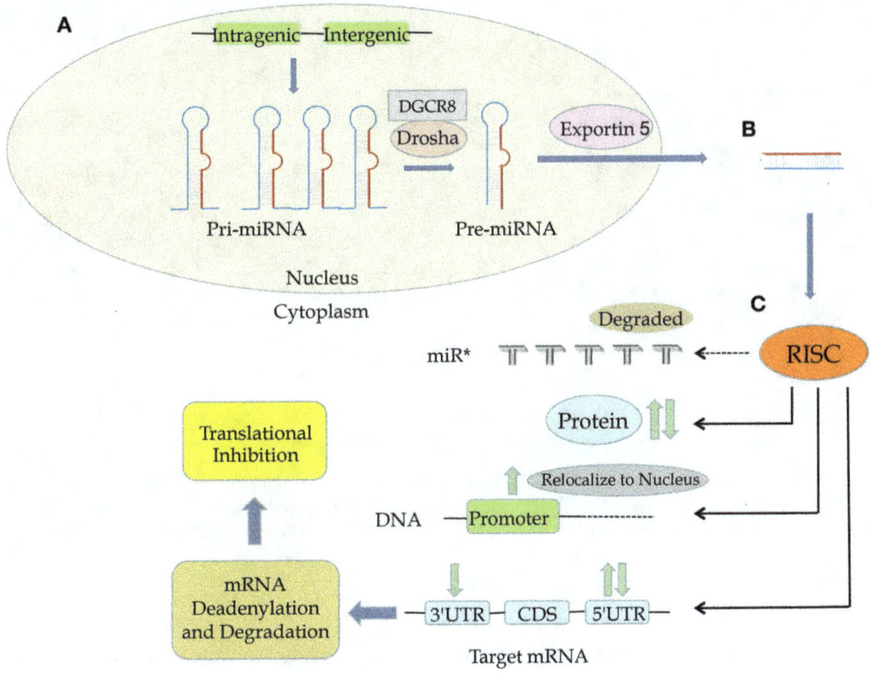

FIGURE 1 | The process and functions of miRNA. **(A)** Both intergenic and intragenic genes encode miRNAs. **(B)** Mature miRNAs are transcribed from pri-miRNA and then then pre-miRNA, translocated from nucleus to cytoplasm by exportin 5, and composed of RNA-induced silencing complex (RISC). **(C)** RISC can target mRNA at 3′UTR, CDS, and 5′UTR as well as DNA promoter sequences and even proteins, leading to upregulation or downregulation of a specific protein.

mir-19b-1, mir-201, and mir-92-1, resides in an 800 base-pair region of the non-coding gene *MIR17HG* (also called *C13orf25*), a genomic region known to be amplified in lymphomas (30). The mir-17-92 cluster is often overexpressed in hematological cancers (31, 32). In contrast, the mir-15a-mir-16-a cluster, which resides in the chromosome 13q14 region (between exons 2 and 5 of the non-coding gene *DLEU2*), is often downregulated in patients with chronic lymphocytic leukemia due to genomic deletion of this region (31, 33).

In addition to structural genetic alterations, epigenetic modulations, including DNA promoter hypermethylation and histone hypoacetylation, have been described in solid tumors (34). For example, miR-127 is downregulated because of promoter hypermethylation in human bladder cancer (34). Usually, hypermethylation of tumor-suppressive miRNAs leads to miRNA silencing, and hypomethylation of onco-miRNAs leads to their activation and to tumorigenesis (35). In addition, long non-coding RNAs (lncRNAs) can target miRNAs, resulting in in tumorigenesis and chemo- and radioresistance. For example, lncRNA FTH1P3 promotes ATP binding cassette subfamily B member 1 (ABCB1) protein expression by targeting miR-206, acting as a miRNA "sponge," leading to the activation of paclitaxel resistance in breast cancer (36). Circular RNAs (circRNAs) also can act as miRNA sponges to regulate miRNA expression. For example, circNT5E was recently reported to directly bind to miR-422a and inhibit its activity, promoting glioblastoma tumorigenesis (37).

The aberrant miRNA expression in cancer can also be caused by downstream miRNA processing. Merritt et al. reported that miRNA expression could be globally suppressed by short hairpin RNAs against Dicer and Drosha, 2 critical ribonucleases involved in miRNA processing (38). This miRNA suppression promotes cellular transformation and tumorigenesis.

The alteration of miRNA expression in cancers can also be caused by aberrant transcription factor activity, which leads to increased or decreased transcription from miRNA genes. The miR-34 miRNA family (comprising miR-34a, miR-34b, and miR-34c) is directly induced by the tumor suppressor p53. In cells with high levels of p53, miR-34 expression is elevated; furthermore, chromatin immunoprecipitation assays revealed that p53 can bind to the promoter of miR-34 (39, 40). The MYC oncoprotein downregulates transcription of tumor suppressor miRNAs such as let-7 and miR-29 family members. MYC can bind to conserved sequences of the miRNA promoter that it suppresses, and the suppression of miRNAs by MYC has been found to facilitate lymphomagenesis (41) (**Figure 2**).

miRNA DYSREGULATION IN NPC INITIATION

The function of miRNAs is largely influenced by the expression of their main targets. Some miRNAs promote tumorigenesis in some cell types and suppress it in others. The classification of a miRNA as an oncogene or a tumor suppressor, therefore, requires knowledge of the type of cell in which it acts. Typically, miRNAs do not cause a specific phenotype by aiming at a single target. Instead, miRNAs target multiple mRNAs concurrently and engage in complex interactions with the machinery that controls the transcriptome. In cancers, miRNAs often are

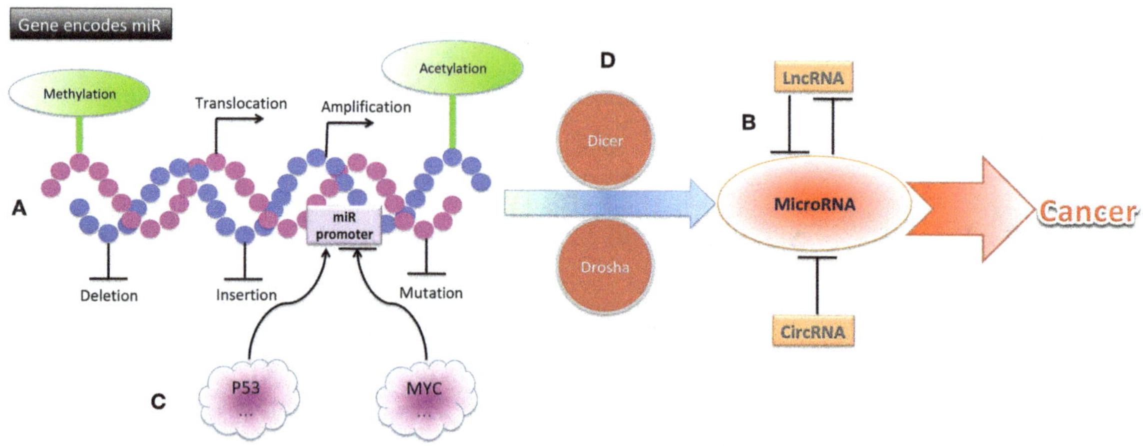

FIGURE 2 | The mechanisms of miRNA dysregulation in cancers. **(A)** Structural gene alterations, including translocation, amplification, deletion, insertion, and mutation contribute to miRNA dysregulation in cancers. **(B)** Epigenetic alterations, including methylation, acetylation, lncRNAs, and circRNAs contribute to miRNA dysregulation in cancers. **(C)** MiRNA promoters can be altered by p53, MYC, and other transcription factors, leading to cancer. **(D)** Alterations of proteins involved in miRNA processing, including Dicer, Drosha, and others, can result in cancer.

dysregulated and function collectively to mark differentiation states or individually as oncogenes or tumor suppressors. In NPC, miRNAs were reported to be expressed aberrantly and exert pivotal effects by altering the expression of their specific mRNA targets (42) (**Table 1**).

Onco-miRNAs in NPC

Tumor suppressor genes are usually inhibited by miRNAs directly, and such miRNAs are considered to be onco-miRNAs. For example, cell cycle inhibitor *CDKN1A* (also called *P21*) is believed to be directly targeted by miR-663 in NPC, leading to the promotion of NPC cell proliferation and tumorigenesis (43). An onco-miRNA, miR-125b, was found to be significantly upregulated in the NPC tissue compared with healthy nasopharyngeal mucosa, and this upregulation was correlated with poor survival outcomes; furthermore, high expression of miR-125b was identified as an independent predictor for shorter survival durations in NPC patients (44). The same study found that miR-125b promoted proliferation and inhibited apoptosis in NPC cells. A direct target of miR-125b, the tumor necrosis factor alpha-induced protein 3 gene *TNFAIP3* (formerly called *A20*), functions as a tumor suppressor in NPC and mediates miR-125b-promoted NPC tumorigenesis by activating the nuclear factor κB (NF-κB) signaling pathway. Together, these findings demonstrate that onco-miRNAs target tumor suppressor genes, leading to NPC initiation.

Tumor-Suppressive miRNAs in NPC

Oncogenes can be suppressed by miRNAs directly, and such miRNAs are considered to be tumor-suppressive miRNAs. For example, the C-X-C motif chemokine receptor 4 oncogene *CXCR4* can be directly targeted by tumor-suppressive miR-9, resulting in the inhibition of NPC pathogenesis. In NPC clinical specimens, miR-9 was observed to be downregulated (45). Interleukin-17 (IL-17), a proinflammatory cytokine, suppresses immune defense, and immune surveillance while promoting tumor growth. A study showed that IL-17 was targeted by miR-135a, resulting in the inhibition of NPC cell proliferation (46). In another study, overexpression of miR-320b was shown to suppress NPC cell proliferation and enhance mitochondrial fragmentation and apoptosis (47). In contrast, silencing miR-320b enhanced NPC tumor growth and inhibited cell apoptosis. The TP53-regulated inhibitor of apoptosis 1 gene, *TRIAP1*, has been found to be directly targeted by miR-320b, which mediates *TRIAP1*'s role in NPC cell proliferation inhibition and apoptosis induction. It has also been reported that miR-326/330-5p clusters can target cyclin D1 gene, *CCND1*, exerting their tumor-suppressive roles on NPC initiation (48). Some tumor-suppressive miRNAs target lncRNAs that function as oncogenes. For example, miR-25 expression was found to be upregulated in NPC cells, and its ectopic expression was shown to suppress NPC cell growth and motility by targeting metastasis-associated lung adenocarcinoma transcript-1 (*MALAT1*), a proto-oncogenic lncRNA (49). The tumor-suppressive miRNAs miR- 451 and miR-539-5p inhibit NPC initiation by targeting the macrophage migration inhibitory factor (*MIF*) and Kruppel-like factor 12 (*KLF12*) genes, respectively (50, 51). Finally, lentivirus can be used as a delivery system to overexpress specific tumor-suppressive miRNAs in NPC, resulting in the inhibition of NPC initiation. For example, lenti-miR-26a was shown to inhibit the tumorigenicity of NPC cells in nude mice significantly, providing a useful strategy for treating NPC patients (52).

miRNA DYSREGULATION IN NPC PROGRESSION

NPC is an aggressive disease that tends to spread locally and metastasize to regional lymph nodes and distant organs. Distant metastasis is the principal mode of treatment failure (53).

TABLE 1 | miRNA dysregulation in NPC initiation, progression and therapies.

miRNA	Target	Mechanism	Function	References
miR-663	*CDKN1A*	Promotes NPC cell proliferation	Onco-miRNA	(43)
miR-125b	*TNFAIP3*	Inhibits NPC cell apoptosis	Onco-miRNA	(44)
miR-9	*CXCR4*	Suppresses NPC pathogenesis	Suppressive miRNA	(45)
miR-135a	*IL-17*	Suppresses NPC cell proliferation	Suppressive miRNA	(46)
miR-320b	*TRIAP1*	Enhances NPC cell apoptosis	Suppressive miRNA	(47)
miR-326/330-5p clusters	*CCND1*	Suppresses NPC initiation	Suppressive miRNA	(48)
miR-25	*MALAT1*	Suppresses NPC cell growth	Suppressive miRNA	(49)
Exosomal miR-23a	*TSGA10*	Promotes NPC angiogenesis	Metastasis promoter	(54)
EBV-miR-BART1/7-3p	*PTEN*	Promotes EMT process	Metastasis promoter	(55, 56)
miR-29c	*TIAM1*	Suppresses NPC metastasis	Metastasis suppressor	(57)
miR-101	*ITGA3*	Inhibits NPC angiogenesis	Metastasis suppressor	(58)
miR-203a-3p	*LASP1*	Inhibits NPC metastasis	Metastasis suppressor	(59)
miR-630	*EZH2*	Inhibits NPC cell invasion	Metastasis suppressor	(60)
EBV-miR-BART6-3p	*MIR3936HG*	Suppresses NPC metastasis	Metastasis suppressor	(61)
miR-324-3p	*WNT2B*	Reduces NPC radioresistance	Radiosensitizer	(69)
miR-519d	*PDRG1*	Sensitizes NPC to IR	Radiosensitizer	(70)
miR-24	*COPS5/SP1*	Enhances NPC radiosensitivity	Radiosensitizer	(15)
miR-19b-3p	*TNFAIP3*	Increases NPC radioresistance	Radioresistant agent	(63)
miR-3188	*mTOR*	Suppresses NPC resistance of 5-FU	Chemosensitizer	(67)

CCND1, cyclin D1; CDKN1A, cyclin-dependent kinase inhibitor 1A; CXCR4, C-X-C motif chemokine receptor 4; IL-17, interleukin-17; MALAT1, metastasis-associated lung adenocarcinoma transcript 1; TNFAIP3, tumor necrosis factor alpha-induced protein 3; TRIAP1, TP53-regulated inhibitor of apoptosis 1; CXCL12, C-X-C motif chemokine ligand 12; EZH2, enhancer of zeste homolog 2; ITGA3, integrin subunit alpha 3; LASP1, LIM and SH3 protein 1; MIR3936HG, a long noncoding RNA; PTEN, phosphatase and tensin homolog; TIAM1, T cell lymphoma invasion and metastasis 1; TSGA10, testis-specific 10; 5-FU, fluorouracil; COPS5, COP9 signalosome subunit 5 (also called JAB1); MTOR, mechanistic target of rapamycin kinase; PDRG1, p53 and DNA damage regulated 1; SP1, specificity protein 1; WNT2B, Wnt family member 2B.

It is known that NPC metastasis is associated with miRNA dysregulation. The functions of miRNAs often are contradictory because they are determined by the cellular environment and the stage of the metastatic process. Therefore, identifying which miRNAs promote or suppress the metastatic process of NPC could lead to the development of new, efficient therapeutic agents to prevent or delay metastasis (**Table 1**).

Metastasis Promoter miRNAs in NPC

Mounting evidence implicates miRNAs in the modulation of angiogenesis, which is essential to the metastatic process. For instance, it has been reported that exosomal miR-23a overexpression promotes angiogenesis in NPC by directly targeting the testis-specific 10 gene, *TSGA10* (54). Furthermore, miR-23a overexpression in pre-metastatic NPC tissue was identified as a prognostic biomarker for early metastasis. In addition, EBV-encoded miR-BART1 has been shown to induce NPC metastasis by regulating pathways that depend on the phosphatase and tensin homolog gene, *PTEN* (55). Another EBV-encoded miRNA, miR-BART7-3p, was shown to promote the epithelial-mesenchymal transition (EMT) and metastasis of NPC cells by suppressing PTEN and consequently activating the PI3K/AKT/GSK-3β signaling pathway (56).

Metastasis Suppressor miRNAs in NPC

The tumor-suppressive miR-29c is also a metastasis suppressor that inhibits NPC cell migration, invasion, and metastasis by targeting the T cell lymphoma invasion and metastasis 1 gene, *TIAM1*, directly (57). In NPC patient samples and cell lines, miR-101 was found to be downregulated, and its ectopic expression significantly inhibited cell migration, invasion, and angiogenesis both *in vitro* and *in vivo*. The prometastatic gene integrin subunit alpha 3 (*ITGA3*) has been identified and validated as a target of miR-101 and shown to mediate the suppressive effects of miR-101 on NPC metastasis. Interestingly, the systemic delivery of lentivirus-mediated miR-101 in NPC suppressed lung metastatic colony formation with no noticeable toxic effects (58). Also, miR-203a-3p was found to be dysregulated and to act as a tumor suppressor in NPC. This miRNA suppresses NPC metastasis by targeting the LIM and SH3 protein 1 gene, *LASP1* (59).

Metastasis suppressor miRNAs can also target or be targeted by lncRNAs in NPC. For example, lncRNA *H19* has been found to be overexpressed in NPC tissue, and *H19* knockdown significantly suppressed invasion NPC cells. *H19* knockdown downregulated the expression of the enhancer of zeste homolog 2 gene, *EZH2*, which is upregulated in NPC and promotes invasion. *H19* does not bind directly to *EZH2* but instead modulates its expression by suppressing the activity of miR-630, which inhibits *EZH2* and interacts with *H19* in a sequence-specific manner. *H19* also suppresses E-cadherin expression and promotes invasion in NPC cells through the miR-630/EZH2 pathway (60). And He et al. demonstrated that EBV-miR-BART6-3p suppressed EBV-associated cancer cell migration and invasion by targeting lncRNA *MIR3936HG* (also known as *LOC553103*) and reversing the EMT process. And *MIR3936HG* knockdown by specific siRNAs was shown to phenocopy the effect of EBV-miR-BART6-3p, while elevated *MIR3936HG* expression enhanced tumor cell migration and invasion to promote EMT (61).

miRNA DYSREGULATION-RELATED SIGNALING PATHWAYS IN NPC

Several signaling pathways are involved in miRNA dysregulation-related processes in NPC. For example, miR-125b was shown to promote NPC tumorigenesis by activating the NF-κB signaling pathway, which plays a critical role in NPC tumorigenesis and progression (44, 62). In addition, miR-19b-3p was found to be upregulated and to be an independent predictor for poor survival outcomes in NPC patients. MiR-19b-3b increased NPC cell radioresistance by targeting *TNFAIP3* and then activating the NF-κB signaling pathway (63).

The PTEN/AKT pathway plays an important role in NPC processes related to miRNA dysregulation. One study found that miR-141 was markedly elevated in NPC tissues and negatively correlated with both patient survival and the expression of the bromodomain containing 7 gene, *BRD7; BRD7* overexpression activated the PTEN/AKT pathway, but restoring miR-141 expression suppressed this activation and partially restored NPC cell proliferation and tumor growth. The BRD7/miR-141/PTEN/AKT axis therefore is important to NPC progression and could provide new treatment targets and diagnostic markers (64). In addition, EBV-encoded miRNAs miR-BART1 and miR-BART7-3p promote NPC metastasis by modulating the PTEN/PI3K/AKT signaling pathway (55, 56). PI3K signaling is also involved in miRNA dysregulation-related processes in NPC. A study of NPC tumor specimens found that tumor-suppressing protein PDCD4 suppresses the pPI3K/pAKT/c-JUN signaling pathway, which in turn modulates miR-374a's binding to *CCND1*, resulting in dysregulation of NPC cell growth, metastasis, and chemoresistance (65). In this study, miR-374a expression was positively correlated with PDCD4 expression and negatively correlated with *CCND1* expression. The PI3K/AKT/mTOR signaling pathway also significantly affects NPC tumorigenesis and development (66). For example, miR-3188 was shown to inhibit NPC cell cycle transition and proliferation, to sensitize cells to chemotherapy, and to extend survival in tumor-bearing mice, and to inactivate p-PI3K/p-AKT/c-JUN signaling by targeting mTOR directly, further suppressing the cell cycle through the p-PI3K/p-AKT/p-mTOR pathway (67).

miRNA DYSREGULATION IN NPC THERAPIES

Radiotherapy and chemotherapy are 2 main treatments for NPC. Mounting evidence shows that miRNAs are dysregulated during radio- or chemotherapy for NPC and may reduce or induce the sensitivity of NPC cells to radiotherapy or chemotherapy (**Table 1**).

miRNA Dysregulation in Radiotherapy

Radioresistance is the main reason for NPC treatment failure (68). Multiple studies have shown that miRNA expression in various cell types changed upon irradiation, as did the specific effects of various miRNAs on cellular radiosensitivity. It has been reported that miR-324-3p reduces NPC radioresistance by directly targeting the well-known oncogene Wnt family member 2B (*WNT2B*), inhibiting the gene's translation (69). Studies have also reported that miR-519d sensitizes NPC cells to radiation by directly targeting the 3′-UTR of *PDRG1* (p53 and DNA damage regulated 1) mRNA (70) and thatiR-24 increases radiosensitivity in NPC by targeting both *COPS5* and *SP1* (specificity protein 1) (15). In contrast, Huang et al. demonstrated that miR-19b-3p upregulation decreases—and downregulation increases—NPC sensitivity to radiation. The researchers also found that miR-19b-3p directly targeted *TNFAIP3*, and the gene's upregulation reversed miR-19b-3p's suppressive effects on NPC cell radiosensitivity. Thus, miR-19b-3p was shown to enhance radioresistance in NPC cells by activating the TNFAIP3/ NF-κB pathway (63). Together, these studies indicate the potential use of miRNAs as radiosensitizing agents in NPC treatment.

miRNAs Dysregulation in Chemotherapy

The importance of miRNAs in chemotherapy response has been demonstrated in multiple human cancers, including cancer of the tongue (71). In NPC, miR-3188 has been found to inhibit cell growth and resistance to fluorouracil by directly targeting the mechanistic target of rapamycin kinase gene, *MTOR*, and regulating the cell cycle (67). Another study showed that the metastasis suppressor miR-29c can also increase NPC cells' sensitivity to both radiotherapy and cisplatin-based chemotherapy (72). The above evidence shows that miRNAs mainly function as chemosensitizers in NPC.

miRNAS AS BIOMARKERS AND NOVEL THERAPEUTIC APPROACHES IN NPC

In the above sections, we showed that miRNAs are dysregulated during NPC initiation, progression, and therapy. In addition, several studies have reported that miRNA dysregulation is associated with the survival of NPC patients, and miRNAs may serve as independent biomarkers for NPC diagnosis, recurrence, and prognosis. Furthermore, a few molecularly targeted drugs have emerged as clinically active against advanced NPC in recent years (73), and the exploration of miRNAs as drugs or drug targets against other cancer types is already underway (29).

miRNAs as Biomarkers in NPC

Several miRNAs show potential as biomarkers in NPC. A recent meta-analysis indicated that increased miRNA expression led to a poor overall survival and increased the likelihood of death of NPC patients (74). The tumor and metastasis suppressor miR-29c has been shown to be downregulated in both the serum and tumor tissue of NPC patients, indicating its promise as a biomarker for NPC diagnosis, prognosis, and recurrence (75). Also, NPC patients were shown to have significantly higher serum levels of miR-663 compared with healthy individuals, and high levels were associated with worse 5-year overall and relapse-free survival outcomes in NPC patients (76). In addition, chemotherapy significantly lowered NPC patients' serum miR-663 levels. These results suggest a critical role for miR-663 as a biomarker of NPC prognosis and response to chemotherapy. Recent studies showed that miR-31-5p was downregulated in present in NPC tissues and cell lines, acting as a tumor suppressive miRNA. And circulating miR-31-5p was identified to be a potential novel and non-invasive biomarker for the early diagnosis of NPC (77). The expression levels of tumor-educated platelet miR-34c-3p and miR-18a-5p are upregulated in NPC, which are promising novel liquid biopsy biomarkers for NPC diagnosis (78). In addition, miR-342-3p was significantly downregulated in NPC specimens and its low expression was significantly correlated with reduced overall survival of NPC patients, indicating miR-342-3p as a biomarker of NPC prognosis (79). All in all, the above results suggest miRNA can be a single biomarker for NPC diagnosis, prognosis, and response to therapy.

Additionally, miRNA signatures have been more and more identified to be novel biomarkers of NPC prognosis and prediction. For example, a two-miRNA signature of miR-548q and miR-483-5p were identified as potential biomarkers of NPC by comparing the plasma miRNA profiles of 31 NPC patients and 19 controls (80). And a three-miRNA signature including miR-548q, miR-630, and miR940 were increased in the plasma of NPC patients compared to those of controls. They are potential novel and useful biomarkers for NPC detection and diagnosis (81). The plasma level of miR-483-5p, miR-103, and miR-29a could be helpful to predict survival in patients with NPC (82). A four-miRNA signature of miR-22, miR-572, miR-638, and miR-1234 were identified to be prognostic biomarkers of NPC to the TNM staging system (83). Recently, a 8-miRNA signature including miR-188-5p, miR-1908, miR-3196, miR-3935, miR-4284, miR-4433-5p, miR-4665-3p, miR-513b, and 16-miRNA signature including miR-1224-3p, miR-1280, miR-155-5p, miR-1908, miR-1973, miR-296-5p, miR-361-3p, miR-425-5p, miR-4284, miR-4436b-5p, miR-4439, miR-4665-3p, miR-4706, miR-4740-3p, miR-5091, miR-513b are promising biomarkers for NPC diagnosis (84). Taker together, miRNAs can be as both single biomarkers and signatures for NPC detection, diagnosis, and prognosis (**Table 2**).

miRNAs as Therapeutic Approaches in NPC

One of the most appealing properties of miRNAs as therapeutic agents is their ability to simultaneously target more than 1 gene, making miRNAs extremely efficient for regulating distinct cell processes relevant to normal and malignant cell homeostasis. In NPC, miRNAs for gene therapy have been delivered using lentiviral vectors. For example, a previous study found that tumor suppressor miR-31-5pinhibited EBV-positive NPC tumorigenesis, and minicircle-oriP-miR-31, a novel EBNA1-specific miRNA delivery system, was constructed and shown to inhibit NPC cell proliferation and migration *in vitro* and to suppress xenograft growth and lung metastasis *in vivo*. The researchers also found that the WD repeat domain 5 gene, *WDR5*, is a target of miR-31-5p. The study proved that targeted delivery of miR-31-5p using a non-viral minicircle vector could serve as a novel therapeutic approach for NPC, indicating a promising miRNA therapy for NPC patients (85). More studies are still ongoing to apply miRNA therapy to patients with NPC.

CONCLUSIONS AND FUTURE DIRECTIONS

The need for novel therapeutic targets and agents for treating NPC patients is urgent, owing to NPC's anatomical location and resistance to both radiotherapy and chemotherapy. Large

TABLE 2 | miRNAs as biomarkers in NPC.

MiR	Expression in NPC	Biomarker	References
MiR-29c	Downregulated in NPC tissue	NPC diagnosis and prognosis	(75)
MiR-663	Upregualted in NPC serum	NPC prognosis and response to chemotherapy	(76)
MiR-31-5p	Downregulated in NPC tissue	NPC diagnosis	(77)
MiR-34c-3p	Upregualted in NPC tissue	NPC diagnosis	(78)
MiR-18a-5p	Upregualted in NPC tissue	NPC diagnosis	(78)
MiR-342-3p	Downregulated in NPC tissue	NPC prognosis	(79)
MiR signatures			
2-miRNA: miR-548q and miR-483-5p		NPC detection	(80)
3-miRNA: miR-548q, miR-630, and miR940		NPC detection and diagnosis	(81)
3-miRNA: miR-483-5p, miR-103, and miR-29a		NPC prognosis	(82)
4-miRNA: miR-22, miR-572, miR-638, and miR-1234		NPC prognosis	(83)
8-miRNA: miR-188-5p, miR-1908, miR-3196, miR-3935, miR-4284, miR-4433-5p, miR-4665-3p, miR-513b		NPC diagnosis	(84)
16-miRNA: miR-1224-3p, miR-1280, miR-155-5p, miR-1908, miR-1973, miR-296-5p, miR-361-3p, miR-425-5p, miR-4284, miR-4436b-5p, miR-4439, miR-4665-3p, miR-4706, miR-4740-3p, miR-5091, miR-513b		NPC diagnosis	(84)

numbers of miRNAs are dysregulated during the process of NPC initiation, progression, and therapy; therefore, miRNAs have been proposed as useful biomarkers to predict prognosis in and therapeutic approaches to cure patients with NPC. The advantages of using miRNAs as drugs antagonizing NPC is that 1 miRNA can target multiple targets and the same target can be targeted by many miRNAs, showing their comprehensive potential roles in the clinic. Based on the previous studies on miRNA dysregulations in NPC, how to use and take the advantages of miRNAs in clinic is to be solved. And due to the fact that miRNAs can regulate many mRNAs, the potential of toxic phenotypes and other off-target effects of miRNA treatment approaches is a major concern. As a result, more and more studies focusing on the toxic effects of targeting miRNAs are required before such therapies can be used safely in NPC patients.

AUTHOR CONTRIBUTIONS

SW was responsible for the writing and editing of the manuscript. F-XC was responsible for modifying the manuscript. WW provided some critical useful suggestions.

ACKNOWLEDGMENTS

We thank Butt, Bryan F from the Department of Scientific Publications at The University of Texas MD Anderson Cancer Center for editorial support.

REFERENCES

1. Wei WI, Sham JS. Nasopharyngeal carcinoma. *Lancet.* (2005) 365:2041–54. doi: 10.1016/S0140-6736(05)66698-6
2. Le QT, Jones CD, Yau TK, Shirazi HA, Wong PH, Thomas EN, et al. A comparison study of different PCR assays in measuring circulating plasma epstein-barr virus DNA levels in patients with nasopharyngeal carcinoma. *Clin Cancer Res.* (2005) 11:5700–7. doi: 10.1158/1078-0432.CCR-05-0648
3. Chan AT, Gregoire V, Lefebvre JL, Licitra L, Felip E, Group E-E-EGW. Nasopharyngeal cancer: EHNS-ESMO-ESTRO Clinical Practice Guidelines for diagnosis, treatment and follow-up. *Ann Oncol.* (2010) 21(Suppl 5):v187–9. doi: 10.1093/annonc/mdq186
4. Lee RC, Feinbaum RL, Ambros V. The *C. elegans* heterochronic gene lin-4 encodes small RNAs with antisense complementarity to lin-14. *Cell.* (1993) 75:843–54. doi: 10.1016/0092-8674(93)90529-Y
5. Ambros V. The functions of animal microRNAs. *Nature.* (2004) 431:350–5. doi: 10.1038/nature02871
6. Lee Y, Kim M, Han J, Yeom KH, Lee S, Baek SH, et al. MicroRNA genes are transcribed by RNA polymerase II. *EMBO J.* (2004) 23:4051–60. doi: 10.1038/sj.emboj.7600385
7. Lee Y, Ahn C, Han J, Choi H, Kim J, Yim J, et al. The nuclear RNase III Drosha initiates microRNA processing. *Nature.* (2003) 425:415–9. doi: 10.1038/nature01957
8. Bohnsack MT, Czaplinski K, Gorlich D. Exportin 5 is a RanGTP-dependent dsRNA-binding protein that mediates nuclear export of pre-miRNAs. *RNA.* (2004) 10:185–91. doi: 10.1261/rna.5167604
9. Chendrimada TP, Gregory RI, Kumaraswamy E, Norman J, Cooch N, Nishikura K, et al. TRBP recruits the Dicer complex to Ago2 for microRNA processing and gene silencing. *Nature.* (2005) 436:740–4. doi: 10.1038/nature03868
10. Betel D, Wilson M, Gabow A, Marks DS, Sander C. The microRNA.org resource: targets and expression. *Nucleic Acids Res.* (2008) 36:D149–53. doi: 10.1093/nar/gkm995
11. Friedman RC, Farh KK, Burge CB, Bartel DP. Most mammalian mRNAs are conserved targets of microRNAs. *Genome Res.* (2009) 19:92–105. doi: 10.1101/gr.082701.108
12. Lal A, Navarro F, Maher CA, Maliszewski LE, Yan N, O'Day E, et al. miR-24 Inhibits cell proliferation by targeting E2F2, MYC, and other cell-cycle genes via binding to "seedless" 3'UTR microRNA recognition elements. *Mol Cell.* (2009) 35:610–25. doi: 10.1016/j.molcel.2009.08.020
13. Orom UA, Nielsen FC, Lund AH. MicroRNA-10a binds the 5'UTR of ribosomal protein mRNAs and enhances their translation. *Mol Cell.* (2008) 30:460–71. doi: 10.1016/j.molcel.2008.05.001
14. Jopling CL, Yi M, Lancaster AM, Lemon SM, Sarnow P. Modulation of hepatitis C virus RNA abundance by a liver-specific MicroRNA. *Science.* (2005) 309:1577–81. doi: 10.1126/science.11 13329
15. Wang S, Pan Y, Zhang R, Xu T, Wu W, Zhang R, et al. Hsa-miR-24-3p increases nasopharyngeal carcinoma radiosensitivity by targeting both the 3'UTR and 5'UTR of Jab1/CSN5. *Oncogene.* (2016) 35:6096–6108. doi: 10.1038/onc.2016.147
16. Eiring AM, Harb JG, Neviani P, Garton C, Oaks JJ, Spizzo R, et al. miR-328 functions as an RNA decoy to modulate hnRNP E2 regulation of mRNA translation in leukemic blasts. *Cell.* (2010) 140:652–65. doi: 10.1016/j.cell.2010.01.007
17. Place RF, Li LC, Pookot D, Noonan EJ, Dahiya R. MicroRNA-373 induces expression of genes with complementary promoter sequences. *Proc Natl Acad Sci USA.* (2018) 115:E3325. doi: 10.1073/pnas.1803 343115
18. Vasudevan S, Tong Y, Steitz JA. Switching from repression to activation: microRNAs can up-regulate translation. *Science.* (2007) 318:1931–4. doi: 10.1126/science.1149460
19. Fabbri M, Paone A, Calore F, Galli R, Croce CM. A new role for microRNAs, as ligands of Toll-like receptors. *RNA Biol.* (2013) 10:169–74. doi: 10.4161/rna.23144
20. Tanaka Y, Kamohara H, Kinoshita K, Kurashige J, Ishimoto T, Iwatsuki M, et al. Clinical impact of serum exosomal microRNA-21 as a clinical biomarker in human esophageal squamous cell carcinoma. *Cancer.* (2013) 119:1159–67. doi: 10.1002/cncr.27895
21. Yang M, Chen J, Su F, Yu B, Su F, Lin L, et al. Microvesicles secreted by macrophages shuttle invasion-potentiating microRNAs into breast cancer cells. *Mol Cancer.* (2011) 10:117. doi: 10.1186/1476-4598-10-117
22. Lu J, Liu QH, Wang F, Tan JJ, Deng YQ, Peng XH, et al. Exosomal miR-9 inhibits angiogenesis by targeting MDK and regulating PDK/AKT pathway in nasopharyngeal carcinoma. *J Exp Clin Cancer Res.* (2018) 37:147. doi: 10.1186/s13046-018-0814-3
23. Ye SB, Zhang H, Cai TT, Liu YN, Ni JJ, He J, et al. Exosomal miR-24-3p impedes T-cell function by targeting FGF11 and serves as a potential prognostic biomarker for nasopharyngeal carcinoma. *J Pathol.* (2016) 240:329–40. doi: 10.1002/path.4781
24. Lo AK, To KF, Lo KW, Lung RW, Hui JW, Liao G, et al. Modulation of LMP1 protein expression by EBV-encoded microRNAs. *Proc Natl Acad Sci USA.* (2007) 104:16164–9. doi: 10.1073/pnas.0702896104
25. Pfeffer S, Zavolan M, Grasser FA, Chien M, Russo JJ, Ju J, et al. Identification of virus-encoded microRNAs. *Science.* (2004) 304:734–6. doi: 10.1126/science.1096781
26. Raab-Traub N. Epstein-Barr virus in the pathogenesis of NPC. *Semin Cancer Biol.* (2002) 12:431–41. doi: 10.1016/S1044579X0200086X
27. Lung RW, Hau PM, Yu KH, Yip KY, Tong JH, Chak WP, et al. EBV-encoded miRNAs target ATM-mediated response in nasopharyngeal carcinoma. *J Pathol.* (2018) 244:394–407. doi: 10.1002/path.5018

28. Calin GA, Sevignani C, Dan Dumitru C, Hyslop T, Noch E, Yendamuri S, et al. Human microRNA genes are frequently located at fragile sites and genomic regions involved in cancers. *Proc Natl Acad Sci USA.* (2004) 101:2999–3004. doi: 10.1073/pnas.0307323101
29. Garzon R, Marcucci G, Croce CM. Targeting microRNAs in cancer: rationale, strategies and challenges. *Nat Rev Drug Discov.* (2010) 9:775–89. doi: 10.1038/nrd3179
30. Ota A, Tagawa H, Karnan S, Tsuzuki S, Karpas A, Kira S, et al. Identification and characterization of a novel gene, C13orf25, as a target for 13q31-q32 amplification in malignant lymphoma. *Cancer Res.* (2004) 64:3087–95. doi: 10.1158/0008-5472.CAN-03-3773
31. Calin GA, Ferracin M, Cimmino A, Di Leva G, Shimizu M, Wojcik SE, et al. A MicroRNA signature associated with prognosis and progression in chronic lymphocytic leukemia. *N Engl J Med.* (2005) 353:1793–801. doi: 10.1056/NEJMoa050995
32. Garzon R, Volinia S, Liu CG, Fernandez-Cymering C, Palumbo T, Pichiorri F, et al. MicroRNA signatures associated with cytogenetics and prognosis in acute myeloid leukemia. *Blood.* (2008) 111:3183–9. doi: 10.1182/blood-2007-07-098749
33. Calin GA, Dumitru CD, Shimizu M, Bichi R, Zupo S, Noch E, et al. Frequent deletions and down-regulation of micro- RNA genes miR15 and miR16 at 13q14 in chronic lymphocytic leukemia. *Proc Natl Acad Sci USA.* (2002) 99:15524–9. doi: 10.1073/pnas.242606799
34. Saito Y, Liang G, Egger G, Friedman JM, Chuang JC, Coetzee GA, et al. Specific activation of microRNA-127 with downregulation of the proto-oncogene BCL6 by chromatin-modifying drugs in human cancer cells. *Cancer Cell.* (2006) 9:435–43. doi: 10.1016/j.ccr.2006.04.020
35. Wang S, Wu W, Claret FX. Mutual regulation of microRNAs and DNA methylation in human cancers. *Epigenetics.* (2017) 12:187–97. doi: 10.1080/15592294.2016.1273308
36. Wang R, Zhang T, Yang Z, Jiang C, Seng J. Long non-coding RNA FTH1P3 activates paclitaxel resistance in breast cancer through miR-206/ABCB1. *J Cell Mol Med.* (2018) 22:4068–75. doi: 10.1111/jcmm.13679
37. Wang R, Zhang S, Chen X, Li N, Li J, Jia R, et al. CircNT5E acts as a sponge of microRNA-422a to promote glioblastoma tumorigenesis. *Cancer Res.* (2018) 78:4812–25. doi: 10.1158/0008-5472.CAN-18-0532
38. Merritt WM, Lin YG, Han LY, Kamat AA, Spannuth WA, Schmandt R, et al. Dicer, Drosha, and outcomes in patients with ovarian cancer. *N Engl J Med.* (2008) 359:2641–50. doi: 10.1056/NEJMoa0803785
39. He L, He X, Lim LP, de Stanchina E, Xuan Z, Liang Y, et al. A microRNA component of the p53 tumour suppressor network. *Nature.* (2007) 447:1130–4. doi: 10.1038/nature05939
40. Chang TC, Wentzel EA, Kent OA, Ramachandran K, Mullendore M, Lee KH, et al. Transactivation of miR-34a by p53 broadly influences gene expression and promotes apoptosis. *Mol Cell.* (2007) 26:745–52. doi: 10.1016/j.molcel.2007.05.010
41. Chang TC, Yu D, Lee YS, Wentzel EA, Arking DE, West KM, et al. Widespread microRNA repression by Myc contributes to tumorigenesis. *Nat Genet.* (2008) 40:43–50. doi: 10.1038/ng.2007.30
42. Chen HC, Chen GH, Chen YH, Liao WL, Liu CY, Chang KP, et al. MicroRNA deregulation and pathway alterations in nasopharyngeal carcinoma. *Br J Cancer.* (2009) 100:1002–11. doi: 10.1038/sj.bjc.6604948
43. Yi C, Wang Q, Wang L, Huang Y, Li L, Liu L, et al. MiR-663, a microRNA targeting p21(WAF1/CIP1), promotes the proliferation and tumorigenesis of nasopharyngeal carcinoma. *Oncogene.* (2012) 31:4421–33. doi: 10.1038/onc.2011.629
44. Zheng Z, Qu JQ, Yi HM, Ye X, Huang W, Xiao T, et al. MiR-125b regulates proliferation and apoptosis of nasopharyngeal carcinoma by targeting A20/NF-kappaB signaling pathway. *Cell Death Dis.* (2017) 8:e2855. doi: 10.1038/cddis.2017.211
45. Lu J, Luo H, Liu X, Peng Y, Zhang B, Wang L, et al. miR-9 targets CXCR4 and functions as a potential tumor suppressor in nasopharyngeal carcinoma. *Carcinogenesis.* (2014) 35:554–63. doi: 10.1093/carcin/bgt354
46. Wang LX, Kang ZP, Yang ZC, Ma RX, Tan Y, Peng XB, et al. MicroRNA-135a inhibits nasopharyngeal carcinoma cell proliferation through targeting interleukin-17. *Cell Physiol Biochem.* (2018) 46:2232–8. doi: 10.1159/000489591
47. Li Y, Tang X, He Q, Yang X, Ren X, Wen X, et al. Overexpression of mitochondria mediator gene TRIAP1 by miR-320b loss is associated with progression in nasopharyngeal carcinoma. *PLoS Genet.* (2016) 12:e1006183. doi: 10.1371/journal.pgen.1006183
48. Song P, Yin SC. Long non-coding RNA EWSAT1 promotes human nasopharyngeal carcinoma cell growth *in vitro* by targeting miR-326/-330-5p. *Aging.* (2016) 8:2948–60. doi: 10.18632/aging.101103
49. Hua WF, Zhong Q, Xia TL, Chen Q, Zhang MY, Zhou AJ, et al. RBM24 suppresses cancer progression by upregulating miR-25 to target MALAT1 in nasopharyngeal carcinoma. *Cell Death Dis.* (2016) 7:e2352. doi: 10.1038/cddis.2016.252
50. Liu N, Jiang N, Guo R, Jiang W, He QM, Xu YF, et al. MiR-451 inhibits cell growth and invasion by targeting MIF and is associated with survival in nasopharyngeal carcinoma. *Mol Cancer.* (2013) 12:123. doi: 10.1186/1476-4598-12-123
51. Sun KY, Peng T, Chen Z, Song P, Zhou XH. Long non-coding RNA LOC100129148 functions as an oncogene in human nasopharyngeal carcinoma by targeting miR-539-5p. *Aging.* (2017) 9:999–1011. doi: 10.18632/aging.101205
52. Lu JA, He ML, Wang L, Chen Y, Liu XO, Dong Q, et al. MiR-26a inhibits cell growth and tumorigenesis of nasopharyngeal carcinoma through repression of EZH2. *Cancer Res.* (2011) 71:225–33. doi: 10.1158/0008-5472.CAN-10-1850
53. Li ZL, Ye SB, OuYang LY, Zhang H, Chen YS, He J, et al. COX-2 promotes metastasis in nasopharyngeal carcinoma by mediating interactions between cancer cells and myeloid-derived suppressor cells. *Oncoimmunology.* (2015) 4:e1044712. doi: 10.1080/2162402X.2015.1044712
54. Bao L, You B, Shi S, Shan Y, Zhang Q, Yue H, et al. Metastasis-associated miR-23a from nasopharyngeal carcinoma-derived exosomes mediates angiogenesis by repressing a novel target gene TSGA10. *Oncogene.* (2018) 37:2873–89. doi: 10.1038/s41388-018-0183-6
55. Cai L, Ye Y, Jiang Q, Chen Y, Lyu X, Li J, et al. Epstein-Barr virus-encoded microRNA BART1 induces tumour metastasis by regulating PTEN-dependent pathways in nasopharyngeal carcinoma. *Nat Commun.* (2015) 6:7353. doi: 10.1038/ncomms8353
56. Cai LM, Lyu XM, Luo WR, Cui XF, Ye YF, Yuan CC, et al. EBV-miR-BART7-3p promotes the EMT and metastasis of nasopharyngeal carcinoma cells by suppressing the tumor suppressor PTEN. *Oncogene.* (2015) 34:2156–66. doi: 10.1038/onc.2014.341
57. Liu N, Tang LL, Sun Y, Cui RX, Wang HY, Huang BJ, et al. MiR-29c suppresses invasion and metastasis by targeting TIAM1 in nasopharyngeal carcinoma. *Cancer Lett.* (2013) 329:181–8. doi: 10.1016/j.canlet.2012.10.032
58. Tang XR, Wen X, He QM, Li YQ, Ren XY, Yang XJ, et al. MicroRNA-101 inhibits invasion and angiogenesis through targeting ITGA3 and its systemic delivery inhibits lung metastasis in nasopharyngeal carcinoma. *Cell Death Dis.* (2017) 8:e2566. doi: 10.1038/cddis.2016.486
59. Jiang N, Jiang X, Chen Z, Song X, Wu L, Zong D, et al. MiR-203a-3p suppresses cell proliferation and metastasis through inhibiting LASP1 in nasopharyngeal carcinoma. *J Exp Clin Cancer Res.* (2017) 36:138. doi: 10.1186/s13046-017-0604-3
60. Li X, Lin Y, Yang X, Wu X, He X. Long noncoding RNA H19 regulates EZH2 expression by interacting with miR-630 and promotes cell invasion in nasopharyngeal carcinoma. *Biochem Biophys Res Commun.* (2016) 473:913–9. doi: 10.1016/j.bbrc.2016.03.150
61. He B, Li W, Wu Y, Wei F, Gong Z, Bo H, et al. Epstein-Barr virus-encoded miR-BART6-3p inhibits cancer cell metastasis and invasion by targeting long non-coding RNA LOC553103. *Cell Death Dis.* (2016) 7:e2353. doi: 10.1038/cddis.2016.253
62. Zhu DD, Zhang J, Deng W, Yip YL, Lung HL, Tsang CM, et al. Significance of NF-kappaB activation in immortalization of nasopharyngeal epithelial cells. *Int J Cancer.* (2016) 138:1175–85. doi: 10.1002/ijc.29850
63. Huang T, Yin L, Wu J, Gu JJ, Wu JZ, Chen D, et al. MicroRNA-19b-3p regulates nasopharyngeal carcinoma radiosensitivity by targeting TNFAIP3/NF-kappaB axis. *J Exp Clin Cancer Res.* (2016) 35:188. doi: 10.1186/s13046-016-0465-1
64. Liu Y, Zhao R, Wang H, Luo Y, Wang X, Niu W, et al. miR-141 is involved in BRD7-mediated cell proliferation and tumor formation through suppression of the PTEN/AKT pathway in nasopharyngeal carcinoma. *Cell Death Dis.* (2016) 7:e2156. doi: 10.1038/cddis.2016.64
65. Zhen Y, Fang W, Zhao M, Luo R, Liu Y, Fu Q, et al. miR-374a-CCND1-pPI3K/AKT-c-JUN feedback loop modulated by PDCD4

suppresses cell growth, metastasis, and sensitizes nasopharyngeal carcinoma to cisplatin. *Oncogene.* (2017) 36:275–85. doi: 10.1038/onc.2016.201

66. Wang F, Lu J, Peng X, Wang J, Liu X, Chen X, et al. Integrated analysis of microRNA regulatory network in nasopharyngeal carcinoma with deep sequencing. *J Exp Clin Cancer Res.* (2016) 35:17. doi: 10.1186/s13046-016-0292-4
67. Zhao M, Luo R, Liu Y, Gao L, Fu Z, Fu Q, et al. miR-3188 regulates nasopharyngeal carcinoma proliferation and chemosensitivity through a FOXO1-modulated positive feedback loop with mTOR-p-PI3K/AKT-c-JUN. *Nat Commun.* (2016) 7:11309. doi: 10.1038/ncomms11309
68. Liu SC, Tsang NM, Chiang WC, Chang KP, Hsueh C, Liang Y, et al. Leukemia inhibitory factor promotes nasopharyngeal carcinoma progression and radioresistance. *J Clin Invest.* (2013) 123:5269–83. doi: 10.1172/JCI63428
69. Li G, Liu Y, Su Z, Ren S, Zhu G, Tian Y, et al. MicroRNA-324-3p regulates nasopharyngeal carcinoma radioresistance by directly targeting WNT2B. *Eur J Cancer.* (2013) 49:2596–607. doi: 10.1016/j.ejca.2013.03.001
70. Xu T, Xiao D. Oleuropein enhances radiation sensitivity of nasopharyngeal carcinoma by downregulating PDRG1 through HIF1alpha-repressed microRNA-519d. *J Exp Clin Cancer Res.* (2017) 36:3. doi: 10.1186/s13046-016-0480-2
71. Sun L, Yao Y, Liu B, Lin Z, Lin L, Yang M, et al. MiR-200b and miR-15b regulate chemotherapy-induced epithelial-mesenchymal transition in human tongue cancer cells by targeting BMI1. *Oncogene.* (2012) 31:432–45. doi: 10.1038/onc.2011.263
72. Zhang JX, Qian D, Wang FW, Liao DZ, Wei JH, Tong ZT, et al. MicroRNA-29c enhances the sensitivities of human nasopharyngeal carcinoma to cisplatin-based chemotherapy and radiotherapy. *Cancer Lett.* (2013) 329:91–8. doi: 10.1016/j.canlet.2012.10.033
73. Lim WT, Ng QS, Ivy P, Leong SS, Singh O, Chowbay B, et al. A Phase II study of pazopanib in Asian patients with recurrent/metastatic nasopharyngeal carcinoma. *Clin Cancer Res.* (2011) 17:5481–9. doi: 10.1158/1078-0432.CCR-10-3409
74. Sabarimurugan S, Kumarasamy C, Baxi S, Devi A, Jayaraj R. Systematic review and meta-analysis of prognostic microRNA biomarkers for survival outcome in nasopharyngeal carcinoma. *PLoS ONE.* (2019) 14:e0209760. doi: 10.1371/journal.pone.0209760
75. Niu M, Gao D, Wen Q, Wei P, Pan S, Shuai C, et al. MiR-29c regulates the expression of miR-34c and miR-449a by targeting DNA methyltransferase 3a and 3b in nasopharyngeal carcinoma. *BMC Cancer.* (2016) 16:218. doi: 10.1186/s12885-016-2253-x
76. Liang S, Zhang N, Deng Y, Chen L, Zhang Y, Zheng Z, et al. Increased serum level of microRNA-663 is correlated with poor prognosis of patients with nasopharyngeal carcinoma. *Dis Markers.* (2016) 2016:7648215. doi: 10.1155/2016/7648215
77. Yi SJ, Liu P, Chen BL, Ou-Yang L, Xiong WM, Su JP. Circulating miR-31-5p may be a potential diagnostic biomarker in nasopharyngeal carcinoma. *Neoplasma.* (2019) 10:181109N847. doi: 10.4149/neo_2018_181109N847
78. Wang H, Wei X, Wu B, Su J, Tan W, Yang K. Tumor-educated platelet miR-34c-3p and miR-18a-5p as potential liquid biopsy biomarkers for nasopharyngeal carcinoma diagnosis. *Cancer Manag Res.* (2019) 11:3351–60. doi: 10.2147/CMAR.S195654
79. Cui Z, Zhao Y. microRNA-342-3p targets FOXQ1 to suppress the aggressive phenotype of nasopharyngeal carcinoma cells. *BMC Cancer.* (2019) 19:104. doi: 10.1186/s12885-018-5225-5
80. Zheng XH, Cui C, Ruan HL, Xue WQ, Zhang SD, Hu YZ, et al. Plasma microRNA profiling in nasopharyngeal carcinoma patients reveals miR-548q and miR-483-5p as potential biomarkers. *Chin J Cancer.* (2014) 33:330–8. doi: 10.5732/cjc.013.10246
81. Zhuo X, Zhou W, Li D, Chang A, Wang Y, Wu Y, et al. Plasma microRNA expression signature involving miR-548q, miR-630 and miR-940 as biomarkers for nasopharyngeal carcinoma detection. *Cancer Biomarkers.* (2018) 23:579–87. doi: 10.3233/CBM-181852
82. Wang HY, Yan LX, Shao Q, Fu S, Zhang ZC, Ye W, et al. Profiling plasma microRNA in nasopharyngeal carcinoma with deep sequencing. *Clin Chem.* (2014) 60:773–82. doi: 10.1373/clinchem.2013.214213
83. Liu N, Cui RX, Sun Y, Guo R, Mao YP, Tang LL, et al. A four-miRNA signature identified from genome-wide serum miRNA profiling predicts survival in patients with nasopharyngeal carcinoma. *Int J Cancer.* (2014) 134:1359–68. doi: 10.1002/ijc.28468
84. Wen W, Mai SJ, Lin HX, Zhang MY, Huang JL, Hua X, et al. Identification of two microRNA signatures in whole blood as novel biomarkers for diagnosis of nasopharyngeal carcinoma. *J Transl Med.* (2019) 17:186. doi: 10.1186/s12967-019-1923-2
85. Wu J, Tan X, Lin J, Yuan L, Chen J, Qiu L, et al. Minicircle-oriP-miR-31 as a novel EBNA1-specific miRNA therapy approach for nasopharyngeal carcinoma. *Hum Gene Ther.* (2017) 28:415–27. doi: 10.1089/hum.2016.136

21

Significance of PET-CT for Detecting Occult Lymph Node Metastasis and Affecting Prognosis in Early-Stage Tongue Squamous Cell Carcinoma

Guo Zhao[1], *Jianli Sun*[1], *Kai Ba*[1*] *and Yunxiang Zhang*[2]

[1] *Department of Oral Medicine, The First Affiliated Hospital of Zhengzhou University, Zhengzhou, China,* [2] *Department of Endodontics, Kaifeng Stomatology Hospital, Kaifeng, China*

Correspondence:
Kai Ba
k.ba@msn.com

Objective: We aimed to clarify the significance of PET-CT for detecting occult lymph node metastasis and for affecting prognosis in early-stage tongue squamous cell carcinoma (SCC).

Methods: Patients with surgically treated primary cT1-2N0 tongue SCC who agreed to undergo a preoperative PET-CT scan were prospectively enrolled. The primary study outcomes were occult neck lymph node metastasis and locoregional control (LRC). The Kaplan-Meier method was used to analyze the LRC rate, and then the factors that were significant in the Kaplan-Meier method were assessed in the Cox model to determine the independent factors.

Results: A total of 135 patients were included, and the median maximum standardized uptake value (SUV max) of the primary tumor was 9.0. When analyzing the PET-CT results, 18 patients were recognized as having neck lymph node metastasis, and 12 patients were proven to have pathologic lymph nodes. A total of 117 patients did not have neck lymph node metastasis reported by PET-CT, and five patients were proven to have pathologic lymph nodes. The sensitivity and specificity of PET-CT for predicting occult metastasis were 70.6 and 94.9%, respectively. In patients with an SUV max $\leq$9.0, the 5-year LRC rate was 95%; in patients with an SUV max >9.0, the 5-year LRC rate was 85%, and the difference was significant. Further Cox model analyses confirmed the independence of the SUV max for predicting LRC.

Conclusion: PET-CT has a high specificity for predicting occult lymph node metastasis, and an SUV max >9.0 is significantly associated with worse LRC in cT1-2N0 tongue SCC.

Keywords: PET-CT, occult lymph node metastasis, early-stage tongue squamous cell carcinoma, tongue squamous cell carcinoma, oral squamous cell carcinoma

INTRODUCTION

Tongue squamous cell carcinoma (SCC) is a common malignancy in the oral cavity, and complete resection is the standard treatment procedure (1, 2). Owing to the wide range of occult lymph node metastasis rates, there is controversy regarding the best neck management. It is important for us to detect patients who are at high risk of neck lymph node metastasis preoperatively.

Current researchers have demonstrated the role of perineural invasion, lymphovascular invasion, depth of invasion, neutrophil-to-lymphocyte ratio, and so on in predicting occult lymph node metastasis (3–6), but the significance of PET-CT for determining occult lymph node metastasis has rarely been discussed. Zhang et al. (7) described that the overall sensitivity and specificity of PET-CT in cT1-2 oral SCC were 21.4 and 98.4%, respectively, with a negative predictive value of 99.1%. Myers et al. (8) demonstrated an estimated overall sensitivity of PET-CT for the N0 neck of 78% with a specificity of 100%. On the other hand, cancer cells use glucose as an energy source, and tumors with strong growth potential and invasiveness are highly likely to take up FDG (9), as indicated by the maximum standardized uptake value (SUV max). Previous authors have depicted the prognostic role of the SUV max in head and neck SCC; however, all these studies included all subsites or analyzed large-volume tumors together with small-volume tumors. Considering that different biological behaviors exist between tongue SCC and SCC at other sites, in the current study, we aimed to clarify the significance of PET-CT for detecting occult lymph node metastasis and affecting prognosis in early-stage tongue squamous cell carcinoma.

PATIENTS AND METHODS

The Zhengzhou University Institutional Research Committee approved our study (No. 201845YZ), and all patients signed informed consent agreements for medical research before the initial treatment. All methods were performed in accordance with the relevant guidelines and regulations.

From January 2010 to December 2018, consecutive patients with primary early stage (cT1-2N0) tongue SCC were prospectively enrolled. The only inclusion criterion was that the patient agreed to undergo a PET-CT examination preoperatively. Clinical pathologic and follow-up data, including age, sex, smoking status, drinking status, pathologic TNM stage based on the AJCC 8th edition, perineural invasion (PNI), lymphovascular invasion (LVI), extracapsular extension (ECS), depth of invasion (DOI), and SUV max of the primary tumor, were recorded in the enrolled patients.

Smokers/drinkers were defined as patients who smoked/drank at diagnosis or who had stopped for <1-year (10, 11). All pathologic sections were reviewed by at least two head and neck pathologists. PNI was considered to be present if tumor cells were identified within the perineural space and/or nerve bundle; LVI was positive if tumors were noted within the lymphovascular channels (12). The pathologic DOI was measured from the level of the adjacent normal mucosa to the deepest point of tumor infiltration, regardless of the presence or absence of ulceration (13). cT1-2 was defined by a maximum tumor diameter of <2 cm or ranging from 2 to 4 cm. Patients were considered cN0 if they had no evidence of nodal metastasis on a clinical exam, ultrasound, or radiographic imaging (not including PET-CT) (9). The cut-off value of the SUV max was set according to the median value (14).

Several PET/CT scanners were used to perform the PET-CT scans (GE Healthcare, Milwaukee, America). Patients fasted for at least 6 h before the PET-CT scan. The procedure was postponed when glucose levels were >200 mg/dL. Each patient received 10–20 mCi of [^{18}F] FDG dose, based on his or her weight. Axial PET and diagnostic CT images were obtained from the calvarial vertex through the upper thighs after urinary voiding. Emission images were obtained after a radiopharmaceutical injection 1 h later. There was no contrast medium used during the CT scan. The images were reconstructed in the thickness of a 2.5 mm slice. The SUV max was measured for both the primary tumor and regional lymph nodes. For every suspicious lesion, the isocontour region of interest centered on the maximum value pixel was drawn automatically with workstation tools generating the SUV max of the region. An SUV max cut-off of 2.5 MBq/g was used for FDG-avid lymph nodes and primary tumors on PET-CT.

In our cancer center, systemic examinations, including ultrasound, CT, and MRI, were routinely performed. PET-CT was selectively suggested, and complete resection of the primary tumor with a margin of at least 1 cm, including the adipose tissue in the mouth floor as well as the sublingual gland and neck dissection (level 1–3), was routinely performed in every patient with any stage of tongue SCC. Adjuvant treatment was suggested if there was neck lymph node metastasis, PNI, LVI, or a positive margin. All patients were regularly followed up with every 3 months within the first 2- years after the operation and every 6 months within the third to fifth years after the operation. If there was suspicion of disease recurrence, active interference was performed.

The primary study outcomes were occult neck lymph node metastasis and locoregional control (LRC). The 4-fold table method was used to analyze the association between PET-CT and occult lymph node metastasis. The survival time was calculated from the date of surgery to the date of the first event of local, regional, or locoregional recurrence or to the latest follow-up. The Kaplan-Meier method was used to analyze the LRC rate, and then the factors that were significant in the Kaplan-Meier method were assessed in the Cox model to determine the independent factors. All statistical analyses were performed using SPSS 20.0, all reported p-value was two-sided, and $p < 0.05$ was considered to be significant.

RESULTS

There were 135 patients (109 males and 26 females) enrolled in total, and the mean age was 54.5 (range: 30–76) years. There were 76 (56.3%) smokers and 55 (40.7%) drinkers. The median SUV max was 9.0 (range: 2.3–29.7). Clinical tumor stages were characterized as cT1 in 57 (42.2%) cases and cT2 in 78 (57.8%) cases. 5 cT1 tumors were corrected into pT2 tumors after operation. PNI and LVI were noted in 18 (13.3%) and 15 (11.1%) patients, respectively. The mean DOI was 6.0 (range: 1.0–9.5) mm. Tumor differentiation was well in 53 (39.3%) cases, moderate in 70 (51.9%) cases, and poor in 12 (8.9%) cases. Negative margins were achieved in all patients.

Occult neck lymph node metastasis was reported in five of the 57 patients with cT1 disease with a rate of 8.8% and in 12 of the 78 patients with cT2 disease with a rate of 15.4%. ECS was reported in three (3/17, 17.6%) patients. The total number of positive lymph nodes was 23.

When analyzing the PET-CT results, 18 patients were recognized as having neck lymph node metastasis, and 12 patients were proven to have pathologic lymph nodes. A total of 117 patients did not have neck lymph node metastasis reported by PET-CT, and five patients were proven to have pathologic lymph nodes. The sensitivity and specificity of PET-CT for predicting occult metastasis were 70.6 and 94.9%, respectively.

The mean follow-up time was 53.9 (range: 6–95) months. Twenty five patients underwent adjuvant radiotherapy, while three patients also received adjuvant chemotherapy. Thirteen patients suffered from disease recurrence: four cases locally, five cases regionally, and four cases locoregionally. Eight patients were successfully salvaged with surgical treatment. In patients with an SUV max ≤9.0, there were three cases of recurrence, and the 5-year LRC rate was 95%. In patients with an SUV max >9.0, there were ten cases of recurrence, and the 5-year LRC rate was 85%; the difference was significant (**Figure 1**, $p = 0.043$). Further Cox model analyses confirmed the independence of the SUV max for predicting LRC (**Table 1**).

DISCUSSION

The most important finding in the current study was that PET-CT had a high specificity for predicting occult lymph node metastasis, and an SUV max >9.0 was significantly associated with worse LRC in patients with early-stage tongue SCC. These results can provide better guidance regarding decision making in terms of neck dissection and can help determine which patients would need adjuvant radiotherapy.

Neck lymph node metastasis is the most important prognostic factor in oral SCC, and neck management for early-stage tongue SCC is a key issue. A few authors who support routine neck dissection depicted that it could be beneficial for accurately staging the neck and identifying patients who require adjuvant therapy as well as improving survival (15). However, some authors have reported that the rate of occult neck lymph node metastasis varies, and a considerable number of patients have been over-treated (16). This controversy prompted the effort to determine the possible predictors for occult lymph node metastasis. Larson et al. (17) aimed to clarify the contribution of adverse pathologic characteristics to clinical outcomes in small tongue SCC and concluded that, even though PNI and LVI occurred, the prevalence of occult lymph node metastasis was very low in small disease with a DOI ≤ 4.0 mm. Wu et al. (18) described that a DOI larger than 4 mm and a stable growth pattern in the invasive front were independent risk factors for occult lymph node metastasis in cT1-2N0 tongue SCC. A similar finding was also reported by Faisal et al. (19): 179 patients with early-stage tongue SCC were divided into three groups according to the AJCC cutoff points in the 8th edition according to depth(group A: 1–5 mm, group B: 6–10 mm, and group C: > 10 mm). The authors noted that the risk of local recurrence and nodal metastasis in group A was 15 and 23%, in group B was 20 and 34%, and in group C was 40 and 53%, respectively. However, all these studies were retrospective, and the analyzed predictors, including DOI, PNI, and LVI, usually remained unknown during the frozen section, which would greatly limit their clinical application.

Cancer cells utilize glucose as energy in general, and PET-CT has been widely used to detect the primary site and metastasized lymph nodes. Additionally, a number of researchers have clarified the role of PET-CT in evaluating neck status. Chaukar et al. (20) previously compared the diagnostic accuracy of staging a cN0 neck among ultrasound, contrast enhanced CT, and PET-CT in 70 oral SCC patients. The authors reported that the PET-CT scan

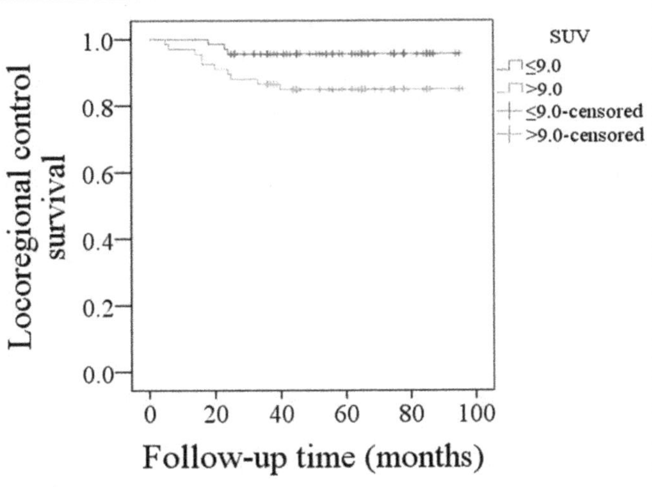

FIGURE 1 | Comparison of locoregional control survival in patients with an SUV max ≤9.0 or >9.0 ($p = 0.043$).

TABLE 1 | Univariate and Cox model analyses of risk factors for the locoregional control survival in patients with cT1-2N0 tongue squamous cell carcinoma.

Variables	Univariate	Cox model	
	Log-rank test	p	HR [95% CI]
Age (<40 vs. ≥40)	0.458		
Gender	0.336		
Smoking	0.478		
Drinking	0.221		
SUV max (≤9.0 vs. >9.0)	0.043	0.034	2.445 [1.226–4.998]
Pathologic tumor stage	0.012	<0.001	3.668 [1.479–9.336]
Pathologic neck lymph node stage	0.024	0.421	4.612 [0.741–9.667]
Perineural invasion	0.089		
Extracapsular extension	0.642		
Lymphovascular invasion	0.031	0.042	2.889 [1.365–4.416]
Tumor differentiation	0.009		
Well			
Moderate		0.097	2.579 [0.947–5.667]
Poor		0.016	3.978 [1.741–8.665]
Radiotherapy	0.116		

had a poor specificity of 54.1% owing to the high false-positive rate, and the CT scan showed the best accuracy with 80.2% with a specificity of 85.4% and sensitivity of 73.6%. The authors concluded this strange finding was contributed in part by the epidemic of chronic granulomatous diseases in India. Currently, more and more researchers are describing a convincing result. Bae et al. (21) enrolled 178 oral SCC patients with negative neck palpation findings, and found the sensitivity for the detection of occult metastasis was higher for PET-CT than that for CT/MRI imaging on a per-patient (69.1% vs. 35.7%), per-level (62.1% vs. 29.3%), and per-side (70.5% vs. 36.4%) basis. Gordin et al. (22) found that PET-CT had a sensitivity of 89% and a specificity of 95% for predicting neck lymph node metastasis in head and neck SCC. A similar finding was also reported by Jeong et al. (23) and Roh et al. (24); however, all these studies included SCCs of all subsites, and small-volume cancers were analyzed together with large-volume cancers. The prevalence of neck lymph node metastasis is significantly associated with tumor stage, but the role of PET-CT in early-stage tongue SCC has rarely been discussed. Zhang et al. (7) might have been the first to report that the overall sensitivity and specificity of PET-CT for predicting occult lymph node metastasis were 21.4 and 98.4%, respectively. This finding was partially consistent with our results. The high specificity found in both studies is possibly attributed to the low occult lymph node metastasis rate. The significant conflict of sensitivity between the two studies might be explained by the following aspects: the different economic status that exists between China and other Western countries might cause differences in oral hygiene, and it is well-known that infectious lymph nodes and inflammation lead to false-positive PET-CT outcomes. The findings of the two studies might suggest that if there is a negative result according to PET-CT, there may be a very high possibility of no occult lymph node metastasis. Some may argue, then, that active observation is an option for early-stage tongue SCC. There have been conflicting results regarding the comparison between elective neck dissection and active observation in cT1-2N0 tongue SCC (15, 16). Another uncommon tool that has been used is sentinel lymph node biopsy (SLNB). Recently, Cramer et al. (25) compared the survival difference between SLNB and elective neck dissection groups; the authors reported that neck dissection was avoided in 63.8% of patients receiving SLNB, the two groups had similar overall survival, and decreases in perioperative morbidity and hospital stay were seen in patients with SLNB. Alex et al. (26) described that SLNB was easily performed with a high success rate, and it had a relatively high specificity and a low false-negative rate. Similar findings were also reported by Holden et al. (27) and Den Toom et al. (28). Both SLNB and PET-CT had high value for predicting nodal metastasis in oral SCC. However, in China, SLNB is not widely used for oral SCC. Although the risk is low, SLNB is invasive. Klode et al. (29) noted that SLNB was much more sensitive than PET-CT for discovering small lymph node metastases in malignant melanoma; however, in cervical cancer patients, Papadia et al. (30) demonstrated that, compared to SLNB, PET-CT represented a "safety net" that helped the surgeon identify metastatic lymph nodes, especially in patients with large tumors. On the other hand, even though our unpublished data showed that PET-CT-guided neck dissection could achieve similar disease control to routine neck dissection, the cost utility as well as the actual applicability of PET-CT remains unknown, and further studies are needed to clarify these questions.

The prognosis of tongue SCC has been frequently analyzed. The widely accepted prognostic factors include tumor stage, neck lymph node stage, PNI, LVI, margin status, and so on (1–3, 5). However, the significance of the SUV max remains unclear. The SUV max is partially related to the malignant grade of tumor cells, reflecting proliferation ability. Hasegawa et al. (31) described that an SUV max >8.0 indicated a higher tumor stage, neck lymph node metastasis, the presence of PNI and LVI, and a higher Ki-67 index. Further survival analysis also confirmed that worse disease-free survival was indicated by an SUV max >8.0. Yokobori et al. (32) reported that patients with T2 stage disease had a higher SUV max than patients with T1 stage disease, and patients with a higher SUV max tended to have a higher frequency of PNI, microvessel density, and expression of LAT1. This finding was consistent with our results, suggesting that the SUV max might be used as a marker of adjuvant treatment in future studies.

The main limitation in the current study might be that it seems to provide the questionable message that PET-CT is suitable for all patients with low-stage oral tongue SCC, which slightly contradicts most recently published guidelines; however, what we wish to demonstrate is that PET-CT is an alternative in select patients. It is also a reliable method for guiding cN0 neck management in early-stage tongue squamous cell carcinoma.

In summary, PET-CT has a high specificity for predicting occult lymph node metastasis, and an SUV max >9.0 is significantly associated with worse LRC in cT1-2N0 tongue SCC.

ETHICS STATEMENT

The studies involving human participants were reviewed and approved by The Zhengzhou University institutional research committee. The patients/participants provided their written informed consent to participate in this study.

AUTHOR CONTRIBUTIONS

All the authors contributed to study design, manuscript writing, study selection, data analysis, study quality evaluating, and manuscript revising. All authors have read and approved the final manuscript.

ACKNOWLEDGMENTS

This study was supported by National Natural Science Foundation of China (Grant No. 81500826).

REFERENCES

1. Fang Q, Li P, Qi J, Luo R, Chen D, Zhang X. Value of lingual lymph node metastasis in patients with squamous cell carcinoma of the tongue. *Laryngoscope.* (2019) 129:2527–30. doi: 10.1002/lary.27927
2. Dai L, Fang Q, Li P, Wu J, Zhang X. Secondary squamous cell carcinoma of the oral cavity after nasopharyngeal carcinoma. *Cancer Res Treat.* (2020) 52:109–16. doi: 10.4143/crt.2019.202
3. Massey C, Dharmarajan A, Bannuru RR, Rebeiz E. Management of N0 neck in early oral squamous cell carcinoma: a systematic review and meta-analysis. *Laryngoscope.* (2019) 129:E284–98. doi: 10.1002/lary.27627
4. Morand GB, Ikenberg K, Vital DG, Cardona I, Moch H, Stoeckli SJ, et al. Preoperative assessment of CD44-mediated depth of invasion as predictor of occult metastases in early oral squamous cell carcinoma. *Head Neck.* (2019) 41:950–8. doi: 10.1002/hed.25532
5. Tam S, Amit M, Zafereo M, Bell D, Weber RS. Depth of invasion as a predictor of nodal disease and survival in patients with oral tongue squamous cell carcinoma. *Head Neck.* (2019) 41:177–84. doi: 10.1002/hed.25506
6. Abbate V, Dell'Aversana Orabona G, Salzano G, Bonavolontà P, Maglitto F, Romano A, et al. Pre-treatment neutrophil-to-lymphocyte ratio as a predictor for occult cervical metastasis in early stage (T1-T2 cN0) squamous cell carcinoma of the oral tongue. *Surg Oncol.* (2018) 27:503–7. doi: 10.1016/j.suronc.2018.06.002
7. Zhang H, Seikaly H, Biron VL, Jeffery CC. Utility of PET-CT in detecting nodal metastasis in cN0 early stage oral cavity squamous cell carcinoma. *Oral Oncol.* (2018) 80:89–92. doi: 10.1016/j.oraloncology.2018.04.003
8. Myers LL, Wax MK, Nabi H, Simpson GT, Lamonica D. Positron emission tomography in the evaluation of the N0 neck. *Laryngoscope.* (1999) 108:232–6. doi: 10.1097/00005537-199802000-00014
9. Arya S, Rane P, Deshmukh A. Oral cavity squamous cell carcinoma: role of pretreatment imaging and its influence on management. *Clin Radiol.* (2014) 69:916–30. doi: 10.1016/j.crad.2014.04.013
10. Ouyang PY, Su Z, Mao YP, Liang XX, Liu Q, Xie FY. Prognostic impact of family history in southern Chinese patients with undifferentiated nasopharyngeal carcinoma. *Br J Cancer.* (2013) 109:788–94. doi: 10.1038/bjc.2013.343
11. Fang QG, Shi S, Liu FY, Sun CF. Squamous cell carcinoma of the oral cavity in ever smokers: a matched-pair analysis of survival. *J Craniofac Surg.* (2014) 25:934–7. doi: 10.1097/SCS.0000000000000710
12. Skulsky SL, O'Sullivan B, McArdle O, Leader M, Roche M, Conlon PJ, et al. Review of high-risk features of cutaneous squamous cell carcinoma and discrepancies between the American Joint Committee on Cancer and NCCN Clinical Practice Guidelines In Oncology. *Head Neck.* (2017) 39:578–94. doi: 10.1002/hed.24580
13. Lydiatt WM, Patel SG, O'Sullivan B, Brandwein MS, Ridge JA, Migliacci JC, et al. Head and neck cancers-major changes in the American Joint Committee on cancer eighth edition cancer staging manual. *CA Cancer J Clin.* (2017) 67:122–37. doi: 10.3322/caac.21389
14. Halfpenny W, Hain SF, Biassoni L, Maisey MN, Sherman JA, McGurk M. FDG PET. A possible prognostic factor in head and neck cancer. *Br J Cancer.* (2002) 86:512–6. doi: 10.1038/sj.bjc.6600114
15. Abu-Ghanem S, Yehuda M, Carmel NN, Leshno M, Abergel A, Gutfeld O, et al. Elective neck dissection vs observation in early-stage squamous cell carcinoma of the oral tongue with no clinically apparent lymph node metastasis in the neck: a systematic review and meta-analysis. *JAMA Otolaryngol Head Neck Surg.* (2016) 142:857–65. doi: 10.1001/jamaoto.2016.1281
16. Otsuru M, Ota Y, Yanamoto S, Okura M, Umeda M, Kirita T, et al. A multicenter retrospective study of elective neck dissection for T1-2N0M0 tongue squamous cell carcinoma: analysis using propensity score-matching. *Ann Surg Oncol.* (2019) 26:555–63. doi: 10.1245/s10434-018-07089-7
17. Larson AR, Kemmer J, Formeister E, El-Sayed I, Ha P, George J, et al. Beyond depth of invasion: adverse pathologic tumor features in early oral tongue squamous cell carcinoma. *Laryngoscope.* (2019) doi: 10.1002/lary.28241
18. Wu K, Wei J, Liu Z, Yu B, Yang X, Zhang C, et al. Can pattern and depth of invasion predict lymph node relapse and prognosis in tongue squamous cell carcinoma. *BMC Cancer.* (2019) 19:714. doi: 10.1186/s12885-019-5859-y
19. Faisal M, Abu Bakar M, Sarwar A, Adeel M, Batool F, Malik KI, et al. Depth of invasion (DOI) as a predictor of cervical nodal metastasis and local recurrence in early stage squamous cell carcinoma of oral tongue (ESSCOT). *PLoS ONE.* (2018) 13:e0202632. doi: 10.1371/journal.pone.0202632
20. Chaukar D, Dandekar M, Kane S, Arya S, Purandare N, Rangarajan V, et al. Relative value of ultrasound, computed tomography and positron emission tomography imaging in the clinically node-negative neck in oral cancer. *Asia Pac J Clin Oncol.* (2016) 12:e332–8. doi: 10.1111/ajco.12255
21. Bae MR, Roh JL, Kim JS, Lee JH, Cho KJ, Choi SH, et al. 18F-FDG PET/CT versus CT/MR imaging for detection of neck lymph node metastasis in palpably node-negative oral cavity cancer. *J Cancer Res Clin Oncol.* (2020). 146:237–44. doi: 10.1007/s00432-019-03054-3
22. Gordin A, Golz A, Keidar Z, Daitzchman M, Bar-Shalom R, Israel O. The role of FDG-PET/CT imaging in head and neck malignant conditions: impact on diagnostic accuracy and patient care. *Otolaryngol Head Neck Surg.* (2007) 137:130–7. doi: 10.1016/j.otohns.2007.02.001
23. Jeong HS, Baek CH, Son YI, Ki Chung M, Kyung Lee D, Young Choi J, et al. Use of integrated 18F-FDG PET/CT to improve the accuracy of initial cervical nodal evaluation in patients with head and neck squamous cell carcinoma. *Head Neck.* (2007) 29:203–10. doi: 10.1002/hed.20504
24. Roh JL, Park JP, Kim JS, Lee JH, Cho KJ, Choi SH, Nam SY, Kim SY. 18F fluorodeoxyglucose PET/CT in head and neck squamous cell carcinoma with negative neck palpation findings: a prospective study. *Radiology.* (2014). 271:153–61. doi: 10.1148/radiol.13131470
25. Cramer JD, Sridharan S, Ferris RL, Duvvuri U, Samant S. Sentinel lymph node biopsy versus elective neck dissection for stage I to II oral cavity cancer. *Laryngoscope.* (2019) 129:162–9. doi: 10.1002/lary.27323
26. Alex JC. The application of sentinel node radiolocalization to solid tumors of the head and neck: a 10-year experience. *Laryngoscope.* (2004) 114:2–19. doi: 10.1097/00005537-200401000-00002
27. Holden AM, Sharma D, Schilling C, Gnanasegaran G, Odell EW, Sassoon I, et al. Biopsy of the sentinel lymph node in oral squamous cell carcinoma: analysis of error in 100 consecutive cases. *Br J Oral Maxillofac Surg.* (2018) 56:615–20. doi: 10.1016/j.bjoms.2018.06.019
28. Den Toom IJ, Heuveling DA, Flach GB, van Weert S, Karagozoglu KH, van Schie A, et al. Sentinel node biopsy for early-stage oral cavity cancer: the VU University Medical Center experience. *Head Neck.* (2015) 37:573–8. doi: 10.1002/hed.23632
29. Klode J, Dissemond J, Grabbe S, Hillen U, Poeppel T, Boeing C. Sentinel lymph node excision and PET-CT in the initial stage of malignant melanoma: a retrospective analysis of 61 patients with malignant melanoma in American Joint Committee on Cancer stages I and II. *Dermatol Surg.* (2010) 36:439–45. doi: 10.1111/j.1524-4725.2010.01479.x
30. Papadia A, Gasparri ML, Genoud S, Bernd K, Mueller MD. The combination of preoperative PET/CT and sentinel lymph node biopsy in the surgical management of early-stage cervical cancer. *J Cancer Res Clin Oncol.* (2017) 143:2275–81. doi: 10.1007/s00432-017-2467-6
31. Hasegawa O, Satomi T, Kono M, Watanabe M, Ikehata N, Chikazu D. Correlation analysis between the SUVmax of FDG-PET/CT and clinicopathological characteristics in oral squamous cell carcinoma. *Odontology.* (2019) 107:237–3. doi: 10.1007/s10266-018-0379-9
32. Yokobori Y, Toyoda M, Sakakura K, Kaira K, Tsushima Y, Chikamatsu K. (18)F-FDG uptake on PET correlates with biological potential in early oral squamous cell carcinoma. *Acta Otolaryngol.* (2015). 135:494–9. doi: 10.3109/00016489.2014.969385

Perineural Invasion in Adenoid Cystic Carcinoma of the Salivary Glands: Where we are and Where we Need to Go

Xiaohao Liu, Xiaojun Yang, Chaoning Zhan, Yan Zhang, Jin Hou and Xuemin Yin**

Department of Oral and Maxillofacial Surgery, Nanfang Hospital, Southern Medical University, Guangzhou, China

***Correspondence:**
Jin Hou
houjin@smu.edu.cn
Xuemin Yin
yinxuemin1983@163.com

Adenoid cystic carcinoma of the salivary gland (SACC) is a rare malignant tumors of the head and neck region, but it is one of the most common malignant tumors that are prone to perineural invasion (PNI) of the head and neck. The prognosis of patients with SACC is strongly associated with the presence of perineural spread (PNS). Although many contributing factors have been reported, the mechanisms underlying the preferential destruction of the blood-nerve barrier (BNB) by tumors and the infiltration of the tumor microenvironment by nerve fibers in SACC, have received little research attention. This review summarizes the current knowledge concerning the characteristics of SACC in relation to the PNI, and then highlights the interplay between components of the tumor microenvironment and perineural niche, as well as their contributions to the PNI. Finally, we provide new insights into the possible mechanisms underlying the pathogenesis of PNI, with particular emphasis on the role of extracellular vesicles that may serve as an attractive entry point in future studies.

Keywords: adenoid cystic carcinoma, salivary glands, perineural invasion, tumor microenvironment, perineurium barrier

INTRODUCTION

There are three main ways by which tumors spread: direct invasion into adjacent tissues, hematogenous metastasis, and lymphatic spread; however, perineural invasion (PNI) is considered a fourth route of dissemination, which can be of great significance in the invasion and metastasis of tumors. PNI has been emerging as a significant pathologic feature of many malignant tumors, including those of the pancreas, prostate, colon, rectum, and head and neck, etc. (1). There is a high incidence of PNI in many of these malignancies, and this feature has become an indicator of poor prognosis and is associated with reduced survival (2).

SACC is one of the most common malignant salivary gland tumors, comprising 10% of all salivary gland neoplasms, which is characterized by PNI, strong invasiveness, and hematogenous metastasis (3). With respect to the primary site of tumor, there are various anatomical locations although most of them arise from the small salivary glands (75.4%). In the major salivary glands, 53.3% of tumors involve the submandibular gland, while 46.7% involve the parotid gland (4). Moreover, SACC comprises 4% of all salivary gland tumors, as well as 7.5% of all epithelial salivary gland malignancies (5). SACC generally has an indolent clinical course; nevertheless, advanced tumors may cause pain and/or nerve paralysis, as SACC has a tendency to directly invade the adjacent nerve sheaths close to the primary tumor and spreads along the nerve, a condition referred to as PNI and perineural spread (PNS), respectively.

The 5-year survival rate is relatively high in SACC patients, in contrast with the poor prognosis associated with other epithelial malignancies (5); however, the recurrence rate is also high in SACC, and closely related to PNI (6). Earlier studies suggested that lymph node involvement is uncommon in SACC, but Amit et al. found that the incidence of occult neck metastases among patients with ACC is 17% by retrospective multicentered study (7). Distant metastases are most frequently detected in the lungs, followed by bones, liver, skin, and breasts. The diagnostic transfer rate of SACC ranges from 25 to 55% (8). Distant metastases from SACC primary tumors can remain asymptomatic for long periods of time (6). Even when the tumor have been completely removed, with no recurrence at the primary tumor site, SACC still has a high tendency to spread to the other body parts over a period of time, which is the major cause of death in patients with SACC. However, outcome in SACC is significantly associated with the involvement of margins. Amit et al. analyzed the data of 507 patients with adenoid cystic carcinoma, and suggested that the positive edge is related to the worst outcome, while the negative edge and the near edge are related to the improved result, but not the distance of the tumor (9).

PNI is significantly correlated with both distant metastasis and unfavorable disease outcomes (10). Notably, in one series of patients with clear surgical margins, 80% of patients harboring PNI eventually progressed to local or distant recurrence, compared with only 27% of patients without PNI (11). Given that microscopic invasion of the cancer cells into the surrounding nerve tissues is assumed to occur via the "path of least resistance" it is often a challenge for a surgeon to detect and determine the resection border during surgery. Due to its microscopic size, CAT (computerized axial tomography), and PET (positron emission tomography) scans may also fail to detect PNI. However, Singh et al. have described that MRI can observe the enlargement and enhancement of the image of nerves that have been invaded by the tumor. This can assess whether the tumor has nerve invasion to a certain extent due to its high soft tissue contrast. Compared with CT, MRI is more sensitive to detect perineural proliferation but CT is complementary to MRI and can be used to assess local skeletal changes (12). There have been several studies concerning the statistical association between margin status and PNI. One such study demonstrated that PNI was the strongest prognostic indicator in their series of patients with SACC; however, no specific *p*-value was presented to support their claims (8). In another study, Jang et al. demonstrated that SACC with PNI subsequently progressed to metastasis, while no distant metastasis was observed in those without PNI (13). Multivariate analysis revealed that PNI was a significant predictive factor in distant metastasis (14). These results indicate that PNI potentiates distant metastatic progression, thus influencing patient outcomes.

Given that PNI is closely related to the prognosis of SACC patients, an in-depth exploration of the underlying mechanisms is needed to identify predictors of this condition, and screen out markers that predict tumor prognosis, which may contribute to the development of novel targeted drugs and reduction in recurrence risk in patients with SACC.

Currently, there are two prominent theories on the pathogenesis of PNI: one is the "path of low resistance" and the other is reciprocal signaling interactions. Due to the anatomical proximity between the salivary glands and some cranial nerves, such as the facial nerve, trigeminal nerve, hypoglossal nerve, and glossopharyngeal nerve, the salivary glands have plenty of neural tissues. Some researchers hypothesize that the tumor cells grow along the eural tissues. Some res" which serves as a conduit for their distant migration, whereas the other researchers believe that there are certain factor-based interactions between tumor cells and nerves, which provide a microenvironment suitable for tumor cell growth and proliferation around the nerves (15). In addition, many recent studies have suggested that cell signaling factors contribute to the interaction between tumor and nerve tissue; for example, by increasing the affinity of tumor cells for neural tissue (8). At present, the occurrence of neurotropic invasion is widely considered to involve a variety of microenvironmental regulatory factors, including chemokines and their receptors, brain-derived neurotrophic factor (BDNF) family proteins and their receptors, nerve growth factor (NGF) family proteins and their receptors, as well as matrix metalloproteinases (MMPs) and PNI-related cells (such as macrophages, astrocytes, and Schwann cells) (16).

In this review, we summarize the current knowledge concerning the characteristics of SACC in relation to the PNI, and then highlight the interplay between components of the tumor microenvironment and perineural niche, as well as their contributions to the PNI. Finally, we provide new insights into the possible mechanisms underlying the pathogenesis of PNI, with particular emphasis on the role of extracellular vesicles that may serve as an attractive candidate pathways in future studies.

ANATOMICAL FACTORS OF SACC PERINEURAL INVASION

PNI is a common clinical manifestation of various tumors, including pancreatic cancer, gastric cancer, prostate cancer, and head and neck cancer (17–20). PNI is distinct from PNS. Specifically, PNI is characterized at the microscopic level by the confined invasion of the tumor mass into nerves, while PNS refers to the clinico-radiological findings of distant distribution via the perineural space, or within the neural sheath and nerve itself (21). In 2009, Liebig et al. proposed that PNI of tumor cells can be defined as tumor cells near peripheral nerve fibers, surrounding them by at least 33%, or tumor cells infiltrating into any layers of nerves–endoneurium, perineurium, and epineurium (1). However, some scholars have divide neural invasion into epineural association, perineural invasion, and endoneural invasion based on the scope of neural invasion. Among them, endoneural invasion is an independent predictor of poor prognosis (22, 23).

The normal peripheral nerve consists of three layers of connective tissue with differing characteristics. The epineurium, the outermost fascial layer, is composed of the dense irregular connective tissues that binds individual nerve fascicles into a nerve trunk; the endoneurium is the innermost layer surrounding axons along with Schwann cells (SCs); the perineurium, the middle layer, is made of layers of flattened cells forming laminar structures wrapping around single nerve fascicles. Epineurium surrounds the entire nerve trunk, thus contributing to the tensile strength of the nerve, but it does not provide a barrier function. The existence of the tight junction (TJ) structures in perineurium and endoneurial vasculature forms the peripheral nerve barrier (24, 25). These structures have been recognized as shielding barriers to the paracellular diffusion of certain molecules and ions (26, 27). Recently, an increasing number of studies have indicated that TJ may act as a barrier against cancer invasion and metastasis (28–30). Therefore, we speculate that a possible explanation of PNI of malignant tumors may be that when tumor cells begin to invade peripheral never, the TJ structure of perineurium must first be disturbed and dismantled to facilitate penetration of the tumor cells.

THE PERINEURAL NICHE AND TUMOR MICROENVIRONMENT IN PNI

A study of neurological invasion, involving nerve cells, tumor cells, and stromal cells, investigated the neurotropic characteristics of prostate cancer and reported that these cell types could respond to secretory or intracellular cytokines, leading to neurologic attacks by tumors, in which axon growth is an important step (1). Axonal growth is complex and involves multiple factors, the most studied of which include chemokines and their receptors, the GDNF family and their receptors, and the NGF family and their receptors, along with matrix metalloproteinases (MMPs) and PNI-related cells (**Table 1**). Schwann cells are closely associated with the process of neural invasion, both prior to and during tumor invasion, and are therefore important for the initiation and development of PNI (16).

TABLE 1 | Mediators in the perineural niche and tumor microenvironment in PNI.

Factors	Interrelated factors	Role in PNI	References
Perineurial cells	Tight junctions	The tight connections in the perineurial cells are the main players of the neural barrier function	(26, 27)
Other PNI-related cells	Schwann cells	Interact with preneoplastic cells	(31)
	TAMs	Positive correlation with PNI	(32, 33)
	Stellate cells	Induce the proliferation of cancer cell and associated with the generation of neuronal plasticity	(34, 35)
Nerve fibers	NGF secretion	Associated with NGF production and lymph node invasion in cancer	(36)
NGF family and receptors	NGF-TRKA	Positive correlations with PNI and poor prognosis in cancer	(37)
	BDNF-TRKB	Significantly correlated with advanced clinical stage, poor prognosis, PNI, vascular invasion, and distant metastasis in SACC; Have a role in the EMT process in SACC	(38, 39)
GDNF family and receptors	GDNF-GFRα1-RET	Induce tumor cell migration	(40)
Chemokines and receptors	CXCL12/CXCR4	Significantly correlated with PNI and increased secretion of MMPs	(41)
	CX3CL1/CX3CR1	Significant positive correlation with PNI and promote tumor migration and invasion	(42)
MMPs	MMP-2 and MMP-9	Degradation of ECM and basement membrane and involved in NGF–TRKA signaling and GDNF–RET pathway	(43)

Perineurial Cells

A transmission electron microscopy study demonstrated that the thickness of the perineurium is ~10-25 microns, and that it consists of 8–15 concentric layers of flat perineurial cells (44). Each perineurial cell layer comprises flattened cells, linked by special connections that provide a barrier to diffusion. In addition, some intraneural blood vessels, with diameters of ~6–10 microns, were found close to the axons; these were composed of 6–8 layers of endothelial cells and formed a blood-neural barrier (BNB) with the perineurium (31). Previous studies have demonstrated that perineurial cells can control the integrity of the BNB by secreting various cytokines and growth factors, such as VEGF, BDNF, GDNF, bFGF, and Angiopoietin-1. Moreover, certain factors secreted by perineurial cells can also contribute to the regulation of the tight junction protein, claudin-5, in BNB endothelial cells, thus strengthening the barrier function of the BNB (32). These findings suggest that various factors in the neural microenvironment may regulate the BNB barrier function by affecting the tight junctions between perineurium cells.

Hence, it is important to fully understand the BNB that may represent the first line of defense against tumor PNI, in order to develop new options for the diagnosis and treatment of tumor PNI.

Other PNI-Related Cells

Schwann cells (SCs) are the most common type of cells in peripheral nerves and, along with glial cells, play a key role in nerve repair and regeneration (33). Recent evidence suggests that the affinity of SCs for specific types of gastrointestinal cancer, as well as their migration in cancer, might precede any invasion of the neural environment, and thus play a role in PNI (34).

Tumor-associated macrophages (TAMs) interact with tumor cells and can modulate tumor growth, proliferation, metastasis, and prognosis via a series of cytokines, which are essential components of the tumor microenvironment (35). Endogenous macrophages also present molecules that participate in the balance and regeneration of peripheral nerves. Moreover, the production of GDNF by endothelial macrophages during PNI is promoted by CSF-1 secretion by pancreatic cancer (PC) cells. Notably, a clinical study has reported a correlation between macrophages and PNI (45).

Stellate cells are myofibroblasts, which can be activated by hypoxia, inflammation, and interactions with precancerous cells and cancer cells. Activated stellate cells promote PNI in pancreatic carcinoma (PC), and are a key contributor to connective tissue hypertrophy (36). The activation of stellate cells promotes the localized growth of PC in co-cultures of tumor cells and pancreatic astrocytes, as well as the propagation of PC cells in an *in-situ* model of PC (46).

Nerve Fibers

Axons, also called nerve fibers, are thread-like projections that carry electrical signals between nerves and receptors in the skin, muscles, joints, and internal organs (47). Emerging evidence has shown that the invasion of tumor is dependent on the axon structure, and denervation can inhibit the growth and metastasis of tumor (48). Pundavela et al. have found that the presence of nerve fibers in breast cancers is relevant to lymph node invasion and the production of biologically active NGF (49) that can stimulate neuron outgrowth (axonogenesis or neo-neurogenesis), thus promoting PNI (50). Further, in order to investigate interactions between nerve fibers and tumor cells, Liu et al. established an *in vitro* model of PNI by co-culturing rat root ganglia (DRG) and human pancreatic cancer cell line (MIA PaCa-2). They found that these cancer cells could stimulate the outgrowth of neurites from DRG. Of note, while these neurites tended to migrate toward pancreatic cancer cell colonies, cancer cells also exhibited a trend of migrating along the contacting neurites simultaneously (37). This indicates that there may exist a reciprocal regulation loop between nerves and cancer cells. Moreover, it has been suggested that higher densities of nerve fibers within tumors were closely associated with poorer clinical outcomes in prostate cancer patients. However, in a mouse model of gastric cancer, the incidence and progression of tumors could be significantly reduced at denervation sites (either surgically or pharmacologically treated) of the stomach (51), again indicating a crucial role of nerves in the growth and progression of tumors (52). Cancer exosomes induced the innervation of the tumor and the exosomes from patients with head and neck cancer had neurite outgrowth activity, while the exosomes from the healthy control group did not (53). Nonetheless, due to the complexity of the tumor microenvironment, the role of nerve fibers in the tumor microenvironment is so far still an understudied research area that warrants further investigation.

NGF Family and Receptors

The nerve growth factor (NGF) family mainly consists of neurotrophin 3 (NTF3), NGF, neurotrophin 4 (NTF4), and brain-derived neurotrophic factor (BDNF) (54). By binding to diverse receptors, NGFs can trigger multiple signaling pathways, which function in the regulation of cell growth, apoptosis, and neuronal formation. Besides, it not only has many important regulatory functions for the survival, growth and differentiation of nerve cells in the peripheral and central nervous system, but also plays a role in regulating the synthesis of neurotransmitters and neuropeptides in sympathetic and sensory nerve cells effect (38). Each NTF binds to tropomyosin-receptor kinases (TRK) receptor with high affinity, or to p75 neurotrophin receptor (p75NTR), with low affinity; NGF binds with high affinity to TRKA; BDNF and NTF4 both bind to TRKB receptors; and NTF-3 binds preferentially to TRKC (39).

Elevated NGF levels have been identified in PC, relative to adjacent normal tissues, with particular over-expression of TRKA in peripheral nerves. Additionally, there is a significant positive correlation between the expression of NGF and TRKA and the incidence of neural invasion, as well as a poor prognosis, in PC and cell co-culture models of PC (55).

BDNF is thought of as "brain fertilizer," due to its potential roles in promoting the survival of existing neurons, as well as inducing the proliferation and differentiation of new neurons and synapses (56). However, BDNF and TRKB have been recently reported to be involved in the malignant progression of multiple cancers, including colon cancer, hepatocellular carcinoma, prostate cancer, and oral squamous cell carcinoma (40, 57). Jia et al. demonstrated that higher expression levels of BDNF and TRKB were significantly correlated with advanced clinical stage, poor prognosis, PNI, vascular invasion, and distant metastasis of SACC (41). Collectively, these findings implicate the involvement of BDNF/TRKB axis in PNI progression of SACC (58). Furthermore, the BDNF/TRKB axis is also reported to have a role in the epithelial-mesenchymal transition (EMT) process in SACC. And the study by Mei Zhang et al. proposed a correlation between PNI and MIF expression that MIF may promote the PNI of SACC by participating in cytoskeletal reorganization and pseudopod formation induced by Schwann-like cell differentiation of EMT and SACC cells (59). Despite the limited number of studies concerning the association between EMT and PNI, EMT is likely to play an invasive critical role in PNI progression, given the enhanced migration and abilities of cancer cells after EMT (42). Notably, there is a significant negative association between TRKB and E-cadherin expression in SACC specimens, supporting a potential role of the BDNF/TRKB axis in EMT during the development of PNI in SACC (58).

Recently, new evidence suggests that the PIK3K/Akt signaling pathway is associated with PNI in ACC. It has been found that NGF can activate PI3K/AKT pathway through phosphorylating AKT in SACC, thereby potentially stimulating scattering and migration of tumor cells which enhances the progression of PNI (60). Additionally, animal experiments have also shown that a high expression of Akt3 serves as a driving factor of salivary gland tumor progression (43). In addition, the NT-3/TrkC axis promotes the progression of PNI and the poor prognosis of SACC by regulating the interaction between SACC cells and SC. Interrupting the interaction between SACC cells and SC by blocking the NT-3/TrkC axis may be an effective strategy for anti-PNI therapy in SACC (61).

GDNF Family and Receptors

The GDNF family, derived from the glial cell line, a group of neurotrophin polypeptides, which is comprises four members: neurturin (NRTN), persephin (PSPN), artemin (ARTN), and glial cell line-derived neurotrophic factor (GDNF). The GDNF family is secreted by neural tissues and binds with relevant receptors to trigger the differentiation of neuronal cells of the central and peripheral nervous systems. It works mainly in a paracrine manner and plays an important role in the development and maintenance of the central and peripheral nervous systems, kidney morphogenesis and sperm formation (42). GDNF, NRTN, ARTN, and PSPN bind to GFRA1 (GDNF family receptor alpha-1), GFRA2 (GDNF family receptor alpha-2), GFRA3 (GDNF family receptor alpha-3), and GFRA4 (GDNF family receptor alpha-4), respectively (42). It has been suggested that PNI may be mediated through the secretion of GDNF by nerves and further activation of tumor cell surface Ret proto-oncogene (RET) receptors. GFRA1 functions as a co-receptor with RET, both of which are required for GDNF interaction. He et al. have found that DRG neurons can release soluble GFRA1 that may enhance RET phosphorylation and tumor cell migration toward GDNF, even when tumor cell expression of GFRA1 is absent (62). Moreover, in another previous study, a high level of GDNF expression was detected in SACC cells and adjacent nerve fibers, which was demonstrated to be associated with an increase in matrix-degradation during PNI progression (63).

Chemokines and Receptors

Chemokines and their receptors have critical roles in the growth and invasion of tumor cells. CXCL12/CXCR4 (C-X-C Motif Chemokine Ligand 12/C-X-C Motif chemokine receptor 4) signal transduction is a candidate for participation in inter-tumor interstitial interaction and has various functions, such as the regulation of cell proliferation, invasion, EMT, metastasis, and angiogenesis in multiple types of malignancy (64). In PC cells, MMP-9 secretion in response to CXCR4 stimulation may contribute to the process of PNI, via enhancement of extracellular matrix (ECM) degradation (65). Furthermore, CXCL12 significantly increases the NGF expression in PC cells and promotes neuronal regeneration by binding to the CXCR4 receptor. An *in vitro* model showed that the elimination of the CXCL12/CXCR4 signaling pathway led to the suppression of chemotactic migration between PC cells and nerve cells; by blocking the CXCL12/CXCR4 pathway, PC cell neurotropism decreased significantly (66). Therefore, CXCL12/CXCR4 signaling is significantly correlated with PNI. Moreover, Thomas et al. performed CXCR4 immunohistochemical staining and semiquantitative scoring on the tumor tissue of 73 head and neck adenoid cystic carcinoma (AdCC) patients and found that high CXCR4 expression in AdCC is associated with an increased risk of local recurrence (67).

CX3CL1 (C-X3-C Motif Chemokine Ligand 1) is found to be abundantly produced and released by neurons. An elevated expression level of its receptor, CX3CR1 (C-X3-C Motif Chemokine receptor 1), has been implicated in the development of PNI and earlier recurrence of numerous cancers, such as PC, gastric cancer, and prostate cancer (68–70). Equally important, both *in vitro* co-culture and *in vivo* PNI models demonstrated that nerve cells, including Schwann cells and neurons, express CCL2 (C-C motif chemokine ligand 2) which capable of inducinge the migration of CCR2 (C-C Motif Chemokine receptor 2) expressing cancer cells toward these nerves, ultimately promoting PNI progression (16, 71, 72). Role of CX3CR1/CX3CL1 axis in primary and secondary involvement of the nervous system by cancer.

Matrix Metalloproteinases (MMPs)

MMPs are a family of endopeptidases responsible for the degradation of the ECM and tissue remodeling. The expression of certain types of collagen has been confirmed in peripheral nerves, including collagen IV, the main component of the basement membrane of Schwann cells (73). MMP2, MMP7, MMP9, and all type IV collagenases secreted in response to NGF or GDNF, are likely to be involved in PNI (74). In addition, the overexpression of MMP2 by myofibroblasts has been documented in SACC, exhibiting high-grade PNI.

These results indicate that nerves can indeed provide an appropriate environment for tumor growth and the reciprocal interaction positively influence the growth of both nerves and tumors. Although the accuracy of a "path of low resistance" theory is still up for debate today, emerging evidence indicates that the PNI phenomenon is more like a process of active invasion rather than simple diffusion.

PNI MODELS

As mentioned above, PNI is very closely correlated with the prognosis of patients with SACC. Although it was discovered over a century ago, we still know little about the molecular mechanisms involved in the PNI process. *In vitro* models of these complicated disease processes are very difficult to create. To gain a comprehensive understanding of the contribution of a series of soluble factors to PNI, some researchers have attempted to create *in vitro* models, using highly controlled experimental settings. For example, Ayala et al. established an *in vitro* model, where murine DRGs were co-cultured with prostate cancer cells in Matrigel (75). Once suspended in Matrigel, the axons from the DRGs could spread in all directions. These axons grew toward tumor colonies and were gradually invaded by cancer, which mimics the clinical observation of the typical centripetalism of PNI spread. Using this model, Ayala et al. first described the symbiosis exhibited between cancers and nerves in PNI, in which both gain a growth advantage when co-cultured (76). Although the use of this model can better mimic the invasion of tumor cells into nearby nerves, it is not able to replicate the highly complex microenvironment of *in vivo* perineural niches. Of note, Deborde et al. used Live-imaging technology to investigate the interactions between cancer cells and Schwann cells *in vitro* coculture and *in vivo* murine models of PNI. They found that neither soluble factors secreted by Schwann cells, nor empty tunnels established by Schwann cells were capable of mediating cancer cell invasion, whereas physical contact between Schwann living cells and cancer cells facilitated invasion process. This model provides a new insight into the analysis of the complex *in vivo* characteristics of Schwann cells in enhancing PNI (77). Currently, a murine sciatic nerve model is widely used to explore PNI; tumor cells are injected into the distal sciatic nerve of mice to establish an *in vivo* PNI model. Under gross observation, the sciatic nerve is seen enlarged; histologically, tumor infiltration of the sciatic nerve can be visualized by hematoxylin and eosin staining and immunohistochemistry of pathological tissue sections. Notably, the effects of PNI can be analyzed by monitoring hind limb motor performance, such as the hind paw width of the mice, as well as sciatic neurological score. More importantly, this model, with the genetic manipulation of mice and/or use of different types of cancer cells, can be applied to study cellular and molecular mechanisms involved in PNI and the effects of therapeutic agents on neural invasion (78). These emerging models of PNI strongly suggested there is an extensive signaling interaction between the nerves and invading tumor cells. Recently, an *in vivo* PNI model has been developed to unravel molecular mechanisms of nerve–tumor interactions. Briefly, rat DRGs are transplanted onto the chick embryo chorioallantoic membrane, followed by the transplantation of human head and neck squamous cell carcinoma (HNSCC) cells adjacent to the DRG. This system can replicate a pro-angiogenic tumor microenvironment observed in carcinogenesis, where the newly formed vasculature provides nourishment for both DRGs and tumor cell grafts (79).

In the past few decades, three-dimensional (3D) printing technology has received widespread attention. Now 3D scaffolds fabricated by 3D bioprinting of biomaterials (bioinks) can be used for the regeneration and reconstruction of complex tissues and organs. Likewise, printed 3D tumor models have also been developed to simulate the *in vivo* tumor microenvironment (80). For instance, using 3D projection printing, an *in vitro* 3D micro-chip in a hydrogel was built, with the objective of simulating 3D vascular morphology of *in vivo* microenvironment, by which the behavior of both cancer and non-cancer cells can be monitored and analyzed (81). In addition, Valentina et al. reported that 3D bioprinting, combined with induced pluripotent stem cells (iPSCs) could effectively control the spatial distribution of cells (e.g., neurons); thus creating a more reliable *in vitro* model (82). Although the applications of this technology in the construction of *in-vitro* 3D tumor and neural tissue models are, so far, in the research stage, they provide some new insights into the study of the underlying mechanisms of PNI pathogenesis and progression.

POSSIBLE MECHANISM OF PNI AND CONCLUSION

Due to its insidious onset, its susceptibility to PNI, and high recurrence rates, SACCs are common malignant neoplasms of head and neck tumors. Furthermore, PNI is closely related to patient prognosis. Although many studies have investigated the mechanisms underlying PNI, the precise details remain unclear. In recent years, researchers have begun to investigate the concept that nerves can reciprocally facilitate cancer invasion and progression (83), representing a paradigm shift in our understanding of the mechanism of PNI. Based on current research, we consider that although anatomical factors, cells, nerve growth factors (NGF, BDNF, etc.), chemokines in the tumor microenvironment are involved in the development of

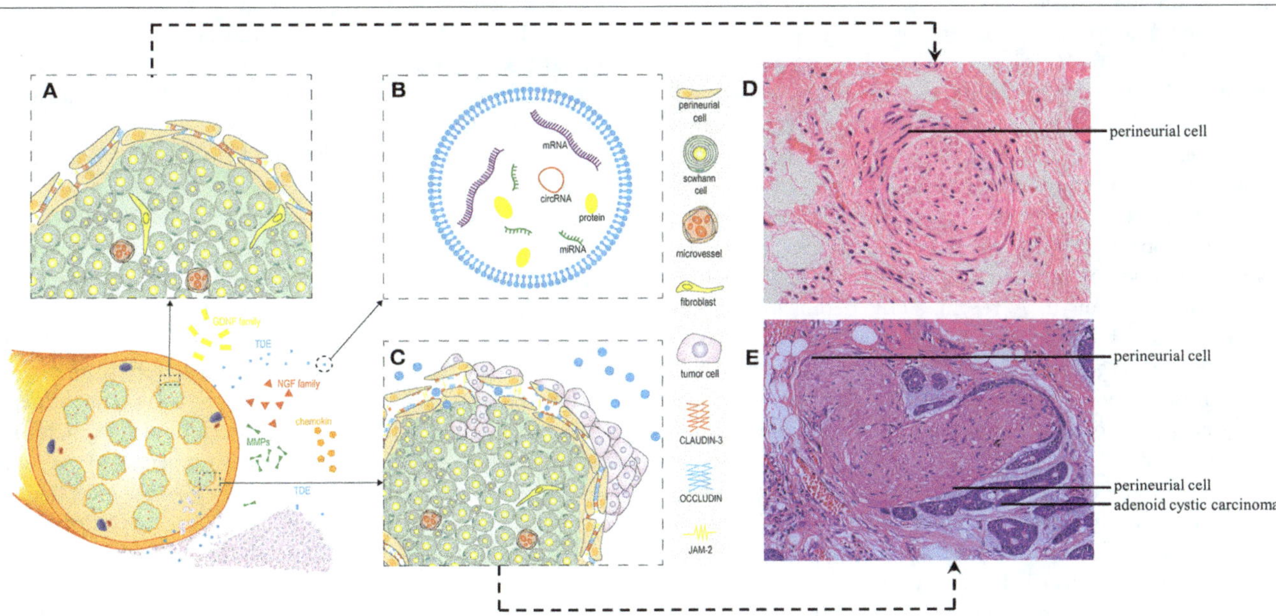

FIGURE 1 | The perineural niche and tumor microenvironment in PNI. **(A)** Diagram showing the architecture and main cellular components of a normal axon. The perineurium that composed of several layers of perineurial cells protects the axon. The perineurium that surrounds individual Schwann cell, micro-vessel, fibroblast. **(B)** Diagram showing the brief structure of tumor derived-exosomes(TDE). TDE contains mRNA, miRNA, protein and other substances, which can be transferred to their target cells, directly or indirectly changing the biological function of recipient cells. **(C)** Diagram showing the architecture and main cellular components of an axon while tumor invades the nerve. After the effect of multiple factors, such as chemokines, GDNF family, NGF family, MMPs and PNI-related cells, the tight connections between the perineurial cells the and the tumor invades the nerve. **(D)** Diagram show the corresponding H&E-stained image of normal nerve. **(E)** Diagram show the corresponding H&E-stained image of tumor infiltrating nerve by the adenoid cystic carcinoma.

PNI, there are other factors that may also contribute to PNI, such as extracellular vesicles (EVs) derived from tumor cells, or other cells in tumor microenvironment and perineural niches (**Figure 1**).

Exosomes, known as the smallest subgroup of EVs, are secreted by cells when multivesicular bodies (MVBs) fuse with the plasma membrane (84). Many previous studies have shown that not only tumor cells produce more exosomes than normal cells, but also tumor-derived exosomes (TDE) containing a diverse set of proteins, mRNA, miRNA, and lipids, can "educate" interstitial cells, endothelial cells, inflammatory cells, and immune cells, in order to regulate the tumor microenvironment and promote tumor growth, invasion, metastasis and angiogenesis (53, 85). Melo et al. (86) found that breast cancer cells can produce mature exosomal miRNAs via a non-cell-dependent pathway, which regulates the phenotype of normal epithelial cells and accelerate their proliferation, and can also be used to generate tumors in nude mice. The development of distant metastases requires primary tumors to break through the basement membrane and penetrate the lymphatic or vascular circulation. Notably, invasive precancerous epithelial cells can overcome this physical constraint by obtaining invasive and migration properties through EMT. Taverna et al. (87) found that exosomal miR-126 derived from chronic myeloid leukemia cells can alter the adhesion and migration ability of recipient cells. Moreover, other studies have confirmed that exosomal miR-105 is specifically expressed and secreted by metastatic breast cancer cells via exosome secretion, and can be transferred to endothelial cells, thereby facilitating cancer metastasis by disrupting the vascular endothelial barrier (88). Hoshino et al. found that tumor-derived exosomes could direct organ-specific metastasis via exosomal integrins (ITGs) (89), based on their intrinsic organotropic homing ability and capacity of initiating pre-metastatic niche formation at foreign sites. Moreover, not only can tumor cells alter the cellular physiology of both surrounding and distant microenvironment through TDE, but other cells in tumor/pre-metastatic microenvironment can also target tumor cells via exosomes, leading to the co-evolution of tumor cells and their microenvironment during tumor dissemination and metastatic outgrowth. A recent study demonstrated that exosomes released by astrocytes could induce an intercellular transfer of PTEN-targeting microRNAs to metastatic tumor cells (90). This finding indicates that exosomes from non-neoplastic cells may also promote the adaptation of disseminated tumor cells to target organs, suggesting the involvement of dynamic bidirectional crosstalk in the pre-metastatic microenvironment. Many previous studies have shown that EVs participate in the dissemination of numerous primary cancer cells, including breast cancer, gastric cancer, colon cancer, liver cancer, malignant melanoma, etc. (91). For instance, one recently published study reported that head and neck tumor-derived exosomes could induce tumor innervation that was enhanced by the exosome-packaged axonal guidance molecule, EphrinB1. This indicates that interventions targeting exosome biogenesis and release may be of therapeutic value against PNI (92). Of particular note, in our previous study, we found that the exosomes derived from the adenoid cystic carcinoma cell line (SACC-83) could be uptaken by human umbilical vein endothelial cells (HUVECs), and destroyed the vascular endothelial barrier (93). Considering that primary tumor-derived EVs can destroy epithelial cell tight junction assembly to induce EMT, and trigger vascular permeability to allow cancer cell dissemination, and "educate" pre-metastatic sites in distant organs, we propose that EVs may also contribute to the disruption of the perineurium barrier and education of the perineural sites into a tumor-promoting microenvironment. It may provide new directions and ideas for further study of PNI pathogenesis in the future. Further, although some research groups have described the involvement of tumor and stroma-derived EVs in the different stages of the metastatic cascade, there is very little information concerning the regulation of tumor cell invasion and metastasis by extracellular vesicles in SACC as well as in PNI.

Of particular note, Galanin is a classic neuropeptide that can function in a variety of physiological processes, such as food intake, nociception, and blood pressure regulation, and it can also act as a growth factor for neurons. Galanin treatment has a tumor-reducing effect in a mouse model of gastrointestinal cancer, and in animal experiments with adenoma formation, galanin appears to be a growth factor that promotes both proliferation and tumor formation (94). In addition, Laminin-5 and insulin-like growth factor-II mRNA binding protein-3 (IMP3) have a good prognostic correlation in various malignancies. Studies have shown that they are also positively expressed in preoperative biopsy specimens of OSCC patients with PNI, implying that preoperative assessment of factors associated with PNI may assist the clinician in the selection of the optimal treatment strategy (95). Nonetheless, whether they can be used as molecular markers of PNI in SACC still needs to be further evaluated.

It's worth mentioning that PNI has been rarely studied in patients with SACC. Emerging evidence for its role as a prognostic factor in SACC is conflicting. Due to the indolent clinical course of SACC, the evaluation of a patient with this malignant tumor is hampered. Furthermore, most previous studies were limited by their small sample size, relatively short follow-up period, mixed pathologies and variable histological sampling of salivary glands, and inadequate reporting of PNI as well (96). Genomic Alterations may also be one of the influencing factors of PNI in SACC. The study found that peripheral nerve invasion was found to be fused with MYB gene with or without copy number changes. MYB-NFIB gene fusion and related GA are associated with ACC peripheral nerve involvement (97). Nonetheless, several studies have found that specific PNI features are indeed closely related to SACC metastasis, locoregional recurrence, long-term survival, and a patient's quality of life (98).

Accordingly, we consider that there are two critical steps in developing strategies for prevention and early therapeutic intervention of PNI: (1) identifying the molecular targets in the microenvironment of perineural niches which are necessary for

PNI development, and (2) finding specific agents against these molecular targets. Therefore, a deeper investigation of underlying mechanisms of PNI should not only clarify the occurrence, proliferation, invasion, recurrence, and metastasis of SACC, but also provide potential targets for the diagnosis and therapy of neurological disorders and diseases.

In conclusion, multiple processes may result in damage at cancer-neural interfaces. There is reciprocity in these interactions, which confers growth and migration advantages to cancer. An in-depth understanding of the molecular mechanism of PNI is essential for developing therapeutic strategies that not only target cancer cells, but also target neural microenvironments as well.

AUTHOR CONTRIBUTIONS

XYi and JH conceived the idea of writing the review. XL wrote the review. XYa assisted to edit. CZ and JZ prepared the Tables and Figures. All authors contributed to the article and approved the submitted version.

REFERENCES

1. Liebig C, Ayala G, Wilks JA, Berger DH, Albo D. Perineural invasion in cancer: a review of the literature. *Cancer Am Cancer Soc.* (2009) 115:3379–91. doi: 10.1002/cncr.24396
2. Bakst RL, Glastonbury CM, Parvathaneni U, Katabi N, Hu KS, Yom SS. Perineural invasion and perineural tumor spread in head and neck cancer: a critical review. *Int J Radiat Oncol Biol Phys.* (2018) 103:1109–24. doi: 10.1016/j.ijrobp.2018.12.009
3. Bjorndal K, Krogdahl A, Therkildsen MH, Overgaard J, Johansen J, Kristensen CA, et al. Salivary gland carcinoma in Denmark 1990-2005: a national study of incidence, site and histology. Results of the danish head and neck cancer group (DAHANCA). *Oral Oncol.* (2011) 47:677–82. doi: 10.1016/j.oraloncology.2011.04.020
4. Cordesmeyer R, Schliephake H, Kauffmann P, Troltzsch M, Laskawi R, Strobel P, et al. Clinical prognostic factors of salivary adenoid cystic carcinoma: a single-center analysis of 61 patients. *J Craniomaxillofac Surg.* (2017) 45:1784–7. doi: 10.1016/j.jcms.2017.08.004
5. Coca-Pelaz A, Rodrigo JP, Bradley PJ, Vander PV, Triantafyllou A, Hunt JL, et al. Adenoid cystic carcinoma of the head and neck–an update. *Oral Oncol.* (2015) 51:652–61. doi: 10.1016/j.oraloncology.2015.04.005
6. Chang CF, Hsieh MY, Chen MK, Chou MC. Adenoid cystic carcinoma of head and neck: a retrospective clinical analysis of a single institution. *Auris Nasus Larynx.* (2018) 45:831–7. doi: 10.1016/j.anl.2017.10.009
7. Amit M, Na'Ara S, Sharma K, Ramer N, Ramer I, Agbetoba A, et al. Elective neck dissection in patients with head and neck adenoid cystic carcinoma: an international collaborative study. *Ann Surg Oncol.* (2015) 22:1353–9. doi: 10.1245/s10434-014-4106-7
8. Dillon PM, Chakraborty S, Moskaluk CA, Joshi PJ, Thomas CY. Adenoid cystic carcinoma: a review of recent advances, molecular targets, and clinical trials. *Head Neck.* (2016) 38:620–7. doi: 10.1002/hed.23925
9. Amit M, Na'Ara S, Trejo-Leider L, Ramer N, Burstein D, Yue M, et al. Defining the surgical margins of adenoid cystic carcinoma and their impact on outcome: an international collaborative study. *Head Neck.* (2017) 39:1008–14. doi: 10.1002/hed.24740
10. Stelow EB, Bishop JA. Update from the 4th Edition of the world health organization classification of head and neck tumours: tumors of the nasal cavity, paranasal sinuses and skull base. *Head Neck Pathol.* (2017) 11:3–15. doi: 10.1007/s12105-017-0791-4
11. Luksic I, Suton P, Macan D, Dinjar K. Intraoral adenoid cystic carcinoma: is the presence of perineural invasion associated with the size of the primary tumour, local extension, surgical margins, distant metastases, and outcome? *Br J Oral Maxillofac Surg.* (2014) 52:214–18. doi: 10.1016/j.bjoms.2013.11.009
12. Singh FM, Mak SY, Bonington SC. Patterns of spread of head and neck adenoid cystic carcinoma. *Clin Radiol.* (2015) 70:644–53. doi: 10.1016/j.crad.2015.01.013
13. Jang S, Patel PN, Kimple RJ, McCulloch TM. Clinical outcomes and prognostic factors of adenoid cystic carcinoma of the head and neck. *Anticancer Res.* (2017) 37:3045–52. doi: 10.21873/anticanres.11659
14. Ju J, Li Y, Chai J, Ma C, Ni Q, Shen Z, et al. The role of perineural invasion on head and neck adenoid cystic carcinoma prognosis: a systematic review and meta-analysis. *Oral Surg Oral Med Oral Pathol Oral Radiol.* (2016) 122:691–701. doi: 10.1016/j.oooo.2016.08.008
15. Bakst RL, Wong RJ. Mechanisms of perineural invasion. *J Neurol Surg B Skull Base.* (2016) 77:96–106. doi: 10.1055/s-0036-1571835
16. Amit M, Na'Ara S, Gil Z. Mechanisms of cancer dissemination along nerves. *Nat Rev Cancer.* (2016) 16:399–408. doi: 10.1038/nrc.2016.38
17. Gupta A, Veness M, De'Ambrosis B, Selva D, Huilgol SC. Management of squamous cell and basal cell carcinomas of the head and neck with perineural invasion. *Australas J Dermatol.* (2016) 57:3–13. doi: 10.1111/ajd.12314
18. Yang YH, Liu JB, Gui Y, Lei LL, Zhang SJ. Relationship between autophagy and perineural invasion, clinicopathological features, and prognosis in pancreatic cancer. *World J Gastroenterol.* (2017) 23:7232–41. doi: 10.3748/wjg.v23.i40.7232
19. Hwang JE, Hong JY, Kim JE, Shim HJ, Bae WK, Hwang EC, et al. Prognostic significance of the concomitant existence of lymphovascular and perineural invasion in locally advanced gastric cancer patients who underwent curative gastrectomy and adjuvant chemotherapy. *Jpn J Clin Oncol.* (2015) 45:541–6. doi: 10.1093/jjco/hyv031
20. Zareba P, Flavin R, Isikbay M, Rider JR, Gerke TA, Finn S, et al. Perineural invasion and risk of lethal prostate cancer. *Cancer Epidemiol Biomarkers Prev.* (2017) 26:719–26. doi: 10.1158/1055-9965.EPI-16-0237
21. Kuhn FP, Hullner M, Mader CE, Kastrinidis N, Huber GF, von Schulthess GK, et al. Contrast-enhanced PET/MR imaging versus contrast-enhanced PET/CT in head and neck cancer: how much MR information is needed? *J Nucl Med.* (2014) 55:551–8. doi: 10.2967/jnumed.113.125443
22. Amit M, Binenbaum Y, Trejo-Leider L, Sharma K, Ramer N, Ramer I, et al. International collaborative validation of intraneural invasion as a prognostic marker in adenoid cystic carcinoma of the head and neck. *Head Neck.* (2015) 37:1038–45. doi: 10.1002/hed.23710
23. Ihsan Ekin D, Helmut F, Ceyhan GO. Generation and impact of neural invasion in pancreatic cancer. *Pancreatic Cancer.* (2012) 295–312. doi: 10.5772/30117
24. Peltonen S, Alanne M, Peltonen J. Barriers of the peripheral nerve. *Tissue Barriers.* (2013) 1:e24956. doi: 10.4161/tisb.24956
25. Pina-Oviedo S, Ortiz-Hidalgo C. The normal and neoplastic perineurium: a review. *Adv Anat Pathol.* (2008) 15:147–64. doi: 10.1097/PAP.0b013e31816f8519
26. Anderson JM, Van Itallie CM. Physiology and function of the tight junction. *Cold Spring Harb Perspect Biol.* (2009) 1:a2584. doi: 10.1101/cshperspect.a002584
27. Pummi KP, Aho HJ, Laato MK, Peltonen JT, Peltonen SA. Tight junction proteins and perineurial cells in neurofibromas. *J Histochem Cytochem.* (2006) 54:53–61. doi: 10.1369/jhc.5A6671.2005
28. Runkle EA, Mu D. Tight junction proteins: from barrier to tumorigenesis. *Cancer Lett.* (2013) 337:41–48. doi: 10.1016/j.canlet.2013.05.038
29. Anderson JM, Balda MS, Fanning AS. The structure and regulation of tight junctions. *Curr Opin Cell Biol.* (1993) 5:772–8. doi: 10.1016/0955-0674(93)90024-K
30. Martin TA, Jiang WG. Loss of tight junction barrier function and its role in cancer metastasis. *Biochim Biophys Acta.* (2009) 1788:872–91. doi: 10.1016/j.bbamem.2008.11.005

31. Reina MA, Lopez A, Villanueva MC, De Andres JA, Maches F. [The blood-nerve barrier in peripheral nerves]. *Rev Esp Anestesiol Reanim.* (2003) 50:80–86.
32. Shanthaveerappa TR, Bourne GH. The 'perineural epithelium', a metabolically active, continuous, protoplasmic cell barrier surrounding peripheral nerve fasciculi. *J Anat.* (1962) 96:527–37.
33. Kanda T. [Blood-nerve barrier: structure and function]. *Brain Nerve.* (2011) 63:557–69.
34. Demir IE, Boldis A, Pfitzinger PL, Teller S, Brunner E, Klose N, et al. Investigation of schwann cells at neoplastic cell sites before the onset of cancer invasion. *J Natl Cancer Inst.* (2014) 106:dju184. doi: 10.1093/jnci/dju184
35. Zeng L, Guo Y, Liang J, Chen S, Peng P, Zhang Q, et al. Perineural invasion and TAMs in pancreatic ductal adenocarcinomas: review of the original pathology reports using immunohistochemical enhancement and relationships with clinicopathological features. *J Cancer.* (2014) 5:754–60. doi: 10.7150/jca.10238
36. Vonlaufen A, Joshi S, Qu C, Phillips PA, Xu Z, Parker NR, et al. Pancreatic stellate cells: partners in crime with pancreatic cancer cells. *Cancer Res.* (2008) 68:2085–93. doi: 10.1158/0008-5472.CAN-07-2477
37. Liu ZS, Wang Y, Li Q, Zhang SL, Shi YR. *In vitro* interaction of human pancreatic cancer cells and rat dorsal root ganglia: a co-culture model. *Zhonghua Zhong Liu Za Zhi.* (2012) 34:259–63. doi: 10.3760/cma.j.issn.0253-3766.2012.04.005
38. Rocco ML, Soligo M, Manni L, Aloe L. Nerve growth factor: early studies and recent clinical trials. *Curr Neuropharmacol.* (2018) 16:1455–65. doi: 10.2174/1570159X16666180412092859
39. Yamashita N, Kuruvilla R. Neurotrophin signaling endosomes: biogenesis, regulation, and functions. *Curr Opin Neurobiol.* (2016) 39:139–45. doi: 10.1016/j.conb.2016.06.004
40. Yang X, Martin TA, Jiang WG. Biological influence of brain-derived neurotrophic factor on breast cancer cells. *Int J Oncol.* (2012) 41:1541–6. doi: 10.3892/ijo.2012.1581
41. Jia S, Wang W, Hu Z, Shan C, Wang L, Wu B, et al. BDNF mediated TrkB activation contributes to the EMT progression and the poor prognosis in human salivary adenoid cystic carcinoma. *Oral Oncol.* (2015) 51:64–70. doi: 10.1016/j.oraloncology.2014.10.008
42. Fielder GC, Yang TW, Razdan M, Li Y, Lu J, Perry JK, et al. The GDNF family: a role in cancer? *Neoplasia.* (2018) 20:99–117. doi: 10.1016/j.neo.2017.10.010
43. Zboray K, Mohrherr J, Stiedl P, Pranz K, Wandruszka L, Grabner B, et al. AKT3 drives adenoid cystic carcinoma development in salivary glands. *Cancer Med.* (2018) 7:445–53. doi: 10.1002/cam4.1293
44. Joseph NM, Mukouyama YS, Mosher JT, Jaegle M, Crone SA, Dormand EL, et al. Neural crest stem cells undergo multilineage differentiation in developing peripheral nerves to generate endoneurial fibroblasts in addition to schwann cells. *Development.* (2004) 131:5599–612. doi: 10.1242/dev.01429
45. Meng F, Li C, Li W, Gao Z, Guo K, Song S. Interaction between pancreatic cancer cells and tumor-associated macrophages promotes the invasion of pancreatic cancer cells and the differentiation and migration of macrophages. *IUBMB Life.* (2014) 66:835–46. doi: 10.1002/iub.1336
46. Apte MV, Wilson JS, Lugea A, Pandol SJ. A starring role for stellate cells in the pancreatic cancer microenvironment. *Gastroenterology.* (2013) 144:1210–19. doi: 10.1053/j.gastro.2012.11.037
47. Ondicova K, Mravec B. Role of nervous system in cancer aetiopathogenesis. *Lancet Oncol.* (2010) 11:596–601. doi: 10.1016/S1470-2045(09)70337-7
48. Boilly B, Faulkner S, Jobling P, Hondermarck H. Nerve dependence: from regeneration to cancer. *Cancer Cell.* (2017) 31:342–54. doi: 10.1016/j.ccell.2017.02.005
49. Pundavela J, Roselli S, Faulkner S, Attia J, Scott RJ, Thorne RF, et al. Nerve fibers infiltrate the tumor microenvironment and are associated with nerve growth factor production and lymph node invasion in breast cancer. *Mol Oncol.* (2015) 9:1626–35. doi: 10.1016/j.molonc.2015.05.001
50. Jobling P, Pundavela J, Oliveira SM, Roselli S, Walker MM, Hondermarck H. Nerve-cancer cell cross-talk: a novel promoter of tumor progression. *Cancer Res.* (2015) 75:1777–81. doi: 10.1158/0008-5472.CAN-14-3180
51. Zhao CM, Hayakawa Y, Kodama Y, Muthupalani S, Westphalen CB, Andersen GT, et al. Denervation suppresses gastric tumorigenesis. *Sci Transl Med.* (2014) 6:115r–250r. doi: 10.1126/scitranslmed.3009569
52. Magnon C, Hall SJ, Lin J, Xue X, Gerber L, Freedland SJ, et al. Autonomic nerve development contributes to prostate cancer progression. *Science.* (2013) 341:1236361. doi: 10.1126/science.1236361
53. Couto N, Caja S, Maia J, Strano MM, Costa-Silva B. Exosomes as emerging players in cancer biology. *Biochimie.* (2018) 155:2–10. doi: 10.1016/j.biochi.2018.03.006
54. Bapat AA, Munoz RM, Von Hoff DD, Han H. Blocking nerve growth factor signaling reduces the neural invasion potential of pancreatic cancer cells. *PLoS ONE.* (2016) 11:e165586. doi: 10.1371/journal.pone.0165586
55. Ma W, Wang C, Su Y, Tian Y, Zhu H. Expression of nerve growth factor and its receptor, tyrosine kinase receptor A, in rooster testes. *Anim Reprod Sci.* (2015) 161:40–46. doi: 10.1016/j.anireprosci.2015.08.001
56. Benarroch EE. Brain-derived neurotrophic factor: regulation, effects, and potential clinical relevance. *Neurology.* (2015) 84:1693–704. doi: 10.1212/WNL.0000000000001507
57. Tanaka K, Okugawa Y, Toiyama Y, Inoue Y, Saigusa S, Kawamura M, et al. Brain-derived neurotrophic factor (BDNF)-induced tropomyosin-related kinase B (Trk B) signaling is a potential therapeutic target for peritoneal carcinomatosis arising from colorectal cancer. *PLoS ONE.* (2014) 9:e96410. doi: 10.1371/journal.pone.0096410
58. Shan C, Wei J, Hou R, Wu B, Yang Z, Wang L, et al. Schwann cells promote EMT and the schwann-like differentiation of salivary adenoid cystic carcinoma cells via the BDNF/TrkB axis. *Oncol Rep.* (2016) 35:427–35. doi: 10.3892/or.2015.4366
59. Zhang M, Li ZF, Wang HF, Wang SS, Yu XH, Wu JB, et al. MIF promotes perineural invasion through EMT in salivary adenoid cystic carcinoma. *Mol Carcinog.* (2019) 58:898–912. doi: 10.1002/mc.22979
60. Alkhadar H, Macluskey M, White S, Ellis I. Nerve growth factor-induced migration in oral and salivary gland tumour cells utilises the PI3K/Akt signalling pathway: is there a link to perineural invasion? *J Oral Pathol Med.* (2020) 49:227–34. doi: 10.1111/jop.12979
61. Li H, Yang Z, Wang W, Wang J, Zhang J, Liu J, et al. NT-3/TrkC axis contributes to the perineural invasion and the poor prognosis in human salivary adenoid cystic carcinoma. *J Cancer.* (2019) 10:6065–73. doi: 10.7150/jca.33635
62. He S, Chen CH, Chernichenko N, He S, Bakst RL, Barajas F, et al. GFRalpha1 released by nerves enhances cancer cell perineural invasion through GDNF-RET signaling. *Proc Natl Acad Sci USA.* (2014) 111:E2008–17. doi: 10.1073/pnas.1402944111
63. Zheng SC, Zhang YR, Luo SY, Zhang LP. [The effect of GDNF on matrix-degrading and cell-adhesion during perineural invasion of salivary adenoid cystic carcinoma]. *Shanghai Kou Qiang Yi Xue.* (2016) 25:212–16.
64. Luo X, Tai WL, Sun L, Pan Z, Xia Z, Chung SK, et al. Crosstalk between astrocytic CXCL12 and microglial CXCR4 contributes to the development of neuropathic pain. *Mol Pain.* (2016) 12:1744806916636385. doi: 10.1177/1744806916636385
65. Jiang YM, Li G, Sun BC, Zhao XL, Zhou ZK. Study on the relationship between CXCR4 expression and perineural invasion in pancreatic cancer. *Asian Pac J Cancer Prev.* (2014) 15:4893–6. doi: 10.7314/APJCP.2014.15.12.4893
66. Xu Q, Wang Z, Chen X, Duan W, Lei J, Zong L, et al. Stromal-derived factor-1alpha/CXCL12-CXCR4 chemotactic pathway promotes perineural invasion in pancreatic cancer. *Oncotarget.* (2015) 6:4717–32. doi: 10.18632/oncotarget.3069
67. Klein NT, van Es RJJ, Valstar MH, Smeele LE, Smit LA, Klein GR, et al. High CXCR4 expression in adenoid cystic carcinoma of the head and neck is associated with increased risk of locoregional recurrence. *J Clin Pathol.* (2020) 73:476–82. doi: 10.1136/jclinpath-2019-206273
68. Zhang M, Zhu ZL, Gao XL, Wu JS, Liang XH, Tang YL. Functions of chemokines in the perineural invasion of tumors. *Int J Oncol.* (2018) 52:1369–79. doi: 10.3892/ijo.2018.4311
69. Lv CY, Zhou T, Chen W, Yin XD, Yao JH, Zhang YF. Preliminary study correlating CX3CL1/CX3CR1 expression with gastric carcinoma and gastric carcinoma perineural invasion. *World J Gastroenterol.* (2014) 20:4428–32. doi: 10.3748/wjg.v20.i15.4428
70. Marchesi F, Locatelli M, Solinas G, Erreni M, Allavena P, Mantovani A. Role of CX3CR1/CX3CL1 axis in primary and secondary involvement of the nervous system by cancer. *J Neuroimmunol.* (2010) 224:39–44. doi: 10.1016/j.jneuroim.2010.05.007

71. Bakst RL, Xiong H, Chen CH, Deborde S, Lyubchik A, Zhou Y, et al. Inflammatory monocytes promote perineural invasion via CCL2-mediated recruitment and cathepsin B expression. *Cancer Res.* (2017) 77:6400–14. doi: 10.1158/0008-5472.CAN-17-1612
72. He S, He S, Chen CH, Deborde S, Bakst RL, Chernichenko N, et al. The chemokine (CCL2-CCR2) signaling axis mediates perineural invasion. *Mol Cancer Res.* (2015) 13:380–90. doi: 10.1158/1541-7786.MCR-14-0303
73. Mehta P, Piao X. Adhesion G-protein coupled receptors and extracellular matrix proteins: roles in myelination and glial cell development. *Dev Dyn.* (2017) 246:275–84. doi: 10.1002/dvdy.24473
74. Jakubowska K, Pryczynicz A, Januszewska J, Sidorkiewicz I, Kemona A, Niewinski A, et al. Expressions of matrix metalloproteinases 2, 7, and 9 in carcinogenesis of pancreatic ductal adenocarcinoma. *Dis Markers.* (2016) 2016:9895721. doi: 10.1155/2016/9895721
75. Ayala GE, Wheeler TM, Shine HD, Schmelz M, Frolov A, Chakraborty S, et al. *In vitro* dorsal root ganglia and human prostate cell line interaction: redefining perineural invasion in prostate cancer. *Prostate.* (2001) 49:213–23. doi: 10.1002/pros.1137
76. Dai H, Li R, Wheeler T, Ozen M, Ittmann M, Anderson M, et al. Enhanced survival in perineural invasion of pancreatic cancer: an *in vitro* approach. *Hum Pathol.* (2007) 38:299–307. doi: 10.1016/j.humpath.2006.08.002
77. Deborde S, Omelchenko T, Lyubchik A, Zhou Y, He S, McNamara WF, et al. Schwann cells induce cancer cell dispersion and invasion. *J Clin Invest.* (2016) 126:1538–54. doi: 10.1172/JCI82658
78. Deborde S, Yu Y, Marcadis A, Chen CH, Fan N, Bakst RL, et al. An *in vivo* murine sciatic nerve model of perineural invasion. *J Vis Exp.* (2018) 56857. doi: 10.3791/56857
79. Scanlon CS, Banerjee R, Inglehart RC, Liu M, Russo N, Hariharan A, et al. Galanin modulates the neural niche to favour perineural invasion in head and neck cancer. *Nat Commun.* (2015) 6:6885. doi: 10.1038/ncomms7885
80. Gu BK, Choi DJ, Park SJ, Kim YJ, Kim CH. 3D bioprinting technologies for tissue engineering applications. *Adv Exp Med Biol.* (2018) 1078:15–28. doi: 10.1007/978-981-13-0950-2_2
81. Huang TQ, Qu X, Liu J, Chen S. 3D printing of biomimetic microstructures for cancer cell migration. *Biomed Microdevices.* (2014) 16:127–32. doi: 10.1007/s10544-013-9812-6
82. Fantini V, Bordoni M, Scocozza F, Conti M, Scarian E, Carelli S, et al. Bioink composition and printing parameters for 3D modeling neural tissue. *Cells.* (2019) 8:830. doi: 10.3390/cells8080830
83. Saloman JL, Albers KM, Li D, Hartman DJ, Crawford HC, Muha EA, et al. Ablation of sensory neurons in a genetic model of pancreatic ductal adenocarcinoma slows initiation and progression of cancer. *Proc Natl Acad Sci USA.* (2016) 113:3078–83. doi: 10.1073/pnas.1512603113
84. Mathieu M, Martin-Jaular L, Lavieu G, Thery C. Specificities of secretion and uptake of exosomes and other extracellular vesicles for cell-to-cell communication. *Nat Cell Biol.* (2019) 21:9–17. doi: 10.1038/s41556-018-0250-9
85. Tkach M, Thery C. Communication by extracellular vesicles: where we are and where we need to go. *Cell.* (2016) 164:1226–32. doi: 10.1016/j.cell.2016.01.043
86. Tran N. Cancer exosomes as miRNA factories. *Trends Cancer.* (2016) 2:329–31. doi: 10.1016/j.trecan.2016.05.008
87. Taverna S, Giallombardo M, Gil-Bazo I, Carreca AP, Castiglia M, Chacartegui J, et al. Exosomes isolation and characterization in serum is feasible in non-small cell lung cancer patients: critical analysis of evidence and potential role in clinical practice. *Oncotarget.* (2016) 7:28748–60. doi: 10.18632/oncotarget.7638
88. Zhou W, Fong MY, Min Y, Somlo G, Liu L, Palomares MR, et al. Cancer-secreted miR-105 destroys vascular endothelial barriers to promote metastasis. *Cancer Cell.* (2014) 25:501–15. doi: 10.1016/j.ccr.2014.03.007
89. Hoshino A, Costa-Silva B, Shen TL, Rodrigues G, Hashimoto A, Tesic MM, et al. Tumour exosome integrins determine organotropic metastasis. *Nature.* (2015) 527:329–35. doi: 10.1038/nature15756
90. Zhang L, Zhang S, Yao J, Lowery FJ, Zhang Q, Huang WC, et al. Microenvironment-induced PTEN loss by exosomal microRNA primes brain metastasis outgrowth. *Nature.* (2015) 527:100–104. doi: 10.1038/nature15376
91. Becker A, Thakur BK, Weiss JM, Kim HS, Peinado H, Lyden D. Extracellular vesicles in cancer: cell-to-cell mediators of metastasis. *Cancer Cell.* (2016) 30:836–48. doi: 10.1016/j.ccell.2016.10.009
92. Madeo M, Colbert PL, Vermeer DW, Lucido CT, Cain JT, Vichaya EG, et al. Cancer exosomes induce tumor innervation. *Nat Commun.* (2018) 9:4215–84. doi: 10.1038/s41467-018-06640-0
93. Hou J, Wang F, Liu X, Song M, Yin X. Tumor-derived exosomes enhance invasion and metastasis of salivary adenoid cystic carcinoma cells. *J Oral Pathol Med.* (2018) 47:144–51. doi: 10.1111/jop.12654
94. Rauch I, Kofler B. The galanin system in cancer. *Exp Suppl.* (2010) 102:223–41. doi: 10.1007/978-3-0346-0228-0_16
95. Tarsitano A, Asioli S, Morandi L, Monti V, Righi A, Morselli LA, et al. Laminin-5 and insulin-like growth factor-II mRNA binding protein-3 (IMP3) expression in preoperative biopsy specimens from oral cancer patients: their role in neural spread risk and survival stratification. *J Craniomaxillofac Surg.* (2016) 44:1896–902. doi: 10.1016/j.jcms.2016.07.012
96. Gomez DR, Katabi N, Zhung J, Wolden SL, Zelefsky MJ, Kraus DH, et al. Clinical and pathologic prognostic features in acinic cell carcinoma of the parotid gland. *Cancer Am Cancer Soc.* (2009) 115:2128–137. doi: 10.1002/cncr.24259
97. Joseph I, Rooban T, Elizabeth J, Rao UK, Ranganathan K. Genomic alterations landscape in adenoid cystic carcinoma of head and neck. *J Orofac Sci.* (2009) 11:73–78. doi: 10.4103/jofs.jofs_40_19
98. Amit M, Eran A, Billan S, Fridman E, Na'Ara S, Charas T, et al. Perineural spread in noncutaneous head and neck cancer: new insights into an old problem. *J Neurol Surg B Skull Base.* (2016) 77:86–95. doi: 10.1055/s-0036-1571834

23

Current Understanding of the Mechanisms Underlying Immune Evasion from PD-1/ PD-L1 Immune Checkpoint Blockade in Head and Neck Cancer

Victor C. Kok [1,2*]

[1] Department of Medical Oncology, Kuang Tien General Hospital Cancer Center, Taichung, Taiwan, [2] Department of Bioinformatics and Medical Engineering, Asia University Taiwan, Taichung, Taiwan

***Correspondence:**
Victor C. Kok
victorkok@asia.edu.tw

Starting in 2014, large phase III clinical trials began to disclose the study results of using programmed death (PD)-1 immune checkpoint inhibitors (ICIs) (pembrolizumab, nivolumab) and PD-ligand (L)1 (atezolizumab, durvalumab, avelumab) ICIs immunotherapy in patients with advanced head and neck squamous cell carcinoma (HNSCC). In the recurrent and metastatic (R/M), cisplatin-refractory setting, nivolumab achieved a 2.2-fold increase of the median 1-year overall survival as compared with investigators' choice of salvage chemotherapy (36.0 vs. 16.6%). A paradigm shift to the winning regimen, pembrolizumab combined with platinum and infusional fluorouracil, has outperformed the past gold standard of cetuximab-based platinum and fluorouracil combination in terms of overall survival (median, 13.6 vs. 10.1 mo) when administered as the first-line treatment for R/M HNSCC. Nevertheless, many patients still did not respond to the PD-1/PD-L1 checkpoint inhibitor treatment, indicating innate, adapted, or quickly acquired resistance to the immunotherapy. The mechanisms of resistance to ICIs targeting the PD-1/PD-L1 signaling pathway in the context of HNSCC are the focus of this review. The past 5 years have seen improved understanding of the mechanisms underlying checkpoint inhibition resistance in tumor cells, such as: tumor cell adaption with malfunction of the antigen-presenting machinery via class I human leukocyte antigen (HLA), reintroduction of cyclin D–cyclin-dependent kinase (CDK) 4 complex to cell cycles, enrichment of CD44+ cancer stem-like cells, or development of inactivating mutation in IKZF1 gene; impairment of T-cell functions and proliferation through mutations in the interferon-γ-regulating genes, suppression of the stimulator of interferon genes (STING) pathway, or resulted from constitutional nutritional iron deficiency state; metabolic reprogramming by cancer cells with changes in metabolites such as GTP cyclohydrolase 1, tetrahydrobiopterin, kynurenine, indoleamine 2,3-dioxygenase, and arginase 1; defective dendritic cells, CD-69 sufficient state; and the upregulation or activation of the alternative immune checkpoints, including lymphocyte activation gene-3 (LAG3), T-cell immunoglobulin and ITIM domain (TIGIT)/CD155 pathway, T-cell immunoglobulin mucin-3 (TIM-3), and V domain-containing Ig suppressor of T-cell activation (VISTA). Several potential biomarkers or biosignatures, which could predict the response or resistance to the PD-1/PD-L1 checkpoint immunotherapy, are also discussed.

Keywords: PD-1/PD-L1 signaling pathway, HNSCC, immune checkpoint blockade, cancer immunotherapy, innate resistance, adapted resistance, immune evasion, head and neck cancer

INTRODUCTION

Scope of Problems

Head and neck cancers encompass a group of malignancies arising from several anatomical mucosal sites, including the nasal cavity, paranasal sinuses, nasopharynx, oropharynx, hypopharynx, larynx and lips, and oral cavity. According to GLOBOCAN epidemiological estimates of incidence and mortality of cancer worldwide, in 2018, there were ~835,000 new cases of cancer arising from the lips, oral cavity, naso-, oro-, and hypo-pharynx and larynx; with the number of deaths in the same year being ~431,000 (1). The majority (95%) of histopathological types of head and neck cancer is squamous cell carcinoma (HNSCC) (2). Virus-related nasopharyngeal carcinoma will be included in this review because of its immunogenicity and encouraging trial outcomes (3, 4). The tumorigenesis can separate head and neck cancers into virus-related (Epstein-Barr virus-related nasopharyngeal carcinoma (NPC) and human papillomavirus (HPV)-positive oropharyngeal HNSCC) cancer and non-viral (HPV-negative) HNSCC, the latter being related to smoking, alcohol, and betel quid consumption in etiology.

Early-stage and locally advanced stage HNSCC should be treated with curative intent incorporating radical surgical resection or radical radiotherapy combined with chemotherapy. More than 65% of previously treated HNSCC will develop local recurrence or distant metastasis (5). It is very challenging for the head and neck cancer team to manage patients with unresectable locally advanced stage, relapsed or metastatic (R/M) HNSCC, mainly because of the high propensity for intrinsic, spatial, and acquired resistance to chemotherapeutic agents, radiotherapy, and anti-epidermal growth factor receptor monoclonal antibodies. The current first-line regimen for R/M HNSCC adopted a new paradigm in 2019, when the results of the randomized controlled trial, comparing pembrolizumab combined with platinum and infusional 5-fluorouracil to the past gold-standard regimen of cetuximab plus the same chemotherapy combination, confirmed an overall survival benefit (hazard ratio, HR, for death at 0.65, 95% confidence interval, CI, 0.53–0.80) favoring the pembrolizumab-based treatment arm (**Table 1**). Pembrolizumab is an anti-programmed cell death (PD)-1 monoclonal antibody, previously known as MK-3475, and subsequently, lambrolizumab (8).

The Rationale of Anti-PD-1/PD-Ligand (L)1 Immunotherapy for R/M HNSCC

One of the hallmarks of cancer is the ability of cancer cells to evade immune destruction (9). PD-1 is a co-inhibitory receptor on the cell surface of cytotoxic T lymphocytes. The ligation of PD-1 and PD-L1 or PD-L2 on tumor cells or antigen-presenting cells (APCs) elicits an immunosuppressive response, which implements subsequent metabolic reprogramming in T cells, decreases effector T cells and memory T cells, and increases Treg and exhausted T cell abundance (10). For the past few years, the abundance of PD-L1 protein in the HNSCC tumor, with its microenvironment sphere, has been the focus of numerous studies (2, 11–17). Observe the oral cavity squamous cell carcinoma (OCSCC) as an example, the prevalence of PD-L1 positivity has been reported in 45-87% of cases, depending on the cut-off value for positivity, whether cytoplasmic staining was counted as positive, and inclusion of the proportion of HPV+ cancer cases (2, 11). The PD-1/PD-L1 axis applies immunosuppressive signals, inducing anergy of cytotoxic T-cells; thus, the blockade of this ligation (analogous to releasing the brake) becomes a strong rationale for anti-PD-1 immunotherapy for R/M HNSCC.

The Recent Development of Anti-PD-1/PD-L1 Monoclonal Antibody-Based Treatment for R/M HNSCC

Table 2 attempts to summarize the recent relevant clinical trials investigating PD-1 or PD-L1 blockade in R/M HNSCC or NPC. Usually, NPC does not belong to the classical HNSCC membership due to unique tumor pathogenesis and different treatment protocols. However, anti-PD-1 therapy for NPC will be shown in this review to give our readers a broader picture of the immunotherapy comparing classical HNSCCs to NPC. The same would apply to HPV-positive oropharyngeal cancer. Overall response rate (ORR), progression-free survival (PFS), duration of response (DoR), and overall survival (OS) are shown if these results are available in the published paper. To date, only the following two anti-PD-1 monoclonal antibodies, pembrolizumab and nivolumab, and two anti-PD-L1 monoclonal antibodies, durvalumab, and atezolizumab (anti-PD-L1), have been tested in

Abbreviations: APOBEC, Apolipoprotein B mRNA editing enzyme, catalytic polypeptide-like; BDSC, Bone marrow-derived stromal cell; BMSC, Bone marrow-derived suppressor cell; CPS, Combined positive score; HNSCC, Head and neck squamous cell carcinoma; ICB, Immune checkpoint blockade; ICP, Immune checkpoint; IDO1, Indoleamine 2,3-dioxygenase-1; IKZF1, IKAROS family zinc finger 1; JAK, Janus kinase; MDSC, Myeloid-derived suppressor cell; MMR, Mismatched Repair; ORR, Overall Response Rate; PD-L1, Programmed death-ligand 1; PFS, Progression-free survival; R/M, Relapsed/metastatic; STAT, signal transducer and activator of transcription; STING, Stimulator of Interferon Genes; TCGA, The Cancer Genome Atlas (program); TIGIT, T-cell immunoglobulin and ITIM domain; Tim-3, T cell immunoglobulin and mucin-domain containing-3; TMB, Tumor mutation burden; TME, Tumor microenvironment; VISTA, V domain-containing Ig suppressor of T-cell activation.

TABLE 1 | Summary of data demonstrating the evolving new paradigms of systemic treatment for R/M HNSCC over 12 years.

Outcomes	Platinum + 5-FU (6)	Cetuximab + Platinum + 5-FU (6)	Pembrolizumab + Platinum + 5-FU (7)*
No. of patients	$n = 200$	$n = 222$	$n = 281$
Overall Response Rate (95% CI)	20% (15–25%)	36% (29–42%)	36.4% (not given)
Progression-Free Survival (mo.)	3.3 (2.9–4.3)	5.6 (5.0–6.0)	HR = 0.84 (95% CI, 0.69–1.02)*
Overall Survival in mo. (95% CI)	7.4 (6.4–8.3)	10.1 (8.6–11.2)	13.6 (not given)
Hazard ratio for OS (95% CI)		0.80 (0.64–0.99)	0.65 (0.53–0.80)

**Results shown here represent the subgroup of patients whose Combined Positive Score (CPS) for PD-L1 was ≥1. The exact figure for progression-free survival was not given in the Abstract.*

R/M HNSCC (**Table 2**). As yet, there is only one published phase I study regarding avelumab, a PD-L1 inhibitor, in R/M HNSCC (27–29).

The efficacy of anti-PD-1 and anti-PD-L1 for R/M HNSCC, regardless of its use at as salvage therapy, in the second-line, or even in the first-line while combined with platinum plus infusional 5-fluorouracil, the ORRs were fairly poor across the board. When used in the first-line combined with PF chemotherapy for R/M HNSCC, the response rate was reported as 36.4% (7). Nearly 64% of the patients' tumors demonstrated either primary or adaptive resistance [cancer cells salvaged themselves by resorting to immunoediting and thus, further created an immunosuppressive tumor microenvironment (TME)] (30) to the combination immunochemotherapy.

This review serves to present the recent research findings with implications on the mechanisms of immune evasion from the anti-PD1 or anti-PD-L1 immune checkpoint blockade.

METHODS

Methodology for the Literature Search

A dynamic PubMed literature search until September 14, 2019, using the Medical Subject Headings and the Boolean search terms, was used to retrieve articles indexed under keywords, such as "head and neck cancer," "head and neck squamous cell carcinoma," "HNSCC," "oral cavity squamous cell carcinoma," "OCSCC," "immunotherapy," "pembrolizumab," "nivolumab," "atezolizumab," "durvalumab," "avelumab," "immune escape," "immune evasion," "resistance," "relapsed or metastatic," "unresected locally advanced," "mechanism," "PD-L1," "PD-1," "immune checkpoint inhibitor," "immunoediting," "tumor microenvironment," "immunosuppressive," and "adapted resistance." The American Society of Clinical Oncology Meeting Abstract database was also searched for the relevant trials. Also, a hand search from the "Similar Articles" inside the PubMed panel was performed to retrieve related articles.

In the EndNote software, "Find Duplicates" function was activated to remove duplicated papers. "Find Full Text" was then activated to download those articles available for download. The Harvard Medical School digital library, "BrowZine," was then used to complete all full-text downloads for the EndNote library. Review articles represented most retrieved articles in the library, and only a few of them would be cited in this review. Whereas, articles with primary research data from innovative experiments and clinical trials would be selected.

RESULTS AND DISCUSSION

HNSCC Cancer Cells Remodel and Shape an Immunosuppressive TME

Within the tumor microenvironment, there exists a plethora of cytokines, and various infiltrating immune cells, such as CD8+ T cells and APCs, including dendritic cells, anti-tumoral M1 macrophages, pro-tumoral M2 macrophages [tumor-associated macrophages (TAM), myeloid-derived suppressor cells (MDSC), cancer-associated fibroblasts (CAFs), and regulatory T cells (Tregs) (**Figure 1**)]. Like the immunosuppressive lymphocytic Tregs, MDSC functions as myeloid regulatory cells (MRC) and is further separated into monocytic-MDSC and polymorphonuclear-MDSC (31). A study by Takahashi and colleagues identified that CAFs stimulate and polarize the increase of CD68+ and CD163+ pro-tumoral macrophages in the TME (32).

Primary Resistance to ICIs in HNSCC

A Birmingham research group developed a 54-gene hypoxia-immune classifier to prognosticate patients with HNSCC, and uncovered that tumors that are high-hypoxia/low-immune are associated with "immune-desert" microenvironmental profiles (33). Hypoxia within a tumor microenvironment will increase the immune-inhibitory PD-L1 generation through the hypoxia-inducible factor (HIF)-1α signaling (33, 34). An immune desert tumor microenvironment promotes immune evasion for cancer cells. These cold tumors respond poorly to single-agent PD-1/PD-L1 immune checkpoint (ICP) immunotherapy. The JAK family of kinases (JAK1/2/3, TYK2) is involved in PD-L1 induction in tumor, stromal, and immune cells (35). A group of investigators from Foundation Medicine Inc., Cambridge, Boston, showed that in a preclinical study focusing on endometrial carcinoma and stomach adenocarcinoma, somatic mutation of JAK1 with loss of function (meaning loss of JAK1-mediated interferon response) results in immune evasion, particularly in microsatellite instability-high (MSI-H) tumors with high total mutational burden (TMB) (35).

TABLE 2 | Summary of clinical trial results of PD-1 or PD-L1 blockade in R/M HNSCC and NPC showing overall response rate (ORR), duration of response (DoR), progression-free survival (PFS), and overall survival (OS).

1st Author/ published year/ (References)/EudraCT No.	Phase of study/Study Name/No. pts	Key immunotherapy drug	Biomarker	Failed treatment previously	Treatment outcomes
Chow/2016/(18)/2012-005771-14	Phase Ib/KEYNOTE-012 Expansion Cohort/*n* = 132	Pembrolizumab at a fixed dose, 200 mg Q3W	Irrespective of biomarker status	57% failed two or more lines of chemo	6-mo. PFS = 23%; 6-mo. OS = 59%. ORR = 22% in PD-L1+ tumors. Duration of response = not reached (range, ≥ 2 to ≥ 11 mo.)
Bauml/2017/(19)/2014-002447-18	Phase II/KEYNOTE-055/*n* = 171	Pembrolizumab	82% PD-L1 positive (CPS ≥ 1%)	75% failed platinum and cetuximab or more	ORR = 16% (95% CI, 11% to 23%). Duration of response = 8 mo. (2+ to 12+ mo.); Median PFS = 2.1 mo., and median OS = 8 mo.
Hsu/2017/(13)/ 2013-004507-39	Phase Ib/KEYNOTE-028/*n* = 27 NPC	Pembrolizumab	Dako 22C3 positive ≥ 1%	70.4% failed three or more lines	ORR = 25.9% (95% CI, 11.1 to 46.3)
Cohen/2019/(20)/2014-001749-26	Phase III/KEYNOTE-040/*n* = 247 (pembro. arm)	Pembrolizumab at a fixed-dose, 200 mg Q3W	PD-L1 tumor proportion score (≥ 50% vs. < 50%)	Failed platinum-containing chemo	ORR = 14·6% (95% CI, 10.4–19.6); Duration of response = 18.4 mo (95% CI 5.8–18.4); Median PFS = 2·1 mo (95% CI 2.1–2.3); Median OS = 8.4 mo. (95% CI 6.4–9.4).
Rischin/2019/(7)/2014-003698-41	Phase III/KEYNOTE-048/*n* = 882 (entire)	Pembrolizumab vs. pembrolizumab + PF vs. cetuximab + PF	CPS for PD-L1 protein expression.	First-line for R/M HNSCC	In the CPS ≥ 1 group, ORR = 36.4% and median OS = 13.6 mo. (in pembrolizumab + PF) vs. ORR, 35.7%; OS, 10.4 mo. (in cetuximab + PF); HR = 0.65, 95% CI, 0.53–0.80).
Ferris/2016/(21); Ferris/2018/(22)/ 2013-003622-86	Phase III/CHECKMATE-141/*n* = 240 (nivo. arm)	Nivolumab 3 mg/kg Q2W	Dako positive ≥ 1%, ≥ 5%, vs. ≥ 10%.	Failed within 6 mo. of platinum therapy	ORR = 13.3% (9.3–18.3); OS = 7.7 mo. (5.7–8.8). 24-mo. OS = 16.9%.
Colevas/2018/(23)/2011-001422-23	Phase Ia/PCD4989g/*n* = 32	Atezolizumab	Responses observed irrespective of HPV or PD-L1 status.	Heavily pretreated	ORR = 22% (95% CI, 9–40%); PFS = 2.6 mo. (0.5–48.4 mo.); Median OS = 6.0 mo (range 0.5–51.6+ mo).
Segal/2019/(24)/not available	Phase I/II expansion/*n* = 62	Durvalumab 10 mg/kg Q2W for 12 mo	32.3% had tumor cell PD-L1 expression ≥ 25%	Failed median of 2 prior systemic treatments (range, 1-13)	ORR = 6.5% (15.0% for PD-L1 ≥ 25%, 2.6% for < 25%); TTP = 2.7 months (range, 1.2-5.5); PFS = 1.4 mo; OS = 8.4 mo. OS rate = 62% at 6 mo and 38% at 12 mo (42% for PD-L1 ≥ 25%, 36% for < 25%).
Siu/2018/(25)/not available	Phase II randomized, open-label/CONDOR/*n* = 67	Durvalumab (10 mg/kg Q2W) monotherapy	PD-L1–low/negative	Failed 1 platinum-containing regimen	ORR = 9.2% (3.46-19.02)
Siu/2018/(25)/not available	Phase II randomized, open-label/ CONDOR/*n* = 133	Durvalumab + tremelimumab (anti-CTLA-4)	PD-L1–low/negative	Failed 1 platinum-containing regimen	ORR = 7.8% (3.78-13.79%)
Bahig/2019/(26)/not available	Phase I-II/*n* = 35 (non-NPC)	Durvalumab (1500 mg Q4W) + tremelimumab (75 mg Q4W × 4 doses) + SBRT to metastases at cycles 2 and 3 of immunotherapy	Biomarker-unselected	Patients with ≥ 2 extracranial metastatic lesions.	Ongoing study
Elbers/2019(27)/not available	Phase I/*n* = 9 (cisplatin-unfit)	Cetuximab-radiotherapy + avelumab (concurrent 10 mg/kg Q2W + 4 months maintenance)	None	Unfit for cisplatin but with an indication for concurrent bioradiotherapy	At 12 (median, 95% CI, 8–26) months follow-up, recurrence occurred in 4/8 patients (50%).
Merlano/2018/(28)/2017-000353-39	Phase Ib-II/CONFRONT/*n* =	Avelumab 10 mg/kg Q2W + Cyclophosphamide 50 mg daily + 8 Gy radiotherapy day 8.	None	Failed at least therapy with platinum, fluorouracil, and cetuximab	Ongoing study.

EudraCT, European Union Drug Regulating Authorities Clinical Trials; NPC, nasopharyngeal carcinoma; SBRT, stereotactic body radiotherapy; CPS, Combined Positive Score.

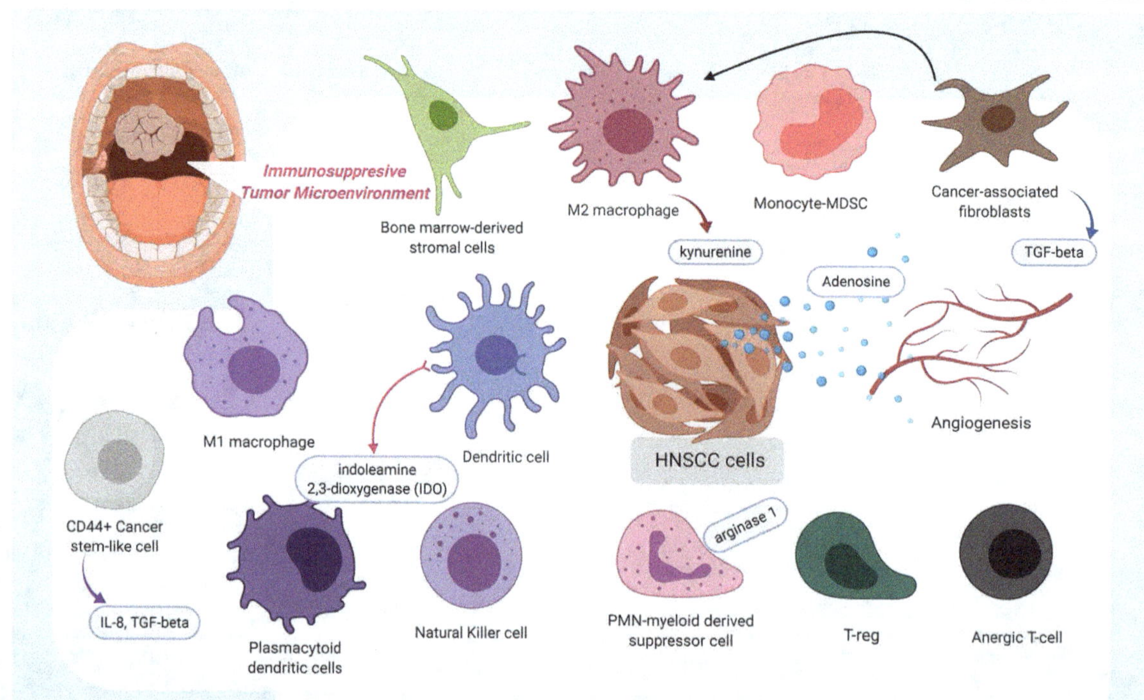

FIGURE 1 | This schematic diagram highlights the immunosuppressive tumor microenvironment (TME) in which a variety of immune cells are polarized to possess pro-tumoral features, stimulated cancer-associated fibroblasts, which release transforming growth factor-β, and even angiogenesis contribute to the immunosuppressive state. Additionally, several molecules, such as kynurenine, adenosine, indoleamine 2,3-dioxygenase, arginase 1, interleukin (IL)-8, and IL-10, were identified to contribute to a pro-tumoral immunosuppressive TME or at extreme, an immune-desert. The figure was created with BioRender.com and was exported under a paid subscription.

Soft tissue infections or deep neck infection in the head and neck region can occur in patients with locally advanced HNSCC. Antibiotic usage around the time of ICI treatment could dampen the effects of PD-1/PD-L1 blockade (36–39), as antibiotics usage for head and neck soft tissue infection will disrupt the integrity of the gut microbiome. A recent study demonstrates that disruptions in the gut microbiome composition, also known as dysbiosis, is one of the mechanisms of primary resistance to ICI therapy (36). Experiments using fecal microbiota transplantation in avatar mice demonstrate that a combination of *A. muciniphila* and *E. hirae* would increase the CCR9- or CXCR3-expressing central memory T cells in the mesenteric lymph nodes and induce dendritic cells to secrete IL-12, a Th1 cytokine essential to elicit immunogenicity during PD-1/PD-L1 blockade (36). However, the actual mechanisms by which the intestinal flora modulate ICP immunotherapy is still unclear.

An immunosuppressive tumor microenvironment can also result from immune modulatory effects of CAF (32), TAM (40), and MDSC (41) (**Figure 1**). In addition, extracellular signals from angiogenesis can also drive immune suppression by directly suppressing APCs and immune effector cells, or by augmenting the effect of Tregs, MDSC, and TAM. Reciprocally, the above-mentioned immune suppressive cells can also drive angiogenesis (**Figure 1**), rendering a vicious cycle of disrupted immune activation (42).

What Does HNSCC Possess to Avoid Immunosurveillance or Destruction via the PD-1/PD-L1 Immune Checkpoint (ICP) Blockade?

To understand the tumor microenvironment of the oral cavity SCC using the infiltrating lymphocyte repertoires as an example, several studies identified considerable antigen-experienced CD4+ and CD8+ cells, Tregs, and PD-1-expressing and Tim-3-expressing T cells, as well as lymphoid follicles with germinal center-like structures (11, 43–48). These immunosuppressive characteristics are indicative of T-cell exhaustion. **Table 2** shows that ~60% of patients with R/M HNSCC would not respond to the PD-1/PD-L1 ICP therapy. This means that even the "release of the brakes" through blocking the ligation of PD-1/PD-L1, cannot adequately allow the cytotoxic T cells to mount an attack of significant proportions on cancer cells, which would prevent tumor shrinkage or induce mixed responses amongst measurable tumor sites. The potential mechanisms being recognized for causing acquired immune escape from the PD-1/PD-L1 ICP in the setting of head and neck cancer are summarized in **Table 3**.

There are currently four areas of research on the molecular resistance mechanisms underlying the selective pressure from PD-1/PD-L1 ICB (**Table 3**). In this review, they are categorized as tumor cell adaption, impairment of T cell functions and proliferation, changes in metabolite- and cytokine-rich tumor

TABLE 3 | Mechanisms of immune escape that are implicated in HNSCC.

Potential mechanisms	HPV+ or HPV-	Component in the immunity against cancer	References
TUMOR CELLS ADAPTION			
Antigen presenting machinery (APM) via class I HLA	No data	Activated CD8+ immunologic pressure could induce transcriptional loss of HLA class one loci; deleterious alterations in *JAK1/2* and β2-microglobulin.	(49–52)
Downregulation of the transporter associated with antigen processing (TAP)-1/2 heterodimer		APM component downregulated by the IFN-γ-phosphorylated STAT1-mediated signaling pathway; results in escaping recognition by tumor antigen-specific cytotoxic T lymphocytes.	(53, 54)
JAK mutation	Both	Leads to loss of sensitivity to IFN-γ signals.	(35)
Cyclin D–CDK4 kinase re-introduction	No data	Destabilizes PD-L1 and controls the PD-L1 abundance in tumor cells.	(55)
Enrichment of CD44+ cancer stem-like cells	No data	Activates immunosuppressive network through cytokine release.	(54)
IKZF1-inactivating mutations	No data	Genomic alterations of the master regulator IKZF1 correlates with low immune recruitment.	(56)
IMPAIRED T-CELL FUNCTIONS AND PROLIFERATION			
Nutritional iron deficiency state	Both	Affects T-cell proliferation	(57–59)
Mutations in interferon-γ-regulating genes	Both	Exhausted "Immune Class" enriched with M2 macrophages, WNT/TGF-β activation	(60, 61)
Suppression of stimulator of interferon genes (STING) pathway	HPV+	Dampens the antitumor immune response.	(62)
Inhibition of STAT1 phosphorylation	Both	Enhanced T-cell exhaustion and accumulation of MDSCs	(63)
CHANGES IN METABOLITE- AND CYTOKINE-RICH TUMOR MICROENVIRONMENTS			
Defective dendritic cells (DC)	Both	Defective cytokine- and STAT-mediated regulation of DC.	(64–66)
CD69-sufficient state	Both	Leads to effector T-cell exhaustion.	(67)
Genetic inactivation of GTP cyclohydrolase 1 (GCP1)	No data	Drastically impairs T-cell maturation.	(58)
Metabolite tetrahydrobiopterin (BH4) inhibited by kynurenine	No data	Will impair T cell function.	(58)
Indoleamine 2,3-dioxygenase-1 (IDO1); Tryptophan metabolite, kynurenine (Kyn) level	Both	IDO1 inhibits T cell proliferation, restricts tumor immune infiltration, and retards antitumor immune responses. Kyn released from ϕ, and myeloid cells activate T-reg cells.	(12, 68, 69)
Cancer-associated fibroblasts secrete TGF-β	Both	Results in restraining CD8+ T effector cells infiltrating into microenvironment. TGF-β1 also decreases the number of dendritic cells in the draining lymph nodes.	(32, 70–73)
Arginase 1 expression on microenvironment myeloid cells	Both	Arg1 leads to L-arginine depletion depriving T cells and NK cells of essential nutrients required for proliferation.	(74)
CD38-upregulation	Both	CD38 inhibits CD8+ T-cell function via adenosine receptor signaling.	(75, 76)
Ectonucleotidases CD39/CD73 axis	Both	CD39 is considered a tumor-specific dysfunction marker. Tregs use the axis to diminish anti-cancer killing.	(76–79)
Polymorphonuclear myeloid-derived suppressor cells (PMN-MDSC) activation	Both	Through the nitric oxide pathway, PMN-MDSCs impair proliferation and expression molecules in activated T cells.	(41)
Nucleotide-binding domain leucine-rich repeat and pyrin domain containing receptor 3 (NLRP3) inflammasome activation	Both	Leads to downstream interleukin (IL)-1β release. NLRP3 inflammasome/IL-1β axis increases MDSCs, Tregs and TAMs creating an immunosuppressive microenvironment.	(80)
ACTIVATION OF AND DEPENDENCE ON ALTERNATIVE IMMUNE CHECKPOINTS			
Lymphocyte activation gene-3 (LAG3) (=CD223) upregulation	More in HPV+	Induces a state of functional exhaustion in effector T-cells.	(81, 82)
T-cell immunoglobulin and ITIM domain (TIGIT)/CD155 pathway activation	Both	Augments TIGIT+ T-regs, a unique T-reg subset, leading to active suppression of anti-tumor immune response and T-cell exhaustion.	(82–85)
T-cell immunoglobulin mucin-3 (TIM-3) upregulation	Both	TIM-3 is considered a tumor-specific dysfunction marker. It dampens effector T-cell functions in the microenvironment.	(44, 48, 77, 86)
V domain-containing Ig suppressor of T-cell activation (VISTA)	Both	Leads to T-cell exhaustion and T-reg recruitment in the microenvironment.	(87, 88)

Investigated mechanisms of acquired immune escape from PD-1/PD-L1 checkpoint blockade relevant to head and neck cancer.

microenvironments, and activation of and dependence on alternative immune checkpoints.

Tumor Cell Adaption

Tumor cell adaption occurs through various processes, namely with modification of molecules causing immune escape via malfunction of the antigen-presenting machinery via class I HLA, reintroduction of cyclin D–CDK4 kinase heterodimers to cell cycles (55), enrichment of CD44+ cancer stem-like cells (54), JAK mutation (35), or development of inactivating mutation in IKZF1 gene, the master regulator of immune infiltrates recruitment (56).

Speckle-type POZ protein (SPOP) is an E3 ubiquitin ligase adaptor protein mediating poly-ubiquitination and proteasome-mediated degradation of several proteins, such as PD-L1 (55, 89). SPOP mutations or copy number variation can act as a tumor suppressor or progressor depending on the different context in different cancer types. In head and neck cancer, TCGA dataset, <2% of patient tumors exhibited mutated or altered SPOP, which was associated with non-significant reduction of the relative risk of relapse or disease progression (relative risk = 0.4, 95% confidence interval, 0.06–2.61) (**Supplementary Table 1**). Recent research identified that cyclin D-CDK4 kinase reintroduction in CAF would destabilize PD-L1 molecules via the cullin 3-SPOP pathway (55). Whereas, loss of function mutations of SPOP will increase the level of PD-L1 and tumor-infiltrating lymphocytes, as observed in mouse models. CDK4/6 inhibitor treatment will theoretically increase PD-L1 levels thus potentiating the ICB treatment (55).

In the milieu of the HNSCC immune microenvironment (**Figure 1**), there exists a kind of CD44+ stem-like cell, whose immunosuppressive capabilities have been demonstrated to be more effective than CD44-negative stem cells to inhibit the effector T-cell population while simultaneously inducing immunosuppressive Tregs and MDSC (54).

Genes function as a master regulator to control the expression of downstream genes by controlling transcription factors. IKZF1 is such a master regulator that could lead to enhanced recruitment of immune infiltrate and tumor sensitivity to ICP inhibitors in several cancer types. Genomic alterations of this gene could negatively affect immunogenicity and tumor response to ICB (56).

Results from genomic studies of HNSCC demonstrate that the immune evasion genetic pathways are different between HPV-negative and HPV-positive HNSCCs (24). The HLA mutations are uncommonly found with <10% prevalence rate in HPV-negative HNSCCs, whereas, the HPV-positive tumors will have more common HLA and Beta2-microglobulin (B2M) mutations and TRAF3 loss (90). B2M is a light chain incorporated with the MHC Class I heavy chain to form a capable antigen-presenting machinery complex. B2M deficiency in tumor cells, which results in defective cell surface HLA Class I complex or subsequent acquired loss of B2M while under immunotherapy, has been recognized as a crucial immune escape mechanism as demonstrated in various solid tumor models (91).

Impairment in T Cell Functions and Proliferation

Potential mechanisms of intrinsic or adaptive resistance rest upon T-cell functions and proliferation, which is the most essential weapon the human body utilizes to destroy cancer cells. T-cell functions and proliferation can be impaired through mutations in interferon-γ-regulating genes, suppression of the Stimulator of Interferon genes (STING) pathway or result from constitutional nutritional iron deficiency states (57–59, 62). It is noted that HPV-antigen expression levels in the tumor microenvironment would enhance cytotoxic T lymphocyte dysregulation (77).

Changes in Metabolite- and Cytokine-Rich Tumor Microenvironments

The other well-known hallmark of cancer is metabolic reprogramming by cancer cells. The tumor extracellular microenvironment contains a vibrant display of metabolites and cytokines released from different cell types aiming to create an immunosuppressive environment for the proliferation of tumor cells. **Table 3** highlights several notable changes in metabolite-rich and cytokine-rich tumor stroma with consequences of dampening anti-cancer immunity. Defective cytokine- and STAT-mediated regulation of dendritic cells (DCs) leads to defective DCs. CD-69 sufficient state will cause effector T-cell exhaustion. The actual mechanism is still elusive; however, it is apparent that CD-69 expressed on leucocytes is responsible for cell retention in the tumor microenvironment and the CD-69 expression on T-cells is associated with the expression of PD-1 and Tim-3 in T-cells (67).

The function of metabolites GTP cyclohydrolase 1 (GCH1) and tetrahydrobiopterin (BH4) has been identified to be able to increase T-cell proliferation and promote their maturation. GCH1 is the first rate-limiting enzyme in the *de novo* BH4-synthesis pathway. Whereas, metabolite kynurenine has been found to activate Treg cells, and the enzyme indoleamine 2,3-dioxygenase (IDO) inhibits T cell proliferation and restricts tumor infiltration. Arginase 1 (Arg1) depletes L-arginine, depriving the essential nutrients that T cells and NK cells need to proliferate. The alterations of these metabolites will adversely impact anti-cancer immunity through various molecular mechanisms.

Activation of and Dependence on Alternative Immune Checkpoints

The fourth group of mechanisms underlying the resistance to PD-1-PD-L1 blockade includes activation of and dependence on alternative immune checkpoints. These alternative immune checkpoints other than PD-L1 include lymphocyte activation gene-3 (LAG3) (=CD223) upregulation, T-cell immunoglobulin and ITIM domain (TIGIT)/CD155 pathway activation, T-cell immunoglobulin mucin-3 (TIM-3) upregulation, and V domain-containing Ig suppressor of T-cell activation (VISTA). The past two decades have seen research identify the G-protein-coupled adenosine receptors mediating downregulation of the inflammatory tumor microenvironment creating an immunosuppressive milieu. Adenosine and adenosine triphosphate (ATP) are the most abundant metabolites within a cell and in the extracellular space, which acts as an autocrine and paracrine messenger. While ATP acts as an accelerator to promote proinflammatory activities, adenosine, via the Gs-coupled A2a and A2b receptors, suppresses various immune cells, including T lymphocytes, NK cells, neutrophils, dendritic cells, and macrophages (75, 76, 78, 92–95).

There are several vital molecules interplaying within the *adenosine receptor signaling*. The molecule, CD73, is an ecto-5-nucleotidase, which will dephosphorylate extracellular AMP to immunosuppressive adenosine (78, 79, 94). As a ubiquitous membranous ectozyme, CD38, cleaves NAD(+) and NADP(+), generating cyclic ADP ribose (cADPR), NAADP, and ADPR, which are directly involved in the calcium signaling essential for a cell (96). Current evidence suggests that one of the significant mechanisms in acquired immune escape from PD-1/PD-L1 inhibition is CD38 upregulation. CD38 promotes adenosine production through the **CD38-CD203a-CD73 axis**. Studies discovered that the tumor cells hijacked and leveraged the adenosine receptor signaling pathway by upregulating the activities of CD38, to develop resistance to PD-1/PD-L1 immunotherapy through inhibition of CD8+ T-cell function. Upregulation of CD38 is induced by tumor-derived soluble mediators, all-trans retinoic acid (ATRA) and IFNβ, in the tumor microenvironment.

Prediction of Response to Anti-PD-1 Immunotherapy in HNSCC

The development of predictive precision oncology aiming to discover and validate biomarkers that can predict the response from PD-1/PD-L1 immunotherapy has evolved relentlessly in the past years. **Table 4** highlights the current discovery of biomarker predictors for immunotherapy response in patients who received PD-1/PD-L1 ICB. The eagerly awaited issues to be solved in predictive biomarker development are to achieve adequate clinical evidence about the discriminative capacity (power) of each biomarker. While the evidence is being investigated through clinical studies, **Table 4** aims to demonstrate some potentially investigated or helpful biomarkers related to the field of HNSCC. These include the combined positive score (CPS) for PD-L1 protein expression, mismatch repair (MMR)-deficient status, apolipoprotein B mRNA editing enzyme, catalytic polypeptide-like (APOBEC)-driven mutations status, the molecular exhausted immune class, molecular active immune class, the interferon-γ signature (6-genes), the expanded immune signature (18-genes), the condition of somatic frameshift events in tumor suppressor genes, the total mutational burden (TMB), and the microenvironment infiltrating arginase 1 (Arg1)+/CD68+ macrophage-mediated immune evasion state.

The immunohistochemistry combined positive score (CPS) for quantifying the PD-L1 expression in a tumor sample has been adopted to predict tumor response to ICB treatment. This score is calculated as the number of PD-L1+ tumor cells, lymphocytes, and macrophages, divided by the total number of viable tumor cells, and multiplying by 100. In various trials, CPS $\geq$ 1% predicts immunotherapy response. The caveat of using CPS at the 1% cutoff to select HNSCC patients for PD-1 ICB is that intratumor heterogeinity should be considered. Rasmussen et al. have prospectively investigated the intratumor heterogeneity in PD-L1 expression in HNSCC in 28 patients with a total of 33 whole surgical specimens (98). With 1% cut off, 52% of the six random core biopsies from each surgical specimen was concordant with CPS. Defining a tumor as positive if just a single-one of the core biopsies was positive using CPS at 1% cut-off, the negative predictive value of a single negative core biopsy was 0% (98).

DNA mismatch repair (MMR) genes, hMLH1 and hMSH2, once inactivated, can accumulate thousands of mutations in simple repeats in genomic DNA and develop microsatellite instability (MSI). A defective MMR system results in both MSI and high tumor mutation burden (TMB-high), which further generates neoantigens to be identified by APCs to mount an effective cytotoxic killing of tumor cells. It has been estimated that MSI is present in ~40% of patients with HNSCC (106). The frequency of MSI in an endemic betel-quid chewing region is about the same as the otherwise non-endemic regions, having a rate of 37.9% (107). Despite the fact that these TMB-high cancers are more immunogenic, unlike those immunogenic-desert tumors, half of the TMB-high patients still do not respond to anti-PD-1 immunotherapy (108). Subsequently, a study looking at the mutational landscape of MSI-high discovered that the extent of immunotherapy response is specifically associated with a mutational load accumulating the insertion-deletion (indel) mutations (99). The authors emphasize that there is a greater impact of frameshifting indel mutations over the more general missense mutations, in eliciting anti-PD-1 immunotherapy response.

Generally speaking, TMB was defined as the total number of somatic, coding, base substitution, and indel mutations counted per megabase (Mb) of genome interrogated (109). In terms of the mutational burden as assessed by real-time gene sequencing, HNSCC exhibits median mutations/Mb of 5.0 with 10.1% (95% CI, 8.5%–11.9%) having > 20 mutations/Mb (109). In a group of 81 patients with HNSCC, higher TMB, as demonstrated by the targeted massively parallel tumor sequencing, predicted PD-1/PD-L1 ICB response ($P < 0.01$) (105).

T Cell-Inflamed Gene Signature

IFN-γ signaling (expanded immune) signature consists of the following 18 genes: *CD3D, CCL5, CD3D, CD3E, IL2RG, CIITA, GZMK, CXCL9, CXCR6, TAGAP, CD2, HLA-E, IDO1, LAG3, NKG7, GZMB, STAT1,* and *CXCL10* (60). Typically, the core IFN-γ gene signature comprises six genes, i.e., *IDO1, CXCL9, CXCL10, HLA-DRA, STAT1,* and *IFNG* (60). In a retrospective analysis of the correlation of the 18-gene signature score (as a continuous variable) with the best of response (BOR) and PFS for 43 patients with HNSCC of the KEYNOTE-012 cohort (18, 110), strong statistical significance ($P = 0.015$ and $P < 0.001$, respectively) was obtained. The 18-gene IFN-γ signature profile derived from the NanoString platform is under development as a clinical-grade companion diagnostic incorporated into the future or ongoing pembrolizumab trials (111).

TABLE 4 | Response prediction to anti-PD-1 immunotherapy in HNSCC.

Gene alterations or signature	Testing platform	Response to anti-PD-1 checkpoint blockade	References
Combined Positive Score (CPS) for PD-L1 protein Expression	Immunohistochemistry on formalin-fixed paraffin-embedded tissue samples	CPS = number of PD-L1+ tumor cells, lymphocytes, and macrophages, divided by the total number of viable tumor cells, and multiplying by 100. In various trials, CPS ≥ 1 predicts response.	(7, 19, 97, 98)
MMR-deficient	Quantification of genomic MSI level (MSI intensity)	Higher insertion-deletion (Indel) load predicts response.	(99)
Apolipoprotein B mRNA editing enzyme, catalytic polypeptide-like (APOBEC)-driven mutations	APOBEC enrichment scores.	Upregulated as an innate immune response particularly in HPV+ tumors. APOBEC3 mutation leads to driver mutation in *PI3KCA*.	(100–102)
Molecular exhausted immune class	Gene expression pattern analyzed by non-negative matrix factorization algorithm	Portends a worse prognosis than active immune class in overall survival.	(61)
Molecular active immune class		Better prognosis (overall survival) than exhausted class. May predict immune responses.	(61)
Interferon-γ signature (6-genes)	NanoString nCounter mRNA	Low signature score did not respond to pembrolizumab.	(103)
Expanded immune signature (18-genes)	NanoString nCounter mRNA	Low signature score did not respond to pembrolizumab.	(103)
Somatic frameshift events in tumor suppressor genes	Targeted massively parallel sequencing	More frequently seen in HPV- responders.	(104, 105)
Total mutational burden (TMB)	Targeted massively parallel sequencing	Predicts response in HPV- HNSCC.	(104, 105)
Microenvironment infiltrating arginase 1 (Arg1)+/CD68+ macrophage-mediated immune evasion	Enzyme-Linked Immunosorbent Assay (ELISA)	Plasma Arg1 level (ng/mL) to predict immune evasion (cutoff to be determined)	(74)

An enriched proinflammatory M1 macrophage signature, enhanced cytolytic activity, abundant tumor-infiltrating lymphocytes, high human papillomavirus (HPV) infection, and favorable prognosis were associated with active immune class (all, $P < 0.05$).

A bioinformatics study using a non-negative matrix factorization algorithm of the RNA sequencing profiles of 522 patients with HNSCC collected in the TCGA identified an immune class (61). This immune class was determined based on the enriched inflammatory response, enhanced cytolytic activity, and active interferon-γ signaling. There are two subclasses within the immune class, namely, the exhausted immune class, with a poor prognosis, and the active immune class, with a favorable prognosis. The active immune class was highlighted to have enriched anti-tumoral M1 macrophage polarization, stronger cytolytic activity, abundant tumor-infiltrating lymphocytes, and higher HPV infection rates (61). The research findings are relevant to the clinical application on selecting patients with active immune signatures for immunotherapy.

Finally, IFN-gamma signaling depends on the integrity of the JAK/STAT pathway. An orthotopic head and neck squamous cell carcinoma model experiment using Stat1 deficient [Stat1(-/-)] mice observed enhanced T-cell exhaustion and accumulation of MDSCs, creating a tumor-permissive microenvironment in Stat1 deficient mice (63).

Based on current research findings, if tumor samples are discovered possessing any of the aforementioned genetic aberrations or signatures indicating a hot immune tumor, a treatment recommendation incorporating the blockade of the PD-1/PD-L1 axis is justified. The status of recommendation on selecting a predictive biomarker will be refined when new evidence or data is available to suggest otherwise.

CONCLUSIONS

Hnsccs have more immunosuppressive tumor microenvironments although the initial research indicated that HNSCCs are amongst the top malignancies ranked from high to low by the neoantigen loads and total tumor burdens. Although a new treatment paradigm has been established placing pembrolizumab + platinum and infusional fluorouracil as the new standard as the first line for R/M HNSCC, ~64% of patients will not benefit from the significant tumor regression criteria, indicating innate, adaptive resistance to the blockade of PD-1/PD-L1 ligation. This review assimilated the research findings after an extensive literature review and presents the potential mechanisms of immune escape from the PD-1/PD-L1 checkpoint inhibition into four aspects as follows: tumor cell adaption, impairment of T-cell functions and proliferation, changes in metabolite- and cytokine-rich tumor microenvironments, and activation of the alternative immune checkpoints. There are no easy methods for immunotherapy response prediction in HNSCC. Even the widely accepted criteria of the combined positivity score for PD-L1 protein expression, commonly adopted in several clinical trials to stratify patients with HNSCC by the degree of immunogenicity, may have a negative predictive value of zero percent if just one core-biopsy was examined, questioning the usefulness of this immunohistochemistry test in unresectable patients.

Targeted massively parallel sequencing and NanoString nCounter mRNA analysis showing the results of total mutational burden or certain immune signatures present promising tests with the potential to discriminate between immune responsive or unresponsive patients with HNSCC, thus requiring further research to confirm their utility in predictive precision immuno-oncology. Every patient with HNSCC contemplating ICI therapy, theoretically, should be considered for several tests, namely TMB, MSI, PD-L1/L2 genome amplification, viral antigens, and next-generation sequencing, to identify actionable targets to combine with ICI therapy.

AUTHOR CONTRIBUTIONS

The sole author of this work performed all aspects related to a review article, such as research idea conception, research strategy planning, literature search, retrieval and selection, extensive analysis of data, drafting the manuscript, drawing figures, creating tables, and finally approved this manuscript for publishing.

ACKNOWLEDGMENTS

The author is grateful that part of this review has been critically reviewed as a Capstone Project Topic Review by an anonymous expert in the field of Harvard Medical School, Boston, in the High-Impact Cancer Research: Cancer Biology and Therapeutics program. A significant amount of time was dedicated to the Capstone Project during the 1 year program. The author of this review took part in the program as a student and this review is a result of these activities.

REFERENCES

1. Bray F, Ferlay J, Soerjomataram I, Siegel RL, Torre LA, Jemal A. Global cancer statistics 2018: GLOBOCAN estimates of incidence and mortality worldwide for 36 cancers in 185 countries. *CA Cancer J Clin.* (2018) 68:394-424. doi: 10.3322/caac.21492
2. Straub M, Drecoll E, Pfarr N, Weichert W, Langer R, Hapfelmeier A, et al. CD274/PD-L1 gene amplification and PD-L1 protein expression are common events in squamous cell carcinoma of the oral cavity. *Oncotarget.* (2016) 7:12024–34. doi: 10.18632/oncotarget.7593
3. Martorelli D, Houali K, Caggiari L, Vaccher E, Barzan L, Franchin G, et al. Spontaneous T cell responses to Epstein-Barr virus-encoded BARF1 protein and derived peptides in patients with nasopharyngeal carcinoma: bases for improved immunotherapy. *Int J Cancer.* (2008) 123:1100–7. doi: 10.1002/ijc.23621
4. Wu TS, Wang LC, Liu SC, Hsu TY, Lin CY, Feng GJ, et al. EBV oncogene N-LMP1 induces CD4 T cell-mediated angiogenic blockade in the murine tumor model. *J Immunol.* (2015) 194:4577–87. doi: 10.4049/jimmunol.1400794
5. Chow LQM. Head and neck cancer. *N Engl J Med.* (2020) 382:60–72. doi: 10.1056/NEJMra1715715
6. Vermorken JB, Mesia R, Rivera F, Remenar E, Kawecki A, Rottey S, et al. Platinum-based chemotherapy plus cetuximab in head and neck cancer. *N Engl J Med.* (2008) 359:1116–27. doi: 10.1056/NEJMoa0802656
7. Rischin D, Harrington K, Greil R, Soulieres D, Tahara M, de Castro G, et al. Protocol-specified final analysis of the phase 3 KEYNOTE-048 trial of pembrolizumab (pembro) as first-line therapy for recurrent/metastatic head and neck squamous cell carcinoma (R/M HNSCC). *J Clin Oncol.* (2019) 37:6000.
8. Hamid O, Robert C, Daud A, Hodi FS, Hwu WJ, Kefford R, et al. Safety and tumor responses with lambrolizumab (anti-PD-1) in melanoma. *N Engl J Med.* (2013) 369:134–44. doi: 10.1056/NEJMoa1305133
9. Hanahan D, Weinberg RA. Hallmarks of cancer: the next generation. *Cell.* (2011) 144:646–74. doi: 10.1016/j.cell.2011.02.013
10. Bardhan K, Anagnostou T, Boussiotis VA. The PD1:PD-L1/2 pathway from discovery to clinical implementation. *Front Immunol.* (2016) 7:550. doi: 10.3389/fimmu.2016.00550
11. Badoual C, Hans S, Merillon N, Van Ryswick C, Ravel P, Benhamouda N, et al. PD-1-expressing tumor-infiltrating T cells are a favorable prognostic biomarker in HPV-associated head and neck cancer. *Cancer Res.* (2013) 73:128–38. doi: 10.1158/0008-5472.CAN-12-2606
12. Foy JP, Bertolus C, Michallet MC, Deneuve S, Incitti R, Bendriss-Vermare N, et al. The immune microenvironment of HPV-negative oral squamous cell carcinoma from never-smokers and never-drinkers patients suggests higher clinical benefit of IDO1 and PD1/PD-L1 blockade. *Ann Oncol.* (2017) 28:1934–41. doi: 10.1093/annonc/mdx210
13. Hsu C, Lee SH, Ejadi S, Even C, Cohen RB, Le Tourneau C, et al. Safety and antitumor activity of pembrolizumab in patients with programmed death-ligand 1-positive nasopharyngeal carcinoma: results of the KEYNOTE-028 study. *J Clin Oncol.* (2017) 35:4050–6. doi: 10.1200/JCO.2017.73.3675
14. Kim HS, Lee JY, Lim SH, Park K, Sun JM, Ko YH, et al. Association between PD-L1 and HPV status and the prognostic value of PD-L1 in oropharyngeal squamous cell carcinoma. *Cancer Res Treat.* (2016) 48:527–36. doi: 10.4143/crt.2015.249
15. Mletzko S, Pinato DJ, Robey RC, Dalla Pria A, Benson P, Imami N, et al. Programmed death ligand 1 (PD-L1) expression influences the immune-tolerogenic microenvironment in antiretroviral therapy-refractory Kaposi's sarcoma: a pilot study. *Oncoimmunology.* (2017) 6:e1304337. doi: 10.1080/2162402x.2017.1304337
16. Ritprajak P, Azuma M. Intrinsic and extrinsic control of expression of the immunoregulatory molecule PD-L1 in epithelial cells and squamous cell carcinoma. *Oral Oncol.* (2015) 51:221–8. doi: 10.1016/j.oraloncology.2014.11.014
17. Vassilakopoulou M, Avgeris M, Velcheti V, Kotoula V, Rampias T, Chatzopoulos K, et al. Evaluation of PD-L1 expression and associated tumor-infiltrating lymphocytes in laryngeal squamous cell carcinoma. *Clin Cancer Res.* (2016) 22:704–13. doi: 10.1158/1078-0432.CCR-15-1543
18. Chow LQM, Haddad R, Gupta S, Mahipal A, Mehra R, Tahara M, et al. Antitumor activity of pembrolizumab in biomarker-unselected patients with recurrent and/or metastatic head and neck squamous cell carcinoma: results from the phase Ib KEYNOTE-012 expansion cohort. *J Clin Oncol.* (2016) 34:3838–45. doi: 10.1200/JCO.2016.68.1478
19. Bauml J, Seiwert TY, Pfister DG, Worden F, Liu SV, Gilbert J, et al. Pembrolizumab for platinum- and cetuximab-refractory head and neck cancer: results from a single-arm, phase II study. *J Clin Oncol.* (2017) 35:1542–9. doi: 10.1200/JCO.2016.70.1524
20. Cohen EEW, Soulieres D, Le Tourneau C, Dinis J, Licitra L, Ahn MJ, et al. Pembrolizumab versus methotrexate, docetaxel, or cetuximab for recurrent or metastatic head-and-neck squamous cell carcinoma (KEYNOTE-040): a randomised, open-label, phase 3 study. *Lancet.* (2019) 393:156–67. doi: 10.1016/s0140-6736(18)31999-8

21. Ferris RL, Blumenschein G, Jr., Fayette J, Guigay J, Colevas AD, Licitra L, et al. Nivolumab for recurrent squamous-cell carcinoma of the head and neck. *N Engl J Med.* (2016) 375:1856–67. doi: 10.1056/NEJMoa1602252
22. Ferris RL, Blumenschein G Jr., Fayette J, Guigay J, Colevas AD, Licitra L, et al. Nivolumab vs investigator's choice in recurrent or metastatic squamous cell carcinoma of the head and neck: 2-year long-term survival update of CheckMate 141 with analyses by tumor PD-L1 expression. *Oral Oncol.* (2018) 81:45-51. doi: 10.1016/j.oraloncology.2018.04.008
23. Colevas AD, Bahleda R, Braiteh F, Balmanoukian A, Brana I, Chau NG, et al. Safety and clinical activity of atezolizumab in head and neck cancer: results from a phase I trial. *Ann Oncol.* (2018) 29:2247–53. doi: 10.1093/annonc/mdy411
24. Segal NH, Ou SI, Balmanoukian A, Fury MG, Massarelli E, Brahmer JR, et al. Safety and efficacy of durvalumab in patients with head and neck squamous cell carcinoma: results from a phase I/II expansion cohort. *Eur J Cancer.* (2019) 109:154-61. doi: 10.1016/j.ejca.2018.12.029
25. Siu LL, Even C, Mesia R, Remenar E, Daste A, Delord JP, et al. Safety and efficacy of durvalumab with or without tremelimumab in patients with PD-L1-low/negative recurrent or metastatic HNSCC: the phase 2 CONDOR randomized clinical trial. *JAMA Oncol.* (2018) 5:195-203. doi: 10.1001/jamaoncol.2018.4628
26. Bahig H, Aubin F, Stagg J, Gologan O, Ballivy O, Bissada E, et al. Phase I/II trial of durvalumab plus tremelimumab and stereotactic body radiotherapy for metastatic head and neck carcinoma. *BMC Cancer.* (2019) 19:68. doi: 10.1186/s12885-019-5266-4
27. Elbers JBW, Al-Mamgani A, Tesseslaar MET, van den Brekel MWM, Lange CAH, van der Wal JE, et al. Immuno-radiotherapy with cetuximab and avelumab for advanced stage head and neck squamous cell carcinoma: Results from a phase-I trial. *Radiother Oncol.* (2019) 142:79-84. doi: 10.1016/j.radonc.2019.08.007
28. Merlano MC, Merlotti AM, Licitra L, Denaro N, Fea E, Galizia D, et al. Activation of immune responses in patients with relapsed-metastatic head and neck cancer (CONFRONT phase I-II trial): multimodality immunotherapy with avelumab, short-course radiotherapy, and cyclophosphamide. *Clin Transl Radiat Oncol.* (2018) 12:47-52. doi: 10.1016/j.ctro.2018.08.001
29. Yu Y, Lee NY. JAVELIN head and neck 100: a phase III trial of avelumab and chemoradiation for locally advanced head and neck cancer. *Future Oncol.* (2019) 15:687–94. doi: 10.2217/fon-2018-0405
30. Sharma P, Hu-Lieskovan S, Wargo JA, Ribas A. Primary, adaptive, and acquired resistance to cancer immunotherapy. *Cell.* (2017) 168:707–23. doi: 10.1016/j.cell.2017.01.017
31. Cassetta L, Baekkevold ES, Brandau S, Bujko A, Cassatella MA, Dorhoi A, et al. Deciphering myeloid-derived suppressor cells: isolation and markers in humans, mice and non-human primates. *Cancer Immunol Immunother.* (2019) 68:687–97. doi: 10.1007/s00262-019-02302-2
32. Takahashi H, Sakakura K, Kudo T, Toyoda M, Kaira K, Oyama T, et al. Cancer-associated fibroblasts promote an immunosuppressive microenvironment through the induction and accumulation of protumoral macrophages. *Oncotarget.* (2017) 8:8633–47. doi: 10.18632/oncotarget.14374
33. Brooks JM, Menezes AN, Ibrahim M, Archer L, Lal N, Bagnall CJ, et al. Development and validation of a combined hypoxia and immune prognostic classifier for head and neck cancer. *Clin Cancer Res.* (2019) 25:5315–28. doi: 10.1158/1078-0432.CCR-18-3314
34. Barsoum IB, Smallwood CA, Siemens DR, Graham CH. A mechanism of hypoxia-mediated escape from adaptive immunity in cancer cells. *Cancer Res.* (2014) 74:665–74. doi: 10.1158/0008-5472.CAN-13-0992
35. Albacker LA, Wu J, Smith P, Warmuth M, Stephens PJ, Zhu P, et al. Loss of function JAK1 mutations occur at high frequency in cancers with microsatellite instability and are suggestive of immune evasion. *PLoS ONE.* (2017) 12:e0176181. doi: 10.1371/journal.pone.0176181
36. Routy B, Le Chatelier E, Derosa L, Duong CPM, Alou MT, Daillere R, et al. Gut microbiome influences efficacy of PD-1-based immunotherapy against epithelial tumors. *Science.* (2018) 359:91–7. doi: 10.1126/science.aan3706
37. Elkrief A, El Raichani L, Richard C, Messaoudene M, Belkaid W, Malo J, et al. Antibiotics are associated with decreased progression-free survival of advanced melanoma patients treated with immune checkpoint inhibitors. *Oncoimmunology.* (2019) 8:e1568812. doi: 10.1080/2162402x.2019.1568812
38. Lalani AA, Xie W, Braun DA, Kaymakcalan M, Bosse D, Steinharter JA, et al. Effect of antibiotic use on outcomes with systemic therapies in metastatic renal cell carcinoma. *Eur Urol Oncol.* (2019). doi: 10.1016/j.euo.2019.09.001. [Epub ahead of print].
39. Zhao S, Gao G, Li W, Li X, Zhao C, Jiang T, et al. Antibiotics are associated with attenuated efficacy of anti-PD-1/PD-L1 therapies in Chinese patients with advanced non-small cell lung cancer. *Lung Cancer.* (2019) 130:10-7. doi: 10.1016/j.lungcan.2019.01.017
40. Sakakura K, Takahashi H, Kaira K, Toyoda M, Murata T, Ohnishi H, et al. Relationship between tumor-associated macrophage subsets and CD47 expression in squamous cell carcinoma of the head and neck in the tumor microenvironment. *Lab Invest.* (2016) 96:994–1003. doi: 10.1038/labinvest.2016.70
41. Raber PL, Thevenot P, Sierra R, Wyczechowska D, Halle D, Ramirez ME, et al. Subpopulations of myeloid-derived suppressor cells impair T cell responses through independent nitric oxide-related pathways. *Int J Cancer.* (2014) 134:2853–64. doi: 10.1002/ijc.28622
42. Rahma OE, Hodi FS. The intersection between tumor angiogenesis and immune suppression. *Clin Cancer Res.* (2019) 25:5449–57. doi: 10.1158/1078-0432.Ccr-18-1543
43. Kato R, Yamasaki M, Urakawa S, Nishida K, Makino T, Morimoto-Okazawa A, et al. Increased Tim-3(+) T cells in PBMCs during nivolumab therapy correlate with responses and prognosis of advanced esophageal squamous cell carcinoma patients. *Cancer Immunol Immunother.* (2018) 67:1673–83. doi: 10.1007/s00262-018-2225-x
44. Liu Z, McMichael EL, Shayan G, Li J, Chen K, Srivastava R, et al. Novel effector phenotype of Tim-3(+) regulatory T cells leads to enhanced suppressive function in head and neck cancer patients. *Clin Cancer Res.* (2018) 24:4529–38. doi: 10.1158/1078-0432.CCR-17-1350
45. Quan H, Fang L, Pan H, Deng Z, Gao S, Liu O, et al. An adaptive immune response driven by mature, antigen-experienced T and B cells within the microenvironment of oral squamous cell carcinoma. *Int J Cancer.* (2016) 138:2952–62. doi: 10.1002/ijc.30019
46. Shayan G, Srivastava R, Li J, Schmitt N, Kane LP, Ferris RL. Adaptive resistance to anti-PD1 therapy by Tim-3 upregulation is mediated by the PI3K-Akt pathway in head and neck cancer. *Oncoimmunology.* (2016) 6:e1261779. doi: 10.1080/2162402X.2016.1261779
47. Linedale R, Schmidt C, King BT, Ganko AG, Simpson F, Panizza BJ, et al. Elevated frequencies of CD8 T cells expressing PD-1, CTLA-4 and Tim-3 within tumour from perineural squamous cell carcinoma patients. *PLoS ONE.* (2017) 12:e0175755. doi: 10.1371/journal.pone.01 75755
48. Oweida A, Hararah MK, Phan A, Binder D, Bhatia S, Lennon S, et al. Resistance to radiotherapy and PD-L1 blockade is mediated by TIM-3 upregulation and regulatory T-cell infiltration. *Clin Cancer Res.* (2018) 24:5368–80. doi: 10.1158/1078-0432.CCR-18-1038
49. Concha-Benavente F, Srivastava R, Ferrone S, Ferris RL. Immunological and clinical significance of HLA class I antigen processing machinery component defects in malignant cells. *Oral Oncol.* (2016) 58:52-8. doi: 10.1016/j.oraloncology.2016.05.008
50. Gettinger S, Choi J, Hastings K, Truini A, Datar I, Sowell R, et al. Impaired HLA class i antigen processing and presentation as a mechanism of acquired resistance to immune checkpoint inhibitors in lung cancer. *Cancer Discov.* (2017) 7:1420–35. doi: 10.1158/2159-8290.Cd-17-0593
51. Ogino T, Shigyo H, Ishii H, Katayama A, Miyokawa N, Harabuchi Y, et al. HLA class I antigen down-regulation in primary laryngeal squamous cell carcinoma lesions as a poor prognostic marker. *Cancer Res.* (2006) 66:9281–9. doi: 10.1158/0008-5472.CAN-06-0488
52. Paulson KG, Voillet V, McAfee MS, Hunter DS, Wagener FD, Perdicchio M, et al. Acquired cancer resistance to combination immunotherapy from transcriptional loss of class I HLA. *Nature Commun.* (2018) 9:3868. doi: 10.1038/s41467-018-06300-3
53. Leibowitz MS, Andrade Filho PA, Ferrone S, Ferris RL. Deficiency of activated STAT1 in head and neck cancer cells mediates TAP1-dependent escape from cytotoxic T lymphocytes. *Cancer Immunol Immunother.* (2011) 60:525–35. doi: 10.1007/s00262-010-0961-7
54. Chikamatsu K, Takahashi G, Sakakura K, Ferrone S, Masuyama K. Immunoregulatory properties of CD44+ cancer stem-like cells in squamous

cell carcinoma of the head and neck. *Head Neck.* (2011) 33:208–15. doi: 10.1002/hed.21420

55. Zhang J, Bu X, Wang H, Zhu Y, Geng Y, Nihira NT, et al. Cyclin D-CDK4 kinase destabilizes PD-L1 via cullin 3-SPOP to control cancer immune surveillance. *Nature.* (2018) 553:91–5. doi: 10.1038/nature25015
56. Chen JC, Perez-Lorenzo R, Saenger YM, Drake CG, Christiano AM. IKZF1 enhances immune infiltrate recruitment in solid tumors and susceptibility to immunotherapy. *Cell Syst.* (2018) 7:92–103.e4. doi: 10.1016/j.cels.2018.05.020
57. Cassat JE, Skaar EP. Iron in infection and immunity. *Cell Host Microbe.* (2013) 13:509–19. doi: 10.1016/j.chom.2013.04.010
58. Cronin SJF, Seehus C, Weidinger A, Talbot S, Reissig S, Seifert M, et al. The metabolite BH4 controls T cell proliferation in autoimmunity and cancer. *Nature.* (2018) 563:564–8. doi: 10.1038/s41586-018-0701-2
59. Hung N, Shen CC, Hu YW, Hu LY, Yeh CM, Teng CJ, et al. Risk of cancer in patients with iron deficiency anemia: a nationwide population-based study. *PLoS ONE.* (2015) 10:e0119647. doi: 10.1371/journal.pone.0119647
60. Ayers M, Lunceford J, Nebozhyn M, Murphy E, Loboda A, Kaufman DR, et al. IFN-gamma-related mRNA profile predicts clinical response to PD-1 blockade. *J Clin Investig.* (2017) 127:2930–40. doi: 10.1172/JCI91190
61. Chen YP, Wang YQ, Lv JW, Li YQ, Chua MLK, Le QT, et al. Identification and validation of novel microenvironment-based immune molecular subgroups of head and neck squamous cell carcinoma: implications for immunotherapy. *Ann Oncol.* (2019) 30:68–75. doi: 10.1093/annonc/mdy470
62. Cadwell K, Wu L, Cao J, Cai WL, Lang SM, Horton JR, et al. KDM5 histone demethylases repress immune response via suppression of STING. *PLoS Biology.* (2018) 16:e2006134. doi: 10.1371/journal.pbio.2006134.
63. Ryan N, Anderson K, Volpedo G, Hamza O, Varikuti S, Satoskar AR, et al. STAT1 inhibits T cell exhaustion and myeloid derived suppressor cell accumulation to promote anti-tumor immune responses in head and neck squamous cell carcinoma. *Int J Cancer.* (2019) 146:1717–1729. doi: 10.1002/ijc.32781
64. Barry KC, Hsu J, Broz ML, Cueto FJ, Binnewies M, Combes AJ, et al. A natural killer-dendritic cell axis defines checkpoint therapy-responsive tumor microenvironments. *Nat Med.* (2018) 24:1178–91. doi: 10.1038/s41591-018-0085-8
65. Chrisikos TT, Zhou Y, Slone N, Babcock R, Watowich SS, Li HS. Molecular regulation of dendritic cell development and function in homeostasis, inflammation, and cancer. *Mol Immunol.* (2019) 110:24-39. doi: 10.1016/j.molimm.2018.01.014
66. Versteven M, Van den Bergh JMJ, Marcq E, Smits ELJ, Van Tendeloo VFI, Hobo W, et al. Dendritic cells and programmed death-1 blockade: a joint venture to combat cancer. *Front Immunol.* (2018) 9:394. doi: 10.3389/fimmu.2018.00394
67. Mita Y, Kimura MY, Hayashizaki K, Koyama-Nasu R, Ito T, Motohashi S, et al. Crucial role of CD69 in anti-tumor immunity through regulating the exhaustion of tumor-infiltrating T cells. *Int Immunol.* (2018) 30:559–67. doi: 10.1093/intimm/dxy050
68. Laimer K, Troester B, Kloss F, Schafer G, Obrist P, Perathoner A, et al. Expression and prognostic impact of indoleamine 2,3-dioxygenase in oral squamous cell carcinomas. *Oral Oncol.* (2011) 47:352–7. doi: 10.1016/j.oraloncology.2011.03.007
69. Platten M, Nollen EAA, Rohrig UF, Fallarino F, Opitz CA. Tryptophan metabolism as a common therapeutic target in cancer, neurodegeneration and beyond. *Nat Rev Drug Discov.* (2019) 18:379–401. doi: 10.1038/s41573-019-0016-5
70. Holmgaard RB, Schaer DA, Li Y, Castaneda SP, Murphy MY, Xu X, et al. Targeting the TGFbeta pathway with galunisertib, a TGFbetaRI small molecule inhibitor, promotes anti-tumor immunity leading to durable, complete responses, as monotherapy and in combination with checkpoint blockade. *J Immunother Cancer.* (2018) 6:47. doi: 10.1186/s40425-018-0356-4
71. Mariathasan S, Turley SJ, Nickles D, Castiglioni A, Yuen K, Wang Y, et al. TGFbeta attenuates tumour response to PD-L1 blockade by contributing to exclusion of T cells. *Nature.* (2018) 554:544–8. doi: 10.1038/nature25501
72. Tauriello DVF, Palomo-Ponce S, Stork D, Berenguer-Llergo A, Badia-Ramentol J, Iglesias M, et al. TGFbeta drives immune evasion in genetically reconstituted colon cancer metastasis. *Nature.* (2018) 554:538–43. doi: 10.1038/nature25492
73. Weber F, Byrne SN, Le S, Brown DA, Breit SN, Scolyer RA, et al. Transforming growth factor-beta1 immobilises dendritic cells within skin tumours and facilitates tumour escape from the immune system. *Cancer Immunol Immunother.* (2005) 54:898–906. doi: 10.1007/s00262-004-0652-3
74. Steggerda SM, Bennett MK, Chen J, Emberley E, Huang T, Janes JR, et al. Inhibition of arginase by CB-1158 blocks myeloid cell-mediated immune suppression in the tumor microenvironment. *J Immunother Cancer.* (2017) 5:101. doi: 10.1186/s40425-017-0308-4
75. Chen L, Diao L, Yang Y, Yi X, Rodriguez BL, Li Y, et al. CD38-mediated immunosuppression as a mechanism of tumor cell escape from PD-1/PD-L1 blockade. *Cancer Discov.* (2018) 8:1156–75. doi: 10.1158/2159-8290.CD-17-1033
76. Mittal D, Vijayan D, Smyth MJ. Overcoming acquired PD-1/PD-L1 resistance with CD38 blockade. *Cancer Discov.* (2018) 8:1066–8. doi: 10.1158/2159-8290.CD-18-0798
77. Krishna S, Ulrich P, Wilson E, Parikh F, Narang P, Yang S, et al. Human papilloma virus specific immunogenicity and dysfunction of CD8(+) T cells in head and neck cancer. *Cancer Res.* (2018) 78:6159–70. doi: 10.1158/0008-5472.Can-18-0163
78. Leone RD, Sun IM, Oh MH, Sun IH, Wen J, Englert J, et al. Inhibition of the adenosine A2a receptor modulates expression of T cell coinhibitory receptors and improves effector function for enhanced checkpoint blockade and ACT in murine cancer models. *Cancer Immunol Immunother.* (2018) 67:1271–84. doi: 10.1007/s00262-018-2186-0
79. Deng W-W, Li Y-C, Ma S-R, Mao L, Yu G-T, Bu L-L, et al. Specific blockade CD73 alters the "exhausted" phenotype of T cells in head and neck squamous cell carcinoma. *Int J Cancer.* (2018) 143:1494–504. doi: 10.1002/ijc.31534
80. Chen L, Huang C-F, Li Y-C, Deng W-W, Mao L, Wu L, et al. Blockage of the NLRP3 inflammasome by MCC950 improves anti-tumor immune responses in head and neck squamous cell carcinoma. *Cell Mol. Life Sci.* (2018) 75:2045–58. doi: 10.1007/s00018-017-2720-9
81. Andrews LP, Marciscano AE, Drake CG, Vignali DA. LAG3 (CD223) as a cancer immunotherapy target. *Immunol Rev.* (2017) 276:80–96. doi: 10.1111/imr.12519
82. Gameiro SF, Ghasemi F, Barrett JW, Koropatnick J, Nichols AC, Mymryk JS, et al. Treatment-naive HPV+ head and neck cancers display a T-cell-inflamed phenotype distinct from their HPV- counterparts that has implications for immunotherapy. *Oncoimmunology.* (2018) 7:e1498439. doi: 10.1080/2162402x.2018.1498439
83. Mandal R, Senbabaoglu Y, Desrichard A, Havel JJ, Dalin MG, Riaz N, et al. The head and neck cancer immune landscape and its immunotherapeutic implications. *JCI Insight.* (2016) 1:e89829. doi: 10.1172/jci.insight.89829
84. Shayan G, Kansy BA, Gibson SP, Srivastava RM, Bryan JK, Bauman JE, et al. Phase Ib study of immune biomarker modulation with neoadjuvant cetuximab and TLR8 stimulation in head and neck cancer to overcome suppressive myeloid signals. *Clin Cancer Res.* (2018) 24:62–72. doi: 10.1158/1078-0432.Ccr-17-0357
85. Wu L, Mao L, Liu JF, Chen L, Yu GT, Yang LL, et al. Blockade of TIGIT/CD155 signaling reverses T-cell exhaustion and enhances antitumor capability in head and neck squamous cell carcinoma. *Cancer Immunol Res.* (2019) 7:1700–13. doi: 10.1158/2326-6066.Cir-18-0725
86. Koyama S, Akbay EA, Li YY, Herter-Sprie GS, Buczkowski KA, Richards WG, et al. Adaptive resistance to therapeutic PD-1 blockade is associated with upregulation of alternative immune checkpoints. *Nat Commun.* (2016) 7:10501. doi: 10.1038/ncomms10501
87. Kondo Y, Ohno T, Nishii N, Harada K, Yagita H, Azuma M. Differential contribution of three immune checkpoint (VISTA, CTLA-4, PD-1) pathways to antitumor responses against squamous cell carcinoma. *Oral Oncol.* (2016) 57:54-60. doi: 10.1016/j.oraloncology.2016.04.005
88. Wu L, Deng WW, Huang CF, Bu LL, Yu GT, Mao L, et al. Expression of VISTA correlated with immunosuppression and synergized with CD8 to predict survival in human oral squamous cell carcinoma. *Cancer Immunol Immunother.* (2017) 66:627–36. doi: 10.1007/s00262-017-1968-0

89. Zhang XJ, Jin Y, Song JL, Deng F. MiR-373 promotes proliferation and metastasis of oral squamous cell carcinoma by targeting SPOP. *Eur Rev Med Pharmacol Sci.* (2019) 23:5270–6. doi: 10.26355/eurrev_201906_18193
90. Hammerman PS, Hayes DN, Grandis JR. Therapeutic insights from genomic studies of head and neck squamous cell carcinomas. *Cancer Discov.* (2015) 5:239–44. doi: 10.1158/2159-8290.CD-14-1205
91. Bernal M, Ruiz-Cabello F, Concha A, Paschen A, Garrido F. Implication of the beta2-microglobulin gene in the generation of tumor escape phenotypes. *Cancer Immunol Immunother.* (2012) 61:1359–71. doi: 10.1007/s00262-012-1321-6
92. Mediavilla-Varela M, Castro J, Chiappori A, Noyes D, Hernandez DC, Allard B, et al. A Novel antagonist of the immune checkpoint protein adenosine A2a receptor restores tumor-infiltrating lymphocyte activity in the context of the tumor microenvironment. *Neoplasia.* (2017) 19:530–6. doi: 10.1016/j.neo.2017.02.004
93. Young A, Mittal D, Stagg J, Smyth MJ. Targeting cancer-derived adenosine: new therapeutic approaches. *Cancer Discov.* (2014) 4:879–88. doi: 10.1158/2159-8290.CD-14-0341
94. Hausler SF, Montalban del Barrio I, Strohschein J, Chandran PA, Engel JB, Honig A, et al. Ectonucleotidases CD39 and CD73 on OvCA cells are potent adenosine-generating enzymes responsible for adenosine receptor 2A-dependent suppression of T cell function and NK cell cytotoxicity. *Cancer Immunol Immunother.* (2011) 60:1405–18. doi: 10.1007/s00262-011-1040-4
95. Ohta A, Gorelik E, Prasad SJ, Ronchese F, Lukashev D, Wong MK, et al. A2A adenosine receptor protects tumors from antitumor T cells. *Proc Natl Acad Sci USA.* (2006) 103:13132–7. doi: 10.1073/pnas.0605251103
96. Malavasi F, Deaglio S, Funaro A, Ferrero E, Horenstein AL, Ortolan E, et al. Evolution and function of the ADP ribosyl cyclase/CD38 gene family in physiology and pathology. *Physiol Rev.* (2008) 88:841–86. doi: 10.1152/physrev.00035.2007
97. Cohen EEW, Bell RB, Bifulco CB, Burtness B, Gillison ML, Harrington KJ, et al. The Society for Immunotherapy of Cancer consensus statement on immunotherapy for the treatment of squamous cell carcinoma of the head and neck (HNSCC). *J Immunother Cancer.* (2019) 7:184. doi: 10.1186/s40425-019-0662-5.
98. Rasmussen JH, Lelkaitis G, Hakansson K, Vogelius IR, Johannesen HH, Fischer BM, et al. Intratumor heterogeneity of PD-L1 expression in head and neck squamous cell carcinoma. *Br J Cancer.* (2019) 120:1003–6. doi: 10.1038/s41416-019-0449-y
99. Mandal R, Samstein RM, Lee KW, Havel JJ, Wang H, Krishna C, et al. Genetic diversity of tumors with mismatch repair deficiency influences anti-PD-1 immunotherapy response. *Science.* (2019) 364:485–91. doi: 10.1126/science.aau0447
100. Faden DL, Ding F, Lin Y, Zhai S, Kuo F, Chan TA, et al. APOBEC mutagenesis is tightly linked to the immune landscape and immunotherapy biomarkers in head and neck squamous cell carcinoma. *Oral Oncol.* (2019) 96:140-7. doi: 10.1016/j.oraloncology.2019.07.020
101. Faden DL, Thomas S, Cantalupo PG, Agrawal N, Myers J, DeRisi J. Multi-modality analysis supports APOBEC as a major source of mutations in head and neck squamous cell carcinoma. *Oral Oncol.* (2017) 74:8-14. doi: 10.1016/j.oraloncology.2017.09.002
102. Gillison ML, Akagi K, Xiao W, Jiang B, Pickard RKL, Li J, et al. Human papillomavirus and the landscape of secondary genetic alterations in oral cancers. *Genome Res.* (2019) 29:1–17. doi: 10.1101/gr.2411 41.118
103. Ayers M, Lunceford J, Nebozhyn M, Murphy E, Loboda A, Albright A, et al. Relationship between immune gene signatures and clinical response to PD-1 blockade with pembrolizumab (MK-3475) in patients with advanced solid tumors. *J Immunother Cancer.* (2015) 3(Suppl. 2):P80. doi: 10.1186/2051-1426-3-s2-p80
104. Georgiadis A, Durham JN, Keefer LA, Bartlett BR, Zielonka M, Murphy D, et al. Noninvasive detection of microsatellite instability and high tumor mutation burden[[Inline Image]] in cancer patients treated with PD-1 blockade. *Clin Cancer Res.* (2019) 25:7024–34. doi: 10.1158/1078-0432.CCR-19-1372
105. Hanna GJ, Lizotte P, Cavanaugh M, Kuo FC, Shivdasani P, Frieden A, et al. Frameshift events predict anti-PD-1/L1 response in head and neck cancer. *JCI Insight.* (2018) 3:98811. doi: 10.1172/jci.insight. 98811
106. Demokan S, Suoglu Y, Demir D, Gozeler M, Dalay N. Microsatellite instability and methylation of the DNA mismatch repair genes in head and neck cancer. *Ann Oncol.* (2006) 17:995–9. doi: 10.1093/annonc/mdl048
107. Lin JC, Wang CC, Jiang RS, Wang WY, Liu SA. Microsatellite alteration in head and neck squamous cell carcinoma patients from a betel quid-prevalent region. *Sci Rep.* (2016) 6:22614. doi: 10.1038/srep22614
108. Le DT, Durham JN, Smith KN, Wang H, Bartlett BR, Aulakh LK, et al. Mismatch repair deficiency predicts response of solid tumors to PD-1 blockade. *Science.* (2017) 357:409–13. doi: 10.1126/science. aan6733
109. Chalmers ZR, Connelly CF, Fabrizio D, Gay L, Ali SM, Ennis R, et al. Analysis of 100,000 human cancer genomes reveals the landscape of tumor mutational burden. *Genome Med.* (2017) 9:34. doi: 10.1186/s13073-017-0424-2
110. Seiwert TY, Burtness B, Mehra R, Weiss J, Berger R, Eder JP, et al. Safety and clinical activity of pembrolizumab for treatment of recurrent or metastatic squamous cell carcinoma of the head and neck (KEYNOTE-012): an open-label, multicentre, phase 1b trial. *Lancet Oncol.* (2016) 17:956–65. doi: 10.1016/s1470-2045(16)30066-3.
111. Wallden B, Pekker I, Popa S, Dowidar N, Sullivan A, Hood T, et al. Development and analytical performance of a molecular diagnostic for anti-PD1 response on the nCounter Dx Analysis System. *J Clin Oncol.* (2016) 34(15_suppl):3034. doi: 10.1200/JCO.2016.34.15_suppl.3034

Permissions

All chapters in this book were first published by Frontiers; hereby published with permission under the Creative Commons Attribution License or equivalent. Every chapter published in this book has been scrutinized by our experts. Their significance has been extensively debated. The topics covered herein carry significant findings which will fuel the growth of the discipline. They may even be implemented as practical applications or may be referred to as a beginning point for another development.

The contributors of this book come from diverse backgrounds, making this book a truly international effort. This book will bring forth new frontiers with its revolutionizing research information and detailed analysis of the nascent developments around the world.

We would like to thank all the contributing authors for lending their expertise to make the book truly unique. They have played a crucial role in the development of this book. Without their invaluable contributions this book wouldn't have been possible. They have made vital efforts to compile up to date information on the varied aspects of this subject to make this book a valuable addition to the collection of many professionals and students.

This book was conceptualized with the vision of imparting up-to-date information and advanced data in this field. To ensure the same, a matchless editorial board was set up. Every individual on the board went through rigorous rounds of assessment to prove their worth. After which they invested a large part of their time researching and compiling the most relevant data for our readers.

The editorial board has been involved in producing this book since its inception. They have spent rigorous hours researching and exploring the diverse topics which have resulted in the successful publishing of this book. They have passed on their knowledge of decades through this book. To expedite this challenging task, the publisher supported the team at every step. A small team of assistant editors was also appointed to further simplify the editing procedure and attain best results for the readers.

Apart from the editorial board, the designing team has also invested a significant amount of their time in understanding the subject and creating the most relevant covers. They scrutinized every image to scout for the most suitable representation of the subject and create an appropriate cover for the book.

The publishing team has been an ardent support to the editorial, designing and production team. Their endless efforts to recruit the best for this project, has resulted in the accomplishment of this book. They are a veteran in the field of academics and their pool of knowledge is as vast as their experience in printing. Their expertise and guidance has proved useful at every step. Their uncompromising quality standards have made this book an exceptional effort. Their encouragement from time to time has been an inspiration for everyone.

The publisher and the editorial board hope that this book will prove to be a valuable piece of knowledge for researchers, students, practitioners and scholars across the globe.

List of Contributors

Shih-Hao Wang
Department of Otolaryngology, Ditmanson Medical Foundation, Chiayi Christian Hospital, Chiayi, Taiwan
Department of Biotechnology, Asia University, Taichung, Taiwan

Hsi-Chin Wu
School of Medicine, China Medical University, Taichung, Taiwan

Khan Farheen Badrealam and Da-Tian Bau
Graduate Institute of Biomedicine, China Medical University and Hospital, Taichung, Taiwan

Yueh-Hsiung Kuo
Department of Biotechnology, Asia University, Taichung, Taiwan
Department of Chinese Pharmaceutical Sciences and Chinese Medicine Resources, China Medical University, Taichung, Taiwan
Chinese Medicine Research Center, China Medical University, Taichung, Taiwan

Yun-Peng Chao
Department of Chemical Engineering, Feng Chia University, Taichung, Taiwan

Hsi-Hsien Hsu
Division of Colorectal Surgery, Mackay Memorial Hospital, Taipei, Taiwan
Mackay Medicine, Nursing and Management College, Taipei, Taiwan

Vijaya Padma Viswanadha
Department of Biotechnology, Bharathiar University, Coimbatore, India

Yi-Hui Chen
Department of M-Commerce and Multimedia Applications, Asia University, Taichung, Taiwan

Pei-Jei Lio and Chung-Jen Chiang
Department of Medical Laboratory Science and Biotechnology, China Medical University, Taichung, Taiwan

Chih-Yang Huang
Department of Biotechnology, Asia University, Taichung, Taiwan
Graduate Institute of Biomedicine, China Medical University and Hospital, Taichung, Taiwan
Cardiovascular and Mitochondria Related Diseases Research Center, Hualien Tzu Chi Hospital, Hualien, Taiwan
Center of General Education, Buddhist Tzu Chi Medical Foundation, Tzu Chi University of Science and Technology, Hualien, Taiwan
Department of Medical Research, China Medical University Hospital, China Medical University, Taichung, Taiwan

Xuehua Xi
Department of Ultrasound, China–Japan Friendship Hospital, Beijing, China

Luying Gao, Ruyu Liu, Xiao Yang, Shenling Zhu, Ruina Zhao, Xingjian Lai, Xiaoyan Zhang and Yuxin Jiang
Department of Ultrasound, Peking Union Medical College Hospital, Chinese Academy of Medical Sciences & Peking Union Medical College, Beijing, China

Bo Zhang
Department of Ultrasound, China–Japan Friendship Hospital, Beijing, China
Department of Ultrasound, Peking Union Medical College Hospital, Chinese Academy of Medical Sciences & Peking Union Medical College, Beijing, China

Qiong Wu
Department of Ultrasound, Peking Union Medical College Hospital, Chinese Academy of Medical Sciences & Peking Union Medical College, Beijing, China
Department of Ultrasound, Affiliated Hospital of Qingdao University, Qingdao, China

Shibao Fang
Department of Ultrasound, Affiliated Hospital of Qingdao University, Qingdao, China

Jingzhu Xu
Department of General Surgery, Peking Union Medical College Hospital, Chinese Academy of Medical Sciences & Peking Union Medical College, Beijing, China

Annette M. Lim and Danny Rischin
Department of Medical Oncology, Peter MacCallum Cancer Centre, Melbourne, VIC, Australia
Sir Peter MacCallum Department of Oncology, Faculty of Medicine, Dentistry and Health Sciences, The University of Melbourne, VIC, Australia

Karda Cavanagh
Department of Cancer Imaging, Peter MacCallum Cancer Centre, Melbourne, VIC, Australia

Rodney J. Hicks
Department of Nuclear Medicine, Peter MacCallum Cancer Centre, Melbourne, VIC, Australia

Luke McLean
Department of Medical Oncology, Peter MacCallum Cancer Centre, Melbourne, VIC, Australia

Michelle S. Goh
Department of Dermatology, Peter MacCallum Cancer Centre, Melbourne, VIC, Australia

Angela Webb
Department of Plastic Surgery, Peter MacCallum Cancer Centre, Melbourne, VIC, Australia

Deguang Kong and Zhisu Liu
Department of General Surgery, Zhongnan Hospital of Wuhan University, Wuhan, China

Anping Li and Kongming Wu
Department of Medical Oncology, The Affiliated Cancer Hospital of Zhengzhou University and Henan Cancer Hospital, Zhengzhou, China

Yu Liu
Department of Geriatrics, Tongji Hospital of Tongji Medical College, Huazhong University of Science and Technology, Wuhan, China

Qiuxia Cui, Jianing Tang and Gaosong Wu
Department of Thyroid and Breast Surgery, Zhongnan Hospital of Wuhan University, Wuhan, China

Kun Wang, Dan Zhang and Yaying Du
Department of Thyroid and Breast Surgery, Tongji Hospital of Tongji Medical College, Huazhong University of Science and Technology, Wuhan, China

Xiangrui Meng and Huilai Zhang
Key Laboratory of Cancer Prevention and Therapy, Department of Lymphoma, National Clinical Research Center for Cancer, Tianjin's Clinical Research Center for Cancer, Tianjin Medical University Cancer Institute and Hospital, Tianjin, China

Huijuan Wang, Jingzhu Zhao, Linfei Hu, Jingtai Zhi, Songfeng Wei, Xianhui Ruan, Xiukun Hou, Dapeng Li, Jun Zhang, Xiangqian Zheng and Ming Gao
Key Laboratory of Cancer Prevention and Therapy, Department of Thyroid and Neck Tumor, National Clinical Research Center for Cancer, Tianjin's Clinical Research Center for Cancer, Tianjin Medical University Cancer Institute and Hospital, Tianjin, China

Weiwei Yang
Department of Otolaryngology-Head and Neck Surgery, Tianjin First Center Hospital, Tianjin, China

Biyun Qian
Department of Epidemiology, School of Public Health, Shanghai Jiao Tong University, Shanghai, China

Yu Wu
Key Laboratory of Cancer Prevention and Therapy, Department of Thyroid and Neck Tumor, National Clinical Research Center for Cancer, Tianjin's Clinical Research Center for Cancer, Tianjin Medical University Cancer Institute and Hospital, Tianjin, China
Department of Head and Neck Surgery, Fujian Cancer Hospital, Fujian Medical University Cancer Hospital, Fujian, China

Yuan Zhang
Department of Head and Neck Surgery, Jiangsu Cancer Hospital, Jiangsu Institute of Cancer Research, Nanjing Medical University Affiliated Cancer Hospital, Nanjing, China

Zhaowei Meng
Department of Nuclear Medicine, Tianjin Medical University General Hospital, Tianjin, China

Lizhao Guan
Department of Biochemistry and Molecular Biology, School of Basic Medical Sciences, Tianjin Medical University, Tianjin, China

Francesca Piludu and Antonello Vidiri
Radiology and Diagnostic Imaging Department, IRCCS Regina Elena National Cancer Institute, Rome, Italy

Simona Marzi
Medical Physics Laboratory, IRCCS Regina Elena National Cancer Institute, Rome, Italy
Marco Ravanelli, Davide Farina and Riccardo Campora
Department of Radiology, University of Brescia, Brescia, Italy

Raul Pellini
Department of Otolaryngology & Head and Neck Surgery, IRCCS Regina Elena National Cancer Institute, Rome, Italy

Renato Covello
Department of Pathology, IRCCS Regina Elena National Cancer Institute, Rome, Italy

Irene Terrenato
Biostatistics-Scientific Direction, IRCCS Regina Elena National Cancer Institute, Rome, Italy

Valentina Ferrazzoli
Department of Biomedicine and Prevention, University of Rome "Tor Vergata", Rome, Italy

Wenli Yang, Minglei Sun, Qiaoyan Jie, Haixia Zhou, Peng Zhang and Juanfang Zhu
Department of Stomatology, The First Affiliated Hospital of Zhengzhou University, Zhengzhou, China

Melvin A. Ambele
Department of Oral Pathology and Oral Biology, Faculty of Health Sciences, School of Dentistry, University of Pretoria, Pretoria, South Africa
Department of Immunology, and SAMRC Extramural Unit for Stem Cell Research and Therapy, Faculty of Health Sciences, Institute for Cellular and Molecular Medicine, University of Pretoria, Pretoria, South Africa

Andre van Zyl
Specialist in Oral Medicine and Periodontics, Private Practice, Stellenbosch, South Africa

Michael S. Pepper
Department of Immunology, and SAMRC Extramural Unit for Stem Cell Research and Therapy, Faculty of Health Sciences, Institute for Cellular and Molecular Medicine, University of Pretoria, Pretoria, South Africa

Marlene B. van Heerden and Willie F. P. van Heerden
Department of Oral Pathology and Oral Biology, Faculty of Health Sciences, School of Dentistry, University of Pretoria, Pretoria, South Africa

Erika Crosetti and Giulia Arrigoni
Head and Neck Oncology Unit, Candiolo Cancer Institute, Fondazione del Piemonte per l'Oncologia - IRCCS (FPO-IRCCS), Candiolo, Italy

Andrea Elio Sprio
Department of Biomedical and Clinic Sciences, University of Turin, Orbassano, Italy

Giovanni Succo
Head and Neck Oncology Unit, Candiolo Cancer Institute, Fondazione del Piemonte per l'Oncologia - IRCCS (FPO-IRCCS), Candiolo, Italy
Department of Oncology, University of Turin, Orbassano, Italy

Chengzhi Xu, Yong Shi and Ming Zhang
Department of Otolaryngology—Head and Neck Surgery, Eye Ear Nose and Throat Hospital, Fudan University, Shanghai, China

Yunbin Zhang
Shanghai Institute of Biochemistry and Cell Biology, Chinese Academy of Sciences, University of Chinese Academy of Sciences, Shanghai, China
Department of Respirology, Shanghai Public Health Clinical Center, Fudan University, Shanghai, China

Yupeng Shen
Department of Otolaryngology—Head and Neck Surgery, Bethune International Peace Hospital, Shijiazhuang, China

Wan-Chun Li
Institute of Oral Biology, School of Dentistry, National Yang-Ming University, Taipei, Taiwan
Department of Dentistry, School of Dentistry, National Yang-Ming University, Taipei, Taiwan
Cancer Progression Research Center, National Yang-Ming University, Taipei, Taiwan

Chien-Hsiang Huang, Yi-Ta Hsieh, Tsai-Ying Chen, Li-Hao Cheng and Chang-Yi Chen
Institute of Oral Biology, School of Dentistry, National Yang-Ming University, Taipei, Taiwan
Department of Dentistry, School of Dentistry, National Yang-Ming University, Taipei, Taiwan

Chung-Ji Liu
Institute of Oral Biology, School of Dentistry, National Yang-Ming University, Taipei, Taiwan
Department of Dentistry, School of Dentistry, National Yang-Ming University, Taipei, Taiwan
Department of Oral and Maxillofacial Surgery, MacKay Memorial Hospital, Taipei, Taiwan
Department of Medical Research, MacKay Memorial Hospital, Taipei, Taiwan

Hsin-Ming Chen
School of Dentistry and Department of Dentistry, National Taiwan University Medical College and National Taiwan University Hospital, Taipei, Taiwan

Chien-Ling Huang
Department of Health Technology and Informatics (HTI), The Hong Kong Polytechnic University (PolyU), Kowloon, Hong Kong

Jeng-Fan Lo
Institute of Oral Biology, National Yang-Ming University, Taipei, Taiwan
Department of Dentistry, School of Dentistry, National Yang-Ming University, Taipei, Taiwan
Cancer Progression Research Center, National Yang-Ming University, Taipei, Taiwan
Department of Dentistry, Taipei Veterans General Hospital, Taipei, Taiwan
Department of Stomatology, Taipei Veterans General Hospital, Taipei, Taiwan

Kuo-Wei Chang
Institute of Oral Biology, School of Dentistry, National Yang-Ming University, Taipei, Taiwan
Department of Dentistry, School of Dentistry, National Yang-Ming University, Taipei, Taiwan
Cancer Progression Research Center, National Yang-Ming University, Taipei, Taiwan
Department of Stomatology, Taipei Veterans General Hospital, Taipei, Taiwan

Katharina Hintelmann, Thomas Berenz, Sabrina Christiansen, Fruzsina Gatzemeier, Agnes Oetting and Thorsten Rieckmann
Department of Otorhinolaryngology, University Medical Center Hamburg-Eppendorf, Hamburg, Germany
Department of Radiotherapy, University Medical Center Hamburg-Eppendorf, Hamburg, Germany

Malte Kriegs, Cordula Petersen and Kai Rothkamm
Department of Radiotherapy, University Medical Center Hamburg-Eppendorf, Hamburg, Germany

Liang Zhou, Duo Zhang, Wei-Jing Tang, Di Tang, Xiao-Ling Shi, Yue Yang and Lei Tao
Department of Otolaryngology, Eye, Ear, Nose and Throat Hospital, Fudan University, Shanghai, China
Shanghai Key Clinical Disciplines of Otorhinolaryngology, Shanghai, China

Christian Betz
Department of Otorhinolaryngology, University Medical Center Hamburg-Eppendorf, Hamburg, Germany

Nina Struve
Department of Radiotherapy, University Medical Center Hamburg-Eppendorf, Hamburg, Germany
Mildred-Scheel Cancer Career Center HATRICs4, University Medical Center Hamburg-Eppendorf, Hamburg, Germany

Chia-Ming Yeh and Mu-Kuan Chen
Institute of Medicine, Chung Shan Medical University, Taichung, Taiwan
Cancer Research Center, Changhua Christian Hospital, Changhua, Taiwan
Department of Otorhinolaryngology-Head and Neck Surgery, Changhua Christian Hospital, Changhua, Taiwan

Chiao-Wen Lin
Institute of Oral Sciences, Chung Shan Medical University, Taichung, Taiwan
Department of Dentistry, Chung Shan Medical University Hospital, Taichung, Taiwan

Chun-Yi Chuang
School of Medicine, Chung Shan Medical University, Taichung, Taiwan
Department of Otolaryngology, Chung Shan Medical University Hospital, Taichung, Taiwan

Yu-Fan Liu
Department of Biomedical Sciences, College of Medicine Sciences and Technology, Chung Shan Medical University, Taichung, Taiwan

Shun-Fa Yang
Institute of Medicine, Chung Shan Medical University, Taichung, Taiwan
Department of Medical Research, Chung Shan Medical University Hospital, Taichung, Taiwan

Chia-Hsuan Chou
Institute of Medicine, Chung Shan Medical University, Taichung, Taiwan

Jian Zhou
Shanghai Institute of Immunology, Shanghai Jiaotong University School of Medicine, Shanghai, China
Department of Otolaryngology, Eye, Ear, Nose and Throat Hospital, Fudan University, Shanghai, China
Shanghai Key Clinical Disciplines of Otorhinolaryngology, Shanghai, China

Lin Zhou, Fei Liu and and Li-Ming Lu
Shanghai Institute of Immunology, Shanghai Jiaotong University School of Medicine, Shanghai, China

Yong Yu and Pentao Liu
Wellcome Trust Sanger Institute, Cambridge, United Kingdom

Maria Karampela and Minna Isomursu
Faculty of Information Technology and Electrical Engineering, University of Oulu, Oulu, Finland

Talya Porat
Faculty of Engineering, Dyson School of Design Engineering, Imperial College London, London, United Kingdom

Vasiliki Mylonopoulou
Department of Applied Information Technology, Division of Human Computer Interaction, University of Gothenburg, Gothenburg, Sweden

Wei-Chun Hu and Wan-Huai Teo
Institute of Oral Biology, National Yang-Ming University, Taipei, Taiwan

Tung-Fu Huang
School of Medicine, National Yang-Ming University, Taipei, Taiwan
Department of Orthopedics and Traumatology, Taipei Veterans General Hospital, Taipei, Taiwan
Department of Exercise and Health Science, National Taipei University of Nursing and Health Sciences, Taipei, Taiwan

Te-Chang Lee
Institute of Biomedical Sciences, Academia Sinica, Taipei, Taiwan

Yujie Liang, Chenyu Guan, Kan Li, Guangsen Zheng, Tao Wang, Sien Zhang and Guiqing Liao
Department of Oral and Maxillofacial Surgery, Guanghua School of Stomatology, Hospital of Stomatology, Sun Yat-sen University, Guangzhou, China
Guangdong Province Key Laboratory of Stomatology, Sun Yat-sen University, Guangzhou, China

Hannah Zaryouh, Ines De Pauw, Hasan Baysal, Filip Lardon and An Wouters
Center for Oncological Research (CORE), Integrated Personalized & Precision Oncology Network (IPPON), University of Antwerp, Antwerp, Belgium

Patrick Pauwels
Center for Oncological Research (CORE), Integrated Personalized & Precision Oncology Network (IPPON), University of Antwerp, Antwerp, Belgium
Department of Pathology, Antwerp University Hospital, Antwerp, Belgium

Marc Peeters and Jan Baptist Vermorken
Center for Oncological Research (CORE), Integrated Personalized & Precision Oncology Network (IPPON), University of Antwerp, Antwerp, Belgium
Department of Medical Oncology, Antwerp University Hospital, Antwerp, Belgium

Xin Hua, Wen Wen, Zhi-Qing Long and Huan-Xin Lin
State Key Laboratory of Oncology in South China, Collaborative Innovation Center for Cancer Medicine, SunYat-sen University Cancer Center, Guangzhou, China
Department of Radiotherapy, Sun Yat-sen University Cancer Center, Guangzhou, China

Shan Liu
Department of Radiation Oncology, Sichuan Cancer Hospital & Institute, Sichuan Cancer Center, School of Medicine, University of Electronic Science and Technology of China, Chengdu, China

Jun-Fang Liao
Department of Radiation Oncology, National Cancer Center/National Clinical Cancer Research Center for Cancer/Cancer Hospital & Shenzhen Hospital, Chinese Academy of Medical Sciences and Peking Union Medical College, Shenzhen, China

Zi-Jian Lu and Ling Guo
State Key Laboratory of Oncology in South China, Collaborative Innovation Center for Cancer Medicine, SunYat-sen University Cancer Center, Guangzhou, China
Guangdong Key Laboratory of Nasopharyngeal Carcinoma Diagnosis and Therapy, Department of Nasopharyngeal Carcinoma, Sun Yat-sen University Cancer Center, Guangzhou, China

Sumei Wang
Guangdong Provincial Key Laboratory of Clinical Research on Traditional Chinese Medicine Syndrome, Guangdong Provincial Hospital of Chinese Medicine, Guangzhou, China
Department of Oncology, The Second Clinical College of Guangzhou University of Chinese Medicine, Guangzhou, China
The Postdoctoral Research Station, Guangzhou University of Chinese Medicine, Guangzhou, China

François-Xavier Claret
Department of Systems Biology, The University of Texas MD Anderson Cancer Center, Houston, TX, United States
Experimental Therapeutic Academic Program and Cancer Biology Program, The University of Texas Graduate School of Biomedical Sciences at Houston, Houston, TX, United States

Wanyin Wu
Guangdong Provincial Key Laboratory of Clinical Research on Traditional Chinese Medicine Syndrome, Guangdong Provincial Hospital of Chinese Medicine, Guangzhou, China
Department of Oncology, The Second Clinical College of Guangzhou University of Chinese Medicine, Guangzhou, China

Guo Zhao, Jianli Sun and Kai Ba
Department of Oral Medicine, The First Affiliated Hospital of Zhengzhou University, Zhengzhou, China

Yunxiang Zhang
Department of Endodontics, Kaifeng Stomatology Hospital, Kaifeng, China

Xiaohao Liu, Xiaojun Yang, Chaoning Zhan, Yan Zhang, Jin Hou and Xuemin Yin
Department of Oral and Maxillofacial Surgery, Nanfang Hospital, Southern Medical University, Guangzhou, China

Victor C. Kok
Department of Medical Oncology, Kuang Tien General Hospital Cancer Center, Taichung, Taiwan
Department of Bioinformatics and Medical Engineering, Asia University Taiwan, Taichung, Taiwan

Index

www.ingramcontent.com/pod-product-compliance
Lightning Source LLC
LaVergne TN
LVHW080946210926
848485LV00004B/780